Handbook of Medical Aspects of Disability and Rehabilitation for Life Care Planning

This textbook is an essential resource for life care planners in understanding and assessing a range of medical disabilities, life care planning as a health care service delivery practice, certification under the International Commission on Health Care Certification, and the path to rehabilitation for mild to catastrophic injuries.

Written by a team composed of expert physicians and doctoral-level practitioners, the book covers the key areas of traumatic injury and resultant disability that life care planners so often face. From acquired brain injury and spinal disorders to amputation, chronic pain, posttraumatic debilitating headaches, and plastic reconstructive surgery, the book provides a road map not only to the treatment options available but also the strategies that can lead to rehabilitation and a possible return to work. Each chapter also discusses possible complications, allowing a holistic perspective on each issue.

Also including chapters on medical cost projection analysis and functional capacity evaluation, this is the complete text for both professionals in the fields of rehabilitation services and life care planning, as well as students training to qualify.

Virgil Robert May III, Rehabilitation Practitioner, Doctor of Rehabilitation, Southern Illinois University, USA.

Richard Bowman, Physical Medicine and Rehabilitation, MD, Certified Life Care Planner, West Virginia, USA.

Steven Barna, Anesthesiology and Pain Medicine (MD) and Certified Life Care Planner (CLCP), Florida, USA.

T0246374

Handbook of Medical Aspects of Disability and Rehabilitation for Life Care Planning

Edited by Virgil Robert May III, Richard Bowman, and Steven Barna

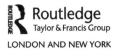

Routledge
Taylor & Francis Group

LONDON AND NEW YORK

First published 2024
by Routledge
4 Park Square, Milton Park, Abingdon, Oxon OX14 4RN

and by Routledge
605 Third Avenue, New York, NY 10158

Routledge is an imprint of the Taylor & Francis Group, an informa business

British Library Cataloguing-in-Publication Data
A catalogue record for this book is available from the British Library

Library of Congress Cataloging-in-Publication Data
Names: May, Virgil Robert, 1950– editor. | Bowman, Richard (Physician), editor. | Barna, Steven, editor.
Title: Handbook of medical aspects of disability and rehabilitation for life care planning / edited by Virgil Robert May III, Richard Bowman and Steven Barna.
Description: Abingdon, Oxon ; New York, NY : Routledge, 2024. | Includes bibliographical references and index.
Identifiers: LCCN 2023041503 | ISBN 9781032271606 (hardback) | ISBN 9781032414928 (paperback) | ISBN 9781003358336 (ebook)
Subjects: LCSH: Life care planning—Textbooks. | Medical rehabilitation—Textbooks.
Classification: LCC RM930.7 .H36 2024 | DDC 362.61—dc23/eng/20231213
LC record available at https://lccn.loc.gov/2023041503

ISBN: 978-1-032-27160-6 (hbk)
ISBN: 978-1-032-41492-8 (pbk)
ISBN: 978-1-003-35833-6 (ebk)

DOI: 10.4324/b23293

Typeset in Times New Roman
by Apex CoVantage, LLC

Contents

Contributors

Kathleen Acer is a clinical psychologist with over 27 years of experience evaluating and treating a wide range of individuals of all ages. Her areas of expertise include the assessment of medical and psychological disability including the formulation of life care plans, forensic examinations, workers' compensations cases, vocational assessments, and fitness-for-duty evaluations. Additionally, Dr. Acer has extensive experience in dealing with individuals with complex medical and psychological trauma.

Sofia Barchuk, DO, is Brain Injury Medicine Fellow, PGY-5, Donald and Barbara Zucker School of Medicine at Hofstra Northwell Physical Medicine and Rehabilitation Specialist, Residency Graduate of the Icahn School of Medicine at Mount Sinai.

Steven Barna is founder of LCPMD, LLC, based out of Tampa, Florida. Dr. Barna is a board-certified, Harvard-trained pain management physician and a Certified Life Care Planner (CLCP). He is an editorial board member for *Pain Physician* and a reviewer for the *Journal of Orthopaedic Trauma*. He has been recognized on Becker's Orthopedic and Spine Review List of 150 Pain Management Physicians to Know. Dr. Barna spent nearly 10 years at Harvard Medical School including roles as assistant professor of medicine and assistant professor of anesthesiology, as well as medical director of the Massachusetts General Hospital Pain Center. He also previously served as assistant professor of orthopedics and sports medicine at the University of South Florida College of Medicine. He is a member of the American Society of Interventional Pain Physicians, North American Spine Society, International Association of Rehabilitation Professionals/International Academy of Life Care Planners Section, and American Academy of Physician Life Care Planners.

Richard Bowman is a board-certified physical medicine and rehabilitation physician. He has a subspeciality board certification in pain medicine through the American Board of Pain Medicine. He was awarded the title "Fellow of the Interventional Pain Practice" from the World Institute of Pain. He has practiced general physiatry and pain medicine in West Virginia since 2001. Dr. Bowman is a founding member, past president, and prior board of directors member of the West Virginia Society of Interventional Pain Physicians (WVSIPP). He received the West Virginia Pain Physician of the Year Award from the WVSIPP in 2016. Dr. Bowman has been a "Certified Examiner of Disability and Impairment Ratings" since 2004. He has litigation testimony experience since 2001. Dr. Bowman became a Certified Life Care Planner in 2016. He serves as a member of the International Commission on Health Care Certification (ICHCC) Board of Commissioners for Life Care Planning. Dr. Bowman has authored multiple studies and textbook chapters in the field of physical medicine and rehabilitation and pain medicine. He has extensive experience in direct clinical instruction of students and residents, didactic instruction, cadaver instruction, and operating room instruction of practicing physicians in the field of interventional pain medicine and didactic instruction of life care planners. Dr. Bowman continues to practice medicine in West Virginia. He continues to provide forensic expert services in the field of life care planning in the United States.

Jennifer Canter is a double-board-certified pediatrician and a professor of pediatrics and a professor of disability and health at New York Medical College. Dr. Canter is also a Certified Life Care Planner and vocational rehabilitation counselor for adults and children. Dr. Canter has a degree in public health with a focus in epidemiology (MPH) from Johns Hopkins University, affording her the additional qualification to synthesize research/evidence-based medicine into her work. Since 2002, Dr. Canter has been the director of clinical and academic programs for forensic/child abuse pediatrics at New York Medical College, The Maria Fareri Children's Hospital, and the Westchester Institute of Development's Child Advocacy Center (CAC). She has an avid research and publication history in traumatic injury and prevention.

Todd S. Capielano is a licensed and certified rehabilitation counselor who has practiced in the private sector of vocational rehabilitation for over 34 years. He has been in the field of vocational rehabilitation since 1985, specializing in vocational evaluations, labor market research, job placement, and career counseling. Todd has been accepted as a vocational expert since 1989 in various courts, including federal, state, civil district courts, and before administrative law judges for Longshore Harbor Workers Compensation Act claims. Additionally, he has served as a vocational expert for the Social Security Administration testifying in thousands of cases since 1992.

Michael Chiou, MD, FAAPMR, Department of Physical Medicine and Rehabilitation, Sunnyview Rehabilitation Hospital, Schenectady, New York.

Kaitlyn Cyncynatus holds a BS in neuroscience from the University of Cincinnati and is a DO candidate at Ohio University Heritage College of Osteopathic Medicine (matriculation 2026).

Robert S. Djergaian did his medical training at Jefferson Medical College (now Sidney Kimmel Medical College) and residency at Thomas Jefferson University Hospital. He is board certified in physical medicine and rehabilitation, formerly a diplomate of the American Academy of Pain Medicine, and is a Certified Life Care Planner. He is currently a clinical assistant professor at the University of Arizona Medical School. His last clinical position was physician director at the Rehabilitation Institute at Banner University Medical Center, Phoenix, Arizona. While in Arizona he served as board president of the Arizona Brain Injury Alliance.

Huma Haider is the founder and CEO of the National Brain Injury Institute, which now serves all 50 U.S. states. They specialize in helping patients get properly diagnosed and treated by providing objective diagnostic proof for patients with mild traumatic brain injuries. She is a pioneer in the adaptation of a proprietary protocol that is now being used throughout the United States in conjunction with a 20-year-old MRI-based diagnostic technology called diffusion tensor imaging (DTI). She is board certified in neurocritical care, anesthesiology, and headache medicine. She is board eligible in internal medicine and has her master's in psychology.

Heather Howe is a 1994 graduate of McGill University's Physical Therapy Program in Montreal, Canada. After graduating, Heather returned to her home province of New Brunswick and began working as a physiotherapist for the Workers Rehabilitation Center treating adults with injuries sustained while on the job ranging from trauma and amputations to complex regional pain syndrome and repetitive strain injuries. After several years of treating the injured worker, Heather moved into the role of case manager for the compensation system, actively managing 80 to 100 claims at any given time. In 2004, Heather decided to make the move to private practice in the field of disability management and held several positions from clinician and educator to manager of clinical services. Heather's area of expertise as a clinician was in the delivery of functional capacity evaluations followed by a workplace accommodation and educating employers on their duty to accommodate both short-term and long-term. In July 2020, Heather completed her certification as a Certified Canadian Life Care Planner (CCLCP). Heather has completed plans for both the plaintiff and defense and has a special interest in the development of plans for individuals with amputations.

Matthew Janzen is a physical medicine and rehabilitation physician specializing in pain management. Dr. Janzen began his medical journey at the University of Minnesota where he obtained his bachelor's of science in genetics and neuroscience before he attended the University of Minnesota Medical School where he received his MD. He spent his intern year after medical school training at Broadlawns Medical Center in Des Moines, Iowa. After his intern year, he spent the next three years completing his physical medicine and rehabilitation residency at Tufts Medical Center in Boston, Massachusetts. Following residency, he completed an interventional pain management fellowship at Deuk Spine Institute in Melbourne, Florida.

Stuart Kahn is double-board certified in physical medicine and rehabilitation and in pain management. He has special interest in the non-surgical treatment of neck, low-back and mid-back pain syndromes.

Alex Karras has devoted his career to assisting his corporate clients navigate a myriad of federal and state regulations, including the Americans with Disabilities Act (ADA), through the development of compliance and training programs for human resources personnel, risk-benefit coordinators, insurance personnel, and physicians, as well as providing litigation oversight in workers' compensation and general liability claims for global corporations and national self-insureds.

Gary E. Kraus has held past positions as assistant clinical professor, Department of Neurosurgery, at the University of Texas Medical School at Houston; chairman of neurosurgery at Memorial Hermann Memorial City Hospital, Houston Texas; and director of neurosciences and gamma knife at West Houston Medical Center. Dr. Kraus is board certified by the American Board of Neurological Surgery, is a fellow of the American Association of Neurological Surgeons, and is certified as a Life Care Planner by the International Commission on Healthcare Certification. He has been listed in "Best Doctors in America," Castle Connolly Top Doctors, Texas Super Doctors, featured in Newsweek among "Best Neurosurgeons in Texas" and "Neurosurgery Leaders in the United States," and is listed in "Who's Who in America."

Jennifer Lambert is a certified pediatric and adult life care planner and vocational evaluator and double-board-certified pediatrician. She is a professor of pediatrics and professor of public health for the Center on Disability & Health at New York Medical College.

Ashley G. Lastrapes has over nine years of experience in private vocational rehabilitation. She earned her PhD in counselor education and supervision from the University of Holy Cross; she holds a master of health science degree in rehabilitation counseling from Louisiana State University Health Sciences Center in 2011 and her bachelor of science degree in psychology from the University of New Orleans in 2009. Dr. Lastrapes is a licensed rehabilitation counselor and licensed professional counselor, as well as a board-approved supervisor in the state of Louisiana. She is also a licensed professional counselor in the state of Texas.

In addition, she holds national certifications as a certified counselor, certified rehabilitation counselor, certified case manager, and Certified Life Care Planner. Dr. Lastrapes is also a vocational expert with the Social Security Administration, Office of Disability Adjudication and Review.

Kathleen Kenney May is a graduate of Indiana University with a bachelor's degree in education and earned her master's degree in rehabilitation administration, counseling, and services from Southern Illinois University – Carbondale. Ms. May worked for several years as a placement and rehabilitation counselor for the Illinois Department of Rehabilitation Services and was recognized by the governor for her work regarding the *International Year of the Disabled*. Upon relocating to Richmond, Virginia, she launched a new department for the Children's Hospital titled the Career Development Department, where she worked with older patients to determine their career goals and interests. Along with her husband, she started May Physical Therapy Services overseeing five outpatient rehabilitation clinics in the Richmond area. Ms. May is currently the business operations administrator for the International Commission on Health Care Certification (ICHCC) and is one of the co-founders of the ICHCC.

Virgil Robert May III received his doctorate in rehabilitation from Southern Illinois University – Carbondale and is currently the president of the International Commission on Health Care Certification (ICHCC). He taught functional capacity evaluation and impairment rating protocols at the University of Florida – Gainesville in UF Health Shands Hospital, the Department of Rehabilitation from the fall of 1992 through the fall semester of 1996. He served as an adjunct professor in the Department of Rehabilitation, Rehabilitation Institute, Southern Illinois University, where he oversaw validation research studies of the NADEP functional capacity evaluation protocols and life care plan certification examination. Dr. May served on the faculty of the National Association of Disability Evaluating Professionals where he instructed physicians, therapists, and vocational evaluators in impairment rating and functional capacity evaluation protocols in major training sites in Canada and the United States. He maintains an outpatient functional capacity evaluation practice in the Richmond, Virginia, area that he has maintained over the past 38 years. He served as a junior partner from 1999 to 2012 in his local therapy business that traded as May Physical Therapy Services, LLC, which offered physical/aquatic therapy services, massage therapy, strength and conditioning training, and work disability/functional capacity evaluations. In addition to the therapy and evaluation businesses, he has consulted with the Coca-Cola Bottling Company, Overnight Transportation, Inc., and the Washington, D.C. Metropolitan Transit Authority regarding analyzing their jobs to ensure compliance with the Americans with Disabilities Act of 1990. Dr. May has lectured in China, Canada, and the United States on measuring work function and has authored over 60 peer-reviewed journal articles and book chapters on industrial rehabilitation and federal/state legislation governing occupational medicine practices. His most recent invited lectures were with the American Rehabilitation Economics Association in October 2021 titled "Functional Capacity Evaluation Explained" and with the University of Wisconsin—Stout Vocational Rehabilitation Institute (SVRI) where he presented his lecture on the "Functional Capacity Evaluation for the Vocational Evaluator and Rehabilitation Case Manager" on January 24, 2022. He holds certification as a Certified Disability Evaluator, Category II, and as a Certified Rehabilitation Provider, Commonwealth of Virginia.

Douglas W. Martin is co-chair of the AMA Guides Editorial Panel and serves as the medical director for the Center for Neurosciences, Orthopaedics, & Spine Occupational Medicine in Sioux City, Iowa. Dr. Martin is a past president of the American Academy of Disability Evaluating Physicians, a member of the American Academy of Family Physicians Commission on Education, and vice chair of the Interstate Postgraduate Medical Association. He was installed as vice president of the American College of Occupational and Environmental Medicine in 2020.

Danielle Melton is board certified in physical medicine and rehabilitation and an associate professor in the Department of Orthopedic Surgery. Dr. Melton received her undergraduate degree in mechanical engineering from Louisiana State University and completed medical school and her residency at Baylor College of Medicine.

Gerard Mosiello is a plastic surgeon in the Department of Cutaneous Oncology at Moffitt Cancer Center. His clinical interests include plastic surgery reconstruction following skin cancer and breast cancer, as well as a variety of cosmetic surgery procedures. Dr. Mosiello received his medical degree from Hahnemann University School of Medicine in Philadelphia, Pennsylvania, graduating with honors.

LeRoy Oddie, CP, MBA, CLCP, is a graduate of the California State University Dominguez Hills prosthetics program and an ABC Certified Prosthetist. Oddie is a ICHCC Certified Life Care Planner and graduated from the Capital University life care planning program, where he guest lectures. Oddie has traveled extensively internationally and domestically lecturing on prosthetics and has authored several texts on prosthetics and life care planning. Oddie is currently employed as a prosthetic specialist with Integrum, Inc.

Tanya Rutherford Owen is a certified rehabilitation counselor, Certified Life Care Planner, and a life care planning fellow. She has served as an adjunct professor and guest lecturer in the Department of Rehabilitation, Education, and Research at the University of Arkansas. She is managing editor of *The Rehabilitation Professional* and *The Journal of Life Care Planning*.

Bharat C. Patel has board certifications in sports medicine, physiatry, pain medicine, electrodiagnostic medicine, and interventional pain management. Fewer than 1 in 10,000 physicians nationwide are quintuple board certified.

Krishn Patel received her bachelors of Science degree from the University of Central Florida, Orlando, Florida.

Reva Payne is the vice president of clinical and medical management for Marker28, a boutique firm specializing in cost compliance and allocation solutions for various cost projections, Medicare Set-Aside, and related services.

Ashley Plonk, RN, BSN serves Health First Hospital in Melbourne, Florida.

Rachel Santiago, MD, FAAPMR, Department of Physical Medicine and Rehabilitation, Sunnyview Rehabilitation Hospital, Schenectady, New York.

Lacy H. Sapp has practiced in the field of vocational rehabilitation since 2000 and has been with Stokes & Associates since 2004. She earned her PhD in counselor education and supervision from University of Holy Cross, her master of health sciences degree in rehabilitation counseling from Louisiana State University Health Sciences Center, and her bachelor of arts degree in psychology with a minor in criminal justice from Southeastern Louisiana University. Dr. Sapp is a licensed rehabilitation counselor, licensed professional counselor, and licensed marriage and family therapist in the state of Louisiana. She holds national certifications as a certified rehabilitation counselor, national certified counselor, and Certified Life Care Planner. She has testified as an expert in her field in both state and federal jurisdictions.

Larry S. Stokes has been in the field of vocational rehabilitation since 1982. He holds a PhD in counseling, specializing in rehabilitation counseling, and a minor in research and statistics from the University of New Orleans. He is a licensed rehabilitation counselor and licensed professional counselor and holds certifications as a rehabilitation counselor, Life Care Planner, and case manager. He has been an adjunct assistant professor in the Counseling and Human Development Department at the University of New Orleans since 1998.

Dana Weldon has practiced in private rehabilitation since 1982 in Canada and the United States in the capacity of a rehabilitation consultant/counselor and Certified Life Care Planner. She has by examination been conveyed certification status as a Certified Rehabilitation Counselor (CRC) through the Commission on Rehabilitation Counselor Certification (CRCC). Dana has successfully achieved the Certified Life Care Planner (CLCP) as well as the Canadian Certified Life Care Planner (CCLCP) status by examination from the International Commission on Health Care Certification.

Aaron M. Wolfson is a licensed psychologist, licensed rehabilitation counselor, and Certified Life Care Planner who has testified as an expert witness in both state and federal jurisdictions. His areas of expertise include chronic pain management, physical rehabilitation, residual earning capacity analysis, and assessment of future medical needs and life care planning.

Claudia von Zweck is an occupational therapist and life care planner in private practice. In addition to her undergraduate degree in occupational therapy, she holds an MSc in epidemiology and PhD in rehabilitation science from Queen's University in Canada. She has an appointment as a clinical assistant professor with the University of British Columbia. Her recent research has addressed a broad range of topics including assistive technology, quality evaluation, COVID-19, and health human resource planning.

Tables

Figures

Preface

Life care planning has evolved into an inspirational process for determining the needs of persons with a chronic, moderate, and/or severe injury or disease process and the costs associated with implementing the life care plan. It is inspirational in terms of the achievements of the field of life care planning in identifying services, medical treatments, rehabilitative programs, and job attainment in the competitive labor market when appropriate, which are documented in the best interest of the injured person.

The inspiration for this book evolved from the International Commission on Health Care Certification's (ICHCC's) review of sample life care plans of candidates sitting for the Certified Life Care Planner and the Canadian Certified Life Care Planner credentials. What was noted was several issues with the description of injury, diagnose(s), and medical treatment applications, as well as rehabilitation programming and duration. It appeared that little effort was made in some plans to apply the medical effects of injury on the individual's ability to perform their activities of daily living, their executive function, joint motion/coordination, mobility, and physical tolerances as impaired by the respective diagnosis/injury. The ICHCC posits that the life care planning process has a strong and essential medical base element for determining the medical and rehabilitative needs of the person with an adventitious injury. In essence, Dr. Joe Gonzales et al., 2015, concluded that "For a life care plan to appropriately provide for all the needs of an individual, the plan must have a strong medical foundation" (p. 4).

To address the medical aspects of the injury/disease process required of the categories of need charts, the editors believed this book would be a great opportunity for practicing life care planners to review and obtain a re-understanding of the medical aspects of injury that they may have learned in their initial academic programs, both at bachelor and graduate levels. The reader will note that we have included chapters explaining the independent medical examination, reports of which life care planners often review. We have included chapters with reviews and explanations of significant body systems, psychological adjustment to disability, disability of the sequelae of immobility, acquired brain injury, traumatic headaches, spinal cord injury, spinal disorders, peripheral neuropathies, amputations, chronic pain, and burn injuries. There are other chapters that include life care planning in general with a sample report, the functional capacity evaluation application to life care planning, legislative guidelines for life care planning services, expert witness guidelines, and the certification process including regulation and accreditation.

The medical dynamics of injury and disease are difficult to comprehend and, in some cases, to understand. We hope that the reader will find the information contained in this book to be applicable to their life care planning practice and most beneficial to the disabled individual about whom they write the life care plan.

Reference

Gonzales, J., Cowen, T., Janssen, C., & Davenport, W. (2015). *Life care plans: A defensive perspective*. The American Academy of Physician Life Care Planners.

Foreword

As a long-time publisher of books and journals for the forensic rehabilitating consulting community, the profession has been witness to and beneficiary of several very useful texts and resources for the practicing rehabilitation consultant and life care planner.

This current text, edited by Dr. V. May, is yet another resource which undoubtedly will add to the literature base of rehabilitation consulting, especially in the area of life care planning. The text, which is targeted to both current practitioners and students in training, consists of 22 chapters addressing a wide range of topics germane to the fields of disability and life care planning. Each chapter/topic was drafted by doctoral-level professionals in areas of rehabilitation and disability, medicine, and law. The text clearly is an attempt to address a wide range of topics that would serve the practicing life care planner with both practical and critical information. Some of these topics include legislative guidelines, pediatrics, provider systems, significant body systems, immobility, brain injury, amputations and spinal disorders, chronic pain, functional capacity evaluations, and guidelines for expert witnesses.

In my opinion, this text paints a broad stroke in providing excellent information from a variety of practicing professionals. The chapters by the various authors provide useful and important information for professionals in the areas of disability, rehabilitation, and life care planning.

Timothy F. Field, PhD
Elliott & Fitzpatrick, Inc.

1 Life Care Planning

History, Process, and the Written Document

Virgil Robert May III and Heather Howe

Life care planning is a health care service delivery system designed to assist individuals who have incurred catastrophic injury or chronic injury sequelae that impair their ability to perform the essential function of their activities of daily living and/or work when applicable. It is a system that utilizes the expertise of health care service providers regarding the diagnosis(es) of the respective injury and the impact on the individual's body systems of that respective diagnosis, the individual's overall mental and physical needs, and the costs of medical/rehabilitative treatments/supplies, medications, environmental/home modifications, to name a few, over their remaining life span.

This chapter is structured to provide the reader with a clear and sound description of this specialized health care delivery system, its roots and how it evolved, organizational efforts among non-medical and medical-based membership organizations, and the essential components of the summary life care plan.

History

The roots of life care planning can be found in the mid-to-late 1970s and is a product of the mindsets of two individuals: 1) Dr. Fred Raffa, an economist and faculty member at the University of Central Florida, and 2) Dr. Paul Deutsch, at the time a vocational rehabilitation counselor who served as an expert witness in personal injury and product liability cases. Dr. Raffa served not only as a faculty member of the University of Central Florida but also as the chairperson of the university's Department of Economics from 1976 until 1980 (The Winter Park Land Trust: Fred Raffa, n.d.). Dr. Raffa continued his economic consultations with personal injury law firms and left the university in 1998 to form the firm Raffa Consulting Economists, Inc.

Dr. Deutsch is retired at this writing and worked as a licensed mental health counselor with a PhD in counseling psychology and counselor education with a specialization in rehabilitation. Dr. Deutsch was a board-certified vocational rehabilitation counselor, board-certified case manager, and a Certified Life Care Planner (CLCP) under the International Commission on Health Care Certification (ICHCC) (LexisNexis Store, n.d.). Dr. Deutsch specialized in working with catastrophic disabilities resulting from either a birth or traumatic onset and is well known in the life care planning field for his knowledge of life care planning practice development and methodological applications.

Dr. Deutsch and Dr. Raffa had the chance to meet on a case referred to them by a plaintiff attorney and found that they had a lot in common in their approach to documenting the needs and costs of catastrophic trauma and forged a working relationship such that in 1981 they published their multivolume LexisNexis Series textbook, *Damages in Tort Actions* (LexisNexis Store, n.d.). Dr. Deutsch is best known for having developed the basic principles, tenets, methodology,

DOI: 10.4324/b23293-1

Table 1.1 Damages in Tort Actions Content Focus

Pain and Suffering	Indemnity
Emotional Distress	Damages Under No-Fault Statutes
Medical Expenses	Libel and Slander
Loss of Earnings and Earnings Capacity	Pre-Impact Terror
Loss of Consortium and Services	Comparative Negligence
Loss of Enjoyment of Life	Releases
Prenatal Injuries	Structured Settlements
Collateral Source Doctrine	Vocational Rehabilitation
Aggravation of Injury	Use of Economic Experts
Expert Witnesses	Illustrative Trial Transcripts, Awards, and Settlements
Jury Instructions	Sample Forms of Pleading
Documentary and Demonstrative Evidence	Practice Manual with Discussion and Analysis
Contribution	Extensive Case Annotations to All Jurisdictions

and processes of life care planning, and their textbook publication reveals the early concept Dr. Deutsch established as the model for today's life care planning methodology and life care plan content development (Deutsch & PA Associates, n.d.). The table of contents of Drs. Raffa and Deutsch best illustrate the roots and early development of life care planning methodology, concepts, and content applications (Table 1.1).

Life Care Planning Evolution

Dr. Deutsch noted that life care planning evolved out of case management with its concepts, methodologies, and tenets within the field of rehabilitation (Deutsch, 2002; Johnson & Weed, 2013). He asserted that the rehabilitation professionals best suited to assume the tasks of providing life care planning services and writing comprehensive medical and rehabilitative plans included rehabilitation counselors, rehabilitation nurses, rehabilitation psychologists, and psychiatrists. However, Dr. Deutsch noted that life care planning was a complex process that required knowledge and expertise from three divergent fields of health care: 1) experimental analysis of behavior, 2) developmental psychology, and 3) case management.

Each of these fields required extensive training and advanced psychology/behavioral analysis degrees and knowledge/experience with case management methodologies and protocols. The experimental analysis of a behavior's primary purpose is to discover all of the variables of which the probability of a response is a function (Skinner, 1966). As Deutsch (2002) concluded from Skinner's (1966) work, the identification of such variables with response to function requires charting to carefully identify, define, analyze, and isolate one's responsive behavior to a stimulus. Thus, he applied such spontaneous, involuntary, and/or self-regulated responses to the category of need that best reflects anatomical change induced by the diagnosis based on the stimulus, allowing the case manager to identify each component of the plan and communicate that need to the patient, family, or any interested third party that required the information (Deutsch).

Dr. Deutsch noted how important developmental psychology is to life care planning by attributing the concept, the actual formatting of the life care plan, and the specified content of the plan to that of developmental psychology (Deutsch, 2002). Developmental psychology is often referred to as life-span psychology, which is the branch of psychology that addresses the changes in one's cognition, motivation, psychophysiological, and social function throughout one's human life span (The Editors of Encyclopedia Britannica, 2017). Given a catastrophic diagnosis of any of the injuries sustained and referred for a life care plan of an adolescent, such as traumatic brain injury or a full-thickness burn (fourth degree), and given the volumes of information provided the guardian/parents and/or family members, it became apparent that when discussion led to future educational, developmental, and behavioral needs, it was obvious that parents could not process all of the information communicated to them. The life care plan evolved to provide parents/guardians and family members information that could be referenced over time, thus providing the family members with a guideline that would suggest critical ages or times when changes had to be made in terms of medical providers, rehabilitative providers, and educational assessments if necessary.

Case management is a health care monitoring process in which health care professionals assuming the role of a case manager become a patient advocate, performing tasks that include supporting, guiding, and coordinating care for patients, families, and caregivers (Case Management Society of America, 2021). Dr. Deutsch (2002) surmised that the life care plan was the tool necessary to assist the case manager in implementing long-term rehabilitation and care of the catastrophically injured individual. Additionally, the plan served as a guideline used by the family to assess the continued medical and rehabilitative needs of the individual; gauge their family member's progress in medical and rehabilitative treatments; and have a better understanding of their family member's functional changes, activities of daily living competency, and their potential for independent living. In essence, Dr. Deutsch attributes the life care plan to establishing the principles of case management among rehabilitation counselors, rehabilitation nurses, rehabilitation psychologists, and psychiatrists that include the standards, tenets, and methodologies that are the foundation of life care planning (Deutsch, 2002, n.d.).

Certification and Membership Organizations

Certification Organizations

Dr. Deutsch (2002) and Dr. Weed (2019) identified several organizations that grew from the life care planning movement that Dr. Deutsch started back in the late 1970s, and these organizations grew rapidly through the early 2000s and became well-established by the second decade into the new millennium. For example, Dr. Virgil Robert May III introduced the field to life care planning certification with the CLCP credential. It was in March 1996 that 80 tests were administered in a group-testing format through the Commission on Disability Examiner Certification. This name was changed in 2002 to the International Commission on Health Care Certification as a result of the interest of Canadian health care practitioners in learning the life care planning service delivery system.

Dr. May designed the ICHCC agency to follow the methodology espoused by Deutsch and Sawyer (1985). Dr. Deutsch's methodology is presented in Table 1.2.

Table 1.2 Life Care Planning Methodology of Dr. Paul Deutsch

- Comprehensive review of records and supportive documentation.
- Clinical interview and history with the patient and, whenever possible, a family member or significant contact who knew the patient premorbidly as well as postmorbidly.
- Interaction with the medical and health-related treatment team to obtain answers to questions not established in the medical records review.
- Research to develop relevant clinical practice guidelines to further establish needs and recommendations as well as support medical and case management foundation.
- Research on relevant research literature to further establish needs and recommendations as well as support medical and case management foundation.
- Where necessary establish further data through staffing with consulting specialists,

However, methodology components have been added to the life care planning process such that the ICHCC has had to make adjustments as well. Weed (2019) identified a methodology to address a step-by-step process in working within the life care planning service delivery system. He addressed the life care planners' responsibilities to include case intake procedures, review of all medical records, supporting documentation that may include depositions of all persons involved in the case, vocational/educational records, employment records, etc.; initial interview arrangements (location, attendees, set time allowed); initial interview materials; consulting with therapeutic team members; preparing preliminary life care plan opinions; obtaining additional sources approved by the referral source; researching costs and sources; finalizing the plan; and appropriate life care plan distribution. The reader will note that all of these specific activities fall within those documented in Dr. Deutsch's methodology.

A second certifying agency evolved 2 years later in 1998 through the work of Kelly Lance, FNP. She assembled a certification board that created the Certified Nurse Life Care Planner (CNLCP) designation exclusive to nurses and whose methodology of practice was taken from the protocols defined by the American Nursing Association's (ANA's) Social Policy Statement. This statement reads as follows:

> Nursing is the protection, promotion, and optimization of health and abilities; prevention of illness and injury; alleviation of suffering through the diagnosis and treatment of human response; and advocacy in the care of individuals, families, communities, and populations.
>
> (May & Moradi Rekabdarkolaee, 2020, p. 28)

Additional influences that were germane to the CNLCP methodology included the Nursing Scope and Standards of Practice, Second Edition; the Nursing's Social Policy Statement: The Essence of the Profession; and The Code of Ethics for Nurses with Interpretive Statements. A suggested definition of nurse life care planning was offered by Howland (2015, as cited in May & Moradi Rekabdarkolaee, 2020, p. 28), in which he defined nurse life care planning as the "protection, promotion, and optimization of health and chronic and complex health conditions". Further assessment by Howland of the nurse life care planner practice methodology included the

> application of advocacy, judgment, and critical thinking skills using the nursing process to develop long-term or lifetime plans of care, including the cost associated with all of a plan's components, which included identified evaluations and interventions, health maintenance, health promotion, and optimization of physical and psychological abilities.
>
> (p. 28)

The third certification agency is found within the American Academy of Physician Life Care Planners (AAPLCP), a membership organization that offers the Certified Physician Life Care Planner (CPLCP) credential. Dr. Joe G. Gonzales (*Gallardo v. Marstiller*, 2022) is the founder and chief executive officer (CEO) of the American Academy of Physician Life Care Planners, who established the academy in 2013 as a professional organization offering membership to board-certified physicians in physical medicine and rehabilitation, as well as other qualified clinical and forensic professionals. The academy's mission is to recognize and espouse the contributions to the life care planning service delivery system made by physical medicine and rehabilitation physicians. Its mission also includes supporting the discipline of life care planning through physician participation, educating physicians of physical medicine and rehabilitation in the process and methodologies of life care planning service delivery, and educating the public as well as the life care planning non-physician community about the central role the life care planning physician assumes in the life care planning service delivery system (American Academy of Life Care Planning Physicians ™, 2023).

Dr. Gonzales's primary goal in establishing his academy was to ensure the life care plan is a document with a strong medical foundation and that physiatrists are uniquely trained and qualified to provide life care planning services to catastrophically and non-catastrophically injured individuals (Gonzales & Zotovas, 2014). He noted that physiatrists previously served as consultants to non-physician life care planners, lending them guidance, support, and signing off on their life care plans. Dr. Gonzales realized more physicians in the first decade of 2000 were entering the field of life care planning and felt a need to organize physicians who desired a practice in life care planning to ensure consistency in the physician methodology in addition to consistent training in this specialty health care service field.

Dr. Stephen Mann (2019) documented that there were just two certifying agencies that certify physician life care planners: 1) the ICHCC and 2) AAPLCP. Dr. Mann noted that the physician life care planners complete any one of the 120-hour training programs that apply to the CLCP credential, having them learn the methodology that Dr. Deutsch developed. After their training, the physician life care planner sits for the CLCP examination before progressing to the Certified Physical Life Care Planner credential administered by the academy.

Membership Organizations

There are four main membership organizations in the field of life care planning, and these include the International Association of Rehabilitation Professionals (IARP), the American Association of Nurse Life Care Planners (AANLCP), the American Academy for Nurse Life Care Planners, the AAPLCP (discussed in the "Certification Organizations" section earlier), and the newest organization, the Association of Certified Life Care Planners (ALCP).

International Association of Rehabilitation Professionals (IARP)

The IARP was established in 1981 as the National Association of Rehabilitation Professionals in the Private Sector (NARPPS). NARPPS began as a private rehabilitation membership organization with a focus on the private rehabilitation movement that began in the late 1960s. The association initially accepted private-sector practitioners but eventually accepted all rehabilitation professionals regardless of their professional setting. NARPPS changed its name to the International Association of Rehabilitation Professionals in 2000 (K. Bailey, personal conversation, January 10, 2023). IARP continues to offer life care planning seminars, webinars, and an annual conference and biannual summits through its merger with the International Academy of Life Care Planners in 2005.

The IARP provides opportunities for members to learn more about various rehabilitation practice applications through their sections, or training venues of different practice settings within health care service delivery systems. IARP offers the following sections:

1. Forensic Section
2. Life Care Planning—IALCP Section
3. Rehabilitation and Disability Case Management Section
4. Social Security Vocational Expert Section (Restricted)
5. Vocational Rehabilitation Transition Services Section

For more information regarding the section opportunities, go to the IARP website at https://rehabpro.org/.

American Association of Nurse Life Care Planners (AANLCP)

Kelly Lance, FNP, is responsible for the creation of this membership organization in 1997. She knew that the nurses who were interested in life care planning would benefit from an organization designed to serve as the educational entity for the planned credential she had in mind, the Certified Nurse Life Care Planner, which came to fruition a year later in 1998 following her assembling the board for this agency (K. Lance, personal conversation, January 8, 2023). Today, the AANLCP has grown to offer a journal and a bimonthly newsletter to its subscribers, as well as webinars with industry leaders, research and coding resources, a robust mentorship program, and an annual conference. The AANLCP states its annual objective is to provide its subscribers with the resources that will help them grow professionally and personally with the connection with other nurse experts as well as establishing a network of support for themselves and their practices. For more information on the AANLCP, please go to their website at www.aanlcp.org/.

American Academy for Nurse Life Care Planners (AANLCP)

The AANLCP was established in 1996, founded by Patricia McCollom, MS, RN (Berens, 2019). Ms. McCollom's goal for this agency was to be a non-profit association that would advance and promote nurses in the life care planning service delivery system. She intended this agency to not just offer the CNLCP credential but also to provide the training and development of educational programs specific to nurse life care planning methodology.

It was soon after that the leadership in life care planning observed the influx of interest from health care practitioners representing numerous disciplines with applications to health care and met with Ms. McCollom to suggest opening her agency to all health care providers so they too could benefit from the network and training her organization offered to its subscribers. Ms. McCollom agreed, as did her advisory board, and the name of her organization changed to the International Academy of Life Care Planners. Due to health issues, Ms. McCollom transferred the agency to the International Association of Rehabilitation Professionals as a special interest section in 2005 (Weed, 2019). Dr. Deutsch (2002) identified the IALCP as establishing the first set of standards in 2000 and was formally published in 2002 (Reavis, 2002). Dr. Deutsch attributed the IALCP to establishing the following standards specific to the life care planner:

- Have a foundation of knowledge and practice.
- Have an appropriate experience base.
- Conduct an active practice, which demonstrates the application of the appropriate professional processes.
- Perform specific methodologies demonstrating advanced practice.
- Participate in professional organizations.
- Participate in community and national organizations. (p. 4)

The Association of Certified Life Care Planners (ACLCP)

This is the newest membership life care planning association, which was established in 2024. The ACLCP has established a strong mission statement for its association, which reads as follows:

> To unite and strengthen the credentials and the professionals holding the Certified Life Care Planner™ (CLCP™) and Canadian Certified Life Care Planner™ (CCLCP™) certifications and to ensure the continued growth, prestige, and high standards of these credentials. The

ACLCP™ will work tirelessly to protect and maintain the dignity, elite standards, and influence of the CLCP™ and CCLCP™ credentials.

Thus, the ACLCP's purpose is to provide all CLCPs and Canadian Certified Life Care Planners (CCLCPs) of the ICHCC a venue to share, express, and formulate ideas and resolution strategies for the amelioration of their CLCP and CCLCP credentials. The ACLCP is designed to provide every member a direct means of access to the ICHCC, and the CLCP/CCLCP credentials in particular, to provide the CLCP/CCLCP with input regarding the credentials' administration protocols, content, and item structure. Such a purpose in the testing process and access to the ICHCC board commissioners and administration allow for a continuation of review and resolution of any credential issues expressed by those practitioners who carry either the CLCP or the CCLCP, or both.

The ACLCP has a focus on research as well as its purpose and will utilize input from only life care planners who hold the CLCP and/or CCLCP credentials. The ACLCP's planned research topics include continued research of life care planners' roles and functions as required by the ICHCC's accreditation board, identifying components of the life care plan and life care planner definitions through scientific study applications and analyses, methodology, and standards and guidelines of practice. The standards and guidelines of practice form the basis of the ICHCC's life care planning credentials, which have been improved upon and validated through the research conducted at Southern Illinois University in 1999–2000 and the more recent research conducted by the ICHCC from 2018 to 2020. The ICHCC feels a need to revisit the role and function of the case manager who provides life care planning services to establish "real-time" standards and guidelines under which additional testing items can be developed and applied, leading to a continuation of a valid test instrument. Thus, such direct CLCP/CCLCP input in the standards and guidelines will improve upon the test validity for testing one's knowledge of life care planning service delivery.

Definitions

Dr. Deutsch knew that as more health care practitioners became involved with life care planning, and to ensure its strength in the competitive health care provider market, the process required a definition. Dr. Deutsch (2002) offered the following as his initial attempt at defining this health care delivery service:

A consistent methodology for analyzing all of the needs dictated by the onset of a catastrophic disability through to the end-of-life expectancy. Consistency means that the methods of analysis remain the same from case to case and does not mean that the same services are provided to like disabilities.

(p. 3)

Life care planning was growing far from where it started in the early 1980s when Dr. Deutsch penned his definition. Dr. Weed (2019), in support of his colleagues, took on the task of rewriting the definition and in 1998 met with a group of rehabilitation consultants and nurses engaged in life care planning at the NARPPS conference (Marcinko, 2019). Their meeting took place in the Forensic Section of the conference supported by the IALCP, the University of Florida with Intelicus, and through a consensus of acceptance, the group published the following definition:

A life care plan is a dynamic document based upon published standards of practice, comprehensive assessment, data analysis, and research, which provides an organized concise plan for current and future needs with associated costs, for individuals who have experienced catastrophic injury or have chronic health care needs.

(p. 7) (Marcinko, p. 32)

The AANLCP published their definition of the life care plan, but it was written more in the form of what the role of the nurse life care planner is and what the plan contained. Their definition reads as follows:

The primary role of the nurse life care planner is to develop a client-specific lifetime plan of care utilizing the nursing process. The plan contains an organized, comprehensive, and evidenced-based approach that estimates current and future healthcare needs. Also included, are the associated costs and frequencies of items and services, which can be utilized as a guide in various applicable sectors (e.g., private, medical-legal, case management).

(Johnson et al., 2022, p. 31)

The AANLCP also wrote a definition of nurse life care planning (Johnson et al.). They added their definition since their methodology is far different from that outlined in the work of Dr. Deutsch. Their definition of life care planning reads as follows:

The specialty practice in which the nurse life care planner utilizes the nursing process for the collection and analysis of comprehensive client-specific data in the preparation of a dynamic document. This document provides an organized, concise plan that estimates for reasonable and necessary, (and reasonably certain to be necessary), current and future healthcare needs with the associated costs and frequencies of goods and services. The nurse life care plan is developed for individuals who have experienced an injury or have chronic healthcare issues. Nurse life care planners function within their professional scope of practice and, when applicable, incorporate opinions arrived upon collaboratively with various health professionals. The nurse life care plan is considered a flexible document and is evaluated and updated as needed.

(p. 31)

The AAPLCP offers the CPLCP credential. Gonzales and Zotovas (2014) offered their definition of the life care plan that reads as follows:

Life care plans are comprehensive documents that objectively identify the residual medical conditions and ongoing care requirements of individuals who are ill or injured, and they quantify the ongoing costs of supplying these individuals with requisite medically-related goods and services throughout their durations of care.

(p. 184)

Dr. Gonzales organized the AAPCLP for physicians trained in physical medicine and rehabilitation and noted that life care planning is actually a seamless extension of physiatry. He offered his definition of life care planning for his association, which reads as follows: Life care planning is a process of applying methodologic analysis to

formulate diagnostic conclusions and opinions regarding physical and/or mental impairment and disability for the purpose of determining care requirements for individuals with permanent or chronic medical conditions.

(Gonzales & Zotovas, 2014, p. 184)

The ICHCC is not supportive of the current definition offered by the IALCP and offered its definition draft copy in 2021 (Johnson et al., 2022; May, 2021). Their definition reads as follows:

The Life Care Plan is defined as a comprehensive document that chronicles the medical and rehabilitative histories of a person who has chronic health care needs and/or who has experienced some form of trauma that has altered the individual's functional capabilities regarding activities of daily living and/or the essential functions of work where applicable. The plan identifies the respective diagnosis(es) related directly to the trauma or the chronic health care condition, the required medical and rehabilitative services, medical supplies, durable medical equipment, medications, support services, the need for barrier-free living environment/ home modifications, and the costs incurred for the individual to achieve as close to premorbid functioning and independence as possible. The plan identifies the costs associated with the maintenance of the maximum level of function achieved (independent vs. dependent) and a detailed projection of potential complications and their associated future costs. The plan further documents the individual's premorbid medical history to assess any potential influences of earlier medical needs on the current trauma.

(p. 1)

The ICHCC's CLCP board of commissioners is charged with establishing a working definition of the life care plan as well as the life care planning service delivery system in general. The ICHCC's board of commissioners, along with the ACLCP, are working to update and redefine the life care plan definition to create a new definition that is more current in life care planning practice.

The purpose of these definitions is to have a model; a baseline specific to the ICHCC certifying agency in the United States and Canada on which to guide CLCPs and CCLCPs into the process of life care planning methodology, concluding with a well-developed, logical, and rational document that identifies the needs and costs the subject with the respective disabling condition will require for the subject's remaining life expectancy.

Regarding the life care plan, the ICHCC accepts the life care planning model espoused by Deutsch and Sawyer (1985), which they detailed in their periodically updated Mathew-Bender textbook from the time of its initial publication through the 1990s. In essence, the ICHCC accepts the premise that the life care plan is a comprehensive document that chronicles the medical and rehabilitative histories of a person who has chronic health care needs and/or who has experienced some form of trauma that has altered the individual's functional capabilities regarding activities of daily living and/or the essential functions of work where applicable. The ICHCC acknowledges that the plan identifies the respective diagnosis(es) related directly to the trauma or the chronic health condition as documented in the medical records and the evaluation records, as well as identifies required medical and rehabilitative services, medical supplies, durable medical equipment, medications, support services, the need for barrier-free living environmental/home modifications, and the costs incurred for the individual to achieve as close to premorbid functioning and independence as possible. Furthermore, the ICHCC notes that the plan details the costs associated with maintenance of the maximum level of function achieved (independent vs. dependent), the subject's premorbid medical history to assess any potential influences of earlier medical needs on the current trauma, and a detailed projection of potential complications and their projected associated future costs if applicable.

The life care plan is a formative guide for the CLCP and CCLCP to determine all of the needs and costs for which the person with an adventitious or disease process disability requires throughout the subject's remaining life span. The AAPLCP defines life care planning as "a process of applying methodological analysis to formulate diagnostic conclusions and opinions regarding impairment and disability to formulate care requirements for individuals with perma-nent or chronic medical conditions" (Gonzales et al., 2015, p. 2). The academy's premise for the life care planning service delivery system is that the primary factors involved in life care planning require the following to be reviewed and extensively investigated:

1. What is the subject's condition (diagnoses and related trauma)?
2. What medically related goods and services does the subject's condition require (medical treatment, rehabilitative programming, barrier-free environmental services, home-dwelling modifications, transportation modifications, etc.)?
3. How much will those goods and services cost over time?

Although appearing to be a rather simple outline of the life care planning process, these points of the process actually blend well with the description of life care planning offered by Deutsch and Sawyer (1985). Taking each of the three factors of the life care planning structure as noted previously, a life care planner can easily be led to identify and include necessary ser-vices, goods, equipment, and other essential factors necessary for ensuring a comfortable and safe quality of life for the subject of the life care plan.

The ICHCC pulled its definition from its website due to the lack of satisfaction among the administration and some of its CLCP commissioners. It was agreed that more time was needed and the definition required some extra thought and rewrites.

Regarding the current definition offered by IARP-IALCP, the ICHCC does not support the definition due to the seventh word in their definition—"dynamic". The ICHCC believes it is the fiducial responsibility of the CLCP to utilize all sources of information before writing the life care plan. Deutsch and Sawyer (1985) pressed upon the reader the need to locate sources regard-ing a diagnosis, potential complications, age-related effects, functional impairments directly related to the diagnosis, and so on. Writing the life care plan is not just a review of the medical records and meetings with direct service providers or with the attending medical provider if possible. There is a need to go to libraries of colleges, universities, and community colleges to research medical and rehabilitative literature specific to the diagnosis. To refer to the life care plan as a dynamic document rather than as a comprehensive document is to suggest that those life care planners who do the minimum will most certainly be called on for something that was necessary but overlooked. This can lead to errors and omission lawsuits that will be extremely costly and could be detrimental to the individual's ongoing practice. The CLCP has an obliga-tion to review all resource materials and discuss questions regarding injury, disability, diagnos-tics, and potential complications with those persons who have expertise in specific areas of the respective case. It is unthinkable that the referral source would like to hear that the CLCP is fin-ished with the life care plan and is sending it out with an invoice, but it remains unfinished. The ICHCC lists the following that justifies the need for the CLCP to research all available sources that address the diagnosis/injury sequelae and the resulting loss of function:

1. Having done due diligence and applied their fiducial responsibility to investigate and research the medical condition and the potential rehabilitative outcomes, the life care plan is complete.
2. Any future injury/sequelae or potential complications should have been identified and addressed in a narrative in the life care plan.
3. Future required care from age-related influence on the anatomical area of injury is unrelated to the CLCP's work provided the potential for age-related effects of trauma were identified and addressed in the plan.

Writing the Life Care Plan: A Case Study

The life care plan is used primarily for the benefit of the person about whom it was written. It also has other insightful influences that may be unknown to the life care planner. The life care plan is a document that easily addresses the life care planner's character and integrity to the referral source. The CLCP is well aware of the ICHCC's ethical principles, one being that of "Do no harm". In doing no harm, the life care planner understands that it is the person with the injury and the resulting disability that are the primary obligations of the life care planning process, not the referral source. I have found upon reviewing life care plans that people tend to write their plans for the referral source and not for the individual subject of the injury. Thus, whether the plaintiff referred or the defense referred, bias is present, and most of the time it shows up in the life care plan. The opposing attorneys can have a "field day" with such biased plans in either the deposition or the witness stand. Regarding two CLCPs working on the same case, one for the plaintiff and one for the defense, theoretically, the life care plans should be identical.

The following life care plan is of an actual injured individual who sustained a distal fibula fracture, a torn anterior talofibular ligament, and a bone chip. The reader will see explanatory text printed in a color that explains the purpose of the respective issue and its place on the Category of Needs chart.

	Initials for Confidentiality
NAME:	*C. P. fddd (Initials)*
REFERRAL SOURCE FILE NUMBER:	23227
DATE OF BIRTH:	02/09/1976
DATE OF INJURY:	10/02/2002
DATE OF EVALUATION:	03/15/2006
DATE OF COMPLETED REPORT:	03/19/2006
REQUESTED BY:	**Shane Maxwell, DO**
COMPLETED BY:	**Heather Howe, CLCP #0200**

Purpose of Referral

C. P. is a 30-year-old Caucasian female who was interviewed in her home on March 15, 2006. Present for the interview was the client and her husband, B. P. Ms. P. was referred for a rehabilitation evaluation by her attorney, Shane Maxwell of Forté Law. The purpose of this evaluation is to assess the extent to which handicapping conditions impede her ability to live independently, to handle all activities of daily living, and to assess the disability's impact on her vocational development status.

Accordingly, I reviewed the provided documentation and interviewed C. and her husband. The interview was conducted on March 15, 2006, at C.'s home at 26 Keefe Court, Richmond, Virginia. Present for the interview was the writer, C. P., and B. P.

The life care plan is a dynamic document based upon published standards of practice, comprehensive assessment, data analysis, and research, which provides an organized, concise plan for current and future needs with the associated costs for individuals who have experienced catastrophic injury or have chronic health care needs (International Academy of Life Care Planners).

The life care plan recommendations included in this report have been identified as a result of what is deemed reasonably necessary, based on provided medical evidence, to preserve and promote C. P. mental and physical well-being.

Acknowledgment of Expert's Duty

I acknowledge that it is my duty to prepare a report and provide evidence in relation to C. P.'s case that is:

1. Fair, objective, and non-partisan
2. Related to matters within my area of expertise; and
3. Providing additional assistance as the court may reasonably require to determine a matter in issue.

Statement of Qualifications

As the author of this report, I am a Certified Life Care Planner, having met the requirements put forth by the International Commission on Health Care Certification. In addition, I am a physical therapist and have been licensed to practice in the state of Virginia since 1994. I hold a Doctor of Physical Therapy degree from the University of Delaware in Newark, Delaware.

Please refer to the enclosed curriculum vita for a full description of my professional training and experience.

Introduction

Demographic Information

Client Name: C. P.; **Address:** 26 Keefe Court, Richmond, VA; **Country:** USA; **Closest Metro Area:** Richmond; **Phone**: 506-384-5214; **Birthdate:** 02/09/1976; **Age:** 30; **Sex:** Female; **Race:** Caucasian; **Marital Status:** Married × 9 yrs; **Birthplace:** Richmond, VA; **Citizen:** Yes; **Bilingual:** No; **Glasses:** No; **Dominant Hand**: Right; **Height:** 5'8"; **Weight (present):** 139 pounds; **Date of Onset:** 10/02/2002.

History: Ms. P. suffered a left ankle fracture of the distal fibula, torn anterior talofibular ligament, and a bone chip resulting from twisting her ankle at work while demonstrating a defensive maneuver as a volleyball coach. She spent 8 weeks on crutches. Despite physical therapy, symptoms persisted. An MRI was ordered, which showed significant scarring. C. was then referred for a second opinion with an orthopedic surgeon who specializes in ankle injuries, and she was referred to an orthopedic specialist. An exploratory laparoscopy was performed as well as a manipulation; however, symptoms worsened, and she was referred to a pain specialist who performed a series of nerve blocks and eventually implanted a spinal cord stimulator. Results were less than satisfactory, and Ms. P. was referred to the Carolinas Pain Institute (CPI) for suspected complex regional pain syndrome. Ms. P.'s treatment consisted of ganglion nerve blocks and a second spinal cord stimulator. Ms. P. continues to receive treatment under the care of Dr. Rauck at the CPI.

Loss of Consciousness or Altered State of Consciousness: No.

Rehabilitation Program(s) [In/Outpatient Since Injury]: Ms. P. received physical therapy rehabilitation on two occasions, initially from November 20, 2002, to August 12, 2002, with Yohan Briggs of Richmond Therapeutics. Ms. P. reported having attended treatments three times per week for the first 2 months and then a reduced frequency. Ms. P. reported that treatment focused on reducing pain, swelling, and improving strength and range of motion. *"I did not find the treatments that helpful but the therapist tried everything and even consulted his colleagues."* A second round of rehabilitation was completed between January 12, 2004, and March 28, 2004, with Graham Black of Max Health Institute. Treatments were scheduled daily over an 8-week period and focused on gait biomechanics, muscle imbalance, balance, and proprioception. Ms. P. reported an initial improvement but then a return of symptoms. *"It was very frustrating to think I was improving and feeling hopeful for me to just get worse again."*

Prior Medical History: Ms. P. noted that she was in good health before this injury without any medical conditions resulting from injuries, illnesses, or diseases. *"I had stitches on my chin when I was 12 and fell off my bike."* Ms. P. denies any prior surgeries except for having her wisdom teeth extracted at the age of 19. Ms. P. is a non-smoker and occasional drinker of alcohol but denies any history of excessive use of alcohol or drug use other than occasional marijuana. Mentally, Ms. P. reported feeling stable all of her life and has never consulted a psychologist, psychiatrist, or counselor for any reason.

Chief Complaint(s)

Current Disability

Disabling Problem(s) (By Client/Family History and Report. No Physical Examination Occurred): *"The way I understand it is I broke my ankle that then triggered a hyperactive response to my nervous system that I now have to try and live with and manage for the rest of my life. The way the doctor explained it to me is that signals travel from my hands and feet up my spinal cord to my brain and that my spinal cord, what should normally be a two-lane country road, is now an eight-lane super highway with bumper-to-bumper traffic. My main problem is pain everywhere. There isn't any part of my body that doesn't hurt at some point in the day. I can't do the things I used to do, and my life revolves around trying to control my symptoms. I don't go out; I've withdrawn from my friends, and my husband barely tolerates me anymore."*

Figure 1.1 shows the pain drawing Ms. P. completed during her functional capacity evaluation (FCE) on 02/15/06:

C. reports being in constant pain every day and at all times. Her day revolves around managing her symptoms and planning ahead. She keeps ice packs in her car when she leaves the house and can only tolerate short periods of activity at one time. Ms. P. is also focused on the next medical treatment that may help rid her of the pain. She has at times doubled her pain medication on bad days and is worried about the potential for dependency on her pain meds.

Anticipated Treatments: Ms. P. remains in therapy at CPI under the medical authorization of Dr. Rauck. Her current medication regimen as managed by Dr. Rauck includes Zanaflex, Lidoderm patches, Clonidine patches, Voltaren, Methadone, Lunesta for sleep, Ultram PRN, and Topamax. She noted that the patches have produced sores on her right dorsal foot, and her left ankle remains discolored, swollen, and warm to the touch. Ms. P. is unaware of any upcoming procedures but sees Dr. Rauck every few months for a review of her medications. It is also noted in the FCE report dated February 15, 2006, that *"She spends little time determining how to become more productive despite her pain, but rather on what treatment strategy is her attending physician going to recommend and will it be effective."*

Psychological Issues

Patient: Ms. P. admits to feeling depressed at times. *"I did not picture this as my life. I had goals and aspirations for my career, having a family someday. My husband and I don't talk about having kids, we just avoid the subject. We both know I couldn't manage a baby like*

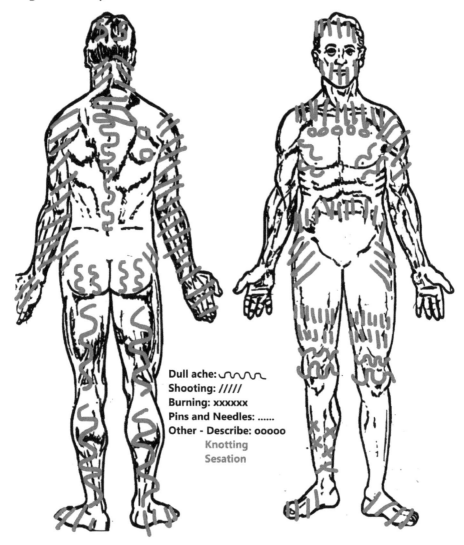

Dull ache: ∿∿∿
Shooting: /////
Burning: xxxxxx
Pins and Needles: ......
Other - Describe: ooooo
   Knotting
   Sesation

Figure 1.1 Pain Drawing Completed During Functional Capacity Evaluation

this." Ms. P. has not been referred for any psychological counseling. When questioned about receiving treatment she reported, *"I am well supported by my family but yeah, it wouldn't hurt, that's for sure."*

Family, Emotional Impact on Spouse/Children: Ms. P. is married without children. Her husband works for his family business and they are making ends meet. She states that her husband has been supportive of her during her disability period and that her brother as well as her parents and in-laws have been supportive. Her parents live in Charlotte, North Carolina, and her in-laws live in Florida. Socially, Ms. P. reported that she has withdrawn somewhat from her friends due to being in constant pain but tries her best to keep in touch. Ms. P. noted that she requires ice packs when she travels outside of the home, keeping a cooler with ice packs in her car.

Physical Limitations

Loss of Tactile Sensation: She has numbness on the scar area on her left ankle and low back where stimulators were implanted. She also presents with allodynia in the lower extremities bilaterally.

Reach: C. has a full range of motion with her upper extremities, but if she has to stretch to reach something, pain is reported in the lower body, hips, knees, and feet.

Lift: Nonfunctional.

Prehensile/Grip: Intact bilaterally.

Sitting: She has pain in her mid to lower back, left hip, and both knees with extended sitting. She can sit for about 1 hour before she has to get up and move around. She does note that when sitting, she is constantly squirming to find a comfortable position.

Standing: She is limited to standing for brief periods only. She notes that when standing, she typically will lean on something, and if a chair is available, she will sit rather than stand.

Walking/Gait: She can walk for short distances but only on even terrain. Walking is always difficult and will increase her pain.

Bend/Twist: She is limited in her ability to bend and twist at the waist and notes that she can no longer swing a golf club.

Kneel: Nonfunctional.

Stoop/Squat: Nonfunctional.

Climb: She is limited in her ability to climb stairs and does require a handrail to hang on to.

Balance: She is frequently off balance and is fearful of falling.

Breathing: She indicates that she used to walk 5 miles a day, but now will get out of breath much easier because she is out of shape due to an inability to exercise.

Headaches: Daily.

Vision: Intact.

Hearing: Intact.

Driving: She can drive, but only short distances in her community, as any greater distance causes increased pain. If she has to drive greater distances, she will have to stop and stretch, whether she is a driver or a passenger.

Physical Stamina (Average Daily Need for Rest or Reclining): Daily on two to three occasions throughout the day. She tires much more easily and attributes some of her fatigue to her medications.

Environmental Influences

Problems with exposure to:

- **Air Conditioning**: Yes, if it's too cold, her pain with increase.
- **Heat:** No.
- **Cold:** Yes, same as air conditioning.
- **Wet/Humid:** Yes, causes joints to ache and pain to increase.
- **Sudden Changes:** Yes, she prefers a predictable and controlled environment.
- **Fumes:** Not that she is aware of.

Table 1.3 Present Medical Treatment

Doctor	Specialty	Phone	Fax	Frequency	Last Seen
Dr. R. Rauck	Anesthesiologist			Monthly	02/20/07

Medication	Strength	Frequency	Tablets	Purpose	Prescribed by
Percocet	7.5 mg	1–2×/day	60	Pain	Rauck
Flexeril	10 mg	3×/day	90	Muscle Relaxant	Rauck
Ambien CR	12.5 mg	1× at night	30	Sleep Aid	Rauck
Zoloft	100 mg	1× /day	30	Anxiety	Rauck
Lisinopril-HCTZ	20 mg	1× /day	30	Blood Pressure	Rauck
Ibuprofen	600 mg	As needed	60	Pain	Rauck

- **Noise:** Yes, increases irritability and feels aggravated.
- **Stress:** Yes.   I Do Not Understand What is Needed Here

Over-the-Counter Medication(s): Zantac 150 mg, 1×/day.
Drugstore and Phone Number: CVS, Mountain Rd.
Assistive Devices: None at this time.

Medical Summary

Date of Medical Summary: 03/19/06
C. P. is a 30-year-old Caucasian female who sustained orthopedic injuries as the result of a workplace trip and fall.

Records Reviewed

- Case file as provided by Dawn Gaide, RN, BSN, of M. Hayes & Associates, 30 East Padonia Road, Suite 201, Timonium, MD, 21093

Diagnosis

Status post left fracture/sprain; status post complex regional pain syndrome, left greater than the right lower foot, type I, with pain complaints spreading throughout her body; status post chronic pain syndrome; status post 13 nerve blocks; status post spinal stimulator implants ×2, laparoscopy of the left foot; status post left ankle manipulation under anesthesia.

Summary

October 2, 2002, according to hospital records provided, Ms. P. suffered a left ankle fracture of the distal fibula, torn anterior talofibular ligament, and a bone chip resulting from twisting her ankle at work while demonstrating a defensive maneuver as a volleyball coach.

October 3, 2002, Ms. P. drove herself to the emergency department of the Bon Secours St. Mary's Hospital due to intense pain and inflammation. An x-ray was completed, and she was consulted by an orthopedic surgeon, Dr. H. Stern, who diagnosed her condition as a fracture/sprain and applied a cast to stabilize her ankle joint.

November 4, 2002, Ms. P. was seen in follow-up by Dr. Stern. According to clinical notes, Dr. Sten recommended that the cast stay on another 2 weeks and that she continue with non-weight bearing.

November 18, 2002, Ms. P. was seen in follow-up by Dr. Stern. According to clinical notes, Dr. Sten removed the cast, prescribed physical therapy, and administered a series of cortisone injections. He also cleared her for partial weight bearing as tolerated and would see her again in 4 weeks.

November 20, 2002, Ms. P. was assessed by a physical therapist, Yohan Briggs of Richmond Therapeutics. According to medical records, his clinical analysis was of ankle instability, reduced strength, reduced range of motion, and pitting edema. He recommended physical therapy treatments three times per week for 8 weeks.

December 20, 2002, Ms. P. was seen in follow-up by Dr. Stern. According to clinical notes, despite having been in physical therapy for 4 weeks, pain and limited range of motion persisted. Though she was now full weight bearing and had stopped using the crutches, walking was painful. Dr. Stern requested an MRI, which revealed a significant amount of scar tissue, and referred her to an orthopedic surgeon, Dr. Zimmer, for a second opinion.

August 21, 2003, Ms. P. was discharged from physical therapy. According to the discharge report of the physical therapist, Yohan Briggs, dated the same, Ms. P. had reached a plateau. Despite a total of 48 treatments, Ms. P. was continuing to experience significant pain in the ankle. Range of motion and strength continued to be limited, and edema persisted. As Ms. P. had received an upcoming consultation date with an orthopedic surgeon, Dr. Zimmer, the decision was made to discontinue treatment until this opinion was received.

September 4, 2003, Ms. P. was consulted by an orthopedic surgeon, Dr. Zimmer. According to his consultation report, surgery was recommended to debride the area of scarring.

October 1, 2003, Ms. P. underwent an exploratory laparoscopy procedure. According to the surgical report, debridement of the scar tissue around the joint was completed as well as exploration of the peroneus brevis, peroneus tertius, and inferior extensor retinaculum tendons to evaluate any tears or separations. It was determined that the tendons were intact.

January 8, 2004, Ms. P. underwent manipulation under anesthesia of the left ankle by Dr. Zimmer. According to the surgical report, following the laparoscopy on October 1, 2003, Ms. P. noted a worsening of symptoms. Following the procedure, Dr. Zimmer referred Ms. P. for rehabilitation at Max Health Institute.

January 12, 2004, Ms. P. was assessed by physical therapist Graham Black of Max Health Institute, who recommended physical therapy treatments at five visits per week over an 8-week period.

March 28, 2004, Ms. P. was discharged from Max Health Institute. According to the discharge report, Ms. P. experienced some relief initially, but symptoms returned and her condition worsened. The physical therapist recommended that she return to Dr. Zimmer.

April 2, 2004, Ms. P. was seen by Dr. Zimmer. According to his consult report, he diagnosed her condition as reflex sympathetic dystrophy and referred her to a pain specialist.

April 12, 2004, Ms. P. was consulted by an anesthesiologist and pain specialist, Dr. Long. According to medical records, Dr. Long confirmed the diagnosis and proceeded with a series of nerve blocks in her lumbar spine. Dr. Long also prescribed oral medication and additional nerve block therapy.

September 22, 2004, Ms. P. continued with significant symptom complaints despite having had nine nerve block injections. Therefore, Dr. Long proceeded with surgery to implant a Precision Spectra dual lead spinal cord stimulator for pain relief. According to the surgery report, there were no complications during the procedure.

November 3, 2004, Ms. P. was seen in follow-up by Dr. Long. According to his clinic note, the results of the implant were not to his or Ms. P.'s satisfaction. As such, Dr. Long referred Ms. P. to a pain management specialist, Dr. Rauck, of the Carolinas Pain Institute and Center for Clinical Research, in Winston-Salem, North Carolina.

April 5, 2005, Ms. P. was consulted by an anesthesiologist and pain specialist, Dr. Rauck. According to his consultation report, Dr. Rauck diagnosed her condition as complex regional pain syndrome, type I, left greater than the right lower foot. He also noted pain complaints spreading throughout her body and severe allodynia from the mid-knee down to her left foot with some sensitivity extending into her groin and left hip. He further noted that she presented with a left foot that is edematous and shiny in appearance with redness and hair loss. Based on his initial findings, Dr. Rauck recommended a second spinal implant and ganglion nerve block treatments.

September 2, 2005, Ms. P. received her fourth ganglion nerve block from Dr. Rauck.

September 21, 2005, Ms. P. underwent surgery to implant an Advanced Bionics dual lead rechargeable stimulator. According to Dr. Rauck's surgical report, there were no complications during the procedure.

February 15, 2006, Ms. P. participated in a functional capacity evaluation with Virgil Robert May III of May Physical Therapy Services, as referred by her attorney. The results of the evaluation indicated that *"Ms. P. is not a candidate for competitive employment, nor is she a candidate for supportive employment or situational work in a sheltered workshop. Her employability and placeability profiles have been compromised such that she no longer qualifies for gainful employment. Her focus is on her symptoms, and her health decline since the onset of her sequela post-ankle fracture, rather than focusing/concentrating on any respective work activity. Thus, she poses a safety risk to herself and to anyone working around her. The Department of Labor's (DOL) lowest Physical Demand Characteristic (PDC) is 'SEDENTARY.' If the DOL had a category for persons who are physically disabled from work, she would meet this respective category's criteria, rather than that of the SEDENTARY PDC.*

"Ms. P. did not complete all of the assigned test activities. She demonstrated a consistent effort throughout this evaluation as evidenced by the data output as applied to her repeated measure test activities detailed in the Raw Data Section. She did not manage and control her symptom response patterns well, such that symptoms influenced her functioning during the tests. Ms. P. was requested to profile her response to physical activities as well as to document the degree of change in the performance of those respective activities. Her profiles are illustrated later.

"To summarize, Ms. P. demonstrated poor control over her symptom response patterns and therefore demonstrated an inability to negotiate her symptoms so that a higher level of task completion could be achieved. Ms. P. exhibited mechanical and strength deficits in range of motion and dynamic activities. Regarding the dynamic lifting study, this test was not offered due to her overt pain behaviors, strength deficits, and the resulting unsafe testing mechanics. Based on the medical records and her performance in this functional study, it is this evaluator's opinion that Ms. P. cannot function independently in the competitive labor market with or without accommodation and worksite modification."

Activities of Daily Living

Sleep Pattern
Arises: 8:00 a.m.
Retires: midnight.
Average Hours Sleep/24 Hours: 5 to 6 hours even with medication.

Sleep Difficulties: She has to take Ambien to sleep. She usually takes this medication every night. She has recently had to increase to two Ambien because one was not helping anymore. She has been on some type of sleep medication since her injury. She reported that without the medication she does not sleep at all.

Independence In

Dressing: She has difficulty washing and dressing her lower body, but she has learned to compensate and do these tasks.
Housework: She can do light chores like washing a few dishes, but heavy cleaning is being done by her mother.
Cooking: Her husband has taken over this task.
Laundry: She can do this independently.
Yard Work: Her husband is responsible for this task and always has been.

Social Activities

Organizations Pre/Post: Very active in the volleyball community pre-injury. Post-injury, she will occasionally watch a game.
Volunteer Work Pre/Post: Helped friends and neighbors, but nothing organized.
Socialization Pre/Post: She feels she has withdrawn from socializing and only goes out on occasion with small groups of friends who are aware of her condition.
Hobbies (Present): No new hobbies.
Hobbies (Previous): Golf, volleyball, and any physical or athletic activities. She no longer participates in these activities.

Personal Habits

Smoking: No.
Alcohol: Social basis only.
Drugs: No.
History of Abuse and/or Treatment Programs: No history of abuse.

Socioeconomic Status

Residence

Primary Residence: C. lives with her husband in a small single-story bungalow in Richmond, Virginia. She has lived in Richmond all her life and has no future plans to leave the city. C.'s parents live in a nearby neighborhood approximately 20 minutes away, while her husband's parents live approximately 45 to 50 minutes away. The house is an older home but was renovated inside and out in 2000. There is one step to access the main entrance.

Income

Disability Policy: No.
W.C.: No.
S.S.D.I.: No.
Wages: Yes.

Current Financial Situation: C. and her husband are making ends meet. She has not worked since her accident while her husband works for the family business. They do have insurance, which he holds through his employment. They managed to pay their medical bills for the first few years but as of last year have amassed debt, which they are making payments on.

Other Agencies Involved

State Vocational Rehabilitation: No.
State Employment Services: No.
Rehabilitation Nurse: No.
Other Agency: No.
Felony Convictions? No.

Education and Training

Highest Grade Completed: High school graduate
Last School Attended: Algonquin College for Entrepreneurship in Travel and Tourism Program
Apprenticeship/OJT: No
Literacy: Yes
Licenses/Certifications: Virginia real estate license issued in 1988, #SA1234567

Military Experience

Branch: Not applicable.
EMPLOYMENT HISTORY
Released to Return to Work: No.
Work History Since Injury: C. has not been able to return to work since her injury. Both real estate sales agent and volleyball coaching require significant walking and on-feet activity. As C. was on crutches for the first 2 months post-injury and then continued having difficulty with pain, swelling, and an ability to bear weight, the various doctors she consulted agreed she was not ready to return to work. C. was earning a 4% commission on real estate sales. In 2001 she earned approximately $100,000.
Employer: Royal LePage; **City/State:** Richmond, VA; **Position:** Sales Agent; **Start Date:** 1988; **End Date:** Present; **Schedule:** Full-time; **Length:** 10 Years; **Wage:** Averages $80,000/ year; **Duties:** Buying and selling of residential properties.

Observations

Orientation: Alert and oriented times three.
Stream of Thought: Clear and rational.
Approach Toward Evaluation: Positive.
Attitudes/Insight: Good.
Appearance: Good.

Tests Administered

As part of the evaluation, C. is asked to complete the following psychometric questionnaires:

Pain, Depression, Anxiety, and Fatigue

The Patient Health Questionnaire (PHQ-9) was used as a measure of depressive symptom severity. C. obtained a score of 4/27 corresponding to the *low range of depressive symptom severity*.

The FFQ-F scale was used to assess the severity of fatigue symptoms. C.'s score was 8/10 corresponding to a *high range of fatigue*.

The Beck Anxiety Inventory is a well-accepted, self-report measure of anxiety used with adults. It assesses the severity of several common symptoms of anxiety that C. may have experienced during the previous month. C.'s score of 21/63 indicates a *clinically significant level of anxiety*.

Self-Reported Limitations

The Disability Index was used to measure the degree to which different activities of the client's life have been affected by her health condition. Her score was 59, placing her in a *severe range of perceived disability*.

The World Health Organization Disability Assessment Schedule is a 36-item self-administered questionnaire that looks at difficulties in a variety of different areas due to health conditions. C. completed this questionnaire and acknowledged the most difficulty ("*Extreme or Cannot Do*") with work tasks. She also acknowledged the "*Severe*" drain on financial resources. C. also reported "*Severe*" difficulty with household responsibilities and "*Severe*" difficulty with standing for long periods (30 minutes).

Cognitive and Emotional Response

The CIEQ-C was used to assess C.'s negative cognitive reactions to her current symptoms. High scores on this scale reflect a tendency to become overwhelmed by distressing symptoms and to focus excessively on symptoms. During this assessment, C. obtained a score of 10/14, corresponding to a ***moderate to high range of catastrophizing beliefs***.

The CIEQ-I was used to assess C.'s perspective on the degree of unfairness that categorizes her current life/health situation. During the assessment, C. obtained a score of 3/10, which corresponds to a ***low range of perceived injustice beliefs.***

The FFQ-K questionnaire was used to assess C.'s worries and concerns that she might engage in an activity that would result in an exacerbation of symptoms. C. scored 4/10, which corresponds to a ***low to moderate level of symptom exacerbation concern***.

Conclusions

The conclusions of this report are based on a comprehensive review of the provided medical and other supporting documentation, along with consideration of principles and independent research conducted by this writer specific to orthopedic injuries, complex regional pain syndrome, and chronic pain. Attention is paid to the clinical practice guidelines for the treatment of these diagnoses promulgated by multiple sources and cited in the life care plan.

C. remains severely impaired secondary to the October 2002 onset of disability. She continues to experience significant physical limitations that affect her ability to fully participate in activities of daily living and her chosen vocation. She will continue to require medical management of her injuries through life expectancy.

It is the opinion of this certified life care planner that the needs and costs outlined in this analysis are reasonable and necessary. In the event of any errors, omissions, or inconsistencies in this information, or should new information become available, this writer reserves the right to modify the conclusions of this report accordingly.

Respectfully Submitted,

A life care plan is a dynamic document based upon published standards of practice, comprehensive assessment, data analysis, and research, which provides an organized, concise plan for current and future needs, with associated costs, for individuals who have experienced catastrophic injury or have chronic health care needs.

(IALCP—International Academy of Life Care Planners, 2003. Definition established during the 2000 Life Care Planning Summit)

Through the development of a comprehensive life care plan, a clear, concise, and sensible presentation of the complex requirements of the patient is identified as a means of documenting current and future medical needs for individuals who have experienced catastrophic injury or have chronic health care needs.

The purpose of this life care plan is to assess the extent to which handicapping conditions impede the patient's ability to live independently, to manage activities of daily living, and to assess the disability's impact on her vocational status. The goals of a comprehensive life care plan are also to improve and maintain the clinical state of the patient, prevent secondary complications, provide the clinical and physical environment for optimal recovery, provide support for the family, and provide a disability management program aimed at preventing unnecessary complications and minimizing the long-term care needs of the patient.

While a life care plan identifies the client's medical, rehabilitation, and social needs, the foundation and rationale for each recommendation must also be detailed along with current costs and availability of services specific to the client's geographical area. The report format should include narrative descriptions, a comprehensive review of the medical and psychological information, the inclusion of references supporting the basis of the medical foundation, the use of charts to delineate the start/stop dates of usage and frequency, annual costs, and lifetime costs.

Foundation: It is noted from C.'s medical file that she participated in rehabilitation from a physical therapist on two occasions. In 2006, 4 years after her injury, she remains in therapy under the care of her anesthesiologist and pain specialist, Dr. Rauck, of the Carolinas Pain Institute. The FCE report also provided photographic evidence of an edematous and discolored left foot, gait and stair climbing patterns. It was the opinion of the FCE evaluator that C. required further medication therapy and pain management medical services. As CRPS is considered a chronic condition, providing a relatively low-cost lifeline does not produce dependence on or excessive use of specialist services, but can be effective in avoiding more expensive crisis management. In accordance with Dr. Rauck and the FCE evaluator, it is considered reasonable and necessary to continue lifelong monitoring for any improvement or deterioration from a physical therapy perspective.

Foundation: It is noted from C.'s medical file that there hasn't been significant involvement from other disciplines such as occupational therapy. Therefore, based on the published guideline on the management of complex regional pain syndrome, it is considered reasonable and necessary to support the recommendation.

Foundation: It is noted from C.'s medical file that before her injury in 2002, she was in good health without any significant prior medical history. In 2006, as per the FCE report, C.'s pain drawing is almost entirely covered by pain sensations. Vocationally, she was a volleyball coach

Table 1.4 Projected Evaluations (Physical Therapy)

Item/Service	Age/Year	Frequency/ Replacement	Purpose balance, mobility, and function.	Cost	Comment	Recommended By
Physical Therapy	Beginning 30/03/2006 Ending Life Exp.	1× /year for 5 years followed by 1× /2–3 years	To assess for changes in the range of motion, strength, weight bearing, gait,	$150 per assessment		Anesthesiologist, Dr. Rauck FCE Evalua-tor, Dr. May Research, Medical Records, CLCP

According to the Royal College of Physicians' 2005 published guidelines for the diagnosis, referral, and management of complex regional pain syndrome in adults, pain is typically the leading symptom of CRPS and is often associated with limb dysfunction and psychological distress. For those in whom pain persists, anxiety, depression, and loss of sleep are likely to develop, even if they are not prominent at the outset. Therefore, an integrated interdisciplinary treatment approach is recommended, tailored to the individual patient. The primary aims are to reduce pain, preserve or restore function, and enable patients to manage their condition and improve their quality of life. The four "pillars" of care are education, pain relief, physical rehabilitation, and psychological intervention.

The role of physical therapy in the assessment of CRPS is to evaluate the state and tolerances of the affected limb and the subsequent impact on function. In accordance with C.'s pain specialist, Dr. Rauck, and FCE evaluator, Dr. May, for further pain management services, annual physical therapy evaluations are recommended.

Source(s): www.rcplondon.ac.uk/guidelines-policy/complex-regional-pain-syndrome-adults

Table 1.5 Projected Evaluations (Occupational Therapy)

Item/Service	Age/Year	Frequency/ Replacement	Purpose	Cost	Comment	Recommended By
Occupa-tional Therapy	Beginning 30/03/2006 Ending Life Exp.	1× /year for 5 years followed by 1× /2–3 years	To assess any changes in inde-pendent functional needs	$150 per assessment		Anesthesiologist, Dr. Rauck FCE Evalua-tor, Dr. May Research, Medical Records, CLCP

According to the Royal College of Physicians' 2005 published guidelines for the diagnosis, referral, and management of complex regional pain syndrome in adults, pain is typically the leading symptom of CRPS and is often associated with limb dysfunction and psychological distress. For those in whom pain persists, anxiety, depression, and loss of sleep are likely to develop, even if they are not prominent at the outset. Therefore, an integrated interdisciplinary treatment approach is recommended, tailored to the individual patient. The primary aims are to reduce pain, preserve or restore function, and enable patients to manage their condition and improve their quality of life. The four "pillars" of care are education, pain relief, physical rehabilitation, and psychological intervention.

The role of occupational therapy in the assessment of CRPS is to assess the state of hypersensitivity of the affected limb, assist in maintaining joint alignment, and aid in regaining independent function through the use of adaptive equip-ment and other functional therapeutic activities. In accordance with C.'s pain specialist, Dr. Rauck, and FCE evaluator, Dr. May, for further pain management services, annual occupational therapy evaluations are recommended.

Source(s): www.rcplondon.ac.uk/guidelines-policy/complex-regional-pain-syndrome-adults

and worked in real estate with additional training in travel and tourism. As per the FCE report, C. is not a candidate for the competitive labor market. All of these changes can have a signifi-cant impact on one's quality of life and a psychological impact on the individual

Table 1.6 Projected Evaluations (Psychology)

Item/Service	Age/Year	Frequency/ Replacement	Purpose	Cost	Comment	Recommended By
Psychology	Beginning 30/03/2006 Ending Life Exp.	1×/Year	To regularly assess cognitive-behavioral pain management strategies.	$100 per evaluation		Anesthesiologist, Dr. Rauck FCE Evaluator, Dr. May Research, Medical Records, CLCP

According to the Royal College of Physicians' 2005 published guidelines for the diagnosis, referral, and management of complex regional pain syndrome in adults, pain is typically the leading symptom of CRPS and is often associated with limb dysfunction and psychological distress. For those in whom pain persists, anxiety, depression, and loss of sleep are likely to develop, even if they are not prominent at the outset. Therefore, an integrated interdisciplinary treatment approach is recommended, tailored to the individual patient. The primary aims are to reduce pain, preserve or restore function, and enable patients to manage their condition and improve their quality of life. The four "pillars" of care are education, pain relief, physical rehabilitation, and psychological intervention.

The role of psychology in the assessment of CRPS is to assess the presence and degree of psychological symptoms such as anxiety, depression, risk of addiction, and coping strategies, among other things as well as the ability of the patient and family to manage stress and adapt to changes in family dynamics. In accordance with C.'s pain specialist, Dr. Rauck, and FCE evaluator, Dr. May, for further pain management services, annual psychological evaluations are recommended.

Source(s): www.rcplondon.ac.uk/guidelines-policy/complex-regional-pain-syndrome-adults

Table 1.7 Projected Evaluations (Dietitian)

Item/Service	Age/Year	Frequency/ Replacement	Purpose	Cost	Comment	Recommended By
Dietitian	Beginning 30/03/2006 Ending Life Exp.	1×/Year	To regularly assess changes in eating habits.	$100 per evaluation		Research, CLCP

According to the Royal College of Physicians' 2005 published guidelines for the diagnosis, referral, and management of complex regional pain syndrome in adults, pain is typically the leading symptom of CRPS and is often associated with limb dysfunction and psychological distress. For those in whom pain persists, anxiety, depression, and loss of sleep are likely to develop, even if they are not prominent at the outset. Therefore, an integrated interdisciplinary treatment approach is recommended, tailored to the individual patient. The primary aims are to reduce pain, preserve or restore function, and enable patients to manage their condition and improve their quality of life. The four "pillars" of care are education, pain relief, physical rehabilitation, and psychological intervention.

The guideline further specifies that general measures such as adequate diet, ensuring adequate hemoglobin level, diabetic control, and cessation of smoking should be emphasized where appropriate. It is noted in the medical record that C. is a non-smoker.

Source(s): www.rcplondon.ac.uk/guidelines-policy/complex-regional-pain-syndrome-adults

Foundation: Though there was little evidence of dietary habits documented in the medical file, this foundation is almost entirely based on the published guideline and therefore supported by <u>research and the CLCP as considered reasonable and necessary</u>.

In accordance with C.'s pain specialist, Dr. Rauck, these medications have been working well and are not forecasted to be changed in the near future. Over the course of her life, C. will require medication to help control the comorbidities associated with her long-term chronic condition. Medication needs vary significantly depending on an individual's medical and lifestyle needs. Common medications used to ameliorate the effects of CRPS include opioids, antidepressants

Table 1.8 Projected Therapeutic Modalities (Physical Therapy)

Item/Service	Age/Year	Frequency/ Replacement	Purpose	Cost	Comment	Recommended By
Physical Therapy	Beginning 30/3/2006 Ending Life Exp	3×/wk for 13 wks 1×/wk for 6 wks 4×/year until age 34 Evaluations annually for the next 5 yrs followed by 1×/2–3 yrs	To control pain, reduce inflam- mation, promote a range of motion and strength	$100/treatment $4500/year $400/year Age 31–34		Anesthesiologist Dr. Rauck, CPI PT, S. Redding Research, Medical Records, CLCP

According to the Royal College of Physicians' 2005 published guidelines for the diagnosis, referral, and management of complex regional pain syndrome in adults, there is currently a lack of evidence to inform the best treatment approach to offer patients with CRPS. Recommended therapeutic approaches can include:

* patient education and support
* general exercises and strengthening
* mirror visual feedback
* graded motor imagery
* gait re-education
* transcutaneous electrical nerve stimulation
* postural control
* hydrotherapy
* edema control strategies
* facilitating self-management of the condition

The guidelines also suggest that it is critical that physical therapy be delivered by a therapist trained in the treatment of the condition. The medical record supports that the patient received such a level of care and continues to receive the appropriate level of care via the Carolinas Pain Institute. The medical record also indicated the previously extended treatment be weaned as recommended by CPI, physical therapist, S. Redding, and supported by anesthesiologist Dr. Rauck. **Needs to be added to the medical record.**

Source(s): www.rcplondon.ac.uk/guidelines-policy/complex-regional-pain-syndrome-adults

https://carolinaspaininstitute.com/

Table 1.9 Projected Therapeutic Modalities (Occupational Therapy)

Item/Service	Age/Year	Frequency/ Replacement	Purpose	Cost	Comment	Recommended By
Occupational Therapy	Beginning 30/3/2006 Ending Life Exp.	1×/wk for 20 wks 4×/yr until age 34 Evaluations annually for the next 5 yrs followed by 1×/2–3 yrs.	To improve skills and use of adaptive equipment to promote independ- ence with ADLs.	$125 per treatment $2500/year $500/year aged 31–34		Anesthesi- ologist, Dr. Rauck, CPI OT, T. MacDonald Research, Medical Records, CLCP

According to the Royal College of Physicians' 2005 published guidelines for the diagnosis, referral, and management of complex regional pain syndrome in adults, there is currently a lack of evidence to inform the best treatment approach to offer patients with CRPS. Recommended therapeutic approaches can include:

* patient education and support
* self-administered tactile and thermal desensitization with the aim of normalizing touch perception
* functional activities
* pacing, prioritizing, and planning activities
* goal setting
* relaxation techniques

(Continued)

Table 1.9 (Continued)

- coping skills
- sleep hygiene
- facilitating self-management of the condition

The guidelines also suggest that it is critical that occupational therapy be delivered by a therapist trained in the treatment of the condition. The medical record supports that the patient received such a level of care and continues to receive the appropriate level of care via the Carolinas Pain Institute. The medical record also indicated the previously extended treatment be weaned as recommended by CPI, occupational therapist of the CPI, T. MacDonald, and supported by anesthesiologist Dr. Rauck. **Needs to be added to the medical record.**

Source(s): www.rcplondon.ac.uk/guidelines-policy/complex-regional-pain-syndrome-adults

https://carolinaspaininstitute.com/

Table 1.10 Projected Therapeutic Modalities (Psychology)

Item/Service	Age/Year	Frequency/ Replacement	Purpose	Cost	Comment	Recommended By
Psychology	Beginning 30/03/2006 Ending Life Exp.	Group therapy 1×/week for 44 weeks/year. Individual counseling 26 hours/year.	Assist in adjustment to disability for C. and her family and to address any changes in family dynamics.	$50/group session $2200/year $125/hr individual $3250/year		Anesthesiologist Dr. Lee, CPI Psychologist, D. Daye Research, Medical Records, CLCP

According to the Royal College of Physicians' 2005 published guidelines for the diagnosis, referral, and management of complex regional pain syndrome in adults, the treatment of chronic pain should include the provision of psychological interventions specific to pain in the form of a group-based multidisciplinary pain management program, for those who require it, based on an appropriate assessment method. In a minority of cases, 1:1 psychological support may be more appropriate. Psychological interventions often follow the principles of CBT; however, alternative methods have also shown efficacy.

*Cognitive-behavioral therapy (CBT) is a broad category of different treatment regimens. However, CBT regimens almost always include cognitive therapy as a core component. Usually, CBT also includes interventions designed to alter behaviors and some combination of operant treatment, coping skills training, relaxation strategies, pacing or activity-rest cycling, exercise and activity management, and pleasant activity scheduling. In accordance with the medical record, anesthesiologist, Dr. Rauck, and treating psychologist of the CPI, D. Daye, ongoing psychological intervention is recommended until life expectancy. **Needs to be added to the medical record.**

Source(s): www.rcplondon.ac.uk/guidelines-policy/complex-regional-pain-syndrome-adults

https://carolinaspaininstitute.com/

Table 1.11 Diagnostic Testing/Educational Assessment

Item/Service	Age/Year	Frequency/ Replacement	Purpose	Cost	Comment	Recommended By
Laboratory Studies: Opioid Compliance	Beginning 30/03/2006 Ending Life Exp	4×/year	To ensure compliance with opioid use	$150/test $600/year		Anesthesiologist, Dr. Rauck, Medical Records, CLCP

Foundation:

Aside from the recommendation made by Dr. Rauck for opioid compliance testing, once the diagnosis of CRPS is confirmed, there was little scientific evidence found to support routine diagnostic testing such as liver function, etc., when not recommended by the primary care physician.

Table 1.12 Wheelchair Needs

Item/Service	Age/Year	Frequency/Replacement	Purpose	Cost	Comment	Recommended By
	Beginning Ending					

Foundation:

According to the medical record, C.'s functional capacity evaluation results indicated significant physical dysfunction in several areas including walking, climbing, bending, and more. However, she was able to demonstrate some function such as walking for 15 min at a speed of 1 mph as compared to the average speed of 2.5 mph according to the American College of Sports Medicine. As the cornerstone in the treatment of CRPS is to use the affected limb as much as possible and avoid "learned disuse" in their attempts to avoid pain, wheelchair needs are not recommended in this plan.

Table 1.13 Aids for Independent Function

Item/Service	Age/Year	Frequency/ Replacement	Purpose	Cost	Comment	Recommended By
Various long-handled items including a reacher, razor handle, sock aid, and nail clipper	Beginning 30/03/2006 Ending Life Exp.	1×/year	Assist with activities of daily living and minimize repetitive bending.	$110		CLCP
Canadian Crutches	Beginning 30/03/2006 Ending Life Exp	1×/2–3 years	To support a more normal gait pattern when ambulating in the community.	$529		CLCP
Bath bench	Beginning 30/03/2006 Ending Life Exp.	1×/5 years	To increase safety as a result of reduced balance.	$29		CLCP

Foundation:

Based on C.'s functional capacity evaluation results, repetitive bending was identified as a functional limitation.

Therefore, the long-handled aids are recommended to assist with activities of daily living. C. also demonstrated a tendency to avoid weighted heel strike during gait. As such, Canadian crutches are being recommended for community use to support a more normal gait pattern. C. also demonstrated reduced balance, and therefore a bath bench is recommended for safety purposes.

Table 1.14 Orthotics/Prosthetics

Item/Service	Age/Year	Frequency/ Replacement	Purpose	Cost	Comment	Recommended By
Orthopedic shoes with custom orthotics	Beginning 30/03/2006 Ending Life Exp.	1×/year	Promote foot positioning and stability	$400 to $500 when purchased together		CLCP

Table 1.15 Home Furnishings

Item/Service	Age/Year	Frequency/Replacement	Purpose	Cost	Comment	Recommended By
Bed sheets of 1500 thread count/sq in (queen sized)	Beginning 30/03/2006 Ending Life Exp.	2 sets in the first year followed by 1×/3 years	To reduce allodynia	$190 first year $95/year		CLCP
Handheld shower head	Beginning 30/03/2006 Ending Life Exp.	1×/5 years	Aid in bathing and shaving	$60–$70		CLCP

Foundation:

Allodynia is documented in the medical file as well as being a common symptom of CRPS.

Table 1.16 Drug/Supply Needs

Item/Service	Age/Year	Frequency/Replacement	Purpose	Cost	Comment	Recommended By
Prescribed Medications	Beginning 30/03/2006	Annual cost	As prescribed for medical care	$1300–$1600 annually	The medications listed are representative of current and future needs. Specific prescriptions may change. Annual costs based on research as referenced later.	Anesthesiologist, Dr. Rauck CLCP
Zanaflex	Ending			$2.93/60 tablets		
Lidoderm patches	Unknown			$5.11/patch		
Clonidine patches				$0.61/patch		
Voltaren				$1.62/100 mg		
Methadone				$0.25/tablet		
Lunesta				$15.69/tablet		
Ultram				$3.58/tablet		
Topamax				$2.64/60 tablets		

and anticonvulsants, corticosteroids, bone-loss medications, sympathetic nerve-blocking medications, and intravenous ketamine.

Several classes of medication have been reported as effective for CRPS, particularly when given early in the disease. However, none are approved by the U.S. Food and Drug Administration (FDA) to be marketed specifically for CRPS, and no single drug or combination is guaranteed to be effective in everyone. Drugs often used to treat CRPS include:

- Acetaminophen to reduce pain associated with inflammation and bone and joint involvement.
- Non-steroidal anti-inflammatory drugs (NSAIDs) to treat moderate pain and inflammation, including over-the-counter aspirin, ibuprofen, and naproxen in sufficient doses.
- Drugs proven effective for other neuropathic pain conditions, such as nortriptyline, gabapentin, pregabalin, and duloxetine. Amitriptyline, an older treatment, is effective but causes more side effects than nortriptyline, which is very similar chemically.

Table 1.17 Home/Facility Care

Item/Service	Age/Year	Frequency/ Replacement	Purpose	Cost	Comment	Recommended By
Private Hire House Cleaning	Beginning 30/03/2006 Ending Life Exp.	Weekly Cleaning	To clean the home.	$75/cleaning $3900/year		CLCP

Foundation:

Based on the results of C.'s FCE:

Ms. C. is not a candidate for competitive employment, nor is she a candidate for supportive employment or situational work in a sheltered workshop. Her employability and placeability profiles have been compromised such that she no longer qualifies for gainful employment . . . .

The Department of Labor's (DOL) lowest Physical Demand Characteristic (PDC) is "SEDENTARY." If the DOL had a category for persons who are physically disabled from work, she would meet this respective category's criteria, rather than that of the SEDENTARY PDC."

According to the National Occupational Classification Career Handbook, Housekeepers 4412.2 are classified at the Medium level of physical demands and therefore beyond C.'s safe functional abilities.

Source(s): https://noc.esdc.gc.ca/CareerHandbook/

Table 1.18 Future Medical Care (Pain Specialty, Anesthesiologist)

Item/Service	Age/Year	Frequency/ Replacement	Purpose	Cost	Comment	Recommended By
Pain Specialty, Anesthesiologist	Beginning 30/03/2006 Ending Life Exp.	1×/year	To assess the ongoing status of CRPS type 1 as well as the proper functioning of the spinal implant.	$350		Anesthesiologist, Dr. Rauck, Research, Medical Records, CLCP

According to the Royal College of Physicians' 2005 published guidelines for the diagnosis, referral, and management of complex regional pain syndrome in adults, pain is typically the leading symptom of CRPS and is often associated with limb dysfunction and psychological distress. For those in whom pain persists, anxiety, depression, and loss of sleep are likely to develop, even if they are not prominent at the outset. Therefore, an integrated interdisciplinary treatment approach is recommended, tailored to the individual patient. The primary aims are to reduce pain, preserve or restore function, and enable patients to manage their condition and improve their quality of life. The four "pillars" of care are education, pain relief, physical rehabilitation, and psychological intervention.

In accordance with C.'s anesthesiologist and pain specialist, Dr. Rauck, annual evaluations are recommended.

Source(s): www.iasp-pain.org; www.rcplondon.ac.uk/guidelines-policy/complex-regional-pain-syndrome-adults

- Topical local anesthetic ointments, sprays, or creams such as lidocaine and patches such as fentanyl. These can reduce allodynia, and skin coverage by patches can provide additional protection.
- Bisphosphonates, such as high-dose alendronate or intravenous pamidronate, that reduce bone changes.
- Corticosteroids that treat inflammation/swelling and edema, such as prednisolone and methylprednisolone.
- Botulinum toxin injections can help in severe cases, particularly for relaxing contracted muscles and restoring normal hand or foot positions.

- Opioids such as oxycodone, morphine, hydrocodone, and fentanyl may be required for individuals with the most severe pain. However, opioids can convey heightened pain sensitivity and run the risk of dependence.
- N-methyl-D-aspartate (NMDA) receptor antagonists such as dextromethorphan and ketamine are controversial unproven treatments.

Source(s): National Institute for Neurological Disorders and Stroke—Complex Regional Pain Syndrome Fact Sheet—www.ninds.nih.gov/complex-regional-pain-syndrome-fact-sheet# :~:text=There%20is%20often%20increased%20sensitivity,pin%20prick%2C%20known%20 as%20hyperalgesia.

Table 1.19 Future Medical Care (Dermatology)

Item/Service	Age/Year	Frequency/ Replacement	Purpose	Cost	Comment	Recommended By
Dermatology	Beginning 30/03/2006 Ending Life Exp.	1×/year for the next 5–7 years	To assess the ongoing status of skin lesions in the prevention of infection	$275		Anesthesiologist Dr. Rauck, Research, Medical Records, CLCP

According to the Royal College of Physicians' 2005 published guidelines for the diagnosis, referral, and management of complex regional pain syndrome (CRPS) in adults, changes in skin innervation, blood flow, interstitial fluid (edema), the trophic constitution of the skin, and skin temperature can increase the risk of skin ulceration. Some of these changes are often present in CRPS. When ulceration occurs, this allows the entry and multiplication of microorganisms, so that patients are at risk of developing cellulitis and deeper tissue infections. In accordance with the medical file documenting the presence of skin lesions on both feet, a dermatology consult is recommended as supported by anesthesiologist, Dr. Rauck. **Needs to be added to the medical record.**

Source(s): www.rcplondon.ac.uk/guidelines-policy/complex-regional-pain-syndrome-adults

Table 1.20 Architectural Renovations

Item/Service	Age/Year	Frequency/ Replacement	Purpose	Cost	Comment	Recommended By
	Beginning Ending					

No recommendations.

Foundation:

No recommendations.

Foundation:

Right ankle range of motion and strength are within normal limits. Subjective complaints affect the whole body. Driving is rated a 7 on the Activity Rating Chart and is associated with burning, shooting, pins and needles, and stabbing pain. In consideration of the addition of hand controls, it is not likely to result in a significant increase in function or tolerance to driving and therefore not supported as a viable recommendation.

Based on observations of the layout of the home, flooring, absence of stairs, etc., made during the interview with the client in her home, there were no supported foundations to justify recommending home modifications.

Table 1.21 Transportation

Item/Service	Age/Year	Frequency/ Replacement	Purpose	Cost	Comment	Recommended By
	Beginning					

Table 1.22 Vocational/Education Plan

Item/Service	Age/Year	Frequency/ Replacement	Purpose	Cost	Comment	Recommended By
	Beginning Ending					

C.'s FCE reported, *"Her employability and placeability profiles have been compromised such that she no longer qualifies for gainful employment."*

Table 1.23 Health and Strength Maintenance

Item/Service	Age/Year	Frequency/ Replacement	Purpose	Cost	Comment	Recommended By
Aquatic center membership	Beginning 30/03/2006 Ending Life Exp.	Annual membership	Promote and maintain activity and exercise	$100		CPI PT, S. Redding Client Interview CLCP
Therapeutic home exercise and desensitization equipment	Beginning 30/03/2006 Ending Life Exp.	1×/3–4 years	To provide emergency roadside assistance	$500 allowance	Based on treating therapists' recommendations	CPI PT, S. Redding CLCP

Foundation:

C. reported having been an active individual before her accident and particularly enjoyed swimming. **Needs to be added to the medical record.** The importance of enjoyable activity is well documented in the treatment of chronic pain and its psychological impact. The importance of activity and exercise are well documented in the treatment of CRPS. The buoyancy of the water supports body weight and removes the pressure off joints, which makes it an ideal environment to move, stretch, and strengthen.

Table 1.24 Future Medical Care/Aggressive Treatment

Item/Service	Age/Year	Frequency/ Replacement	Purpose	Cost	Comment	Recommended By
Battery replacement surgery for spinal cord stimulator	Beginning 30/03/2016 Ending Life Exp.	1×/10 years	Replacement of rechargeable battery system.	$15,727	Patients must remember to charge the system daily.	Anesthesiologist, Dr. Rauck, CLCP

A 2005 study published in the *Ochsner Journal* by B. Kashy et al. of select patients with severe CRPS-1 who were unresponsive to all forms of pain treatment showed that they may benefit from amputation as a last option for relief of suffering; however, larger studies are needed to prove the efficacy of amputation. According to the medical record, as a result of insufficient medical research and a lack of clearly defined criteria to assess amputation as a last resort, anesthesiologist, Dr. Rauck does not support amputation as a future medical care option.

Source: Kashy, B. K., Abd-Elsayed, A. A., Farag, E., Yared, M., Vakili, R., & Esa, W. A. S. (2015). Amputation as an unusual treatment for therapy-resistant complex regional pain syndrome, type 1. Ochsner Journal, 15(4), 441–442.

Table 1.25 Potential Complications

For information purposes only. No prediction of the frequency of occurrence is available.

Complication	Cost	Comment
Lead migration	Cost varies according to extent of the complication	Lead migration is the most common complication of spinal cord stimulation implantation.
Systemic complications	Cost varies according to extent of the complication	A 2012 study by Robert Schwartzman, MD, and published online in the *Journal of Neuroscience & Medicine* examined how CRPS affected the systems of cognition; constitutional, cardiac, and respiratory complications; systemic autonomic dysregulation; neurogenic edema; musculoskeletal, endocrine, and dermatological manifestations; and urological and gastrointestinal function.
Substance abuse	Cost varies according to extent of the complication	As per the medical record.
Psychological/psychiatric crisis management	Cost varies according to extent of the complication	As per the medical record.

References

American Academy of Life Care Planning Physicians™ (AAPLCP). (2023). *About the AAPLCP*. https://aaplcp.org/About/About.aspx

Berens, D. (2019). A journey through the history of life care planning research: The journal of life care planning and the foundation for life care planning research. *Journal of Life Care Planning*, *17*(3), 61–69.

Deutsch, P. M. (2002). Historical perspective of life care planning. *Top Spinal Cord Injury Rehabilitation*, *7*(4), 1–4.

Deutsch, P. M. (n.d.). *Frequently asked questions—life care planning*. Paul M Deutsch and Associates, PA. www.paulmdeutsch.com/FAQs-life-care-planning.htm#top

Deutsch, P. M., & Sawyer, H. (1985). *Guide to rehabilitation*. Mathew Bender.

Deutsch, P. M., & PA Associates. (n.d.). *Paul M Deutsch, PhD, CRC, CCM, CLCP, FIALCP*. http://paulm-deutsch.com/FAQs-life-care-planning.htm

Gallardo v. Marstiller, 596 U.S. ___, 142 S. Ct. 1751. (2022). www.supremecourt.gov/DocketPDF/20/20-1263/193414/20210922152244871_Brief%20of%20American%20Academy%20of%20P hysician%20Life%20Care%20Planners%20as%20Amicus%20Curiae%20In%20Support%20of %20Neither%20Party.pdf

Gonzales, J, Cowen, T., Janssen, C., & Davenport, W. (2015). *Life care plans: Sustaining medical damages in personal injury torts*. The American Academy of Physician Life Care Planners.

Gonzales, J., & Zotovas, A. (2014). Life care planning: A natural domain for physiatry. *American Academy of Physical Medicine and Rehabilitation*, *6*, 184–187. http://dx.doi.org/10.1016/j.pmrj.2014.01.011

Johnson, C., Cary, J., & Robert, E. (2022). A comparison of the definition of a life care plan: The impact on life care planners. *Journal of Life Care Planning*, *20*(3), 25–43.

Johnson, C., & Weed, R. (2013). The life care planning process. *Physical Medicine and Rehabilitation Clinics of North America*, *24*(3), 403–417. https://doi.org/10.1016/j.pmr.2013.03.008. Epub April 26, 2013.

LexisNexis Store. (n.d.). *Damages in tort actions*. https://store.lexisnexis.com/search?query=Raffa

Marcinko, D. (2019). International academy of life care planning. *Journal of Life Care Planning*, *17*(3), 31–35.

May, V. R. (2021). *Life care plan definition* [Unpublished manuscript].

May, V. R., & Moradi Rekabdarkolaee, H. (2020). The international commission on health care certification life care planner role and function investigation. *Journal of Life Care Planning*, *18*(2), 3–67.

Reavis, S. (2002). Standards of practice. *Journal of Life Care Planning*, *1*(1), 49–57.

Skinner, B. F. (1966). What is the experimental analysis of behavior? *Journal of the Experimental Analysis of Behavior*, *9*(3), 213–218.

Weed, R. (2019). A brief history of life care planning. *Journal of Life Care Planning*, *17*(3), 5–14.

The Editors of Encyclopedia Britannica. (2017, May 29). Developmental psychology. In *Encyclopedia Britannica*. www.britannica.com/science/developmental-psychology

The Winter Park Land Trust: Fred Raffa. (n.d.). *info@winterparklandtrust.org*. www.winterparklandtrust.org/fred-raffa-bio

2   Disability Legislation in the United States and Canada

Tanya Rutherford Owen[1]

Every individual with a disability has a unique manifestation of their medical condition. Where this manifestation meets the restrictions of one's environment is frequently conceptualized as impairment. With this impairment, the individual must function within the larger society and all of that society's systems. It is when the aforementioned impairment interacts with the majority society and results in discrimination or marginalization that disability-related legislation is born.

As was the case with women's suffrage and civil rights legislation, disability-related legislation (and related judicial decisions) is in response to interactions that hindered or violated rights. When examining modern disability policy creation in America, most often disability-related legislation emerged through the collective efforts of individuals with disabilities demonstrating through education, resistance, and, when necessary, controversial tactics to make changes. Because disability does not affect the majority of the American population, policies that encourage inclusion and accessibility have historically been overlooked by most members of American society. In the history of America, it is only in our recent past that disability was conceptualized not through the medical model (i.e., a condition inherent in the individual) but a social model (i.e., disability results from barriers in the society and environment).

Disability legislation shapes not only the behaviors of the institutions within the society writ large but can also have a profound impact on specific functions, including medical service delivery, upon which many individuals with a disability rely. Therefore, the importance of the role of disability legislation in the lives of people with disabilities cannot be overstated. In this chapter, we will examine relevant pieces of legislation in the United States and Canada that impact individuals with disabilities. This chapter is certainly not intended to be an exhaustive accounting of all disability legislation. Most importantly, however, we discuss how the process of legislation shapes the lives of and is shaped by the lives of individuals with disabilities.

Demographics in Disability in the United States

No chapter can be written about the demographics of people with disabilities without mentioning the difficulty of actually defining the word "disability". The World Health Organization (WHO) defines disability as follows: "Disability is the umbrella term for impairments, activity limitations, and participation restrictions, referring to the negative aspects of the interaction between an individual (with a health condition) and that individual's contextual factors (environmental and personal factors)" (World Report on Disability, 2011, p. 4). According to the WHO, there are over a billion people worldwide living with some form of disability (Disability, 2021; Disability and Health, 2020).

In the United States, there are various definitions of disability. The Americans with Disabilities Act of 1990 (ADA) definition of disability is likely the most widely recognized definition.

DOI: 10.4324/b23293-2

The ADA (1990) and the subsequent ADA Amendments Act (2008) define disability as "an impairment that substantially limits one or more major life activities, a record of such an impairment, or being regarded as having such an impairment" (ADA Amendments Act of 2008, 2009, para. 4).

In terms of collecting data about people with disabilities, the American Community Survey (ACS), administered by the U.S. Census Bureau, is likely the most widely used data collection device in the United States. The ACS identifies an individual as having a disability if they answer yes to any of the following areas of impairment:

1. **Hearing difficulty:** Deaf or having serious difficulty hearing
2. **Vision difficulty:** Blind or having serious difficulty seeing, even when wearing glasses
3. **Cognitive difficulty:** Because of a physical, mental, or emotional problem, having difficulty remembering, concentrating, or making decisions
4. **Ambulatory difficulty:** Having serious difficulty walking or climbing stairs
5. **Self-care difficulty:** Having difficulty bathing or dressing
6. **Independent living difficulty:** Because of a physical, mental, or emotional problem, having difficulty doing errands alone such as visiting a doctor's office or shopping (How Disability Data Are Collected, 2017, para. 4)

Based on the ACS data, which was last published in 2018, there were approximately 40,585,700 individuals, or 12.6% of the non-institutionalized American population, who met the definition of disability outlined earlier (Erickson et al., 2021). These individuals were most likely to be within the 75+ age category (Erickson et al.). The most commonly reported type of disability was an ambulatory disability, which was reported in 6.8% of the population (Erickson et al., 2021). With over 40 million Americans affected by disability, it is not surprising that policies that pertain to disability have developed throughout the evolution of the United States.

Disability Policy Making in Action: A Case Study

In 1952, Ed Roberts was a 13-year-old football player and mediocre student who lived in northern California. That is, until his family was infected by the poliomyelitis virus, commonly known as polio, and from which Ed was the only member of his family who did not fully recover. The virus left Ed with an inability to move, or even breathe, on his own. With his life consisting of confinement to an iron lung for 18 hours per day, Ed first attempted to control his life by refusing to eat, and his weight, as a result, plummeted from 120 to 50 pounds within seven months (Shapiro, 1994). Renewed by a sense that he could control his own life, he shifted his focus to his ability to gain an education, as his mind had not been affected by the virus. By his senior year of high school, Ed returned to school in his wheelchair, only to be denied his diploma when the principal and assistant superintendent declared that his inability to complete driver's education and gym prohibited him from satisfying graduation requirements. Where the iron lung machine and the wheelchair had been Ed's mechanism for physical recuperation, they would not be enough for him to accomplish what his classmates would. That is, until his mother who was a former labor organizer, complained to the officials in the school district (and school board) and it was determined that the driver's education requirement would be dropped and his physical rehabilitation sessions could count as Ed's gym requirement (Shapiro).

After high school, Ed studied for two years at San Mateo Community College while continuing to live at home. Rather than applying to the University of California at Los Angeles

(UCLA), which had a program for World War II veterans with disabilities, Ed (with the encouragement of his academic advisor at San Mateo) set his sights on the University of California Berkeley (UC Berkeley) because it had a better program in Ed's area of study, political science (Shapiro, 1994). However, his rehabilitation counselor through California's Department of Rehabilitation did not support Ed's pursuit of a four-year degree because she did not believe that he would work. Like his mother had done for him two years prior, Ed and officials from San Mateo Community College appealed the counselor's decision, but when they were unsuccessful, they made Ed's case to the local newspaper, which was successful in having the rehabilitation agency relent.

Overcoming that barrier, however, Ed still had to face gaining admittance to UC Berkeley. "We've tried cripples before and it didn't work" (Shapiro, 1994, p. 45) was what Ed was told, and the school's lack of accessibility was seen not only in the classrooms and cafeteria but also in the fact that there was no dormitory with flooring strong enough to hold Ed's 800-pound iron lung, on which he still relied to breathe. By now, Ed knew not to take no for an answer and continued to seek out people within the Berkeley system who would champion his cause. He found one and with him came a proposed solution that allowed Ed to live in the university's hospital while attending classes on campus. With time, Ed benefited from a power wheelchair, which allowed him the freedom to be without an attendant for some periods of time. By 1967, there were 12 students on the Berkeley campus with significant disabilities. In this culture, Ed finished his undergraduate and master's degree and began work toward his doctorate. During his time at Berkeley, Ed petitioned for students with disabilities to remain in rehabilitation programs (when they were threatened with dismissal) by using the media and gathering support from students and university officials when needed. He, and his cohort of the group they called the "Rolling Quads", petitioned the city to include curb cutouts on the city streets—and were successful. With these experiences of success, the group of students still living in the hospital decided that they wanted to institute a program to help students with disabilities live independently, and through his connection with Jean Wirth, the counselor from San Mateo who encouraged him to apply to Berkeley, they acquired federal funding to establish the Physically Disabled Students Program (PDSP) on the Berkeley campus in 1970 (Shapiro). One key component of this program, whose goal was to assist students in finding accessible housing among other resources that promoted independent living, was that the staff of PDSP were counselors with disabilities. Ed placed at the center of the program's goal quality of life for the person with the disability, a radical departure from the medical model of disability centered more on symptom control and disease prevention. Hence, Ed Roberts is known as the father of the independent living movement. By 1972, the Center for Independent Living (CIL) was incorporated, and this program served both students and non-students with disabilities in their quest to be independent, self-sufficient, and integrated into the community as a whole. By 1975, Ed Roberts was appointed director of California's Department of Rehabilitation—the same program that 15 years prior refused to pay for Ed's education because he would likely never work!

As director of California's Department of Rehabilitation, Ed Roberts showed up to support a group of protestors who in 1977 took over the offices of Joseph Maldanado in San Francisco in response to his boss's (Joseph Califano) unwillingness to sign necessary regulations about Section 504 of the Rehabilitation Act. Section 504 states:

> No otherwise qualified handicapped individual in the United States shall solely on the basis of his handicap, be excluded from the participation, be denied the benefits of, or be subjected to discrimination under any program or activity receiving federal financial assistance.
>
> (Section 504, Rehabilitation Act of 1973, n.d., para. 1)

Developing and signing regulations of the act was not done by 1977, four years after the law was signed by President Richard Nixon, despite a judge's order that this be done. It was only through over 100 individuals with disabilities and protestors conducting a 25-day sit-in (the longest at a federal building in history) that the regulations were signed by Secretary Califano. At the same time, Secretary Califano signed the regulations for the Education of All Handicapped Children Act, which was passed in 1975 but whose provisions were blocked along with the Section 504 provisions.

Shapiro (1994) concludes, "The San Francisco sit-in marked the political coming of age of the disability rights movement" (p. 68). This particular protest was unique in that it was led by people with disabilities, for people with disabilities. This group of protestors involved individuals with multiple types of disabilities, which was in contrast to prior movements that were more homogeneous in their disability-specific focus. In this group, individuals with wide-ranging disabilities, including people from the gay community in San Francisco, spoke with one voice. This group garnered support from local stores and restaurants that donated food to those involved in the sit-in. They received support from other civil rights groups in San Francisco, including members of the Black Panther Party. Through their use of solidarity, use of the media, and determination to see their cause through, this collective effort of people with disabilities succeeded in gaining further access to the communities in which they belonged.

For Ed Roberts, his journey began as one person whose life was unexpectedly impacted by disability. For a preteen whose life had been by all accounts uneventful, Ed, after the onset of polio, believed that he knew what was best for his own life. He was encouraged to fight discriminatory behavior in his environment when he found it, first by his mother, next by educators, and then, most importantly, by forming a community of like-minded students with disabilities who wanted, like all Americans, to have control over their destiny and equal access to their community. While Ed's story is a singular one, the collective fights waged by those in his orbit who used the media, circulated petitions, provided education initiatives, and organized demonstrations led to changes in disability policies one piece of legislation at a time. Over a lifetime, the legislative impact of Ed Roberts is still seen in the lives of children and adults with disabilities over 25 years after his death.

Mechanisms for Policy Development in America

In the story of Ed Roberts, it becomes evident that disability policy is the by-product of friction between person and environment. On a singular level, the conflict between a person with a disability and their environment leads to exclusion, similar to what Ed Roberts experienced when his principal asserted that he could not become a high school graduate without completing driver's education. In this case, Ed and his mother protested this decision, and after enough encounters within the school system, a policy exception was made for Ed. While this allowed Ed to graduate from high school, it did not change the policy that was inherently discriminatory against any individual who was physically unable to complete driver's education due to ambulatory impairments, vision impairments, or other reasons. The fight for a waiver of graduation requirements, or similar fights made on behalf of a small number of individuals with disabilities, are typically made, as in Ed Roberts' case, at a local level.

Local Agency Services

Currently, local advocacy for individuals with disabilities in the community can be performed by local agencies. An example of a local disability-related agency is a center for independent living. These agencies are typically not-for-profit agencies designed to assist individuals with disabilities in advocacy, service, and the public education system. Like Roberts and others who staffed the Center for Independent Living in Berkley, an agency like this may assist an individual with acquiring attendant care to assist with activities of daily living. They may assist with coordinating transportation for individuals with disabilities who cannot drive themselves to travel within the local community. They may assist parents who desire to explore residential options for their adult children with disabilities. They may assist with providing day programs for individuals with disabilities within the community.

State Agency Services

At the next level of service, provision is the state government. An example of state-level agencies that provide services for individuals with disabilities includes the vocational rehabilitation offices located in each state. These agencies were created through 1920 legislation, the Smith Fess Act (Rubin & Roessler, 2008). These offices are found in every state and are funded through state and federal funds. The focus of services offered by the state's vocational rehabilitation office includes services to assist people with disabilities in obtaining and maintaining employment. For Ed Roberts, it was his local California vocational rehabilitation office that sponsored educational training. Services are tailored to the individual's needs but may involve evaluation, training, provision of equipment, job placement assistance, and/or coordination of necessary medical treatment to facilitate employment. The majority of these services are provided at no charge to the individual with a disability.

Federal Agency Services

Another avenue for government-related service provision for individuals with disabilities is through the federal government. One example of this service provision includes the Social Security Disability Insurance (SSDI) program. The SSDI program was established through the 1956 Amendments to the Social Security Act, and it provides benefits to Americans with disabilities between the ages of 50 and 65 who qualify for the program. In 2019, it was estimated that 8.5 million Americans receive such benefits (Chartbook: Social Security Insurance, 2021). The Social Security Disability program provides monthly stipends for living expenses and is also a mechanism for individuals with disabilities to obtain healthcare coverage through Medicare before age 65 after a designated waiting period. Additionally, through the Ticket to Work program, recipients of SSDI benefits are automatically qualified for no-cost vocational rehabilitation services.

Court Decisions

In the United States, the judiciary is the branch of government left to interpret the policies generated through state and federal legislation. If there are questions about the intent of legislation or applicability of legislation, the courts are called upon to answer these questions. One clear example of the roles of the branches of government in creating disability policies in the United States is the series of decisions referred to as the *Sutton* trilogy, issued after the passage of the ADA in 1990. The three cases creating the Sutton trilogy will be outlined briefly next.

1999 Sutton v. United Airlines

Twin sisters, Karen Sutton and Kimberly Hinton (the Suttons), filed suit against United Airlines after not being hired by United as commercial pilots due to their uncorrected vision, which was worse than 20/100. They filed suit under the ADA, noting that they had physical impairments (i.e., vision impairment) that substantially limited one or more major life activities or they were regarded as having such impairment. The sisters wore glasses that corrected their vision, and they functioned in day-to-day activities. The U.S. Supreme Court, in a 7–2 decision, held that under the ADA, decisions about impairment must be made on an individual basis, and in the case of the Suttons, they were not protected under the ADA because with glasses, they had no impairment and therefore were not disabled (*Sutton v. United Air Lines, Inc.*, 1999).

1999 Murphy v. United Parcel Service

Vaughn Murphy was hired by United Parcel Service (UPS) as a mechanic, which involved him operating commercial vehicles. He was mistakenly medically cleared to drive and began his work. However, UPS subsequently dismissed Mr. Murphy after they learned that his hypertension exceeded acceptable Department of Transportation limits. Mr. Murphy sued UPS, claiming that he was discriminated against under the ADA. However, in their 7–2 decision, the U.S. Supreme Court decided that Mr. Murphy was not considered disabled under the ADA because, with hypertension medication, he could function normally and was therefore not disabled (*Murphy v. United Parcel Service*, 1999).

1999 Albertson's v. Kirkingburg

Hallie Kirkingburg was hired by Albertsons to work as a commercial truck driver. Before employment, he was erroneously certified as meeting Department of Transportation vision standards. Two years later, this mistake was found and Mr. Kirkingburg was told that a waiver was needed for him to continue in his truck driver work, but before obtaining such, his employment was terminated. Upon obtaining such a waiver, Albertsons would not rehire him. Mr. Kirkingburg sued Albertsons claiming discrimination under the ADA. The U.S. Supreme Court, in a 7–2 decision (1999), stated that not all individuals with a physical difficulty are disabled under the ADA and each individual must prove that they are disabled by showing that such a physical difficulty substantially limits one or more life activity. In doing so, they must consider how an alleged disability can be mitigated through aids (e.g., glasses), medications, etc.

The impact of these decisions significantly eroded the applicability of the ADA on the lives of Americans it was intended to protect. In essence, by 1999 in the United States, an individual who underwent bilateral lower extremity amputations could be deemed not "disabled" under the ADA, if they effectively functioned with two lower extremity prosthetics. Therefore, between 1999 and 2008, the protections once believed to be inherent in the ADA preventing discrimination against Americans with disabilities were less robust, a problem only rectified by the U.S. Congress passing the Americans with Disabilities Amendments Act in 2008. Within this piece of legislation, the applicability of protection against disability-based discrimination was more widespread and self-evident.

Disability Policy in Private Systems

Whereas U.S. state or federal government disability policies typically apply throughout the entire agency within which the policy is adopted, disability policy in the private sector has been less unified. In terms of employment of individuals with disabilities, for example, one employer may implement a policy promoting employment, training, or promotion for individuals with disabilities; however, this policy only applies to this employer (n = 1). Certainly, a disability-related policy developed and adopted by Employer X in St. Louis, Missouri, would have no impact on Employer Y in Los Angeles, California. As a result, disability policy in the private sector is often a patchwork of policies with no uniform implementation guidelines. In terms of employment of individuals with disabilities, therefore, the result is higher unemployment for individuals with disabilities when compared to their counterparts without disabilities. A review of January 2021 data published by the U.S. Bureau of Labor Statistics reveals that the unemployment rate for individuals with disabilities ages 16+ was 12.0%, compared with 6.6% for individuals without disabilities (Table A-6. Employment Status of the Civilian Population, 2021). Additionally, the employment population ratio for individuals with disabilities in January 2021 ages 16+ was 19.6%, compared with 66.4% for individuals without disabilities (Table A-6. Employment Status of the Civilian Population, 2021). Finally, in a 2008 survey of American employers, only 19.1% of companies in the United States reported employing individuals with disabilities (Domzal et al., 2008). It is undisputed that decades of employment-related anti-discrimination legislation targeted at federal and state agencies have not translated to favorable employment of people with disabilities in the private sector.

Disability Legislation/Policy Over the Decades

When examining disability within any culture, from ancient Greece to modern-day America, the perception of disability is shaped by and reflective of that culture's values. Rubin and Roessler (2008) posit that this lens as it pertains to a disability is shaped by the perceived threat of the disability to society at large, the cause of the disability, and who is perceived to be responsible for the disability. Throughout American history, disability-related services have been provided through religious and non-profit groups at a local level, through various state governments, and through the U.S. government.

This section contains pieces of pertinent disability-related legislation that were passed in the United States from Colonial America to the present. Examining disability-related service provision in the context of legislation reveals what group of people, at what time, perceived themselves to be responsible for providing services to people with disabilities. While the pieces of legislation each intended to provide different services for individuals with disabilities, it is critical to understand the disability-related cultural mores of each time period. Within this context, one can see how the various pieces of disability legislation were developed. In a larger scenario, over the decades, themes emerged surrounding how the lives of individuals in the United States who have disabilities are affected by and affect society's perceptions of how people with disabilities are treated.

Early Disability Legislation

All societies have consisted of individuals who have disabilities, either disabilities that are congenital or acquired over one's lifespan. How these individuals are treated within their society is often a reflection of the common beliefs about disability. Thankfully, this treatment has evolved from Greek and Roman societies, which committed infanticide for children who were perceived to have a disability, to our modern American society, where most people agree that such treatment is barbaric. Emerging from acts of infanticide, disability in the Middle Ages was perceived "as either God's punishment or the result of demonic possession" (Rubin & Roessler, 2008, p. 4). Unfortunately, relics from this belief can still be observed in the treatment of individuals with disabilities in modern America.

Similar to the Spartans, who valued physical prowess over other human qualities, colonists in early America relied heavily upon their physical capacities for survival. As a result, early

America banned individuals with physical, mental, or emotional disabilities from entering the county (Rubin & Roessler, 2008). American society also adopted views of disability from the Middle Ages whereby individuals with disabilities were perceived to be the result of God's punishment, with many of the remedies for illness or disability aimed at driving out an illness through extreme and usually painful means. By 1752, the Quakers established the first hospital, and between 1765 and 1783, three medical schools opened in America (Rubin & Roessler), which over time helped to improve the types and quality of medical treatment provided in the American colonies.

However, even in 19th-century America, cultural beliefs in Social Darwinism and a laissez-faire approach to economics resulted in rehabilitation-related services receiving almost no support from the federal government and only minimum state support (Rubin & Roessler, 2008). Disability-related movements during this period were primarily aimed at protecting Americans against perceived societal burdens or economic burdens for caring for people with disabilities. Again, however, relics of religion-infused perceptions of individuals with disabilities remained, resulting in religious-based humanitarian groups providing services to some individuals with disabilities, that is, individuals who were perceived to be less "fortunate".

The turn of the 20th century ushered in the Progressive Era. Core to this group's belief was the role of government in controlling society's evils (Rubin & Roessler, 2008), and as a result, legislation providing funding for disability-related services could result in the improvement in the lives of people with disabilities. During this time, the role of the federal government increased: first under the leadership of President Theodore Roosevelt and later under Progressive presidents Taft and Wilson. These presidents perceived the role of government as one that moved America toward a place where most Americans had access to mechanisms for progress and social betterment (Rubin & Roessler).

1908 Federal Employers Liability Act (FELA)

This legislation established a federal system for workers who sustain injuries or die in the course of their employment on the railroad. This legislation was passed by the U.S. Congress under President Theodore Roosevelt after the 1906 FELA was declared unconstitutional by the U.S. Supreme Court (Federal Employees Liability Act, 2021).

1910 New York Workers Compensation

In 1910, New York became the first of the 46 United States to pass workers' compensation legislation. This provided coverage to New York workers injured in the course of their employment. By 1921, similar laws were passed by 42 states. By 1948, when Mississippi passed a workers' compensation law, all 48 contiguous states in the United States had some type of workers' compensation coverage (Rubin & Roessler, 2008). These laws were perceived to be under the purview of the state government, rather than the federal government.

1917 Smith-Hughes Act

This legislation provided federal funding to states to promote vocational education in agricultural, industrial trades, and home economics. The result of the Smith-Hughes Act (formally the National Vocational Education Act) expanded vocational courses and enrollment in vocational programs. With time, the act was criticized for reinforcing class- and race-based inequalities (Steffes et al., 2021).

1918 The Soldiers Rehabilitation Act

This legislation, also known as the Smith-Sears Vocational Rehabilitation Act, expanded the role of the Federal Board of Vocational Education to provide vocational rehabilitation services for veterans who sustained injuries during World War I if their disability presented a barrier to employment. Employment through vocational rehabilitation training had to be a feasible possibility (Rubin & Roessler, 2008).

1920 The Smith-Fess Act

The Smith-Fess Act of 1920 expanded funding of vocational rehabilitation services to all citizens with physical disabilities in all states. While vocational rehabilitation programs existed in eight states prior to the Smith-Fess Act, this legislation established funding for programs in all states. Funds were provided to states based on their populations (at a 50% federal and 50% state ratio) and were to be used for vocational guidance, education, placement services, and occupational adjustment (Rubin & Roessler, 2008).

1935 Social Security Act

Signed into law by President Franklin D. Roosevelt, this act provided benefits to retired Americans over age 65 who were blind and had physical disabilities, as well as benefits for children. The language of H.R. 7260 was as follows:

> An act to provide for the general welfare by establishing a system of Federal old-age benefits, and by enabling the several States to make more adequate provisions for aged persons, blind persons, dependent and crippled children, maternal and child welfare, public health, and the administration of their unemployment compensation laws; to establish a Social Security Board; to raise revenue; and for other purposes.
>   (The Social Security Act of 1935, n.d., para. 1)

This act also made the federal-state vocational rehabilitation program a permanent program, which could only be discontinued by congressional action.

1936 Randolph-Sheppard Act

Representative Jennings Randolph (from West Virginia) and Senator Morris Sheppard (from Texas) sponsored this bill, which mandated a priority for individuals with blindness to operate vending facilities on federal properties (20 U.S. Code § 107-Operation of Vending Facilities, n.d.; Randolph Sheppard Vending Facility Program, 2020). The goal was to focus on improving employment opportunities for individuals with visual disabilities.

1943 Barden-LaFolette Act

This act, also referred to as the vocational rehabilitation amendments, offered a comprehensive definition of vocational rehabilitation and expanded services to individuals with psychiatric and intellectual disabilities. It established separate agencies to provide services to individuals who were blind. It expanded vocational rehabilitation services to include physical restoration as a goal of service. It required that states submit written plans as to how monies would be spent on the state/federal vocational rehabilitation program (A Brief History of Legislation, n.d.).

Disability Acts in the 1950s–1960s

Undoubtedly, World War II had a significant impact on how Americans viewed disability and what disability-related legislation was passed in this era. During the war, individuals with disabilities were often needed to work in positions vacated by soldiers who left to fight in the war. Additionally, many soldiers returned from war after sustaining physical or psychological injuries and, unlike soldiers from previous wars, had access to improved medical care, which allowed them to live significantly longer with their disabilities. It was not until 1947 that the American Medical Association (AMA) created a specialty, physical medicine and rehabilitation, for physicians interested in the long-term management of the medical needs for individuals with disabilities (Rubin & Roessler, 2008). Along with improved medical treatment, funding for vocational rehabilitation also grew during this time, attributable in part to Presidents Eisenhower, Kennedy, and Johnson, causing many to term this the "Golden Era of Rehabilitation" (Rubin & Roessler).

1954 Vocational Rehabilitation Act Amendments

The Vocational Rehabilitation Act Amendments were passed to expand vocational rehabilitation services by increasing federal funding and increasing services to individuals with mental illness or "mental retardation". The act increased federal funding to state vocational rehabilitation services and expanded monies for additional rehabilitation centers and the training of rehabilitation professionals through university programs (A Brief History of Legislation, n.d.; Vocational Rehabilitation Act Amendments, 1954).

1956 Social Security Act Amendments

This act expanded Social Security benefits to individuals aged 50–64 who were deemed to have medical conditions that were permanently and totally disabling. Additionally, benefits were extended to adult children of retired or deceased workers if they had disabilities that began before age 16. Finally, this act lowered the retirement age for widows to 62 (Special Collections-Chronology, n.d.).

Vocational Rehabilitation Act Amendments of 1965

This act further expanded vocational rehabilitation services through funding for service provision by eliminating the requirement of demonstrating an economic need to qualify for any vocational rehabilitation service and by extending the time allowed to determine eligibility for a recipient. Additionally, services could be provided to individuals with "behavior disorders". Through this legislation, federal funding was increased from 50/50 funding to 75 (federal)/25 (state). With extended time allowed for eligibility, vocational rehabilitation counselors had more time to determine if individuals with more severe disabilities could benefit from vocational rehabilitation services (A Brief History of Legislation, n.d.; The History of Vocational Rehabilitation, 2015–2021).

1968 Architectural Barriers Act

This act required that buildings leased or purchased after 1968 by the federal government be made accessible to the public, which included building and bathroom access according to Uniform Federal Accessibility Standards (UFAS) (24-CFR § 570.614-Architectural Barriers Act, n.d.).

Major Developments in the 1970s–1980s

The 1960s in America inspired hundreds of thousands of Americans to become involved in the civil rights movement. As a result, President Lyndon B. Johnson signed the Civil Rights Act of 1964, which was designed to end segregation in public places and prevent employment discrimination based on race, color, religion, sex, or national origin (Legal Highlight: The Civil Rights Act of 1964, n.d.). Excluded from any protected class in this act, however, were Americans with disabilities.

Until this time in American culture, disability was conceptualized as a medically determined impairment residing within the individual. However, in the 1970s, this model was abandoned by some in favor of a biopsychosocial model, which beckoned for societal reform rather than individual treatment of a disease or impairment (Hogan, 2019). The legislation passed in America during the 1970s reflected this shift in attitude, with a focus on removing societally placed barriers for individuals with disabilities to more fully participate in daily activities. During the 1980s, legislative acts were passed with a continued emphasis on the removal of environmental barriers for people with disabilities. Included under this umbrella was the ongoing move toward the inclusion of individuals with disabilities in the workplace.

1973 Rehabilitation Act of 1973

This act, signed by President Richard Nixon (after two vetoes), prohibited discrimination against individuals with disabilities by any program administered by the federal government or receiving federal funds. The act defined a person with a disability as "a person who has a physical or mental impairment that substantially limits one or more major life activities, has a record of such impairment or is regarded as having such an impairment" (Information and Technical Assistance on the Americans with Disabilities Act, n.d., para. 2). In terms of agency creation, the act established the Rehabilitation Services Administration (RSA) and the Client Assistance Demonstration Projects which were designed to advise individuals of their rights under the Rehabilitation Act. The act comprised several sections, including:

- Section 501 of the act focused on the hiring of individuals with disabilities within the federal government.
- Section 502 created a board (the Architectural and Transportation Barriers Compliance Board [ATBCB]) to enforce standards from the 1968 Architectural Barriers Act.
- Section 503 prohibited discrimination in hiring based upon disability by federal contractors or subcontractors.
- Most would consider the most impactful portion of this piece of legislation to be Section 504(a) which states:

   No otherwise qualified individual with a disability in the United States, . . . shall, solely by reason of his or her disability, be excluded from the participation in, be denied the benefits of, or be subjected to discrimination under any program or activity receiving Federal financial assistance or under any program or activity conducted by any Executive agency or by the United States Postal Service

   (Section 504, Rehabilitation Act of 1973, n.d., para. 1).

- Section 508 addressed accessibility in communications and technology. In terms of vocational rehabilitation services, this act prioritized services to individuals with the most severe disabilities first (A Brief History of Legislation, n.d.).

1975 Education of All Handicapped Children Act

Under this act, public schools that accepted federal funds were required to provide equal access to education for children with disabilities. Through this act, schools, in cooperation with parents, were required to develop an educational plan for children with disabilities. The goal of the plan is to provide to the child as closely as possible the educational experience provided by the school to children without disabilities (Education for All Handicapped Children Act, 2021).

1978 Rehabilitation Act Amendments

Under this act, the National Institute of Handicapped Research was created. In 1986, the institute was renamed the National Institute on Disability Rehabilitation Research (NIDRR), and in 2014 the National Institute on Disability, Independent Living, and Rehabilitation Research (NIDILRR). This act also created (within the vocational rehabilitation system) independent living rehabilitation services for individuals with severe disabilities. The centers could provide attendant care, independent skills training, job placement, housing, transportation assistance, and other services designed to assist individuals with disabilities in living independently (Rubin & Roessler, 2008; Parallels in Time: A History of Developmental Disabilities, 2021).

1980 Social Security Disability Amendments of 1980

President Carter signed into law these amendments to the Social Security Act that established a maximum family disability benefit. It also created incentives for work-related activities by individuals receiving benefits, for example, a 15-month "re-entitlement" period for individuals who attempted work but were unsuccessful in retaining their employment (Social Security Disability Amendments, 1980; Ticket to Work, n.d.).

1982 Telephone Communications for the Disabled Act

This act required that the Federal Communications Commission (FCC) (within one year) establish regulations to ensure reasonable access to telephone service by persons with impaired hearing (H.R. 7168-Telecommunications for the Disabled Act of 1982, n.d.).

1984 Voting Accessibility for the Elderly and Handicapped Act

This act required that for federal elections occurring after December 31, 1985, a reasonable number of voter registration and polling places must be made accessible for individuals with disabilities unless their state provides the opportunity for mail-in voting (Rubin & Roessler, 2008; Chapter 201-Voting Accessibility for the Elderly and Handicapped, n.d.).

1986 Air Carrier Access Act of 1986

This act prohibited discrimination against individuals with disabilities by airline carriers who operated at federally funded airports. Enforcement of this act was given to the Department of Transportation (Rubin & Roessler, 2008).

1986 Rehabilitation Act Amendments

This act encouraged vocational rehabilitation services to expand the use of rehabilitation engineering services for individuals with disabilities, given the advancements in technology in this area. Another significant component of the act was the funding for employment-related services for individuals with severe disabilities, including supported employment programs designed to integrate individuals with disabilities into the competitive labor market (H.R. 4021-Rehabilitation Act Amendments of 1986, n.d.; Rubin & Roessler, 2008).

1988 Fair Housing Amendments Act

This act mandated building standards for new multifamily housing construction to provide accessibility for individuals with disabilities. This act expanded discrimination classes in the 1968 Fair Housing Act to include individuals with disabilities. This was the first federal law extending discrimination protection in the private sector to individuals with disabilities (Rubin & Roessler, 2008; Fair Housing Act, 2015a).

The 1990s and Disability Policy

The 1990s in America was a time of focus on the economy. President George H.W. Bush, whose goal for the United States was to be a "kinder and gentler nation", lost the 1992 presidential race to President Bill Clinton, whose strategist James Carville became famous for his quote, it's "the economy stupid". With that, the focus on legislation passed in this era was largely focused on employment and economic impact.

1990 Americans With Disabilities Act

Perhaps no other piece of disability-related legislation in America is more widely recognized than the ADA. The passage of the ADA in 1990 reflected the culmination of hundreds of years of efforts to improve access of individuals with disabilities to American society. While historically most disability-related legislation applied to government activities (specifically state or federal agencies), the ADA was the first large-scale piece of legislation designed to prevent discrimination based on disability in the private sector. The ADA codified the definition of disability, following the same one that the Rehabilitation Act of 1973 (Section 504) had, which is "a physical or mental impairment that substantially limits one or more major life activities; a person who has a history or record of such an impairment; or a person who is perceived by others as having such an impairment" (Information and Technical Assistance on the Americans with Disabilities Act, n.d., para. 2).

There are five titles of the ADA, each of which is designed to prohibit discrimination in various sectors.

Title I: Employment Practices. This title is intended to protect qualified individuals with disabilities from employment discrimination if the individual can perform the essential functions of a job with or without accommodation. It applies to American employers with 25 or more employees (effective 1992) and 15 or more employees (effective 1994) (Rubin & Roessler, 2008).

Title II: State and Local Government Services. This title is intended for state and local government services, including transportation providers, to provide access for individuals with disabilities to their programs, benefits activities, and services provided by such entities (A Guide to Disability Rights Laws, 2020).

Title III: Public Accommodations and Commercial Facilities. This title is intended for private entities to provide individuals with disabilities access to private entities such as, but not limited to, hotels, restaurants, professional offices, private schools, etc. (Rubin & Roessler, 2008).

Title IV: Telecommunications. This title of the ADA amended the Communications Act of 1934 to mandate that dual-party relay systems become available for telephone services by 1993 to increase access for individuals with speech and hearing disabilities while using telephone systems (Rubin & Roessler, 2008; A Guide to Disability Rights Laws, 2020).

Title V: Miscellaneous. This title of the ADA contains miscellaneous provisions not classified elsewhere in the act, including the prohibition against retaliation and provisions addressing the relationship of the ADA to other laws (An Overview of the Americans with Disabilities Act, 2021b).

1998 Workforce Investment Act (WIA) and Rehabilitation Act Amendments of 1998

This five-title act was designed to support workforce development through job training and adult education and literacy. This act established a one-stop delivery system of employment-related services to job seekers. In Title IV of the act, vocational rehabilitation services were integrated into the one-stop system. In Title III of the act, the U.S. Employment Services was integrated into the one-stop system (Bradley, 2013).

1999 Ticket to Work and Work Incentives Improvement Act of 1999 (TWWIIA)

The goal of this act was to increase the number of individuals receiving Social Security benefits who successfully return to employment. The act extended Medicare coverage to 93 consecutive months for individuals who return to work and enhanced incentives for individuals with disabilities to return to work through the Ticket to Work Program and through funding community work incentive coordinators to assist individuals in using these incentives (Ticket to Work, n.d.).

1999 Olmstead v. L.C., 527 U.S. 581

Unlike other disability-related legislation described in this section, *Olmstead v. L.C.* was the U.S. Supreme Court decision about the issue of the rights of individuals with disabilities to live within the community. The issue decided by the court was whether the state of Georgia could keep two women with disabilities institutionalized after their treatment providers determined that they could move to a community-based program. Specifically, had the state violated the rights of women afforded them under Title II of the ADA? The Court determined that public entities should provide community-based (rather than institutionally based) services when the individuals do not oppose such service provision when the services are appropriate for the individual(s) and when the community-based services can be reasonably accommodated (*Olmstead v L.C.* 138 F.3d 893 27 [1999], n.d.-b).

Disability Acts 2000 to Present

As the dawn of the 21st century was upon us, the role of technology in our lives was at the forefront. People around the world braced for Y2K, where many believed that a potential calendar code problem would crash computer systems worldwide. Along with the worldwide attention on the centrality of computer use in our lives, in America, the 2000s brought a time of the large-scale terrorist attack on September 11, 2001, and subsequent wars. In 2008, the Americans with Disabilities Amendments Act (ADAAA) was signed by President George W. Bush, amending the legislation signed by his father, President George H.W. Bush, in 1990. By 2008, America faced a financial crisis and recession that prompted widespread government activity. By 2010, the Affordable Care Act (commonly referred to as Obamacare) was passed in the U.S. Senate by a vote of 60–39.

2008 Americans With Disabilities Amendment Act

After 18 years of judicial and regulatory decision-making on ADA-related provisions, President George W. Bush signed the ADAAA of 2008. Through these decisions and regulations, the definition of disability had been interpreted narrowly, and the intent of this act was to expand the definition of disability with a more inclusive interpretation (Notice Concerning the Americans with Disabilities Act (ADA), n.d.). The ADAAA retained the definition of disability in the 1990 ADA (described previously in this chapter) but rejected several decisions by the U.S. Supreme Court and ADA regulations promulgated by the Equal Employment Opportunity Commission (EEOC) that directed that the definition of disability should be construed narrowly. Specifically, the ADAAA required that the EEOC revise how "substantially limits" is defined in their guidelines and clarified that the ADAAA covered episodic disabilities that substantially limit activities when active. The ADAAA expanded the definition of "major life activities" to include major bodily functions and specified other, not previously delineated activities such as reading and walking. The ADAAA also changed the "regarded as" prong of the definition of disability (Notice Concerning the Americans with Disabilities Act (ADA), n.d., para. 3).

2010 The Patient Protection and Affordable Care Act

While not specifically designed for individuals with disabilities, the Affordable Care Act, otherwise known as "Obamacare", prohibited insurers from excluding individuals with pre-existing medical conditions. It also expanded coverage to individuals who receive Medicaid benefits and reduced the cost of healthcare coverage in general to lower-income individuals (Health Coverage Rights and Protections, n.d.). These provisions were particularly relevant and impactful for healthcare services for people with disabilities.

2011 New Americans With Disabilities Act

This 2011 set of regulations specifically implemented the ADA in terms of places of public accommodations. This act adopted the 2010 ADA Standards for Accessible Design and were applied to over 7 million places of public accommodations (Justice Department's New ADA Rules, 2015b).

2014 Workforce Innovation and Opportunity Act (WIOA)

This act is intended to assist individuals seeking employment, training, and/or other services with successful return-to-work efforts. It is also intended to meet employers' needs in filling job vacancies with properly trained workers. Through this act, students with disabilities receive transition services (i.e., planning for post–high school life) completed before employment, with 15% of federal funds for vocational rehabilitation specifically designated for such services (WIOA Programs, n.d.).

Canadian Disability Legislation

While the majority of this chapter has focused on disability policy within the United States, what follows is an outline of several important pieces of Canadian legislation pertaining to

Canadian citizens with disabilities. In 2017, it was estimated that over 6 million Canadians, or 22% of the population, had a disability (Morris et al., 2018). In contrast to the strong role that the federal government has placed in shaping disability policy in America, in Canada, one will find that many provinces have borne the responsibility of regulating protections against disability-related discrimination practices. Burns and Gordon (2010) note in a review of disability-related literature that three times as much literature was found regarding U.S. disability-related legislation when compared to Canadian literature. A brief discussion of some, but not all, Canadian disability-related legislation is presented next.

Canadian Government Legislation

1977 The Canadian Human Rights Act

This statute prohibits discrimination or harassment based upon 11 designated classes of protection, of which disability is one. This statute applies throughout Canada to any federally regulated activity, including private-sector agencies, that are regulated by the Canadian government. Companies in the private sector that are federally regulated, such as banks and broadcasters, are also covered by this human rights law (Canadian Human Rights Act R.S.C., 2021a).

1982 The Canadian Charter of Rights and Freedoms

Specifically, within Section 15 of the Canadian Charter of Rights and Freedoms, entitled Equality Rights, it is noted that every individual is afforded equal protection under the law, "without discrimination based upon race, national or ethnic origin, colour, religion, sex, age or mental or physical disability" (Guide to the Canadian Charter of Rights, 2020, Section 15).

1998 The Employment Equity Act

The purpose of this act is to reduce barriers by potential employees perceived to have disadvantages (e.g., women, Aboriginal people, people with disabilities) in employment. Not only does the act encourage equity in hiring, it also encourages accommodations as a means of achieving equity. This act applies to industries that are federally regulated in Canada (Employment Equity Act S.C., 2021b).

2019 The Accessible Canada Act (Bill C-81)

The purpose of this act is to create a barrier-free Canada by 2040 both by preventing new barriers and targeting and removing existing barriers to full societal participation by individuals with disabilities throughout Canada. Barriers may be identified in employment, transportation, community access, communication, and other areas, and the act applies to both public (Canadian government) and private entities regulated by the federal government. The definition of disability contained in the act is:

> any impairment, including a physical, mental, intellectual, cognitive, learning, communication, or sensory impairment—or a functional limitation—whether permanent, temporary, or episodic in nature, or evident or not, that, in interaction with a barrier, hinders a person's full and equal participation in society.
>
> (Accessible Canada Act, 2020, para. 3)

Provincial Government

Canadian provinces and territories each have human rights acts under which individuals are protected from discrimination and harassment. Many of these include specific mention of individuals with disabilities as a protected class. Some Canadian provinces, including Quebec, Ontario, Manitoba, Nova Scotia, and British Columbia, have laws protecting against disability-related discrimination. Some of these are outlined next.

2000 Quebec's Act Respecting Equal Access to Employment in Public Bodies

The purpose of this act is to promote equal access to employment for certain groups discriminated against, including women, minority groups, Aboriginal people, and individuals with disabilities. This applies to employers in Quebec who employ 100 or more employees (Act Respecting Equal Access to Employment, 2020).

2005 The Accessibility for Ontarians With Disabilities Act (AODA)

The AODA requires that organizations follow accessibility standards in the areas of information and communications (including website accessibility), customer service, transportation, employment, and public space design. This act applies to individuals and organizations in both public and private sectors in Ontario. The goal of the province is to be completely accessible by the year 2025 (Accessibility for Ontarians with Disabilities Act, 2012–21).

2013 The Accessibility for Manitobans Act

This act was created to prevent and/or remove barriers that exist for individuals with disabilities, with a focus on barriers in customer service, information and communication, transportation, employment, and the built environment. This act applies to private and public sectors (The Accessibility for Manitobans Act, n.d.-a, n.d.-b).

2017 The Nova Scotia Accessibility Act

This act was created to further the goal of making Nova Scotia accessible by 2030. The act seeks to remove or prevent barriers for individuals with disabilities in areas identified as:

> (i) the delivery and receipt of goods and services, (ii) information and communication, (iii) public transportation and transportation infrastructure, (iv) employment, (v) the built environment, (vi) education, and (vii) a prescribed activity or undertaking Under the Act, small businesses can apply for grants to assist in making accessibility improvements.
> (Nova Scotia, n.d.; Accessibility Act, 2017)

2018 British Columbia Accessibility Act

The purpose of this act is to achieve accessibility by preventing and/or removing barriers for individuals with disabilities within the following areas: the delivery and receipt of goods and services, information and communication, public transportation and transportation infrastructure, employment, the built environment, education, and a prescribed activity or undertaking. It is the goal of the province of British Columbia to achieve full accessibility by 2024 (Bill M 219–2018 British Columbia Accessibility Act, n.d.)

Areas for Growth in Disability Policy and Legislation

With the passage of time, most would agree that both the United States and Canada have become more accessible to individuals with disabilities. However, there remain numerous areas where ongoing legislative work is required to improve accessibility. Some of these areas include improving employment opportunities for people with disabilities, increasing full access to technology that has become central to many of our lives, and the ability of people with disabilities to continue to make important decisions for themselves, including choices about sexuality, and seeking to close loopholes that allow ongoing disability-based discrimination.

Even with the passage of the ADA (1990) and the ADAAA (2008), there remain important exemptions from the laws that continue to perpetuate restrictions in terms of access by individuals with disabilities. Currently, in the United States, religious exemption continues to be a controversial topic in discrimination enforcement. Under Title I of the ADA, an individual with a disability is protected from employment-based discrimination by a religious entity if that entity employs at least 15 individuals (An Overview of the Americans with Disabilities Act, 2021b). Under Title III of the ADA, which addresses accessibility to public accommodations, disability discrimination by private businesses is prohibited. However, religious entities, including their physical facilities and their programs, are exempt from ADA provisions, even if they are open to the general public. The result of this exemption is that commonly visited religious entities, including schools, food banks, hospitals, daycare centers, etc., are not required to be accessible to individuals with disabilities in the United States (Religious Entities Under the Americans with Disabilities Act, 2021a). The practical result of this is that a child with a disability who attends a religious-based daycare or school may encounter barriers to the learning environment without recourse to have those barriers removed to gain access to equal educational opportunities.

Yet another area where individuals with disabilities in America continue to face restricted access, despite the passage of laws intended to prohibit such, is in the realm of employment. After the passage of the Individuals with Disability Education Act in 1975, the graduation rate of children from high school has increased, although it still remains lower than the graduation rate of children without disabilities. However, as these individuals transition from school-based settings to employment-based settings, their participation declines. This is reflected in the U.S. Bureau of Labor Statistics January 2021 report of employment participation rates for individuals with disabilities at approximately 20%, compared to 66% for individuals without disabilities (Erickson et al., 2021).

While a full explanation of this is beyond the scope of this chapter, it certainly has ties to disability policy creation in America. Through the Social Security Disability program, once a person is deemed "disabled" through the Social Security Administration, the regulatory provisions of the administration make it complex for a person to return to work without risking loss of income and, perhaps more importantly, access to medical care afforded through the program. This can be of critical importance for individuals with disabilities. According to the U.S. Social Security Administration, less than one half of 1% of individuals who receive SSDI or Supplemental Security Income (SSI) return to work (Liu & Stapleton, 2011). Despite efforts by the administration to reduce this complexity and enable workers to successfully return to work, the practical effect of the poor return-to-work rate is financially dooming over 10 million Americans who rely on these benefits to live without further independently acquired income (Annual Statistical Report on the Social Security Disability Insurance Program, 2016). Additionally, individuals with disabilities can continue to be paid less than minimum wage for their work if their employer obtains a certificate through the U.S. Department of Labor's Wage and Hour Division. While some states have outlawed this practice, it remains a widespread practice that negatively impacts the employment of people with disabilities.

Yet another area of limitations for individuals with disabilities is the ongoing limited access to technology. While there are historical fights for physical community access for people with disabilities dating back to the 1960s in America, Burns and Gordon (2010) note that until approximately 2005, there had not been discussion about accessibility in terms of computer technology. In more recently passed disability-related legislation in Canada, accessibility to websites is specifically noted in the goals of the legislation (Accessibility for Ontarians with Disabilities Act, 2005). Some courts have decided that community access does not include website access, including a 2002 U.S. District Court decision in *Access Now, Inc. vs. Southwest Airlines*. In this decision, the court ruled that Southwest Airlines' website was not a place of public accommodation and covered under Title III of the ADA because it did not physically exist but was a virtual construct. However, by 2006, in *National Federation for the Blind v. Target Corporation*, the court decided that websites and/or Internet access are covered under Title III of the ADA (*National Federation for the Blind v. Target Corporation*, 2021). The issue of providing equal access to technology has received growing attention following the outbreak of COVID-19 in 2020, which underscored why inequitable access to technology is a critical civil rights issue.

Conclusion

In America, how one defines the word "disability" has been the subject of multiple legal decisions, conferences, articles, books, and likely thousands of conversations related to disability. The ADA (1990) defined disability with what some argue were unenforceable (or unenforced) regulations, and through a series of legal decisions, the U.S. Supreme Court limited that definition. In 2008, the U.S. Congress passed the ADAAA, which allowed a broader interpretation of the definition of disability. The ACS collected data based upon one definition of disability until 2008 and yet another definition of disability after 2008 (How Disability Data are Collected From the American Community Survey, 2017). The U.S. Social Security Administration uses yet another definition of disability when it administers its disability adjudication system. Therefore, unlike other civil rights movements, where the definition of what it means to be a woman or what it means to be a certain race is typically not at the center of the conversation, the lack of an agreed-upon definition of disability has resulted in a splintering of the disability community. Unlike other civil rights protections, disability has been treated differently. It is only when disability is conceptualized as a diagnostic lens, as race and gender are, that legal and other systems will best be able to understand and therefore prevent and combat disability discrimination.

Not only has the lack of an agreement on the word "disability" been problematic in the quest for equal protection under the law, but so too has the splintering within the disability community. While some communities of people with disabilities have a strong, central identity, others do not. For example, individuals with hearing impairments have long had (since 1817 in America) educational institutions specifically available for the education of students who were Deaf or hearing impaired, but the advent of cochlear implants in the 1980s resulted in strong mixed reactions within the Deaf and hard of hearing community. While some individuals pursued the medical device, others objected to such a pursuit, based upon rejection of the premise that deafness was something to be "fixed". The National Association of the Deaf in 1991 issued a position paper on cochlear implants, stating that they deplored the Food and Drug Administration (FDA) for approving such a device. Over time, this controversy has continued and reflects that the disability community is simply not a homogenous group of individuals and there are both within-group and between-group differences.

Despite the differences that have existed and will continue to exist, there have been examples of this heterogeneous group of individuals coalescing to effect change for the entire community.

Perhaps there is no better example of this than the groups of Americans who converged to usher into law the ADA of 1990. By all accounts, the passage of the ADA by a 91–6 margin in the Democrat-controlled U.S. Senate and signed by a Republican president, George H.W. Bush, would not have occurred without the collective efforts of a diverse group of individuals with disabilities championing this legislation. Recall that provisions of Section 504 of the Rehabilitation Act of 1973 were only signed after a series of sit-ins at Health, Education, and Welfare offices by individuals with disabilities to put pressure on then-Secretary Joseph Califano Jr. to sign the provisions. The fight between the 1973 passage and the 1977 signing was fought by a diverse group of individuals with disabilities, some in wheelchairs, some with cerebral palsy, some with deafness, and some with AIDS—all of whom joined forces and effected change in terms of societal inclusion and improved access. Likewise, when the passage of the ADA stalled, most notably due to concerns about the cost of public transportation, protestors participated in the March 1990 "Capitol Crawl", with individuals with mobility limitations abandoning their assistive devices and climbing the 78 stairs to the steps of the U.S. Capitol (Disability History: The Disability Rights Movement, 2019). The result of years of work, protest, and education resulted in the passage of the ADA four months later.

Using this model of inclusion and activation, individuals in the disability community have worked tirelessly at the local community, state, and federal levels to push for nationwide protection against discrimination. As seen earlier in this chapter, in his struggle to obtain an education, Ed Roberts learned multiple lessons, and they included the following:

1. Having parents who not only advocate for you but include you in the fight was critical.
2. Money is always in the equation.
3. Individuals with disabilities are in the best position to determine what is important to their lives.

Anyone who has participated in the fight for equal rights would likely argue that the importance of advocacy cannot be understated. Through this advocacy, it is common to find that changes in attitudes and language occur more quickly than do the changes that require financial investment (Burns & Gordon, 2010). Throughout the history of disability-related legislation in both Canada and the United States, voices for inclusion are typically tempered by voices for cost containment. For example, while the ADA of 1990 significantly impacted future discourse concerning disability-related accessibility, with no accompanying cost, many private-sector employers in America (who perceived an associated cost for hiring people with disabilities) were less willing to change their hiring practices in terms of inclusivity. When there is pushback against inclusion and access, it is often out of fear (whether well-founded or not) that the inclusion requirement will place a financial burden on covered entities.

Over time, one observes that individuals with disabilities have become increasingly involved in the development of legislation that impacts their lives. With the rise of the independent living movement in the 1970s in America, the collective voice of individuals with disabilities became a growing wave of influence subsequently heard in the development of post-1970s legislation. Person by person, community by community, changes have been demanded of societies that have long histories of excluding people with disabilities from participation. While there are many fights left to fight, the arc of history, through advocacy, legislative acts, and court decisions, has bent toward inclusion.

Note

1 Special thanks to Dr. Brent Williams for his assistance in this project.

References

A Brief History of Legislation. (n.d.). *Colorado state university student disability center*. https://disability-center. colostate.edu/disability-awareness/disability-history/#:~:text=1943%20%E2%80%94%20The%20Vocational%20Rehabilitation%20Amendments,include%20physical%20restoration%2C%20and%20each

Access Now v. Southwest Airlines 227 F. Supp. 2d 1312. (2002). https://law.justia.com/cases/federal/district-courts/FSupp2/227/1312/2529905/

Accessibility Act. (2017, April). *Nova scotia legislature*. https://nslegislature.ca/legc/bills/62nd_3rd/1st_read/b059.htm

Accessibility for Ontarians with Disabilities Act, 2005, S.O. 2005, c. 11. (2012–21). *Queen's printer for Ontario*. www.ontario.ca/laws/statute/05a11

Accessible Canada Act. (2020, November). *Government of Canada*. www.canada.ca/en/employment-social-development/programs/accessible-canada/act-summary.html#h2.02

Act Respecting Equal Access to Employment in Public Bodies. (2020, October). *Publications Quebec*. http://legisquebec.gouv.qc.ca/en/ShowDoc/cs/A-2.01

ADA Amendments Act of 2008 Frequently Asked Questions. (2009, January). *Office of federal contract compliance programs*. www.dol.gov/agencies/ofccp/faqs/americans-with-disabilities-act-amendments

A Guide to Disability Rights Laws. (2020, February). *United States department of justice*. www.ada.gov/cguide.htm#anchor62335

An Overview of the Americans with Disabilities Act. (2021b, February). *ADA national network*. https://adata.org/factsheet/ADA-overview#:~:text=Title%20V%20%2D%20Miscellaneous%20Provisions,of%20drugs%2C%20and%20attorney's%20fees

Annual Statistical Report on the Social Security Disability Insurance Program. (2016). *Social security office of retirement and disability policy*. www.ssa.gov/policy/docs/statcomps/di_asr/2016/sect01.html#:~:text=In%20December%202016%2C%20there%20were,disabled%20widow(er)s

Bill M 219–2018 British Columbia Accessibility Act. (n.d.). *Queen's printer*. www.bclaws.gov.bc.ca/civix/document/id/lc/billsprevious/3rd41st:m219-1

Bradley, D. H. (2013). *The workforce investment act and the one-stop delivery system*. Congressional Research Service 7-5700. https://fas.org/sgp/crs/misc/R41135.pdf

Burns, K. K., & Gordon, G. L. (2010). Analyzing the impact of disability legislation in Canada and the United States. *Journal of Disability Policy Studies*, 20(4), 205–218.

Canadian Human Rights Act R.S.C., 1985, c. H-6. (2021a, February). *Government of Canada*. https://laws-lois.justice.gc.ca/eng/acts/H-6/page-1.html

Chapter 201: Voting Accessibility for the Elderly and Handicapped. (n.d.). *United States house of representatives*. https://uscode.house.gov/view.xhtml?path=/prelim@title52/subtitle2/chapter201&edition=prelim

Chartbook: Social Security Insurance. (2021, February). *Center on budget and policy priorities*. www.cbpp.org/research/social-security/chart-book-social-security-disability-insurance#:~:text=The%20Social%20Security%20Administration%20

Disability. (2021). *World health organization*. www.who.int/health-topics/disability#tab=tab_1

Disability and Health. (2020, December). *World health organization*. www.who.int/news-room/fact-sheets/detail/disability-and-health

Disability History: The Disability Rights Movement. (2019, December). *National park service*. www.nps.gov/articles/disabilityhistoryrightsmovement.htm

Domzal, C., Houtenville, A., & Sharma, R. (2008). *Survey of employer perspectives on the employment of people with disabilities: Technical Report*. CESSI.

Employment Equity Act S.C. 1995, c. 44. (2021b, February). *Government of Canada*. https://laws-lois.justice.gc.ca/eng/acts/E-5.401/page-1.html#h-215135

Erickson, W., Lee, C., & von Schrader, S. (2021). *Disability statistics from the 2018 American community survey (ACS)*. Cornell University Yang-Tan Institute (YTI). www.disabilitystatistics.org/

Fair Housing Act. (2015a, August). *United States department of justice*. www.justice.gov/crt/fair-housing-act-2

Federal Employers Liability Act (FELA). (2021, February). *Encyclopedia.com*. www.encyclopedia.com/history/encyclopedias-almanacs-transcripts-and-maps/federal-employers-liability-act-1908

Guide to the Canadian Charter of Rights and Freedom. (2020, June). *Government of Canada*. www.canada.ca/en/canadian-heritage/services/how-rights-protected/guide-canadian-charter-rights-freedoms.html

Health Coverage Rights and Protections. (n.d.). *HealthCare.gov*. www.healthcare.gov/health-care-law-protections/

Hogan, A. J. (2019). Social and medical models of disability and mental health: Evolution and renewal. *Canadian Medical Association Journal, 191*(1), 16–18. https://doi.org/10.1503/cmaj.181008

How Disability Data are Collected from the American Community Survey. (2017, October). *United States census bureau.* www.census.gov/topics/health/disability/guidance/data-collection-acs.html

H.R. 4021-Rehabilitation Act Amendments of 1986. (n.d.). *Congress.gov.* www.congress.gov/bill/99th-congress/house-bill/4021

H.R. 7168-Telecommunications for the Disabled Act of 1982. (n.d.). *Congress.gov.* www.congress.gov/bill/97th-congress/house-bill/7168?s=1&r=43#:~:text=Telecommunications%20for%20the%20Disabled%20Act%20of%201982%20%2D%20Amends%20the%20Communications,by%20persons%20with%20impaired%20hearing.&text=Directs%20the%20FCC%20to%20establish%20the%20necessary%20technical%20standards

Information and Technical Assistance on the Americans with Disabilities Act. (n.d.). *ADA.Gov.* www.ada.gov/ada_intro.htm

Justice Department's New ADA Rules Go Into Effect on March 15, 2011. (2015b, August). *United States department of justice.* www.justice.gov/opa/pr/justice-department-s-new-ada-rules-go-effect-march-15-2011

Legal Highlight: The Civil Rights Act of 1964. (n.d.). *U.S. department of labor.* www.dol.gov/agencies/oasam/civil-rights-center/statutes/civil-rights-act-of-1964#:~:text=In%201964%2C%20Congress%20passed%20Public,religion%2C%20sex%20or%20national%20origin

Liu, S. L., & Stapleton, D. C. (2011). Longitudinal statistics on work activity and use of employment supports for new social security disability insurance beneficiaries. *Social Security Bulletin, 71*(3). www.ssa.gov/policy/docs/ssb/v71n3/v71n3p35.html#:~:text=Despite%20such%20historic%20opportunities%20and,rolls%20and%20return%20to%20work

Morris, S., Fawcell, G. Brisebois, L., & Hughes, J. (2018, November). *Canadian survey on disability reports: A demographic, employment and income profile of Canadians with disabilities aged 15 years and over, 2017.* Statistics Canada. https://www150.statcan.gc.ca/n1/pub/89-654-x/89-654-x2018002-eng.htm

Murphy v. United Parcel Service, Inc. 527 US 516 (1999). Retrieved February 28, 2021, from www.oyez.org/cases/1998/97-1992

National Federation of the Blind v. Target Corporation. (2021). Disability Rights Advocate. https://dralegal.org/case/national-federation-of-the-blind-nfb-et-al-v-target-corporation/

Notice Concerning the Americans with Disabilities Act (ADA) Amendments Act of 2008. (n.d.). *United States equal opportunity employment commission.* www.eeoc.gov/statutes/notice-concerning-americans-disabilities-act-ada-amendments-act-2008

Nova Scotia. (n.d.). *Accessibility services Canada.* https://accessibilitycanada.ca/legislation/nova-scotia/

Olmstead v. L.C. 138 F.3d 893 27 (1999). (n.d.-b). Cornell Law School. www.law.cornell.edu/supct/html/98-536.ZS.html

Parallels in Time: A History of Developmental Disabilities. (2021). *The Minnesota governor's council on developmental disabilities.* https://mn.gov/mnddc/parallels/six/6c/3.html#:~:text=Under%20the%201978%20amendments%2C%20centers,%3B%20recreational%3B%20and%20job%20placement

Randolph Sheppard Vending Facility. (2020, November). *United States department of education, program.* https://www2.ed.gov/programs/rsarsp/index.html

Religious Entities Under the Americans with Disabilities Act. (2021a, February). *ADA national network.* https://adata.org/factsheet/religious-entities-under-americans-disabilities-act

Rubin, S. E., & Roessler, R. (2008). *Foundations of the vocational rehabilitation process.* PRO-ED.

S. 6–94th Congress: Education for All Handicapped Children Act. (2021, February). *GovTrack.us.* www.govtrack.us/congress/bills/94/s6

Section 504, Rehabilitation Act of 1973. (n.d.). *United States department of labor.* www.dol.gov/agencies/oasam/centers-offices/civil-rights-center/statutes/section-504-rehabilitation-act-of-1973

Shapiro, J. P. (1994). *No pity, people with disabilities forging a new civil rights movement.* Three Rivers Press.

Social Security Disability Amendments of 1980. (1981). Legislative history and summary of provisions. *Social Security Bulletin, 44*(4), 14–31.

Special Collections-Chronology. (n.d.). *Social security administration.* www.ssa.gov/history/1950.html#:~:text=August%201%2C%201956%20The%20Social,the%20retirement%20age%20for%20widows

Steffes, T., Duigan, B., & Lotha, G. (2021). *Smith Hughes act.* www.britannica.com/topic/Smith-Hughes-Act

Sutton v. United Air Lines, Inc. (n.d.). Oyez. Retrieved February 28, 2021, from *www.oyez.org/cases/1998/97-1943*

Table A-6. Employment Status of the Civilian Population by Sex, Age, and Disability Status, Not Seasonally Adjusted. (2021, February). *United States bureau of labor statistics*. www.bls.gov/news.release/empsit.t06.htm

The Accessibility for Manitobans Act. (n.d.-a). *The legislative assembly of Manitoba*. https://web2.gov.mb.ca/bills/40-2/b026e.php

The Accessibility for Manitobans Act. (n.d.-b). *Manitoba*. www.accessibilitymb.ca/index.html

Ticket to Work. (n.d.). *Social security administration*. https://yourtickettowork.ssa.gov/about/history.html#:~:text=The%20Ticket%20to%20Work%20and%20Work%20Incentives%20Improvement%20Act%20of,wished%20to%20return%20to%20work.&text=The%20SSI%20program%20provides%20cash,have%20limited%20income%20and%20resources

The History of Vocational Rehabilitation. (2015–2021). *South Carolina vocational rehabilitation department*. https://scvrd.net/history

The Social Security Act of 1935. (n.d.). Social security administration. www.ssa.gov/history/35act.html

20 U.S. Code § 107—Operation of Vending Facilities. (n.d.). *Legal information institute*. www.law.cornell.edu/uscode/text/20/107

24 CFR § 570.614—Architectural Barriers Act and the Americans with Disabilities Act. (n.d.). *Cornell law school*. www.law.cornell.edu/cfr/text/24/570.614

Vocational Rehabilitation Act Amendments. (1954). *Social security administration, social security bulletin*. www.ssa.gov/policy/docs/ssb/v17n10/v17n10p16.pdf

WIOA Programs. (n.d.). *United States department of labor*. www.dol.gov/agencies/eta/wioa/about#:~:text=The%20Workforce%20Innovation%20and%20Opportunity,compete%20in%20the%20global%20economy

World Report on Disability. (2011, December). *World health organization*. www.who.int/teams/noncommunicable-diseases/disability-and-rehabilitation/world-report-on-disability

3   Third-Party Provider Systems

Larry S. Stokes, Aaron M. Wolfson, Todd S. Capielano,
Lacy H. Sapp, and Ashley G. Lastrapes

Third-party provider systems are responsible for services to workers with injuries and disabilities under various laws, both state and federal. These systems include entities such as the Social Security Administration and the various workers' compensation systems. Evaluating work ability is central to determining the need and scope of potential services regardless of the specific rules governing compensation or rehabilitation. Health care providers are important collaborators and should be familiar with the rules, policies, and processes of the various systems. In this chapter, we will discuss these third-party payor systems and the processes, procedures, and policies of these systems, which include state workers' compensation, federal workers' compensation programs, and Social Security Disability Insurance. We will also discuss the health care professional's role in each process. We begin with a brief history of disability and rehabilitation within the context of work to present the roots of what has become the modern systems. Even though the rules, processes, and administration may change through the years, the goal remains the same—the care and rehabilitation of the injured or disabled worker.

Disability and Work

Work defines how one contributes to their society, community, and family and is often critical in organizing personal identity. If a person cannot work because of a disability, then subsequent challenges may occur in their lives. Beyond the actual physical, cognitive, or emotional impairments produced by a disability, the person must also persist in maintaining gainful, competitive employment. If the individual cannot meet performance requirements for their occupations, they may require subsequent medical treatment, job restructuring, training, or alternative job placement. If the person with a disability is barred from employment because of the assumptions or fears of those who withhold employment, then community reeducation is indicated (Obermann, 1965). Third-party systems are designed to aid in the continuation of employment and assure that critical treatment, rehabilitation, and compensation are available for workers with injuries or disabilities.

In addition to work being a means of financial compensation, there is a satisfaction in belonging to a group or team, achieving goals, and being productive. Work, particularly after the onset of a disability, can eliminate the feeling of rejection and combat low self-worth. Unfortunately, having a disability has too often been equated with a lack of capability. The use of various terms can describe different aspects of the disability experience. The World Health Organization (WHO) divides disability into three dimensions: impairment, activity limitation, and participation restrictions. Impairment refers to a loss of a structure or function, such as a loss of a limb. Activity limitation refers to the loss of ability such as the ability to walk or see. Participation restrictions refer to the inability to engage in normal activities such as work, recreation, or

DOI: 10.4324/b23293-3

socialization. Obermann (1965) describes the term impairment as a deviation in one's ability. He adds that the term disability is a loss of function, while the term handicapped is the inability to meet the standards required for productivity.

Another term used in reference to disability is economic impairment. Economic impairment refers to the difference between the individual's pre-disability wage-earning capacity and the individual's post-disability wage-earning capacity. Economic impairment is the analysis of the difference or loss of wage-earning capacity when that person is not employed or employed in occupations other than they were before the disability, due to a disability or handicap. Many impaired, handicapped, or disabled persons are productively employed; however, some remain underemployed or unemployed. Vocational rehabilitation is meant to reduce the economic loss and assist an impaired, handicapped, or disabled individual to return to a productive life in the workforce. In addition to the economic loss of wage-earning capacity, consideration must be given to medical expenses incurred because of a disability.

Rehabilitation is a process that requires integrated services by various specialists on the treatment team. These specialists can include a vocational rehabilitation counselor; physician; nurse; case manager; social worker; speech, physical, and occupational therapists; home health care; and others. Another important contributor to the team is the third-party benefits administrator or claims professional. The rehabilitation process is truly collaborative, and assistance can come from families, friends, and other helpers as well. While medical professionals assist the individual in overcoming medical, physical, and mental limitations, vocational rehabilitation counselors work with the individual to help define or acquire vocational skills, identify jobs, and assist in returning the individual to the workforce. This process might include assessment of intelligence, achievement, interest, aptitudes, particular skills, and services needed to assist the individual in attaining employment through education, training, job identification, and placement. If return to employment is not possible or delayed, systems exist to compensate the injured worker.

The Use of the *AMA* Guides to the Evaluation of Permanent Impairment in Rehabilitation

The AMA's *Guides to the Evaluation of Permanent Impairment*, 6th ed., defines impairment ratings as "a loss of use or derangement of any body part, organ system, or organ function" (Rondinelli, 2008). The goal of this resource is to provide an impairment rating guide that is authoritative, fair, and equitable to all parties (Rondinelli). In developing the *Guides*, an evidence-based foundation and a modified Delphi panel approach were used for consensus building. The *Guides* is a treatise on evaluating impairment.

Typically, the four basic points of consideration regarding the severity of an illness or injury include: (1) what is the problem (diagnosis); (2) what symptoms and resulting functional difficulty does the patient report; (3) what are the physical findings pertaining to the problem; and (4) what are the results of the clinical studies. The latest edition encourages attention to and documentation of the functional consequences of impairment. The methodology applies terminology and an analytical framework based on the WHO's International Classification of Functioning, Disability, and Health (ICF). Five impairment classes permit the rating of the patient from no impairment to the most severe impairment.

The ICF model is intended to describe and measure the health and disability of individuals and consists of three components: (1) body functions and body structures: physiological functions and body parts, which can vary from the normal state to loss or deviations, which are referred to as impairments; (2) activity: task execution by the individual and activity limitations or difficulties carrying out such activities; and (3) participation: involvement in life situations and participation restrictions or barriers to experiencing such involvement. These components comprise functioning and disability in the model.

The following definitions used in the *Guides* are relevant for this chapter:

Impairment: a significant deviation, loss, or loss of use of any body structure or body function in an individual with a health condition, disorder, or disease.

Disability: activity limitations and/or participation restrictions in an individual with a health condition, disorder, or disease.

Impairment Rating: consensus-derived percentage estimate of a loss of activity reflecting the severity of a given health condition and the degree of the associated limitations in terms of activities of daily living.

Practical Application of the Guides to the Evaluation of Permanent Impairment

The *Guides* note that whole-person impairment is the result of an impairment evaluation noted in a percentage based on ranges from normal (0%), to totally dependent on others for care (90+%), to approaching death (100%). Only permanent impairment may be rated according to the *Guides*, and only after maximum medical improvement (MMI) status has been reached. Future impairment cannot be rated. Subjective complaints alone are generally not ratable under the *Guides*. There are potential exceptions to this principle, such as pain. The examiner's role in performing an impairment evaluation is to provide an independent, unbiased assessment of the individual's medical condition, functional ability, and limitations. The *Guides* note that although treating physicians may perform impairment ratings on their patients, it is recognized that these are not independent and therefore may be subject to scrutiny.

The *Guides* note that in many cases, the physician may need to obtain additional consultant input such as a functional evaluation performed by physical, occupational, or speech therapists, as well as by trained rehabilitation professionals in functional capacity evaluations (FCEs). Additionally, a psychological assessment performed by a psychologist or rehabilitation counselor trained in the evaluation of work demands may best match the individual to an acceptable and safe work setting within the functional parameters of the individual's disability. Specifically, an FCE is the ideal assessment tool for determining the most compatible work setting and essential functions of the respective job that are within the individual's adjusted functional worker trait factors (May, 1999; May et al., 1998). These functional tests initially examined and evaluated the ability of a worker to perform physical job match conditions as described by the U.S. Department of Labor in *Selected Characteristics of Occupations as Defined in the Revised Dictionary of Occupational Titles* (1993) and *The Revised Handbook for Analyzing Jobs* (1991). Functional examination/evaluation has emerged as a valid and effective tool to support a safe return to work, activities of daily living, or leisure activities after an injury or illness.

Legal vs. Medical Probability

Legal terminology defines the association between an event and an outcome as "probable" if it is more likely than not. If the probability of a causal relationship is greater than a 50% chance, then it is noted as "probable." A "possible" causal relationship exists between a cause and event when the likelihood of the relationship is equal to or less than 50%. The *Guides* note a contrast in the standards in the scientific and medical literature in which the likelihood that an association between the potential cause and effect might be greater than 95% for the relationship to be considered "probable." Under that standard, everything else is only "possible."

The *Guides* note that causality is an association between a given cause (an event capable of producing an effect) and an effect (a condition that can result from a specific cause) with a reasonable degree of medical probability. It is noted that in many cases patients have pre-existing pathology that may have contributed to their current clinical condition. An aggravation is a circumstance or event that permanently worsens a pre-existing or underlying condition. The *Guides* note that the terms "exacerbation," "recurrence," or "flare-up" imply worsening of a condition temporarily, which subsequently returns to baseline. Exacerbation does not equal aggravation.

Apportionment is an allocation of causation among multiple factors that caused or significantly contributed to the resulting impairment. Apportionment requires a determination of the percentage of impairment directly attributable to pre-existing as compared with resulting conditions and directly contributing to the total impairment rating derived.

The *Guides* are referenced in legal proceedings as a basis for the determination of anatomical impairment, and expert testimony is presented to assist the trier of fact to determine the factors of the case to find causation and determine damages. The admissibility of expert testimony was discussed in the *Frye* case, which established the general acceptability by the scientific community for admissibility of an expert witness's scientific opinion, which includes medical opinions (*Frye*, 1923). The U.S. Congress established Rule 702 of the Federal Rules of Evidence (United States, 1975), which states that "if scientific, technical, or other specialized knowledge will assist the judge or jury to understand the evidence or to determine a fact and issue, a witness qualified as an expert by knowledge, skill, experience, training, or education may testify about these issues in the form of expert testimony." There have been decisions over the past years, including *Daubert v. Merrell Dow Pharmaceuticals* (*Daubert*, 1993) and its progeny, *General Electric v. Joiner*, (*General Electric*, 1997), and *Kumho Tire Company v. Carmichael* (1999), which set standards for the federal courts regarding the admissibility of scientific and expert testimony. In these standards, the judge is responsible for ensuring that the evidence offered in expert testimony is reliable. Although these are federal rules, they are at times applied in civil jurisdictions and administrative legal proceedings. The *Daubert* test asks whether there is a scientific theory, if that theory has been tested, if there is a known error rate, and if the theory has been subject to peer review. Additionally, in the *Kumho Tire Company v. Carmichael* case, the *Daubert* test has been extended to other kinds of expert testimony, including medical testimony (*Daubert*).

State Workers' Compensation and Rehabilitation

A system of compensation for personal injuries is not a modern idea. Historical evidence documents compensation systems for injured parties that have been around since recorded history. From the early days of master/servant relationships, there has been a tendency for a master to help support their servants (Obermann, 1965). Injured or wounded soldiers were supported by their kings or leaders. Historical documents indicated that the concept of compensation was discussed and instituted approximately 2000 years BC. The U.S. version of workers' compensation laws has roots in Germany under sickness and accident laws, including workers' accident insurance and public aid for those who were not able to return to work because of a disability. Early discussions of vocational rehabilitation led to the development of modern-day programs for injured workers.

One such modern-day program is state workers' compensation. State workers' compensation is a system where an injured employee is entitled to benefits, including medical care and wage replacement. These benefits are designed to assist the employee to return to gainful employment. The benefits are paid to the employee by the employer or the employer's worker's compensation insurance carrier. Employers are responsible for benefits provided to an employee who is injured in the course of employment, and most employees are covered from the day they start employment. Employees who experience injuries in the course of their employment may be entitled to wage replacement benefits if the employee is unable to return to work or if they can work but in a lesser-paying job.

Compensation and rehabilitation services are designed to help return injured workers to the workforce. To protect themselves against losses, most employers purchase commercial insurance policies. Workers' compensation laws vary among states. The main emphasis under workers' compensation programs has been directed toward medical treatment, although some states provide for the vocational rehabilitation of injured workers.

A worker can be considered an employee if employed full-time, part-time, or seasonally. Some state laws contain exceptions, such as domestic employees, real estate salespersons, uncompensated officers and directors of organizations, and public officials. Also, volunteer workers can be exempt from being covered under workers' compensation laws.

A worker's pre-existing condition does not prevent recovery under workers' compensation law because the employer takes the worker as he finds them. The worker is entitled to no less protection than a previously unimpaired worker if they have a pre-existing condition which is aggravated by work-related activity. Some states have adopted legislation or programs, such as the Second Injury Fund, to encourage the hiring of a person with an impairment, handicap, or disability back into the workforce. Second Injury Fund programs protect employers by providing compensation for further loss from additional impairment for subsequent injuries or exacerbation of previous injuries.

The state workers' compensation system is one of the only systems we have for compensating most injured workers for their losses incurred while working. The compensation for these losses can be handled either through a claim for compensation or, in some cases, civil lawsuits ending in litigation. These lawsuits are intended to identify and quantify the damages to a person both medically and in their physical, psychological, and vocational handicapping conditions that result in economic loss. To that end, pre-injury wage-earning capacity can be compared to post-injury wage-earning capacity to quantify economic damages or losses.

Workers' compensation laws in the various states cover both mental and physical injuries from either accidents or occupational diseases. Typically, a mental injury must be the result of a physical injury or sudden, unexpected, or extraordinary stress related to employment. A personal injury accident is an unexpected, actual, identifiable event, with or without fault, that directly produces an injury. An occupational disease is a disease or illness which is due to causes and conditions related to employment, in which the employee is exposed to substances that cause disease.

To be compensable, an event must arise out of and be within the course and scope of the employee's job, work, or employment. Generally, the fault of the employer or employee does not affect the compensability of an injury. Most states have exceptions for causation when there is a willful intention for an employee to injure himself or someone else or by the employee's intoxication or being under the influence of drugs or alcohol. In these situations, and usually pending post-accident urine drug screening, the employee may not be entitled to benefits. Many states have adopted a random mandatory drug and alcohol examination, as well as mandatory drug and alcohol examination after a reported accident with injury.

An example of a compensable state worker's compensation claim involves a construction worker who smashes a finger. The injury is compensable if the accident occurs on the job and while performing his or her duties as a construction worker. Some incidents such as automobile accidents driving to or from work or being assaulted on the job are not so clearly compensable if there is ambiguity regarding whether the worker was actually performing work-related activities. Similarly, if claimants fail to disclose pre-existing conditions at the time of hire, subsequent manifestations of those conditions, even if they develop during work, may not be compensable. There must be a documented causal connection between the work incident and the subsequent disabling condition.

State Workers' Compensation Medical Treatment

When an employee is entitled to state workers' compensation benefits, all necessary medical, surgical, hospital services, medicine, or related allied health professional treatment, such as psychological services and rehabilitation counseling, are to be provided by the employer. Medical treatment can include evaluations, routine care, surgery, laboratory tests, imaging, equipment and supplies, prosthetic and orthotic devices, and transportation and mileage costs to and from medical services. Health care providers include hospitals, clinics, physicians, dentists, registered or licensed nurses, pharmacists, optometrists, podiatrists, chiropractors, physical therapists, psychologists, mental health counselors, rehabilitation counselors, social workers, or other health care providers. Some states requiring workers' compensation insurance have allowed the injured employee to select their physician, paid for by the employer or its carrier. An employee can select a treating physician in any field or specialty. Likewise, an injured employee can choose the facility where laboratory tests or diagnostic imaging takes place. The injured worker may be able to choose a physical therapist and pharmacy. However, the employer has the right to a second medical opinion, independent medical opinion, or another medical opinion.

An employee must submit for an examination by a qualified physician or other allied health professional paid for by the employer if requested. If the injured employee refuses to undergo an examination by a second medical opinion physician, compensation benefits can be affected. An injury may cause an injured worker to need surgery, although the injured worker cannot be compelled to have the surgery. There is typically no time limit under which an employee is entitled to medical treatment if the treatment is found to be reasonable and related to the work injury.

Employers, as well as injured workers, are entitled to medical reports outlining the findings of the evaluation and treatment recommendations. Under certain workers' compensation laws, the records of health care providers are released, often without regard to the patient/physician privilege. Some states use medical treatment guidelines for injured workers that are meant to ensure that treatment recommendations are generally accepted by the medical community as usual and necessary. If treatment is recommended outside of the guidelines, exceptions can be granted to deviate from the guidelines. Some states have also adopted a fixed reimbursement schedule based on usual and customary charges for services to establish a reasonable payment for medical services.

State Workers' Compensation Classifications of Disability

Temporary Total Disability (TTD). This classification is determined when an individual is unable to perform any type of gainful work activity for some time, but the disability will only be temporary. For instance, if the injured worker undergoes a surgical procedure such as a meniscus repair, there will be a time of convalescence and rehabilitation when the individual is incapable of performing gainful work. During this time, the worker is considered TTD.

Permanent Total Disability (PTD). The PTD classification means that the worker cannot go back to any occupation and is disabled from working and earning wages in the labor market throughout the worker's life expectancy. PTD is rare and is primarily seen when attempts to vocationally rehabilitate the injured worker have been exhausted. The injury and subsequent limitations are severe to the extent that the injured worker is unable to maintain or sustain work in any capacity. For example, an injured worker may have spine impairments involving multiple or failed spine surgeries, continued pain without relief from treatment, and limitations outlined by a physician that is less than a full range of sedentary physical demand level work with the need to alternate positions at will and require frequent breaks throughout the day. Furthermore, this individual may have only performed unskilled work and does not have transferable skills or computer knowledge and only a limited education. Through vocational rehabilitation efforts, it is the opinion of the vocational rehabilitation counselor that there is no work suitable for this injured employee in his or her geographic area.

Temporary Partial Disability. This classification is the short-term period in which the worker has limitations but can perform some of the functions of their job, with or without modification. These workers can stay on the job and perform their tasks in a modified or light-duty manner, such as having a helper; lifting, carrying, pushing, or pulling lighter weights; alternating sitting, standing, and walking; or using assistive devices, such as lifts.

Permanent Partial Disability (PPD). This classification is applied if an injury does not result in total disability but leaves the injured employee with lasting impairments.

Once the worker reaches MMI, permanent work restrictions are determined. MMI represents a point in time in the recovery process after an injury when further formal medical or surgical intervention cannot be expected to improve the underlying impairment. If the impairments are considered permanent, the classification is changed from temporary partial to permanent partial disability.

State Workers' Compensation Injuries Requiring Special Consideration

Most accidents with injury involve neurological or orthopedic sequelae; however, other types of injuries include claims for cardiovascular, mental, repeated trauma, and occupational disease. To be compensable under state workers' compensation, the cause must be determined to be related to work or working conditions.

For example, a truck driver involved in an accident while driving the company truck may result in a back injury. If subsequently the worker becomes depressed and anxious and seeks psychological treatment, this would be classified as compensable if it is determined to be related to the original injury.

In *mental* disability claims, a mental injury is not necessarily caused by a physical injury but results from emotional stress. Again, to be compensable, the employee must show mental stress as a result of unexpected stress related to employment. If our same truck driver from the earlier example does not sustain physical injuries during the accident but becomes depressed and anxious—for example, let us assume he has flashbacks and nightmares and becomes fearful of driving—the truck driver may be diagnosed with post-traumatic stress disorder. This is considered a mental disability and can be compensable.

Medical treatment of repetitive physical trauma can be compensable in lieu of an identifiable single event if the work could produce such conditions. An employee can be awarded workers' compensation benefits if they can establish that the condition was the result of repeated trauma. For example, carpal tunnel syndrome is compensable if linked to repetitive work movements. Similarly, if a cashier experiencing back pain without an identifiable injury can establish that the condition arose out of and in the course of employment, the claim can be compensable.

Occupational diseases can be caused by chronic exposure to noxious or dangerous conditions at work, which can result in a worker's disability. For example, toxic mold disease is considered an occupational disease if it develops because of repeated exposure causing impairments. The occupational disease or illness must be due to conditions particular to an occupation, process, or employment in which the employee is exposed to such conditions that would cause the disease or illness.

State Workers' Compensation Indemnity Benefits

In addition to medical treatment, the injured worker is eligible for other benefits, including replacement of lost wages, or *indemnity benefits*. A typical workers' compensation benefit for lost wages is calculated utilizing an average weekly wage. Average weekly wages are based on the wages at the time of the accident.

Worker's compensation indemnity benefits vary among the states but are typically 66 2/3% of the worker's average weekly wage, depending on the maximum rate. Many states have adopted maximum and minimum compensation rates, which are set by their respective legislatures. If the employee's average weekly wage and compensation benefit exceeds the maximum allowable, the employee would only get the maximum allowable indemnity benefit. A typical calculation for minimum and maximum compensation rates would be based on statewide average weekly wages. If a worker earns weekly wages at a rate less than the minimum compensation, the employee may get his actual wages.

The employer has a reasonable basis to contest an employee's right to the benefits under certain conditions and has to facilitate an examination by a physician upon the report of a work injury. Some states have adopted penalties for employers for unreasonable acts, such as failure to pay timely benefits, authorize a choice of physician or change of physician, pay travel expenses and mileage, authorize treatment, and unlawful discrimination. The claimant can likewise be penalized for misrepresentation concerning wages and benefits, medical history, the extent of a disability, post-accident earnings, and post-accident injuries. Some states have developed fraud units to investigate such claims.

An injured employee receiving compensation benefits may also receive benefits from federal assistance programs, unemployment compensation, or disability insurance policies; however, compensation from the varying programs may be affected. For example, if an employee who is receiving state workers' compensation indemnity benefits is approved for benefits from the Social Security Administration, the Social Security Administration is likely to apply for an offset against workers' compensation. The Social Security Administration would then only be responsible for providing the excess amount of funds to the injured worker. Unemployment compensation requires the worker to certify that he or she can work to qualify for benefits. If the worker certifies that he or she can work, they are not considered disabled and are not likely to qualify for workers' compensation benefits. If the workers' compensation carrier or employer is made aware that the worker is receiving unemployment benefits, they will more probably than not terminate indemnity benefits. Disability insurance benefits will be discussed later in this chapter; however, this situation is much like unemployment compensation systems whereby if a worker can work, they are not considered disabled and entitled to benefits.

Federal Acts of Worker Health Support and Protection

At the turn of the century, the American industrial revolution saw an explosive period of productivity growth in the country with a monumental shift from agricultural work to work based on emerging technologies. The U.S. Congress began taking legislative action to both protect industrial workers and provide necessary medical and financial benefits for injured workers. This process took parallel forms as both state and federal laws emerged to accommodate the country's changing workforce. Federal actions to protect certain types of workers include the following and will be explored in this chapter. The Federal Employees Compensation Act (FECA) was formed to protect federal workers. The Federal Employers Liability Act (FELA) was passed to protect vulnerable railroad workers. Section 27 of the Merchant Marine Act, called the Jones Act, was passed to shield our nation's seamen. Other measures such as the Longshore and Harbor Workers' Compensation Act (LHWCA), the Occupational Safety and Health Act (OSHA), the Federal Coal Mine Health and Safety Act (FCMHSA), and the Veterans Readjustment Assistance Act all added new levels of protection for American workers on a federal level.

The Federal Employees Compensation Act

As discussed, most occupations are covered by state workers' compensation laws that dictate benefit eligibility, claims processes, and guidelines for access to medical care and indemnity benefits. Several classes of employees are exempt from state workers' compensation systems and are covered by federal legislation. The federal government enacted the first law in 1882 to cover federal employees involved in "life-saving agencies" (Nordland, 1991). In 1908, Congress passed FECA as a general-purpose program to protect essentially all federal employees and their dependents from the consequences of workplace injury or death. Before this action, employers generally operated on the *assumption of risk* doctrine, which held that certain occupations were entitled to higher levels of compensation due to the inherent risks of the job. Employees assumed this risk when they agreed to work in these occupations.

Contributory negligence was another defense for employers to avoid liability. If through some action, the employee was responsible for the accident in whole or in part, then contributory negligence could be established. Most state workers' compensation systems adopt a "no-fault" approach to industrial accidents and work injuries; however, matters handled in state and federal court venues typically require proof that the employer's negligence was a proximate cause of the subsequent injuries. Along those lines, the *fellow servant doctrine* allowed avoidance of liability if the employer could prove that a fellow employee was responsible, in whole or in part, for their co-worker's injuries. Somewhat surprisingly, the charge to adopt a federal protection system was taken up by both labor unions and employers. The labor unions wanted better and more defined protection for injured workers. Even though relatively few workers were victorious in the court systems, those who were successful were generally awarded large financial awards that employers found unacceptable (Nordland, 1991).

In 1908, FECA provided partial coverage for injured workers that entitled them to one year of pre-injury wages, with an available one-year extension at a lower rate of compensation. The act was updated in 1916 to amend benefits and establish the Federal Employees Compensation Commission, which was later absorbed by the Department of Labor after World War II. Congress amended the act significantly in 1949 to include many of the components and policies that are still in place today. For example, a schedule for award benefits was established to provide a set amount of compensation as a percentage of functional loss due to an injury. The amendments assured that personal attendant services would be covered and allowed for vocational rehabilitation. Most importantly, it made FECA an exclusive remedy through the Office of Workers' Compensation Programs (OWCP) to help return federal workers to gainful employment. The establishment of the OWCP assumed that quick diagnosis and intervention were critical to limit the severity of disability and to minimize lost time. Additionally, workers with ongoing disabilities, including psychological injury, could return to partial or full employment if offered adequate rehabilitation (Maffeo, 1990).

The Federal Employees' Compensation Program manages claims and benefits, pays medical expenses, and pays indemnity benefits to federal employees who sustained a work-related injury or disease (Barnes et al., 2020). FECA also covers eligible survivors of a federal employee who died due to a work-related injury or disease. Additional assistance includes vocational rehabilitation, which can aid in the worker's return to the workforce when medically released for work activities (Nordland, 1991; Maffeo, 1990).

Medical benefits under FECA include services, appliances, and supplies prescribed or recommended by physicians which are likely to cure, give relief, reduce the degree or period of disability, or aid in lessening the amount of monthly compensation. Authorized medical treatment, medications, hospitalization, and transportation needed to secure these services are also provided. Although there is not a specific list of covered medical conditions, musculoskeletal-type injuries such as the neck and back and injuries to the extremities are the most common occupational injuries experienced in the workplace. Common occupational diseases and illnesses include hearing loss, asbestos-related illnesses, coronary/vascular disease, psychiatric conditions, pulmonary illnesses, and cumulative trauma or repetitive motion diseases. Generally, a claim for disability or death benefits under FECA must be made within three years of the date of the injury or death. Injured employees have the right to select their medical provider, although the provider must be authorized by the OWCP to render care.

Compensation for wage loss is not payable unless medical evidence has been submitted that supports the injury/disability. Physicians are asked to document various aspects of the individual's condition, including any history or evidence of concurrent or pre-existing injury or disease or physical impairments, diagnostic findings, diagnosis, treatment rendered and recommended, period of total disability or partial disability, and projected timeframe as to when the patient can resume light-duty work or regular work activity. The physician and supervisor of an employing agency may also be required to document whether the injured employee is suitable for work activity. The supervisor completes the physical job requirements section of the form regarding the injured worker's job of injury as it relates to the exertional and non-exertional activities including lifting/carrying; sitting; standing; walking; climbing; kneeling; bending/stooping; twisting; pushing/pulling; simple grasping; fine manipulation; reaching; operating a vehicle and machinery; temperature extremes; environmental exposure to chemicals, fumes, and dust; and general noise levels. Durational requirements of these activities are either marked as performed on a "continuous, intermittent, or not at all" basis, with the number of hours each activity is performed per day. The physician endorses whether the employee can perform regular work activities as described and whether the employee can perform full-time or part-time work, including the number of hours per day the employee can work. If the physician's opinion is that the employee cannot perform regular work duties, the physician outlines which of the essential job requirements the injured worker can perform and at what duration the duties can be performed.

Medical information concerning impairment and disability is necessary as it relates to the ability of the employee to potentially return to his or her job of injury full-time, part-time, or in a light-duty/modified capacity. Similar to the state workers' compensation system for the classification of disability and impairment, the classifications include *Temporary Total Disability (TTD), Permanent Total Disability (PTD), Total Partial Disability (TPD), and Permanent Partial Disability (PPD)*. There are available forms to assess the classification of disability that include psychiatric/psychological conditions, cardiovascular/pulmonary conditions, or musculoskeletal conditions. Furthermore, some forms specify the physical requirements of the worker's job of injury and physical capacities to perform those functions. The work capacity evaluation forms succinctly outline the functional capacities of the worker. The exertional activities such as sitting, standing, walking, lifting, carrying, pushing, and pulling are addressed as well as non-exertional activities such as stooping, climbing, twisting, reaching, kneeling, and squatting. The forms also list the number of hours per day the individual can perform these activities.

Compensation for the classifications of disability is based on the difference between the wages earned at the time of injury and what wages the injured worker can earn after the injury. These post-injury wages are generally established by a certified vocational rehabilitation counselor, who has been engaged by the OWCP to provide vocational rehabilitation services to the injured worker. If there is a difference in what an injured worker was earning at the time of injury compared to what he or she can earn post-injury, this is considered a loss of wage-earning capacity.

Under federal guidelines, injuries can be unscheduled or scheduled. Unscheduled injuries are injuries typically to the trunk of the body and are neurological or psychological. Scheduled injuries typically reference injuries to limbs or the face. Regarding scheduled injuries, such as the loss of a limb, the injured worker is entitled to a scheduled benefit award once MMI is reached. This award is in addition to any other FECA disability benefits received even if he or she has returned to full-time work. Scheduled awards are given for permanent partial impairment to specific body parts. The Division of Federal Employees' (2022) compensation bases scheduled awards on a percentage of disability, ranging from 1% to 100% impairment, and the number of corresponding weeks associated with the body part "member" as it relates to the percentage of impairment. For example, an arm that has a permanent impairment rating of 20% has a scheduled award of 62.40 weeks, whereas an arm with a 100% total impairment is based on 312 weeks. The AMA's *Guides to the Evaluation of Permanent Impairment* are used as a basis for schedule award determinations.

Regarding unscheduled injuries, if an employee is unable to work full-time at the job of injury but can work either part-time or at a job in a lower pay category, the employee is considered partially disabled and eligible for a monthly indemnity benefit equal to two-thirds of the difference between the employee's pre-disability and post-disability monthly wage. If the employee has at least one dependent or a spouse, they are entitled to a monthly benefit equal to 75% of the difference between the employee's pre-disability and post-disability monthly wage. The OWCP continues to pay benefits until the worker medically recovers, is found not to be entitled to benefits, or is determined to have recaptured previous wage-earning capacity. If it is determined that the employee will be unable to return to his or her job of injury in any capacity, the employee is entitled to vocational rehabilitation services provided by a Department of Labor OWCP-certified vocational rehabilitation counselor.

Under FECA guidelines, vocational rehabilitation services are provided to assist the injured employee in returning to gainful employment consistent with any limitations outlined by the physician(s), work experience, transferable skills, and educational attainment. An injured federal worker referred to a certified rehabilitation counselor by the OWCP has statutory obligations to cooperate with job placement or training efforts. The rehabilitation counselor develops a rehabilitation plan with the injured worker that encompasses goals such as direct job placement with specific job goals, on-the-job training, or formal retraining such as computer classes or other job-specific training.

Compensation may be reduced or terminated if the employee fails to participate or to make a good faith effort to participate in a vocational rehabilitation program to obtain gainful employment. The primary objective of vocational rehabilitation is to return the injured worker to a job as close in earnings as possible to his or her pre-injury earnings. When the case is referred for vocational rehabilitation, the counselor is generally required to contact the employer of the injury to determine if the injured worker has the opportunity and ability to return to work in the same or modified capacity with or without accommodation. If job placement is with the employer of the injury, the counselor develops the rehabilitation plan to assist the injured worker in maintaining or sustaining employment with the employer of the injury. Follow-up services are generally provided for 90 days once the worker has returned to work to ensure a successful return to work.

If it is determined that the employer of injury cannot accommodate the injured worker in a modified/alternative job, the next step is to develop a rehabilitation plan for alternate job placement. The rehabilitation counselor assesses the injured worker's current placement potential with or without additional training. A comprehensive vocational assessment is conducted, which includes a vocational interview to obtain pertinent background information such as education, training history, work history, hobbies, interests, and occupational goals of the injured worker. Vocational testing may be warranted to further assess the injured worker's achievement and/ or intellectual capacities, aptitudes, and vocational/career interests. Included in the vocational assessment is a transferable skills analysis that takes into consideration the injured worker's work experience and functional limitations to determine if they possess skills and work-related abilities that will transfer to suitable alternate employment options with direct placement, on-the-job training, or formal retraining. The latter is considered primarily when additional education or skills are required to increase the injured worker's employability or wage-earning capacity.

One of the outcomes of the 1916 FECA was the establishment of the Department of Labor's OWCP, which administers claims to employees who have incurred qualified injuries or occupational illnesses or diseases. The OWCP oversees four disability compensation programs. These programs include the general program, the Coal Mine Workers' Compensation Program (Federal Black Lung Benefits Act), the Federal Employees' Compensation Program, and the LHWCA Compensation Program.

The Federal Employers Liability Act

Around the same time, FECA was adopted, Congress passed FELA in 1908 as the exclusive remedy for claims involving railroad workers. For context, in 1907, there were 4,534 deaths of railroad employees on the job. The following year, there were more than 12,000 deaths. At the turn of the century, the average life expectancy of a railroad switchman was seven years (Lewis Jr., 1961). The adoption of FELA was meant to supersede all state workers' compensation laws and was designed to allow for a more reasonable standard of liability than existing common law. The act held that instead of the proximate cause standard, the employee must only demonstrate that the railroad's negligence played a part, no matter how small, in the accident. Two additional acts were passed that provided additional opportunities to clarify liability regarding railroad occupations. The first, the Safety Appliance Act, provided safety standards for some railroad equipment. The second, the Locomotive Inspection Act, provided for regular locomotive inspection and surveillance. Violation of either of these two acts relieved the employee of the burden of proving negligence, only causation. Currently, there are no caps on damages recovered from all past, present, and probable future harm associated with the railroad employer. Damages include pain, suffering, and mental anguish (Orne, 2015).

There are several common criticisms of FELA. First, critics cite the overwhelming costs due to attorney and administrative fees. Second, the current system breeds divisiveness between employee and employer due to the need to establish negligence. The heightened adversarial nature of the system often complicates efforts for injured workers to return to previous employment. Another cited criticism is that ultimate damage awards are large and unpredictable due to a lack of monetary caps. Finally, delays in the awarding of settlements take months to years, postponing the relief sought by injured railroad workers.

Jones Act

Just as America's railroad workers were being protected, U.S. seamen were afforded protection under the Merchant Marine Act of 1920, or more specifically section 27, referred to as the Jones Act (Papavizas, 2020). The Jones Act holds that a seaman who suffers a personal injury can sue their employer for unseaworthiness. This is a strict liability claim, not a workers' compensation claim, that requires proof that the vessel or a crewmember was not fit. The seaman is also entitled to *maintenance and cure*, which entitles a seaman who becomes injured or sick while in service to the ship to receive day-to-day living expenses and medical care. Maintenance refers to the room and board of the injured seaman while recovering from injury. It includes expenses such as rent, mortgage, utilities, food, and the like. Maintenance is paid weekly or biweekly. Many times, companies pay a standard per diem rate for maintenance until such time that it has been medically determined that the individual has reached maximum medical benefit. Cure refers to compensation for the cost of medical care and services to treat the injury or illness up until the time maximum medical care has been determined.

In the case of untimely death, no claim can be made for lost earnings. The courts have expanded maintenance and cure to cover seamen on shore leave and have expanded the duration of cure to extend until the seaman reaches maximum improvement (Friedell, 2017).

Longshore and Harbor Workers' Compensation Act

In 1927, Congress expanded protection to inland maritime workers by passing the LHWCA and subsequently included amendments in 1972 and 1984. This is a federal program that covers certain private-sector maritime workers. The LHWCA was based on a Supreme Court ruling that it was unconstitutional to apply state workers' compensation laws and statutes to maritime workers who are injured on navigable waters of the United States. There are instances in maritime law where there is potentially more than one remedy in a jurisdiction that can be concurrent or mutually exclusive (Simet, 1962). Concurrent state jurisdiction is decided by each state. For example, a worker injured in a dry dock may file a state workers' compensation claim and later file under the LHWCA. Generally, it is up to the courts to decide the jurisdiction of these types of concurrent claims (Szymendera, 2020).

Unlike concurrent jurisdiction for state workers' compensation claims and LHWCA claims, LHWCA and Jones Act claims are mutually exclusive, and an injured worker cannot file a claim under both acts. In 1920, the Merchant Marine Act was passed regulating maritime commerce in U.S. ports and waters. Under this act, the Jones Act provision deals with cabotage (coastal shipping). The Jones Act establishes certain legal remedies for injured maritime workers (seamen) to obtain appropriate medical care and compensation following an injury. The Jones Act is not a workers' compensation program, but rather allows injured sailors to file suit against their employers as well as ship owners based on claims of negligence or unseaworthiness (Szymendera, 2020).

Employers covered by state or federal workers' compensation allow protection from being sued by injured employees. There is, however, an instance under the LHWCA in which a third-party claim can be filed. This is considered a 905(b) claim, which refers to a specific amendment in the LHWCA that allows a third-party claim to be filed against the vessel owner. For a 905(b) claim to be filed, the employer must also be the owner and operator of a vessel on which the employee was injured and the injury must be caused by the employer's negligence as the vessel owner (Szymendera, 2020).

In determining whether the claim falls under the Longshore Act, the injured worker must meet both the *situs* and *status* test. The *situs* test refers to the physical location where the accident or injury occurred. Locations include adjoining piers, wharves, dry docks, railways, and other adjoining areas near the water used to load, unload, repair, or build a vessel. The *status* test refers to the actual type of work performed by the injured worker at the time of the accident or injury. These include but are not limited to work performed as longshoremen or shipbuilder occupations such as welders, pipefitters, crane operators, and the like. Where there is an unclear status of the worker, these cases many times are resolved by a trier of fact, an administrative law judge, or a staff member of the U.S. Department of Labor.

Employers typically purchase workers' compensation insurance or self-insure to pay claims related to injury or job-related illness (Szymendera, 2020). The act is administered by the U.S. Department of Labor, OWCP, Division of Federal Employees' Longshore and Harbor Workers' Compensation (DFELHWC). The LHWCA provides medical benefits for injured workers to cover the cost of treatment due to covered injury or illness. This can include prescription drugs, procedures, and travel to and from medical appointments. Claimants are free to choose their doctor, provided the clinician has not been disbarred from LHWCA programs for violations. The LHWCA applies to any firm with workers who work full-time or part-time on navigable waters of the United States plus adjoining areas including piers, wharves, dry docks, terminals, building ways, marine railways, or other areas used for loading, unloading, repairing, or building vessels. The indemnity benefits and medical benefits are paid by the employer's insurance carrier or by an approved OWCP self-insured employer (Congressional Research Service, 2020).

Under the LHWCA, disability is defined as

> incapacity because of injury to earn the wages which the employee was receiving at the time of injury in the same or any other employment; but such term shall mean permanent impairment, determined (to the extent covered thereby) under the *Guides to the Evaluation of Permanent Impairment* promulgated and modified from time to time by the American Medical Association, in the case of an individual whose claim is described in Section 10(d)(2).
>
> (DFELHWC, United States Department of Labor, 2022)

The LHWCA uses various classifications of disability similar to those discussed under state workers' compensation, including TTD, PTD, TPD, and PPD. In addition to a disability acquired during one's natural work-life expectancy, a worker can become *disabled after retirement* if an illness does not manifest until after the worker has left the workforce. In these instances, the claimant is entitled to two-thirds the national average weekly wage times the percentage of impairment according to the AMA impairment tables. Finally, *survivor benefits* are cash payments to the surviving spouse and minor children that extend until the spouse remarries or dies and when the children reach age 18 or 23 if full-time students. Decisions regarding eligibility and benefits are made by the Department of Labor. If eligibility is uncontested, benefits are paid in full. If eligibility is contested, both parties meet for an internal conference with an administrative law judge. All decisions can be appealed to the benefits review board through the Department of Labor.

Under the LHWCA, workers' compensation indemnity benefits are calculated after the average weekly wage of the worker has been established. There are three methods for calculating the employee's average annual earnings under the LHWCA based on whether the injured worker was engaged in employment all or most of the year, less than all or most of the year, or exceptional conditions to employment (e.g., seasonal, intermittent, discontinuous, and other employment, which amounts to less than a full work year). Once the average weekly wage has been determined, the payment of PTD benefits, TTD benefits, and scheduled PPD benefits are paid at a rate of two-thirds of the average weekly wage of the injured worker. Non-scheduled PPD benefits are paid to the injured worker at a rate of two-thirds of a difference between the average weekly wage and the employee's post-accident wage-earning capacity.

Medical care provided under the LHWCA must be reasonable and necessary. The injured worker has the right to choose his or her treating physician under the act. If the injured worker at some point wants to change treating physicians, prior approval from the employer or the Department of Labor is first required. In cases where a treating physician is recommending surgical intervention, the employer may recommend obtaining a second medical opinion to the secretary of labor or district director. Generally, the treating physician's opinion is usually given more weight than a second medical opinion or an independent medical examination. In cases where the injured worker has two alternative yet valid medical opinions in terms of treatment, it is the right of the injured worker to choose his or her course of treatment. Where an independent medical examination or defense medical examination is obtained by the carrier/employer, the results of these examinations generally form the basis of the employer/carrier's defense in a longshore claim as to whether they will deny the claim, continuing paying the claim, or potentially suspend further benefits.

While it is considered mandatory that the injured worker complies with vocational rehabilitation under other systems, under the LHWCA, any vocational rehabilitation services provided by the OWCP are voluntary. An injured longshore worker may request vocational rehabilitation services through the Department of Labor; if approved and authorized, a certified rehabilitation counselor under contract with the Department of Labor may be assigned to assist the injured worker in developing a rehabilitation plan and returning to gainful work activity.

Injured workers under LHWCA are not required by law to cooperate or engage with vocational rehabilitation that is obtained by the employer/insurance carrier. When a vocational rehabilitation counselor is engaged by the employer/insurance carrier, the goal is primarily to determine an injured worker's vocational outlook, wage-earning potential because of the injury, and any subsequent limitations outlined by the medical evidence.

The DFELHWC also administers the *Non-appropriated Fund Instrumentalities Act, Defense Base Act,* and *Outer Continental Shelf Lands Act* (United States, 2022). The Non-appropriated Fund Instrumentalities Act provides workers' compensation benefits to civilian employees injured while working for non-appropriated fund instrumentalities within the U.S. armed forces. Examples include employees of military bases such as commissaries, schools, daycare centers, and similar facilities. The Defense Base Act was enacted in 1941. This act provides workers' compensation benefits to civilian employees working outside the United States on U.S. military bases or under a contract with the U.S. government for public works or national defense. Individuals are generally employed by U.S. government contractors and subcontractors in overseas employment that may include war zone areas. The Outer Continental Shelf Lands Act was enacted in 1953. This act provides workers' compensation to workers who sustain injuries occurring as the result of operations "arising out of or in connection with any operations conducted on the outer Continental Shelf which are submerged lands lying seaward of state coastal waters (3 miles offshore) which are under U.S. jurisdiction." A Special Fund was also established at the DOL for cases in which the employer cannot pay to cover second injuries (Sturley & Ammerman, 2020).

Occupational Safety and Health Act

The ultimate passage of the 1970 Occupational Safety and Health Act (OSHA) also had its roots in the turn-of-the-century industrialization. There was growing anger over basic protections like limited hours for the workday and basic workplace safety. Deadly fires sweeping across New York City sweatshops prompted local legislation regulating factory inspections. In 1912, the Public Health Service (PHS) was assigned responsibility for occupational-related diseases, and in 1913, the U.S. Department of Labor was formed. By 1941, 24 states had established PHS offices to monitor industrial hygiene. These actions culminated in OSHA, whereby the government established an agency with a broad mandate to protect the majority of the nation's workers (Steiger, 1974). Concurrently, the National Institute for Occupational Safety and Health (NIOSH) was established within the Department of Health, Education, and Welfare to provide OSHA with the best scientific evidence on how to protect workers (Rosner & Markowitz, 2020). Operationally, states were free to enforce federal safety standards and impose fines. The variability in enforcement and fines ultimately led to uneven adherence to regulations, which changed when the agency began targeting high-risk violators (Bradbury, 2006).

Federal Coal Mine Health and Safety Act

Almost simultaneous to the passage of OSHA, the 1969 FCMHSA was enacted in response to a mine disaster where an underground explosion killed 78 coal miners. The passage of the act also followed a precipitous rise in the rates of pneumoconiosis, or "black lung." The act established the current federal exposure limit for respirable coal dust created by the Coal Workers' Health Surveillance Program (CWHSP), which is administered by NIOSH. According to the law, coal workers are entitled to free regular chest x-rays. If unable to work due to injury or illness, miners are entitled to payments equivalent to 50% of the minimum monthly payments to a federal employee in grade GS-2 who is disabled. The act also provided dependent benefits (Suarthana et al., 2011).

Federal Acts Available to Veterans

Efforts to protect our country's military veterans also began to take shape during the turn of the century. The War Risk Insurance Act of 1917 established rehabilitation and vocational training for veterans with dismemberment, sight, hearing, and other permanent disabilities. The Vocational Rehabilitation Act of 1918 authorized the Federal Board for Vocational Education to provide rehabilitation training to any honorably discharged veteran of World War I, and a 1919 law established medical care for veterans with the PHS. The Veterans Administration (VA) was established in 1930, and benefits for military veterans were consolidated primarily in this department. The VA became responsible for medical services, disability compensation, and life insurance retirement payments. Perhaps the most substantial effort to protect and benefit veterans was the GI Bill of Rights, which aided in the transition of 16 million World War II veterans. The GI Bill, more formally known as the Servicemen's Readjustment Act, provided up to four years of education or training plus a monthly subsistence allowance. It also provided federally guaranteed home, farm, and business loans with no down payment. The act also provided unemployment compensation for veterans who had served a minimum of 90 days (Department of Veterans Affairs, undated).

Subsequent congressional action strengthened the country's commitment to its veterans. The Veterans Preference Act of 1944 gave veterans hiring preference where federal funds were spent. Each major U.S. military engagement seems to have spurred additional coverage to keep up with the changing needs of veterans. The Veterans' Readjustment Assistance Act of 1952, also known as the "Korean GI Bill," provided unemployment insurance, job placement, home loans, and other benefits. This act limited educational benefits initially enjoyed by World War II veterans. The Ex-Servicemen's Unemployment Compensation Act of 1958 established a permanent system of unemployment benefits that for the first time covered peacetime veterans. Post–Vietnam era veterans were addressed by the Veterans' Readjustment Benefits Act, called the "Vietnam GI Bill."

Social Security Administration

The Social Security Administration (SSA) regulates two programs that provide benefits based on disability: (1) the Social Security Disability Insurance (SSDI) program (title II of the Social Security Act) and (2) the Supplemental Security Income (SSI) program (title XVI of the Social Security Act). The Social Security Act and SSA regulate and establish rules for deciding if an individual is disabled. The SSA's criteria for determining if someone is disabled are not necessarily the same as the criteria applied in other government and private disability programs. (Blue Book, 2008; Disability Benefits, 2019; Red Book, 2020).

Disability and Substantial Gainful Activity

According to the SSA, disability is the inability to engage in a substantial gainful activity (SGA) due to any medically determinable physical or mental impairment resulting in death or lasting for no less than 12 months. A medically determinable impairment is a physical or mental impairment that results from anatomical, physiological, or psychological abnormalities shown by medically acceptable clinical and laboratory diagnostic techniques. Medical evidence consisting of signs, symptoms, and laboratory findings must establish a physical or mental impairment. The disability determination services (DDS), a network of Social Security field offices, initially processes most disability claims. The DDS or an administrative law judge in SSA's Office of Hearings and Appeals may decide unfavorable determinations (Blue Book, 2008; Red Book, 2020).

SSA representatives in field offices typically obtain applications for disability benefits either in person, by telephone, or by mail. The field office receives data regarding the individual's impairments and verifies nonmedical eligibility requirements, including age, employment, marital status, or Social Security coverage information. The field office then sends the case to DDS for evaluation of disability. The definition of disability is the same for all individuals applying for disability benefits under title II or an adult applying under title XVI. SGA is used to describe a level of work activity and earnings. Gainful work activity could include work performed for pay or profit, work generally performed for pay or profit, or work intended for profit. SGA is one of the factors used in determining the eligibility for disability benefits. (Blue Book, 2008; Red Book, 2020).

Once approved for disability benefits, the SSA disability program periodically reviews medical impairments to determine if the individual continues to have a disability. This continuing disability review (CDR) occurs every three years unless it is expected that the medical condition will improve. If improvement is expected, the first review will generally be at 6 to 18 months after the date the individual becomes disabled. If the medical condition is not expected to improve, the CDR happens once every seven years. For SSI, the CDR is initiated once every three years for a child, unless the child is disabled due to low birth weight. The CDR is usually conducted by age one if the disability is determined based on low birth weight (Blue Book, 2008).

Social Security Disability Insurance—Title II

Purpose, Origin, and Qualifying Criteria

Title II of the Social Security Act became law in July 1956. Title II provides payment of disability benefits to insured individuals under the Social Security Act by their contributions to the Social Security trust fund through the Social Security tax on their earnings and certain disabled dependents of insured individuals. To meet the criteria for SSDI benefits, one must have (1) worked in jobs coved by Social Security, (2) have a medical condition that meets Social Security's definition of disability, and (3) have been unable to work for one year or more because of disability. Typically, SSDI benefits will continue until the individual can work again regularly (Blue Book, 2008).

Population Served. Three basic categories of individuals can qualify for benefits under the SSDI program. The first category includes a disabled insured worker under the age of 65. The second category includes individuals disabled since childhood or before the age of 22 who are dependent on a deceased insured parent or parent entitled to SSDI disability or retirement benefits. The third category includes a disabled widow or widower, age 50 to 60, of a deceased spouse insured under Social Security (Blue Book, 2008).

Process of Benefits Award. The individual would have to have worked in jobs covered by Social Security and have a medical condition that meets the Social Security definition of disability to qualify for Social Security disability benefits. Benefits are not payable for short-term or partial disability, which means that the disability must have lasted or will last for at least one year or will result in death. In addition to meeting the definition of disability, the individual must have worked long enough and recently enough to be eligible for benefits. Social Security work credits are based on yearly earnings or self-employment income. An individual can earn up to four credits each year. The number of work credits for qualification changes from year to year and will depend on the individual's age. Once approved for benefits, SSA usually continues benefits until the individual can work regularly. There is a return-to-work incentive during the trial work period that provides continued benefits and health care coverage when transitioning back to work (Blue Book, 2008).

The ticket to work program allows individuals with disabilities to plan their employment and return to work. The program is free and voluntary. It assists those individuals with disabilities receiving SSA benefits to obtain vocational rehabilitation services, employment services, and support services to prepare them for work and maintain employment. This incentive shifts the focus of the disability programs from keeping disability benefits to the rehabilitation of the individual with the disability and assisting in return to work (Red Book, 2020).

For SSDI benefits, SGA is used to decide if the benefits continue after returning to work and completing a trial work period (TWP). A TWP is an SSDI incentive that allows individuals with a disability to return to work without being penalized. During a TWP, the beneficiary can earn wages while maintaining their benefits. Through this trial period, a beneficiary receiving Social Security disability benefits may test their ability to work and still be considered disabled. The TWP consists of at least 9 months of work (not necessarily consecutive) in a continuing 60-month period. (Blue Book, 2008; Red Book, 2020).

There is a higher level of SGA for legally blind individuals. For example, in 2021, the level of SGA for the non-blind population was $1,310.00 per month and SGA was $2,190.00 per month for those with blindness. The beneficiary can perform work and continue to receive benefits as long as their monthly income does not exceed the SGA income levels. The SGA level is typically adjusted every year based on increases in the national average wage index (Disability Determination Under Social Security and (Red Book, 2020).

Supplemental Security Income—Title XVI

Purpose, Origin, and Qualifying Criteria

Title XVI became law in 1972 and provides for SSI payments to individuals, including children under 18, who are disabled and have limited income and resources. SSI also pays monthly benefits to individuals who are blind or age 65 or older. (Blue Book, 2008).

Unlike the SSDI program, SSI benefits are not based on prior work or a family member's previous work. To receive SSI, the individual must be disabled, blind, or at least 65 years of age and have limited income and resources. The individual must also be a U.S. citizen or a qualified alien; reside in one of the 50 states, the District of Columbia, or the Northern Mariana Islands; and not be absent from the United States for a full calendar month or 30 or more consecutive days (Understanding SSI-2020 Edition). Under title XVI, a child under the age of 18 is disabled if they have a medically determinable physical or mental impairment or a combination of impairments that causes marked and severe functional limitations. These impairments can cause death or last for a continuous period of no less than 12 months (Blue Book, 2008).

Population Served. Under the SSI program, there are two basic categories under which a financially needy person can get payments based on disability: (1) an adult age 18 or over who is disabled and (2) a child under 18 who is disabled (Blue Book/Disability Evaluation Under Social Security, 2008). SSI defines income as anything able to be used for food or shelter, including earned and unearned income (A Guide to SSI, 2021).

Process of Benefits Award. Earned income includes wages, net earnings from self-employment, certain royalties and honoraria, and money from sheltered workshops. Unearned income includes all income that a person does not earn, such as Social Security benefits, workers' compensation, pension payments, unemployment, support, maintenance, annuities, rent, and other income. In 2021, limited income was less than $814.00 per month per individual or $1,211.00 per month per couple. Since a larger portion of earned income is not counted, a person who received SSI can earn up to $1,673.00 per month or $2,467.00 per month per couple and still receive SSI. Although work is encouraged for people who already receive SSI, a person applying for SSI while working cannot have much earned income because workability affects the disability decision. For example, a person applying for SSI disability benefits who is not blind and earning more than $1,310.00 per month will not likely be approved for SSI benefits. A person who is blind making $2,190.00 per month probably will not be approved for SSI benefits either (A Guide to SSI, 2021).

For SSI benefits received based on disability, different standards apply to determine if the eligibility of benefits should continue. SGA is only considered when the initial claim is filed unless the disability is blindness, and the SGA is not considered. For SSI, SGA is not considered after the person becomes eligible for SSI; however, it must be determined if the individual meets non-disability requirements, including income and resources (Red Book, 2020).

Administrative Law Hearing Process

The administrative law hearing process occurs after the initial and second (reconsideration) application for benefits has been denied. The next step in the appeals process is a hearing with an administrative law judge. The individual may seek representation, and therefore, the individual or their representative can request a hearing. The administrative law judge may have other witnesses testify, such as a medical doctor or vocational expert, at the hearing. Hearings are generally recorded and informal. At the hearing, the administrative law judge asks the individual and the vocational and medical experts questions for testimony while under oath. The administrative law judge decides based on the evidence and testimony at the hearing. After the hearing, the administrative law judge administers a written decision. Given an unfavorable decision, the individual is provided 60 days after receiving the notice to request an appeal (The Appeals Process, 2018).

Current Status and Number of Awards

In December 2019, there were 9,765,096 individuals, including disabled workers, disabled children, and disabled widowers, receiving Social Security disability benefits; most (85.8%) were disabled workers. The number of disabled beneficiaries increased from 1,812,786 in 1970 to 9,765,096 in 2019. The number of disabled workers drives this increase. In December 2019, the largest number of disabled worker beneficiaries was aged 60 to 64. Disability benefits convert to retirement benefits when the individual reaches the full retirement age, 65 to 67. In 2019, the musculoskeletal system and connective tissue diseases were the primary reason disabled workers and disabled widowers received benefits. Intellectual disabilities were the principal reason for disability among disabled children (Annual Statistical Report, 2019).

Return to Work/Stay at Work

The U.S. Department of Labor's Office of Disability Employment Policy (ODEP) has developed policies, programs, and practices to encourage the continued employment of workers with impairment or disability. This agency also developed collaborative policies for stay-at-work and return-to-work efforts. The collaboration includes community practice to provide input related to stay-at-work and return-to-work issues. These policies and practices are meant to shorten long-term work disability and job loss through injury or illness and provide recommendations to agencies and other stakeholders. Health care services under workers' compensation should include an emphasis on return-to-work and stay-at-work options. The goal should be better health outcomes and return to employment for workers in a compensation system as soon as possible and nearly as practical to their pre-injury work and wages. There are differences among the states in their workers' compensation laws, administration process, and claims resolution. Each state's workers' compensation system should meet the needs of its workforce, employers, and economic system. Vocational rehabilitation during medical rehabilitation should be a part of each state's workers' compensation program. Many states have implemented cost-containment measures, including managed care, fee schedules, treatment guidelines, and formularies.

According to the Workers' Compensation Research Institute, most states have implemented medical fee schedules; 30 have adopted treatment guidelines, 21 have utilization review regulations, and most allow for managed care. Sixteen states have medical directors. Work-related disability management and outcomes can be successful when employers and the system support injured workers through rehabilitation to recovery. Best practices indicate that to prevent an injury from turning into a disability, the system should include the utilization of efficient and effective medical care, along with employer and insurer collaboration, and an emphasis on return to work through rehabilitation. Assisting injured workers to return to work can relieve some of the demands of the workers' compensation, medical system, and Social Security Disability system. Some states have adopted initiatives to help injured workers return to work. To track progress and establish evidence for success, a program should establish factors that can be researched to determine its utility. Some of the factors include diagnosis, patient satisfaction, time to return to work, medical cost, indemnity cost, employer satisfaction, and medical provider satisfaction. The challenge for policymakers is to take a systematic approach and develop policies that support workers' compensation stay-at-work and return-to-work programs. To do this, they must include multiple stakeholders, including the injured worker, employer, insurance carrier, health care provider, rehabilitation counselors, and the state itself.

It may be helpful to define a few terms to assist the reader in understanding the system.

- **Provider:** An individual or organization that provides health care services, including medical, physical, behavioral, pharmacological, and rehabilitative health care services.
- **Return to work:** A focus on supporting workers who sustain injuries or develop health conditions or illness to return to jobs they held before the injury, if possible, or a modified position with their employer, a different position with the employer, or a position with another employer through transferable skills.
- **Stay at work:** A focus on supporting workers who sustain injuries or develop an illness to remain in the jobs they held at the time of their injury with their employer, either in the position they held at the time or modified or other positions. The goal here is to stay at work and not leave the workforce.
- **Work disability:** An inability to perform the essential functions of a job or maintain employment due to a health condition.
- **Social Security Disability Insurance:** A Social Security program that pays monthly benefits to citizens who become disabled before reaching retirement age and are unable to work.
- **Evidence-based medicine (EBM):** The conscientious, explicit, judicious, and reasonable use of modern best evidence in making decisions about the care of individual patients. An EBM integrates clinical experience and patient values with the best available research information.
- **Evidence-based practice:** The use of systematic decision-making processes or provision of services that have been shown through available scientific research to consistently improve outcomes. The evidence-based practice relies on data collected through experimental research. Evidence-based practice also considers individual client characteristics and clinician expertise.

As demonstrated earlier, there exists a robust third-party system and network of mandated policies to protect employees injured at work. At the heart of the process is the notion that employees can expect a safe work environment and are entitled to medical and pecuniary benefits if they happened to become injured during the course and scope of their normal employment.

Despite changes to the laws mentioned previously to remove some of the adversarial components of the system, third-party reimbursement systems can tend to engender skepticism and distrust. It is important as medical providers to be fully aware of how actions, treatment plans, and documentation can impact an injured worker's treatment arc. It is advisable for direct service providers to seek out and consult with third-party administrators and claims adjusters, if necessary, to ensure a smooth and equitable continuum of care post-injury

References

Annual Statistical Report on the Social Security Disability Insurance Program, 2019. (2020). www.ssa.gov/policy/docs/statcomps/di_asr/2019/di_asr19.pdf

The Appeals Process. (2018, January). 5-10041, ICN 459260. www.ssa.gov/pubs/EN-05-10041.pdf

Barnes, C., El-Hodiri, N., & Kniss, M. (2020). *Comparisons of benefits in retirement and actions needed to help injured workers choose best option* (pp. 1–66). Federal Employees' Compensation Act. GAO-20-523.

Blue Book/Disability Evaluation Under Social Security. (2008). www.ssa.gov/disability/professionals/bluebook/

Bradbury, J. C. (2006). Regulatory federalism and workplace safety: Evidence from OSHA enforcement, 1987–1995. *Journal of Regulatory Economics*, *29*, 211–224.

Daubert v. Merrell Dow Pharmaceutical, Inc., 509 U.S. 579. (1993).

Disability Benefits. (2019, July). *Social security administration*. 5–10029, ICN 456000. www.ssa.gov/pubs/EN-05-10029.pdf

Friedell, S. (2017). Interplay of the Jones act and the general maritime law. *Journal of Maritime Law & Commerce*, *48*(4), 371–402.

Frye v. United States, 293 F. 1013 (D.C. Cir. 1923).

General Electric v. Joiner. (1997). 522 U.S. 136.

Isernhagen, S. (2009). Introduction to functional capacity evaluation. In E. Genovese & J. Galper (Eds.), *American medical association guide to the evaluation of functional ability* (pp. 1–18). American Medical Association.

Kumho Tire Company v. Carmichael, 526 U.S. 137. (1999).

Lewis Jr, T. J. (1961). Federal Employers Liability Act. *SCLQ*, *14*, 447.

May, V. (1999). The NADEP work disability evaluation model. In R. V. May & M. F. Martelli (Eds.), *The national association of disability evaluating professionals (NADEP) guide to functional capacity evaluation with impairment rating applications*. NADEP Publications.

May, V., Taylor, D., Brigham, C., & Washington, C. (1998). Functional capacity evaluation, impairment rating, and applied certification processes. *Neuro Rehabilitation*, *11*(1), 13–27.

Nordland, W. (1991). The federal employees' compensation act. *Monthly Labor Review*.

Obermann, C. E. (1965). *A history of vocational rehabilitation in America*. T. S. Denison & Company, Inc.

Orne, K. (2015). It's about time: Modernizing the federal employer's liability act of 1908. *Arizona State Law Journal*, *47*(1), 343–366.

Papavizas, C. (2020). The story of the Jones act (merchant marine act, 1920). *Tulane Maritime Law Journal*, *44*(3), 459–485.

Red Book a Summary Guide to Employment Supports for People with Disabilities Under the Social Security Disability Insurance (SSDI) and Supplemental Security Income (SSI) Programs. (2020, January). 64–030, ICN 436900. www.ssa.gov/pubs/EN-64-030.pdf

Rondinelli, R. D. (Ed.). (2008). *Guides to the evaluation of permanent impairment* (6th ed.). American Medical Association.

Rosner, D., & Markowitz, G. (2020). A short occupational safety and health in the United States. *Public Health Then and Now*, *110*(5), 622–628.

Roy, E. (2003). Functional capacity evaluation and the use of validity testing. *The Case Manager*, *14*(2), 64–69.

Simet, D. P. (1962). Concurrent Jurisdiction in Maritime Death—Faith in a Sea Fable?. *Buffalo Law Review*, *11*(2), 405.

Steiger, W. (1974). OSHA: Four years later. *Labor Law Journal*, *25*(12), 723–728.

Sturley, M., & Ammerman, M. (2020). Recent developments in admiralty and maritime law at the national level and in the fifth and eleventh circuits. *Tulane Maritime Law Journal, 44,* 513.

Suarthana, E., Laney, A., Storey, E., Hale, J., & Attfield, M. (2011). Coal workers' pneumoconiosis in the United States: Regional differences 40 years after implementation of the 1969 federal coal mine health and safety act. *Occupational and Environmental Medicine, 68*(12), 908–913.

Szymendera, S. (2020). *The longshore and harbor workers' compensation act (LHWCA): Overview of the workers' compensation for certain private-sector maritime workers* (pp. pp. 1–12, Version 9). Congressional Research Service Report R41505.

United States. (1975). *The federal rules of evidence.* Matthew Bender.

United States Department of Labor. (1991). *The revised handbook for analyzing jobs.* Employment and Training Administration.

United States Department of Labor. (1993). *Selected characteristics of occupations defined in the revised dictionary of occupational titles.* Employment and Training Administration.

United States Department of Labor. (2022). *Division of federal employee's longshore and harbor workers' compensation 2000.* www.dol.gov/agencies/owcp/dlhwc/lhwca#906

4   Independent Medical Evaluations

Douglas W. Martin

The unique recipe of mixing the art and science of medicine with the needs of the insurance and legal community is what makes the provision of a quality independent medical evaluation so difficult.

Interestingly, if you utter the words "independent medical evaluation (IME)" to medical students, residents, or fellows, you will typically get a blank stare. These evaluations are typically not on the radar screen within formal medical education curricula, and the common physician does not hear about them until they are well into establishing their practices. But this fact is often lost upon those who rely upon these evaluations to establish certain medical opinions within the context of a claim and for those who seek out experts who can effectively communicate this information (Martin, 2018).

An IME is an evaluation conducted by a third-party physician, usually in the context of a medicolegal or insurance claim. Several systems utilize IMEs including workers' compensation, personal liability, Veterans' Administration, and Social Security disability. There are no Accreditation Council on Graduate Medical Education (ACGME)–accredited training programs on IMEs that are available to physicians, but several organizations provide continuing medical education activities whereby skills can be acquired.

What Is an Independent Medical Evaluator?

An independent medical evaluator is usually a physician who performs a health care evaluative service as a third party at the request of an advocate who participates in a medicolegal or insurance claim. The phrase "independent medical examination" is also sometimes used. However, for obvious reasons, it reflects a narrower scope of practice in that an actual examination of an individual claimant occurs. It is preferred, therefore, to use the phrase "independent medical evaluation" as this would also encompass activities, such as file reviews, where a physical examination does not take place (Martin, 2017).

These services are usually requested by employers or insurance carriers within the workers' compensation benefits system but are also commonly performed in legal cases where there has been a claim of injury or illness caused by one party upon another (Demeter & Washington, 2003).

Within our U.S. legal system, decision-makers such as judges, juries, and commissions, commonly referred to as "triers of fact", are responsible for determining whether an injury has occurred that is compensable by some form of monetary award. Thus, the independent medical evaluator is often looked upon to offer a professional opinion as to not only whether an injury or illness has occurred but also whether it is a temporary or permanent issue. In the case of a permanent medical problem, it is necessary within the claim process to determine the severity and

DOI: 10.4324/b23293-4

extent of the medical issue so that a reasonable monetary award can be decided to compensate the injured party. In the case of longer-term or more catastrophic injuries and illnesses, IMEs can also help determine what resources will be necessary to provide long-term care to the individual in question. This is critical so that a fair and justified reserve amount of money can be set aside by an insurance carrier or other stakeholder to cover the medical needs of the injured party.

There are other reasons that an IME might be requested. Within the workers' compensation benefits system, an injured party may be undergoing medical treatment that the employer or employer's insurance carrier is questioning. Often, IMEs are requested in this situation when the treating physician has requested advanced diagnostic testing or where a treatment such as surgery is of high cost. Given that the costs of care within the workers' compensation system are higher for the same medical diagnoses compared to the general medical population, these IMEs are often directed due to a concern of cost/benefit analysis insofar as the question arises as to whether a test or treatment is necessary to effectuate a good outcome, which is almost always measured in terms of a successful return to work (Novick & Rondinelli, 2000).

IMEs may be requested in long-term disability (LTD) claims. Usually, the issue arises out of an LTD claim that has been submitted by a covered person to an insurance carrier. LTD insurance is quite common in the United States and is often offered as an employment benefit to workers. When illness or catastrophic injuries prevent the individual from returning to work, LTD policies provide some residual level of income, typically for the remainder of the person's work life.

In reviewing LTD claims, insurance carriers will rely heavily upon the medical records submitted by the claimant's treating physicians. And it is the norm that these records can provide enough information for the claim reviewer to decide when the medical issues rise to the level where the LTD policy terms would apply. However, there are some instances where the medical condition either is unclear or is controversial and the medical records do not allow an easy determination of coverage. Also, there are situations where there may be questions about the severity of functional limitation for a given medical condition and whether the level of functional limitation is permanent, can be mitigated to allow a successful return to work, or can be accommodated in other ways by an employer. In these situations, an IME can be requested to address any or all of these questions.

Since personal injury lawsuits are common in the United States, the IME physician can play a crucial role in providing an unbiased opinion regarding the extent of a claimed injury and the impact that the injury may have on future earnings capacity. Frequently, the litigants within a personal injury case will be especially focused on the level of "pain and suffering" since monetary damages can be awarded within these types of lawsuits and not in others. As a physician, the IME provider can also communicate opinions regarding future care needs and the impact of pain upon function, which are often lynchpins in determining the number of monetary awards given in these claims.

Obviously, the IME physician needs to understand the motivation of the claimants within a personal injury lawsuit. It is commonplace for evaluators to witness anger, skepticism, and a variety of other negative emotions as part of this process. Although these emotions can be a part of all litigated medical claims, they may be heightened within these types of lawsuits. Also, it is important to understand the impact these emotions can play not only in a mental health context but also when mental health problems manifest themselves into actual physical maladies, frequently referred to as "somatization".

It must be understood by all stakeholders that there is no formal training on the proper provision of an IME in either medical schools or residency programs. The non-medical stakeholder may be surprised at this. However, the traditions and standard practices of the ACGME and the

American Board of Medical Specialties (ABMS) do not contain recommendations on IMEs within their regulations, and no ABMS specialty board certification organization (the American Board of Family Medicine, the American Board of Preventive Medicine, the American Board of Physical Medicine and Rehabilitation, for example) contains a requirement or even a suggestion that IME parameters be taught.

Thus, there is a dichotomy in that the legal need for having an IME does not mesh with the non-existent importance paid to it within the formal medical education process. Some physicians are fortunate to join practices where a colleague or partner is performing this service, and in those situations, a mentoring process occurs. Other physicians may receive inquiries from attorneys or insurance carriers regarding whether they would be willing to provide IME services but may have no idea what the specifics entail.

A variety of entities provide continuing medical education (CME) courses on the subject. The currently available organizations that provide these educational opportunities are as follows:

- International Academy of Independent Medical Evaluators (www.iaime.org)
- American Board of Independent Medical Examiners (www.abimc.org)
- American College of Occupational & Environmental Medicine (www.acoem.org)
- SEAK (www.seak.com)

Medicolegal Systems and the IME Provider

The purpose of having an IME performed within any medicolegal context is to have on record a professional medical report which serves as an expert opinion that one side or the other can use to advocate for their argument or claim. Within these contexts, the more definitive the opinion is, the more weight and value it has to the side who is attempting to prove an argument or claim. However, it is imperative to note that the IME opinion must be expressed within the limits of medical knowledge, and since medicine is both art and science, there are often areas where consensus does not exist. This explains why, for example, medical opinions can differ from one IME provider to another.

An IME report may be a requirement of a court or other trier of fact when litigation is pending, or attorneys may desire a written report to assist in settlement negotiations prior to hearings or trials. As such, it is critically important that the IME physician understand the context within which the claim lies, as there may be specific jurisdictional rules that dictate not only what sort of evaluation is to occur but also what sort of information is essential to communicate that is then used to satisfy the questions that the disability system requires (Demeter & Washington, 2003).

When contemplating the position and purpose of IMEs, ethics frequently come into play. From the physician's perspective, it is often of considerable debate as to how the role of patient advocacy can influence decision-making, especially regarding disability certification. A patient advocate's true and traditional role is to always do what is in the patient's best interest. But a more contemporary view that many physicians practice is to always do what the patient wants. The problem with these two views is that in areas of disability determination, they can be at odds with each other.

When there is a dispute regarding these issues that surround the treating physician's viewpoint, it becomes critical that the IME physician remain impartial. However, many argue that an IME provider cannot ever really be unbiased, given that they know in full from whom their fees are provided. It remains challenging for any service industry provider, whether medical or otherwise, to set aside customer satisfaction issues when payment for a function has a certain expected outcome.

This is a fact not lost upon the courts and judges. Many judges refuse to allow the characterization of these evaluations as "independent" and instead rule that they must be referred to as "defense medical evaluations" or "plaintiff medical evaluations", making a point that it is the counselor or who they represent who is paying the bill for these services and not the court itself, which has directed them to occur. Having said that, there are a few instances in the individual state workers' compensation programs where an IME can indeed be requested by the court but for which the payment for the IME is the responsibility of one side or the other or, in some cases, shared.

Regardless, the prudent IME physician should exercise caution and avoid being stereotyped as "defense" or "plaintiff" friendly. Unfortunately, many stakeholders in medicolegal systems can readily identify IME physician outliers whose opinion can be counted on despite the specifics of an individual case. Unfortunately, these outlier physicians may taint the public's perception of IME providers and can create an unbecoming phraseology for doctors of medicine. Such statements and phrases as "his opinion is bought and paid for", "he wouldn't find anything wrong even if I were dead", "the disabling doctor", and "defense whore" echo in the halls of insurance companies and attorney offices across the country (Martin, 2018).

As such, there is a place for the physician performing IMEs willing to make objective and fair determinations. When an IME physician uses sound medical judgment, is comprehensive in their assessment of a medical problem, and applies consistently evidence-based decision-making, there is little reason to be concerned about the validity and acceptance of their opinions.

Group or private LTD insurance is quite common in the United States, and group policies are quite commonly offered as part of a worker's benefits package by the employer. As they are actual contracts, contract law governs how programs are administered. Typically, if an employee becomes disabled, they are covered by a short-term disability policy for 90 days. If the disability extends beyond that time frame, LTD provisions become available.

LTD benefits are usually paid only if the employee is unable to perform the functions of any occupation, and the language regarding the specificity of how this is interpreted is included within each specific policy. Although less common currently, there continue to be individual LTD insurance policies with higher premiums that are considered "own occupation" policies, meaning that benefits are paid when an individual cannot return to their specific prior occupation but may be able to work in other capacities. There are also LTD policies that pay benefits when an individual has a loss of income, comparing a prior job that they can no longer do to a current job that they can do but that has lower pay.

LTD policies traditionally pay 60% of the individual's prior wage and have a maximum cap with cost-of-living allowances. Additionally, most LTD policies contain a provision that the insured must also concurrently apply for Social Security disability. The Social Security Disability Insurance (SSDI) entitlements may offset a portion of the wage benefits paid by the LTD carrier.

IME physicians play a role in the LTD decision process, usually via the performance of a file review, where an independent evaluator looks at the applicant's medical record and is asked if the medical evidence supports the claim for LTD. Usually, each LTD insurance carrier has internal medical professionals who perform initial and confirmatory reviews. Commonly, the worker may appeal via the LTD policy language if the claim is denied. Often, this appeal will trigger the request for an independent review.

In some cases, an actual independent examination may be requested. This is typically done when the medical records do not provide a clear picture of the claimant's health status or when there are questions about the legitimacy of specific diagnoses. Commonly, LTD coverage disagreements arise when there are claims of controversial diagnoses or when there are chronic conditions that have episodic exacerbations. Also, mental health claims create the need for IMEs because they are often challenging to analyze based solely on treatment records.

Lastly, IME physicians may become involved with LTD claims as expert witnesses when a denial of a claim and its appeal has occurred and the claimant has filed suit against the LTD carrier. Sometimes, these lawsuits involve "bad faith" claims for which the claimant attempts to show that the LTD acted outside the typical norms during the decision process. These lawsuits are usually quite contentious, are of potentially high monetary value, and require an IME physician with experience in fitness for duty and knowledge of the bio-psycho-social-economic BPSE) model of evaluation.

Medical Record Review

A prior analysis of the treatment records gives the IME physician a chronological view of the treatment of the medical condition from the start to the present. It allows the IME physician the ability to drill down on more questionable portions of the record. It narrows the IME physician's history to those questions posed to the examinee that will clearly examine the pertinent issues. Many times, it is interesting to find that the information that the examinee believed they heard from their treating providers is not consistent with what is communicated in the medical record. It is often the role of the IME physician to determine if this discrepancy exists. When there is a disparity in the record compared to the history given by the examinee, is this a simple mistake? Is it because the examinee is fabricating the information? Is the treating physician purposefully not disclosing information in the written record that was verbalized to their patient? These are all questions the IME physician may be asked to attempt to resolve, at least to the best of their ability. One could not opine on this matter without previously reviewing the medical records relevant to the case at hand (Blair, 2014).

Specific attention should be paid to the timeline when major diagnostics or interventions were performed. Noting the dates of magnetic resonance imaging (MRI) scans and surgical procedures may be particularly important. In cases where fitness for duty or return to work is debatable, the IME physician should note when treating physicians have changed their recommendations on work status and the rationale (if it is discussed) for temporary or permanent restrictions.

It is always important to look for inconsistencies in the record. Most often, one can predict where the contentious issues of a claim reside by identifying where inconsistencies exist. When inconsistencies are found, it should serve as a reminder to the IME physician to expand the history, taking on those subjects during the examination.

In musculoskeletal claims, close attention may be paid to physical and occupational therapy notes. Often, emphasis on these records is not rendered at the level they deserve. Commonly, you will see the physical therapist (PT) or occupational therapist (OT) comment upon activity or work issues at appointments that are either cursorily addressed or not addressed at the physician appointments. One also can obtain a clearer picture of function from the OT and PT documentation than in other medical encounter documentation. Lastly, OT and PT evaluations are exceptionally helpful in identifying trends over a series of visits and painting a picture regarding delayed recovery or maximum recovery.

To additionally help the IME physician, it is beneficial to keep in mind that eventually, the evaluator will be relating the story in written format in the IME report. Storytelling is often an art form, but when combing through the records, the evaluator should determine if a relevant story can be relayed based upon the records contained. If a cohesive story can be relayed, a respectable job was completed. If not, something may have been missed and should trigger an additional review to fill in the missing information. Sometimes, a cohesive story may not be feasible to tell. This is when completing the puzzle by asking the right questions of the claimant during the history-taking portion of the examination becomes critical.

Taking an IME History and Conducting the Examination

Every IME should be approached with a particular set of core principles (the "4 Cs"; Martin, 2018) which include:

- Clarification of Purpose
- Complete Preparation
- Content
- Communication

Clarification of Purpose

Clarification of purpose refers to the preparatory measures that need to occur before the examination. This includes verifying the purpose of the evaluation with the requestor. Although it might seem that this is an unnecessary step, often, it is true that the requesting party has not thought through the entire claim or case. In some situations, the conversation between the IME physician and requesting party can shed new light on certain aspects of a claim that the requesting party has not considered. Additionally, the requesting party may be new to the IME process; they may be an entry-level claims examiner who has been trained as to when an IME should be requested but has little experience in what the process entails or exactly how the information can be helpful to them as a claims evaluator.

Clarification of purpose also refers to the importance of confirming the mechanical aspects of the appointment, including those informational items such as time, date, and location of appointment. It also includes a verification and acknowledgement of the business parameters that are germane to the process, such as scheduling rules, no-show issues, payment, report deadlines, and other items.

At this time, an understanding of the report standard is also confirmed. In most situations, there is no "set" format that a report must follow, and if the requesting party is new to the IME examiner, it may be helpful to send an example report and ask if the format is acceptable. In other jurisdictions, such as some state workers' compensation systems, the IME report must follow a rigid format. In a rigid format report setting, there is little room for creativity with the report document; however, the learned IME physician often devises unique ways of staying within the format requirements but also implementing changes that not only add to the value of the information contained within the report but also indicate to the requesting party that special attention has been paid to their claim. Examples of these types of changes include the use of color, varying the font on subheadings, offsetting of paragraphs, and the use of pictures or drawings.

It is useful during the report clarification phase to also understand whether the purpose of the examination is for employability or disability determination. IME reports tend to be a bit different depending upon the focus. In an employability determination, the usual vein of discussion and decision-making is oriented toward what the individual being examined can do. In contrast, in a disability determination, attention is typically turned toward what the individual cannot do.

It is also a good idea to understand who the reader of your report will be (there may be a whole host of individuals) and, more importantly, what level of expertise the reader possesses.

It is essential to understand that some readers will have little, if any, medical background, and for those readers, staying away from medical terminology or providing a glossary is helpful.

One way to think about the clarification of purpose is to remember that the report should be considered a legal document that will be available in perpetuity unless the rules or statutes that govern the circumstance dictate otherwise. Careful preparation by the IME physician will help avoid uncomfortable issues that might come up in the future. For example, one might be surprised in a deposition if an opposing attorney has brought with them a report you prepared from 10 years prior, particularly if your style or methods were not the same as they are currently. While it is certainly acceptable for IME physicians to be on a path of continuous quality improvement, they should also be aware and prepared for these sorts of things, and being consistent in the approach, including clarifying the purpose of the IME, will go a long way to minimizing worry about potential inconsistencies.

Complete Preparation

Preparation for the IME begins with a comprehensive review of all pertinent records. These include not only the medical records but also any non-medical records when deemed appropriate and relevant to the questions that need to be answered. A review of records will also lead the IME physician to focus on certain critical areas and help them to develop questions that will be asked during the history-taking part in the IME.

The IME physician will be asked to look at laboratory data. It must be emphasized that the IME physician should be familiar with various laboratory reports and their meanings. Reference ranges that are specific to certain blood tests, for example, may be different from one laboratory to the next. The sensitivity and specificity of each laboratory test, while not listed within the context of the laboratory report, is often an important point in many claims. The IME physician, if dealing with these issues, should have a good understanding of the biostatistics that are involved.

Frequently, radiographic reports will be a part of the medical record to review. It is important that the IME physician obtain the studies if made available, which is becoming easier in the digital age of radiology where computed tomography (CT), MRI, and plain film x-rays can be shared on computer systems or copied onto a CD or flash drive. Radiologists can make mistakes. Especially when reviewing MRI scans, there is quite a variation in radiology terminology from one radiologist to the next. One radiologist's disc "bulge" may be the other's disc "herniation". Terms such as "encroachment," "stenosis", "impingement", "insult", "narrowing", "crowding", constriction", and "compression" are used to describe exiting nerve root anatomy but may have a variety of meanings.

Complete preparation also demands that the IME physician take thought and consideration regarding exactly how the examination will occur. Since the IME evaluation is quite different from the traditional physician-patient encounter, the IME physician may feel uneasy about the closing of the evaluation encounter if there is no discussion about the diagnosis or treatment plan. It is helpful for the IME physician to develop a verbal script of sorts to follow. Many IME physicians have written templates that they use for history taking, and indeed many of these are available commercially. Other IME physicians have developed their own templates. Others prefer to write questions during the review of records before the examination so that they remember to ask those questions during the evaluation itself. Regardless, it is recommended that some type of format be followed.

It is also helpful for the IME physician to think about how they will conclude the examination. Since it may seem odd to not have a discussion with the examinee about their diagnosis and what is recommended for treatment, it is incumbent upon the IME physician to conclude the evaluation so that both the doctor and the claimant come away with an understanding of the role the IME physician plays while also being comprehensive about the process.

Content

Content refers to the actual process of conducting the proper history and physical examination. As is typically the case with any medical encounter, the history is typically taken first.

The timing and circumstances of the onset of symptoms are critical to understand. The IME physician should spend a substantial amount of time on this during the documentation of the medical history. If there is a traumatic event, the location and position of the body and all outside external forces and conditions may be explored for thorough understanding. The severity of the trauma may be explored not just in terms of the examinee's perception but what occurred regarding the specific event in question. For example, much more detail should be obtained concerning a slip and fall injury other than just asking when it happened and upon what the person slipped. The mechanics of what the person was doing when the slip happened (walking, running, sliding, etc.); whether they were carrying anything when they fell; whether they slipped forward, backward, or sideways; and what they impacted on the way down (something other than the ground?) may be explored. Understanding the terrain of the ground (slippery, unsteady, uneven) can be important for causality, just as it is important to determine if the person tried to break their fall (fall on an outstretched hand, impacted their knees before their torso, etc.). The severity of the fall can often be estimated by asking about what happened immediately after the fall. Did the person immediately stand back up? Did they require help to get up? Did they have to remain down and call for help? Finally, asking whether the fall was witnessed by anyone can be important, as the witness could help with verifying the accuracy and validity of the historical information given by the examinee.

A unique factor in the IME history is that the IME physician can review the medical record with the examinee. The physician should discuss with the examinee the important findings from prior physical or mental health exams and explore the examinee's understanding of their significance. Such is also the case with any results from prior tests. It may be surprising to some IME physicians how misinformed the examinees sometimes are regarding these important items.

The historical trend of symptoms should also be explored and noted. As with any medical condition, attention should be paid to those activities or factors that alleviate and aggravate symptoms. A discussion should occur, using the prior medical records as a backdrop, regarding what medical treatments have been helpful and which have not. While addressing treatment outcomes, it is also important to understand the examinee's compliance with the recommended treatment plans. If there is information within the record that shows that compliance was an issue, the subject should be explored during the exam to understand the reasons as to why compliance was a problem.

If the usual progression or resolution of symptoms for a diagnosed condition does not follow what is typical for the given condition, the IME physician should try to figure out why the problem has not resolved or progressed. Is there a misdiagnosed condition? Is there an alternative explanation for the continued or worsening symptoms in the face of a condition that typically improves with time and minor medical involvement? Such possibilities that may be explored by the IME physician include the likelihood of medically unexplained symptoms (MUS), which can be part of what is now called somatic symptom disorder. While the issue of somatic symptom disorder and its caveats far exceed the focus of this chapter, the possibility of this disorder will lead the IME physician to explore important historical items such as adverse childhood experiences; prior spousal, sexual, or other forms of abuse; prior claims behavior; and the context within which a claim has been made. Once the history is obtained, the physical or mental examination is completed.

The physical exam can be considered to begin the moment that the evaluator begins observing the examinee. This includes looking out the window and watching them walk into the clinic and down the hallway. Seasoned IME examiners, when possible, derive considerable benefit from having their office windows turned toward their office parking areas and offices that provide sight lines down hallways. You may be surprised many times as to how the examinee's gait patterns and behaviors can change in these various areas. You may also be surprised as to how canes and other assistive walking devices are forgotten in exam rooms or thrown into automobile trunks after at the end of appointments. It is also useful to observe the interaction of the examinee with individuals other than you. Do they treat everyone the same? Do they put on a different tone and demeanor for you as the examiner only to show something completely different to your office staff? These types of differences can shed significant light on the claim behavior of the examinee and the validity of their complaints.

If the examinee must disrobe for the examination, it is preferable to wait to do this until after the history is complete. The IME physician should ensure that there is adequate privacy and dignity by providing suitable attire for the examination, such as a gown, shorts, tank top, or other forms of draping. It is also important to have a chaperone when appropriate since we are not dealing with a typical medical encounter but one that is outside those constraints. The IME physician should take necessary steps to avoid any potential issues with claims of inappropriate examinee contact. When a chaperone is used, it should be documented in the report.

Many IME physicians have established a practice of using a chaperone for the entire IME process, including the history and the physical examination. This methodology has benefits in that the chaperone can not only serve as a witness to the events if there were ever to be a challenge to certain portions of the evaluation process, but they may also serve other functions such as a scribe for history taking and aid with certain portions of the examination.

Just as it was discussed that templates and forms can be helpful for the history, so too can they be helpful for the physical examination. Many IME physicians use preprinted forms that are organ specific; in other words, they may use physical exam worksheets for the upper extremity, spine, vision, and hearing, for example. Such worksheets can facilitate the recording of certain observations and measurements and may ensure a more complete exam by prompting recollection of certain physical examination tests that might otherwise be forgotten.

The IME physician should have a standard approach to concluding the examination. As the physical examination is typically the final part of the IME encounter with the physician, it is prudent to ask the examinee how they are doing and whether there is anything else that they would like to be checked.

Communication

An integral part of communication, and an exercise that has become an important part for some in the IME process, is to ask the examinee to complete an exit interview or satisfaction survey after the examination but prior to leaving the office. The best way to accomplish this is to discuss the survey with the examinee and give it to them to complete once the physical examination is completed and before they leave the examination room. The easiest method to accomplish this is for the IME physician to have this survey with them and to review the importance of its completion immediately once the examination has concluded, as there is a much better completion rate when the examinee knows the survey must be filled out before leaving.

Such satisfaction surveys can ask questions regarding the adequacy and clarity of communication from the IME physician's office about directions to the office, the quality of the interaction with the office staff, and the physical appearance of the office itself. However, these satisfaction surveys can provide a quite different function for the IME physician, since it serves as a record against which future accusations that the IME was not comprehensive can be measured or can provide a defense against claims that "the doctor hurt me" during the exam. Thus, exit interviews or surveys can ask questions such as whether the examinee felt the exam was comprehensive, whether any part of the examination caused pain, or whether enough time was spent by the IME physician. Finally, an overall rating regarding the examinee's experience can be obtained and can be used in any promotional items that the IME physician may elect to use.

The Written Report

The IME physician may be a great history-taker, might be stellar in the differential diagnostic process, and might even be recognized as an expert in their field, but if they are unable to write a quality IME report, they will not be seen as helpful. It is often the case that requesting parties have no knowledge about an IME physician other than the quality of the report that they generate (Freeman, 1998).

The simple truth is that physicians typically do not write well. When you think about their formal education process, this might seem a bit difficult to understand, but when you drill down and understand what it entails, it really should not surprise anyone. Physicians tend toward science majors in college, and these bachelor's degree programs at most might require two semesters of English. In medical school, there is no requirement to be able to write well, as medical data is now communicated in short factoids. Sometimes, there is a struggle to even find a complete professionally written sentence in a student chart note. The problem is that this "habit" typically goes uncorrected. Electronic health records (EHRs) do not help. The plethora of EHRs that are available do not even require the medical student, resident, or practicing physician to write anything in favor of clicking a series of boxes that generate pre-determined verbiage. If there is no need for the writing of a sentence, let alone a paragraph, laziness prevails. If there is no ability to practice and improve, writing skills deteriorate.

But the stakeholders who engage in medicolegal claims place a premium upon the written report, where details are pivotal. The ability to clearly communicate a medical history so that anyone reading the report can understand exactly what happened in an injury case becomes not only necessary but critical. Following the thought processes and understanding of how the IME physician has come to their conclusion is held at such a high premium that requesting parties search long and hard to find physicians who possess the ability to write in this manner.

It must be understood that the IME report is a script that may form a foundation for later testimony. Thus, an increased focus on accuracy and clarity is paramount. Also, IME reports will often become permanent records that will exist in perpetuity. The IME physician should know and prepare for the fact that there is a repository of their reports that are being kept in a file somewhere by someone. Legal service companies exist that provide this type of service.

The essential components of a quality IME report can vary but should typically include the following:

- Introduction
- Results of Clinical Evaluation
- Clinical Impressions
- Assessment of Current Health Status

- Medical Management Plan
- Synthesis of Information
- Conclusions and Recommendations (Nierenberg et al., 2005)

Each of these components is best identified within the report by the use of subheadings. Given that IME reports are longer than most medical records, the use of subheadings is beneficial, as it makes certain sections of information easily identifiable. Also, since the report may be read by different people responsible for distinct parts of claim administration, the use of subheadings helps those individuals focus on their relevant tasks. For example, the litigator might be interested in the causation section. The nurse case manager might want to look at the medical management plan. The insurance company actuary might only be looking at the indemnity costs of disability payments or wage replacement benefits.

Introduction

The introduction will typically include the identifying information of the examinee, which consists of their name, date of birth, and last four digits of their Social Security number. In some situations, the Social Security number identifier may not be necessary, and in other situations the examinee may not wish to disclose this information if it is not required to do so. If the claim has been given a case or a file number, it is appropriate to also include this information.

Within the introductory section, the referral source should be identified to include the specific name of the requesting party as well as the agency or entity that they represent. The purpose of the evaluation should be specifically stated, which should include the type of benefit system that the examination is being conducted under as well as any applicable jurisdictional rules that apply.

At some point, a listing of all records and radiographs that have been presented for review should be included. It may be best to include this list in an appendix that is attached at the end of the IME report as opposed to placing this at the beginning of the report, since an extensive list tends to turn off the reader early on if presented in this manner.

Results of the Clinical Examination

The next portion of the report should include the history and physical examination. When recording the history, some IME physicians prefer to use a sublabel such as "History of Present Illness" or "History of Current Condition". Any such title is appropriate.

Stylistically, the history should tell a story as it is related by the examinee. The narrative of the events should follow the standard approach for all medical histories in that pertinent positives and negatives are to be investigated and recorded.

IME physicians take different approaches regarding how they record the history as it pertains to what is recorded in the past medical records. Some physicians do not include any references to the past records in the history section, preferring to record only the information obtained from the examinee. These reports usually will then include a review of the past records in a different section of the IME report. One of the criticisms of this type of report is that there is a lengthy list of summaries of the medical encounters that can go on for pages and pages. While it is certainly a good idea to review the past records in detail, this approach can be unnecessary and could be construed as negative in that most requesting parties are well aware of what has occurred previously and do not need to have this degree of detail recounted in an IME report.

Instead of this approach, the examiner may consider a distinctive style that incorporates a mixture of what the examinee is reporting to them and what is included in the past medical record. Admittedly, this methodology is more complicated and requires an artistic skill set of writing that is not necessarily easy to master. However, in reviewing this with a host of stakeholders, this method is preferred by me because it is easier to follow and reads more like a story being told. This "mixture method" also affords the IME physician the ability to identify not only where the information is coming from (the examinee, the records, or both) but, more importantly, allows a simplistic method to manage those situations where the history from the examinee does not agree with what is included within the past records. When such disagreement exists, the IME physician should explore this further with the examinee to understand the discrepancy. If an explanation is given by the examinee, it should be included here, even if the explanation makes little sense from a medical standpoint.

The history should also include a review of systems and a listing of current medications and allergies. It is crucial to obtain a detailed occupational history, especially when evaluating a disability claim. Family history and social history are just as important. The IME physician should take extra effort to understand the biopsychosocial dynamic of the injury or illness claim. Investigating a history of adverse childhood events, spousal abuse, or substance abuse can often lead to a better understanding of claim behavior. It is also known that one of the strongest predictors of disability claims is the presence of a spouse who is also receiving disability benefits. An understanding of prior workers' compensation claims, including any prior impairment ratings or permanent physical activity restrictions, should be documented in this section. Lastly, a listing of all prior surgeries should be included.

Most IME reports also include a subheading for the physical and/or mental examination results. The IME physical examination must be detailed and thorough, and this should be reflected in the way that it is recorded within the report.

It should be known that the physical examination during an IME may start before the examinee enters the office. Some IME physicians are fortunate to have their office windows face the parking lot, and observations of gait patterns and methods of getting in and out of a vehicle and how they either are consistent with or different from those patterns while in the office are noteworthy. It is relevant to describe how the examinee gets in and out of the chair and off and on the examination table. I have, on a few occasions, observed claimants who had severe knee problems kick start their motorcycles with the "injured" leg quite aggressively and normally.

In this subsection, there should also be a place to discuss the relevant diagnostic tests or radiographs that have been presented as part of the prior records. Most IME physicians will discuss these in a separately identifiable part of the report.

Clinical Impressions

The clinical impressions portion of the report is the location where the diagnoses are listed. It is best to list these numerically. This is not the place to use descriptive or causal language, as those topics are dealt with in a different section of the report. As an example, a diagnosis should not be listed as "lower back strain leading to chronic pain due to the 2015 motor vehicle accident" but simply "low back strain". Many physicians elect to also include the relevant International Statistical Classification of Diseases and Related Health Problems (ICD-10) code, and that is an optional practice.

Assessment of Current Health Status

This section typically includes an area describing the prognosis. The IME physician should indicate whether the medical conditions being evaluated are stable, declining, or improving. It is insufficient to simply report this without also going on to explain the medical basis for the opinion. If there are informational items that are missing or diagnostic tests that need to be done to answer this question better, these should be described in detail and the rationale as to why they are necessary.

There are times when the medical condition being evaluated will have a natural and expected deterioration over time. These are most often encountered in illnesses or diagnoses that involve the internal organ systems. The question sometimes comes up as to how these deteriorating medical problems are addressed within disability systems. The answer is that there are usually protocols involved where a claimant can refile for additional benefits if the condition worsens over time. Thus, it is helpful for the IME physician to comment upon the likelihood of a progressive deterioration of a condition within the report, as it helps the requesting party plan for these contingencies in the future.

The IME physician needs to understand that there are now several scientific studies that have addressed health status in individuals who are not working. Such "worklessness" has been shown to worsen (or even increase the incidence of) several chronic medical conditions including diabetes, cancer, coronary artery disease, and a variety of mental health conditions. When assessing an individual who has been out of work or one who might not be working into the future, it is relevant to include this vital information.

Medical Management Plan

This section deals with the recommendations for future further evaluations and a treatment plan. It is extremely helpful to the requesting party for the IME physician to describe maintenance care recommendations in detail, listing the frequency of need for physician or other ancillary health care provider visits, the duration of medication need, and the requirements of replacement of prosthetic or medical care devices (ambulatory assistive devices, braces, etc.).

It is also helpful to discuss the time frames that will be required to accomplish the treatments that are being recommended. If surgery is being suggested, normal post-surgical healing periods should be included along with any expected post-surgical care processes. Surgical complications should be discussed if they are unique or pertinent to the decision process or if the surgery is controversial or optional. Also, it is helpful to include expectations of future health care needs if surgery is declined or does not occur for a different reason.

If certain therapies are being suggested, the number of treatments and time frames over which they should occur should be included. If a mental health issue is being addressed, it may be appropriate to discuss the differences between options for care between psychiatrists, psychologists, or other mental health providers.

The reason it is important to include this level of detail is that the requesting party is often in need of making appropriate set-aside determinations or plans for future incurred medical expenses. Obviously, there can be great differences in cost when comparing a surgical case versus one that can be managed with conservative care.

Synthesis of Information

This section of the report often will include the "meat" or "crux" of the issues that the IME physician is being asked to address. Depending upon what the focus of the IME is, there may be extended discussions regarding causation (Melhorn et al., 2014), impairment (Rondinelli, 2008), disability, or return to work (Talmage et al., 2011) recommendations. With comprehensive IMEs, each of these might be included, and it is suggested that they each be given their section and subheading.

There are times when the IME physician may not have enough medical information to answer a question that is posed. The evaluator must be honest when this occurs and not rush to judgment. If additional tests are needed, they should be explained as to what they will help determine. If a different specialty evaluation is needed, the specific issues that the specialist should address should be described.

Within this section, the IME physician must review and analyze all the available documentation and ask whether it fits with the examinee's story or not. Many times, there will be inconsistencies, and the evaluator should not only describe these but also attempt to determine the reasons why.

In cases of long-term disability determination, the IME physician should expressly state if the examinee meets the requirements of disability that are stated within the policy. Of course, this requires that the examiner have a good knowledge of what those requirements are. Since there can be variability between disability systems, a detailed working understanding is paramount.

Conclusion and Recommendations

The concluding section of the IME report includes concluding remarks and specific answers to the questions that have been prepared by the requesting party. It is recommended that the IME report repeats and lists the questions verbatim and that clear and complete answers be given.

It is critical that all the IME physician's opinions be given "within a reasonable degree of medical certainty", which is the legal standard that usually must be met for most of those opinions to be considered and entered as part of legal testimony.

Lastly, the IME physician is wise to include disclaimers at the end of the report. These disclaimers allow the IME physician latitude in changing their opinion if additional medical records are found that were not previously presented or if new medical facts are obtained. They also reinforce the fact that there is not a doctor-patient relationship and that the opinions given in the report are not intended to necessarily be acted upon because the IME physician is not the treating doctor. The disclaimers also point out that the IME physician opinions are not intended to substitute for a legal opinion or for an administrative act to be made or enforced. These last points are critical to avoid the situation where an IME physician is accused of being a "judge and jury" regarding the claim that is being evaluated.

The IME report should always be signed by the IME physician after proper proofreading and correction. It is not acceptable to send a report without a signature or to use a stamp that states "sent unreviewed (or unsigned) to avoid delay". Such practices do not project professionalism and credibility and are to be avoided.

Stylistic Issues and Artistic Points

The written report projects your credibility. Requesting parties may know nothing about you other than what they receive in the mail. Whether that sounds crass or not is irrelevant, because the report that you submit will be read by many individuals. The report's quality is the single most important driver in marketing your performance as an IME physician.

Do not think for a minute that IME physicians operate in a bubble. Claims adjusters, nurse case managers, attorneys, and other stakeholders that utilize IMEs talk among themselves. They do it informally as well as formally. If one does an excellent job with IME reports, it is highly likely that one will receive requests from other parties. Word-of-mouth advertising will take care of itself.

So, what makes a good IME report read well? It should be written in a style that will stimulate the reader. Many claims examiners or attorneys may be reading your report as the tenth one during that day. The idea is that the IME reports should tell a story and move the reader forward. As you read the report, you should get the sensation and the feeling that you want to get to the next section eagerly.

But when writing IME reports, the physician should understand the level of expertise of the reader. Writing at a level that only physicians would be able to understand would be pointless. Although it is acceptable to include proper medical terminology in the physical exam and diagnostic section, the history and discussion sections should be written using lay terminology that most in the public would be able to understand. If medical terms must be used, consider defining them in a glossary.

It is often asked what tone the report should have. This is an excellent question, and there are different opinions on the question because it depends upon how the report is going to be used. Some IME requestors might want a report that has a certain degree of "shock value" if it is going to be used to argue for or against a contentious topic. Nevertheless, in general, it is best to write in a relaxed tone. If there is a feeling when reading the report that someone is shouting at you, chances are the verbiage is too aggressive.

In addition to the traditional teaching points of paying attention to sentence and paragraph length, verb tense consistency is critical. One way of determining whether your report is easy to read is to read it aloud yourself. If something does not sound right, it needs to be revised.

Analogies usually are not useful in IME reports, as the specificity of the medical issues typically precludes their utility. However, there may be a role for them in the discussion section if the IME physician feels that it could drive a point home.

These examinations do not establish a physician-patient relationship. The report should never use the term "patient", as there could be a question that this relationship has been established when other measures have been taken to preclude it. Additionally, other sections of the report should avoid discussions of treatment that are in the active voice. For example, in discussing a potential treatment for peripheral neuropathy, the writer should not say "This examinee should be treated by starting oral gabapentin", but rather "One of the considerations in additional treatment for peripheral neuropathy is gabapentin", thus avoiding any inference of treatment from the IME physician.

The report should avoid redundancies. IME doctors have a lot of trouble with this. State your point once and then move on. Junk words or the use of the "phrase of the day" is unnecessary. The use of clichés or "doctorisms", which are phrases commonly used within our profession that the lay public does not understand, should obviously not be used.

File Reviews

Independent file reviews are IMEs conducted without taking a history or performing an examination. File reviews are in most cases a bit narrower in scope than IMEs, focusing upon only one or two critical questions that the requesting party needs to know about.

Obviously, meticulously focusing on the medical records presented becomes the focal point for the file reviewer. Establishing a trend regarding the care that is given from the time of diagnosis until the time of maximum medical improvement (MMI) or the current time is helpful.

File reviews are simpler when the questions posed are oriented toward asking about whether a treatment for a condition is reasonable and necessary or whether additional medical care is warranted. They are more difficult when questions are asked about causation or disability because the reviewer cannot ask their own questions, which are commonly necessary to fill in gaps in the information that is provided in the record.

With questions regarding causation, the file reviewer is often left to ponder whether the history recorded in the file is accurate and often wishes that more detail exists. In many cases, there is insufficient information within the medical records to allow a file reviewer to determine causation "within a degree of reasonable medical certainty", and the file review report should explain what would be necessary to make a proper determination.

Peer review or pre-certification reports are a type of independent file review where there is a specific request regarding the appropriateness of the medical care being provided to a claimant. Often, there are questions regarding medications, injections, or surgical procedures that are being recommended. In these cases, it is often requested that the independent file reviewer have a discussion with the treating physician regarding the recommendation to obtain a better understanding of the rationale for the intervention. The file reviewer should approach this discussion with an open mind, but at the same time understand what has been documented and what has not been documented within the medical record. The file reviewer should have a good understanding of evidence-based practice guidelines and what they state regarding the intervention in question. The file reviewer may ask the treating physician if they are aware of EBM guideline perspective and delve into issues of why the recommendation is being made if it deviates from these guidelines. It should be noted that in some situations, the treating physician may not be aware of the medical guidelines and the issues, and this is an opportunity for the file reviewer to at least introduce them as a process of education. There are times that a treating physician may be quite resistant to a peer review discussion and be angry that another physician (or a party who has hired them) is challenging their recommendations. Thus, independent file reviewers who must perform peer review discussions should have a bit of "thick skin" when it comes to these interactions.

References

American Board of Independent Medical Examiners. Retrieved June 15, 2022, from www.abime.org

American College of Occupational and Environmental Medicine. Retrieved June 15, 2022, from www. acoem.org

Blair, B. (2014, January 9). *IME bootcamp* (Paper presentation). Proceedings of the 27th Annual Meeting and Scientific Session of the American Academy of Disability Evaluating Physicians (AADEP), San Antonio.

Demeter, S. L., & Washington, R. J. (2003). The impairment-oriented evaluation and report. In S. L. Demeter & G. B. J. Andersson (Eds.), *Disability evaluation* (2nd ed., pp. 111–124). Mosby.

Freeman, G. (1998, March 31). *Tips for writing reports* (Paper presentation). Conference Proceedings of the American Academy of Disability Evaluating Physicians (AADEP) Comprehensive Training Course, Chicago.

International Academy of Independent Medical Evaluators. Retrieved June 15, 2022, from www.iaime.org

Martin, D. W. (2017, April 24) *The independent medical examination* (Paper presentation). Conference Proceedings of the 102nd American Occupational Health Conference, American College of Occupational and Environmental Medicine, Denver, CO.

Martin, D. W. (2018). *Independent medical evaluation: A practical guide*. Springer International Publishing.

Melhorn, M., Talmage, J., Ackerman, W., & Hyman, M. (Eds.). (2014). *AMA guides to the evaluation of disease and injury causation* (2nd ed.). AMA Press.

Nierenberg, C., Brigham, C., Direnfield, L. K., & Burket, C. (2005, November–December). Standards for independent medical examinations. *AMA Guides Newsletter*, *10*(6), 1–9.

Novick, A. K., & Rondinelli, R. D. (2000). Impairment and disability under worker's compensation. In R. D. Rondinelli & R. T. Katz (Eds.), *Impairment rating and disability evaluation* (pp. 141–158). Saunders.

Rondinelli, R. (Ed.). (2008). *AMA guides to the evaluation of permanent impairment* (6th ed.). AMA Press.

SEAK, Inc. Retrieved June 15, 2022, from www.seak.com

Talmage, J. B., Melhorn, J. M., & Hyman, M. H. (Eds.). (2011). *AMA guides to the evaluation of work ability and return to work* (2nd ed., pp. 47–68). AMA Press.

5 Significant Body Systems

Kaitlyn Cyncynatus and Steven Barna

Body Systems

Nervous System

General Overview

The nervous system is divided into two distinctive systems: the central nervous system (CNS) and the peripheral nervous system (PNS). Both divisions receive and process sensory information that will be distributed throughout the processes of the body. The CNS predominantly consists of the brain and spinal cord, while the PNS is composed of cranial and spinal nerves. The brain in the CNS can further be divided into the cerebrum, cerebellum, and brainstem.

The main functions of the nervous system are to transmit sensory information to the brain, where the information will be perceived through distinct, specified areas throughout the brain and transmitted to target areas of the body. The *afferent system* relies on specialized receptor cells that receive and relay sensory information from the environment and within its body system to the brain. Each distinct area of the brain has specified afferent receptors that are sensitive to different signals. Once the brain receives the afferent signals, the *efferent system* sends signals through the brainstem and spinal cord out through the peripheral nerves to elicit a motor response. The transmission between the afferent (in) and efferent (out) systems requires intricate communication throughout the entire nervous system.

The most fundamental functional unit of the nervous system is the *neuron*. The neuron is responsible for the molecular transfer of signals within the brain and the transmissions of communication from the brain to the rest of the body. The neuron consists of four distinct features: the dendrites, cell body (soma), axon, and the axon terminal branches. Dendrites are short, delicate processes located on most of a neuron's anterior portion. Dendrites receive chemical or electrical signals from terminal axonal branches of other neurons and transmit signals toward the cell body. The cell body, or soma, contains the nucleus of the neuron and is responsible for maintaining the cell's overall health. The junction between the cell body and the axon is a region known as the axon hillock that houses the trigger zone.

Neuronal dendrites receive electrical impulses from surrounding neurons that will potentially reach a threshold level that will trigger an influx of ions that causes a depolarization event (see Figure 5.1 for structure illustration). Signals will transduce away from the cell body through the axon, or "nerve fiber," during depolarization, and the conduction of neuronal signals—saltatory conduction—down the axon is a quick "all-or-nothing" process that includes chemical "jumps" between the *nodes of Ranvier* down the axon toward the terminal branches. Axons are encased in a sheath of fat-like insulation material known as *myelin*. Myelin allows for smooth, quick

DOI: 10.4324/b23293-5

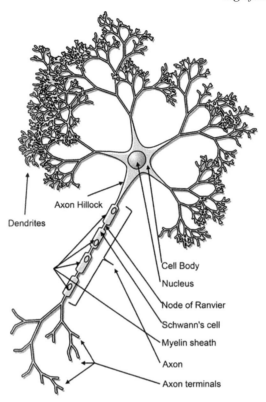

Figure 5.1 Illustration of Key Neuronal Structures

signal transductions down the axon. Once the electrical impulse (action potential) reaches the axonal terminal branches, a chemical signal is released as *neurotransmitters* such as dopamine or acetylcholine. The *synapse* is the transfer of chemical signals through the release of neurotransmitters from the axon terminal branches of one neuron to the receptor dendrites of a nearby neuron. Since the nervous system extends much longer than a single neuron, the efferent and afferent systems rely on chains of neurons for consistent communication throughout the body.

The nerve cell bodies are typically grouped as gray matter, while the myelinated axon tails are designated as white matter. Within the brain, the nerve cell bodies, known as nuclei, can be visualized as the cortex of the brain and are also located deep within the cerebrum. Conversely, the myelinated neuronal tails that create the axonal tracts underlying the gray matter are the white matter, making up the majority of the brain. In the spinal cord, the gray matter is located spanning down the center of the cord, as an H-shape, while the white matter is the outermost portion encasing the gray matter. The gray matter located within the periphery is termed ganglia.

Central Nervous System

The CNS is incased by a variety of protective barriers. All aspects of the CNS float in a liquid of cerebrospinal fluid which protects and acts as a medium of nutrient and waste exchange between the blood and the CNS. The cerebrospinal fluid cushions the brain through internal cavities, termed ventricles, within the cerebrum and brainstem. The cerebrum, cerebellum, and brainstem are protected by the skull, while the spinal cord is protected by the vertebral column. There are also additional membranous layers of coverings that encase and protect the CNS called the *meninges*. These coverings of the *meninges* from the outermost layer are *dura mater*, *arachnoid mater*, and *pia mater*. The cerebrospinal fluid occupies the *subarachnoid space*, or the spaces between the arachnoid mater and pia mater.

Cerebrum

The cerebrum consists of the highest total area of the brain. The cerebrum is separated between two symmetrical hemispheres, the left and the right. The left and right hemispheres have some specialized tasks, such as the left brain being more language-oriented while the right brain is more emotion-focused. Typically, there is one dominant hemisphere that is opposite of the dominant writing hand. However, the two hemispheres communicate through intricate innervations that allow for higher thinking and complex movements. Both hemispheres receive sensory information (afferent) and initiate motor (efferent) responses, as well as have identical anatomical structures. The connective tissue between the two hemispheres is the *corpus callosum*, which allows for the communication of signals between the hemispheres. The hemispheres operate contralaterally, meaning the left hemisphere innervates efferent responses to the right side of the body while the right hemisphere innervates to the left side. The brainstem is the structure of the brain that processes this contralateral control.

The cerebrum has evolved to compact such a large surface area of nerve cells within the size limitations of the skull (see Figure 5.2 for cerebrum anatomy illustration). The brain is not smooth, but instead, the cerebrum consists of copious convoluted folds. These folds are convoluted gyri. Between the gyri lies an intervening furrow, the shallow *sulcus*, while a very deep sulcus is a *fissure*. The outermost layer of the cerebrum is the *cortex*, which consists solely of gray matter. Venturing medially into the cerebrum leads to white matter, tracts, and nuclei (deep gray matter) where synapses occur. Besides strictly separating the cerebrum into two hemispheres, the brain is also divided into four lobes: *frontal lobe*, *parietal lobe*, *temporal lobe*, and *occipital lobe*. Each lobe constitutes different functions, and the cortex will vary depending on the function; all lobes are named after the regions of the skull they reside under.

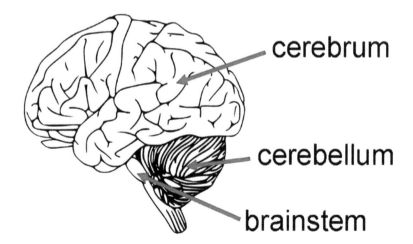

Figure 5.2 Illustration of the Cerebrum

Frontal Lobe

The frontal lobe is the anterior-most portion of the brain. It is located just above the temporal lobe and anterior to the parietal lobe. The frontal and parietal lobes are separated by the central sulcus, while the frontal and temporal lobes are separated by the lateral sulcus. It was the last lobe to evolutionarily develop and has multiple highly processed functions involving memory, attention, motivation, and fine muscle and motor controls. The *motor strip* is located on the posterior end of the frontal lobe. The nerve cells that initiate fine, isolated extremity movements are termed Betz cells, and they are referred to as the *upper motor neurons*. Betz cells are spatially organized in the precentral gyrus, and their axons pass downward to the spinal cord to the *internal capsule* and then the *pyramidal tract*. These upper motor neurons will communicate with lower motor neurons located within the peripheral areas of the body and dictate efferent skeletal muscle movements. The upper motor neurons initiate and terminate all of the movements of the lower motor neurons through the corticospinal tract, where signals will travel through the brainstem and contralaterally propagate to the opposite side of the body. The frontal lobe takes the longest time to fully develop, and therefore is also responsible for higher intellectual roles such as abstract thinking, judgment, and planning for the future. Due to the involvement of these higher processes, the frontal lobe plays a key role in the formation of a personality. Therefore, damage to the frontal lobe before the age of 20 can significantly alter the development of a personality. The prefrontal cortex, responsible for cognitive control functions, and Broca's area, responsible for producing speech, are also notably located in the frontal lobe.

Parietal Lobe

The parietal lobe is located on the top of the head posterior to the frontal lobe. The primary somatosensory cortex is the management relay center for the integration of the body's sensory information such as taste, touch, hearing, sight, and smell. The postcentral gyrus is also located within the parietal lobe and receives and relays afferent information about spatial coordination regarding pain (nociceptors); temperature (thermoreceptors); form, shape, and texture; pressure (mechanoreceptors); and position (proprioceptors).

Temporal Lobe

The temporal lobe is inferior to the parietal lobe and posterior to the frontal lobe. This lobe is primarily responsible for processing auditory information. It is also one of the centers for dreams, memory, and emotions. Located within the left temporal lobe is another essential language processing area named Wernicke's area. Wernicke's area is responsible for language comprehension and works closely with Broca's area in the frontal lobe to comprehend and develop language.

Occipital Lobe

The occipital lobe is the most posterior lobe, and it rests above the cerebellum. The primary function of the occipital lobe is to receive and process visual information. The significant nerve located in this lobe is the optic nerve, which is the bundle of nerves that interprets visual stimuli from the eyes.

Basal Ganglia

The basal ganglia are aggregates of gray matter located within the cerebral hemispheres. Gray matter in the brain constitutes clusters of cell bodies with little to no myelinated axons, while white matter is located deeper in the brain with predominantly long myelinated axons with fewer cell bodies. The differences in color between the cortex and deeper within the brain are due to the difference in color as a result of the myelin sheaths. Myelin sheaths constitute fatty insulation that results in a whiter color versus the unmyelinated gray-colored cell bodies. Myelinated axons allow neurons to send action potentials at a faster velocity compared to unmyelinated neurons. While the frontal lobe is responsible for the specific, fine movements, the basal ganglia regulate motor sequencing, motor skills, and complex actions, but also modulation of higher-order cognitive functions and mood regulation (Riva et al., 2018). The basal ganglia receive afferent information directly from the thalamus and the cerebral cortex and synapse communication signals to the brainstem and spinal cord through the *extrapyramidal system*. The extrapyramidal system is an essential feedback system controlling body movement. The *internal capsule* lies close to the basal ganglia, which contain important efferent motor tracts descending from the frontal lobe descending through the spinal cord.

Thalamus

The thalamus is an egg-shaped structure that is a part of the diencephalon and is located deep and centrally within the cerebral hemispheres. The diencephalon is composed of four components: the dorsal thalamus, ventral thalamus, hypothalamus, and epithalamus. The thalamus is composed primarily of gray matter (cell bodies) and is the main relay center for sensory and motor messages from periphery receptors to the sensory areas of the postcentral gyrus of the parietal cortex. The thalamus works closely with the hypothalamus and pituitary gland to relay hormonal signals through the bloodstream Herrero et al., 2002).

Hypothalamus

The hypothalamus is also one of the four components of the diencephalon. Hypo, meaning under or beneath, means the hypothalamus is located directly below the thalamus. It has a role in the endocrine system as a collection of ganglia that intricately communicates with the pituitary gland. It has a variety of crucial functions:

1. It controls the autonomic system and hence regulates the parasympathetic and sympathetic functions.
2. It is part of the pathway by which emotions influence body functions.
3. It secretes hormones influencing the posterior pituitary gland for maintaining body water control.
4. It secretes hormones that influence the anterior pituitary gland's release of sex, thyroid, and adrenal stimulating hormones.
5. It is part of the arousal mechanism for maintaining the waking state.
6. It is an essential part of the mechanism for regulating appetite.
7. It is crucial for the maintenance of normal body temperature.

Pituitary Gland

The pituitary gland is a pea-sized structure that is located on the base of the hypothalamus. The hypothalami-hypophysial pathway relies on communication from the hypothalamus to the pituitary gland to relay hormones through the endocrine system. Capillaries surround the pituitary gland to allow for the direct transfer of hormones throughout the body to the bloodstream. The pituitary gland is the master gland of hormone release. The pituitary gland is divided into the front (anterior) and back (posterior) pituitary. The hypothalamus communicates directly to the posterior pituitary gland through a stalk of blood vessels and nerves, sending nerve impulses to communicate with the anterior pituitary (Daniel & Prichard, 1966). Some of the main hormones released from the anterior pituitary gland are:

1. Follicle-stimulating hormone (FSH)
2. Luteinizing hormone (LH)
3. Growth hormone (GH)
4. Thyroid-stimulating hormone (TSH)

Additionally, some of the main hormones that are made in the hypothalamus and are stored or released from the posterior pituitary are:

1. Antidiuretic hormone or vasopressin (ADH)
2. Oxytocin

Language Areas

The language function is a collaborative communication system between multiple lobes of the cerebral hemisphere. The receptive functions include the integration of visual and auditory afferent input, while the efferent motor output utilizes an expressive function. The language areas are located in the left cerebral hemisphere; however, language requires association between the frontal, parietal, and temporal lobes. *Wernicke's area* is centered over the parietal and temporal cortex and is the main receptive function. Wernicke's area receives audio or visual information and allows the brain to interpret and encode language. Conversely, *Broca's area* is located just anterior to the temporal lobe and is the main expressive function. Broca's area controls and manages speech production. Damage to Wernicke's area blocks interpretation of language but allows for normal communication, while damage to Broca's area allows for an incomplete interpretation of language and inappropriate speech responses. *Association areas* are interconnections between areas of the cortex within a single hemisphere or between hemispheres that allow for higher mental and emotional processes.

Cerebellum

The cerebellum, or the "little brain", is the posterior-most portion of the brain. It is located directly under the occipital lobe. The cerebellum consists of its cortex of gray matter with sulci and gyri, right and left hemispheres with a central section, and almost all information to and from the cerebellum is processed by the midbrain of the brainstem. The cerebellum is responsible for the maintenance and function of posture and coordination. Working closely with the cerebral cortex, the cerebellum allows for smooth and accurate motor movements and consists of a motor plan. The motor plan utilizes unconscious muscle feedback to adjust and plan for smooth movement and adjustments. The cerebellum has three main functions:

1. Maintenance of equilibrium and balance of the trunk. Afferent input comes from the vestibular portion of the eighth cranial nerve. Efferent messages leave the cerebellum and connect with the reticular formation of the brainstem concerned with vestibular functions (equilibrium).
2. Regulation of muscle tension, spinal nerve reflexes, and posture and balance of the limbs. Afferent information arrives from the muscles and tendons of the limbs. Efferent messages synapse in the brainstem to influence the extrapyramidal system to affect fine motor control.

3. Regulation of the coordination of fine limb movements originally initiated by the frontal lobe. Afferent information comes from the cerebral cortex via the pons of the brainstem. Efferent information goes back to the cerebral cortex via the thalamus for fine motor control.

Brainstem

The brainstem sits between the cerebrum and the spinal cord. This structure is the connection between the cerebrum, spinal cord, cranial nerves, and cerebellum. The brainstem is composed of three parts in the order of the *midbrain* (cerebral peduncles), the *pons*, and the *medulla oblongata*. The midbrain regulates motor movement such as eye movements as well as auditory and visual processing. The pons collaborates with the midbrain to control eye reflexes such as pupil and eye movements, especially during rapid eye movement (REM) sleep. Finally, the medulla is the most important structure of the brainstem. The medulla works closely with the pons to regulate the respiratory rhythm of breathing. The medulla also regulates throat reflexes such as vomiting, sneezing, coughing, and swallowing as well as cardiac functions and the diameter of small arteries, otherwise understood as blood pressure.

Nerve fibers between the cerebrum and spinal cord must pass through the brainstem, and cell masses termed the *reticular formation* are also associated with the brainstem. The reticular formation initiates and maintains wakefulness and alertness. Long tracts of axons from the cerebrum (motor tracts and somatosensory tracts) travel through the brainstem to go to the spinal cord. All structures of the brainstem work intricately with cranial nerves III–XII. All nerve cell nuclei are located within the brainstem. Unlike the cross-communication method between the different cerebral hemispheres, the left cranial nerves control the left body movements, while the right cranial nerves control the right body movements.

The early years of the development and study of medicine as a science and as a practice focused on the description and classification of the cranial nerves (Porras-Gallo et al., 2019). Anatomists realized the importance of the cranial nerves due to these nerves' characteristics of anatomy for which Porras-Gallo et al. gave much credit to the influence of these nerves in the rationality of medicine coupled with social, cultural, religious, and philosophical factors (p. 381). The relevance of the cranial nerves is underscored in human anatomy. These nerves carry information from sensory organs to the brain, with instructions for the muscles of all of the organs in the face, neck, heart, and abdomen (Trejo, 2019). In essence, the cranial nerves' relevancy encompasses everyone's senses of smell, facial sensations, vision, hearing, swallowing, breathing, and heartbeats. A listing of the 12 cranial nerve functions within our body systems is listed as follows, and the 12 cranial nerves are illustrated in Figure 5.3:

1. Olfactory: Sense of smell.
2. Optic: Sense of vision.
3. Oculomotor: Movement of the eye up, down, and in toward the nose; constriction of the pupil.
4. Trochlear: Movement of the eye down and out.
5. Trigeminal: Muscles of mastication; sensation of skin and face, teeth, and lining of mouth and nose.
6. Abducens: Movement of the eye outwards.
7. Facial: Muscles of facial expression; taste to the anterior two-thirds of the tongue; salivary glands secretion.
8. Vestibulocochlear (acoustic).

   a. Vestibular portion: Equilibrium and balance.
   b. Cochlear portion: Sense of hearing.

12 Cranial Nerves

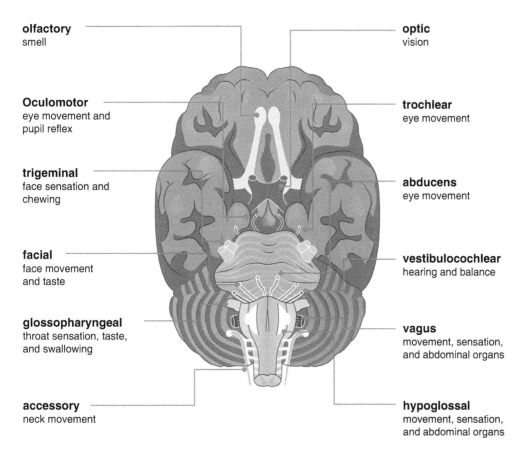

olfactory
smell

optic
vision

Oculomotor
eye movement and
pupil reflex

trochlear
eye movement

trigeminal
face sensation and
chewing

abducens
eye movement

facial
face movement
and taste

vestibulocochlear
hearing and balance

glossopharyngeal
throat sensation, taste,
and swallowing

vagus
movement, sensation,
and abdominal organs

accessory
neck movement

hypoglossal
movement, sensation,
and abdominal organs

Figure 5.3 The 12 Cranial Nerves

9. Glossopharyngeal: Swallowing and speech sounds; taste to the posterior one-third of the tongue.
10. Vagus: Swallowing and speech sounds; heart rate; gastrointestinal movement.
11. Spinal accessory: Neck muscles (trapezius and sternocleidomastoid).
12. Hypoglossal: Tongue movement; speech; swallowing movement (Johnson, 2019).

Spinal Cord

Afferent and efferent information must travel to and from the spinal cord through distinct nerve fiber tracts at various levels throughout the spinal cord. Afferent information received from the periphery will enter from the trunk and extremities and travel through the somatosensory nerve tracts in the spinal cord to reach the cerebrum, cerebellum, and brainstem. Similarly, efferent impulses will travel from the cerebrum, cerebellum, and brainstem through the distinct nerve tracts to the spinal cord. The spinal cord is protected by the vertebrae of the spine. The spinal cord has five distinct nerve areas running down the back end of the body. From top to bottom the nerve areas of the spine include the cervical nerves (C1–C8), thoracic nerves (T1–T11), lumbar

SPINAL CORD

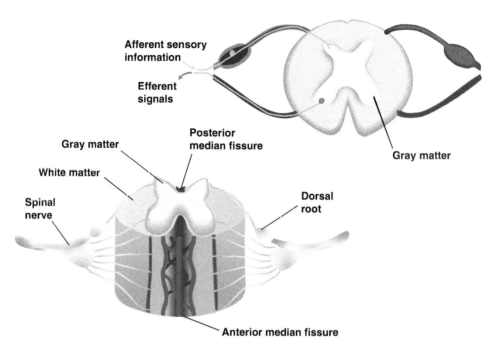

Afferent sensory
information

Efferent
signals

Gray matter

White matter

Spinal
nerve

Posterior
median fissure

Gray matter

Dorsal
root

Anterior median fissure

Figure 5.4 Spinal Cord, Nerves, and the Brain

nerves (L1–L4), sacral nerves (S1–S3), and coccygeal nerves. All nerves integrated within the vertebrae maintain different functions.

The spinal cord also consists of well-defined areas of gray matter where synapses occur for the transmission of these impulses. (See Figure 5.4 for spinal cord and brain anatomy illustration.) Unlike the architecture of the cerebrum where the gray matter is located only on the cortex and deep within the cerebrum, in the spinal cord the gray matter is flipped and surrounded by the cerebrum. The ventral or *anterior horns* are the anterior projections of this gray matter and are the location of the final synapse for efferent impulses leaving the spinal cord. Conversely, the dorsal or *posterior horns* are the posterior projections of the gray matter and are the location of many initial synapses for afferent information entering the spinal cord.

Three main tracts are located within the spinal cord—the *spinothalamic tract*, which carries pain (nociceptors) and temperature (thermoreceptors) impulses to the thalamus for synaptic relay to the postcentral gyrus of the parietal lobe; the *posterior columns*, which carry position sense and pressure sense impulses to the thalamus, also for relay to the parietal lobe; and the *corticospinal* or pyramidal *tract*, which carries impulses from the precentral gyrus through the internal capsule of the frontal lobe to initiate muscle activity. These upper motor neurons synapse in the anterior horns with cells of the *lower motor neurons* whose axons leave the spinal cord via spinal nerves.

The spinal cord is also associated with basic reflexes that utilize autonomic motor movements. Reflexes either involve a direct motor movement due to quick sensory information transcending through motor neurons or a cascade of communication through interneurons to initiate a motor response. Reflexes such as the traditional "knee-jerk" reaction take place unconsciously through the spinal cord to elicit a fast motor response.

Peripheral Nervous System

Somatic Nervous System

Within the spinal cord, the PNS is composed of a collection of nerves innervated throughout the spinal level. Spinal nerves each have two roots (anterior [providing motor innervation] and posterior [providing sensory innervation]) that act as an intermediary between the sensory information of the CNS and motor movements of the periphery (Kaiser & Lugo-Pico, 2021). The anterior roots contain the axons of the cell bodies in the anterior horn within the spinal cord, while the posterior root has cells bodies outside, but close to, the spinal cord in the sensory nerve ganglia, therefore consisting of a total of two axons. There are 30 pairs of spinal nerves that correspond with each vertebra (8 cervical, 12 thoracic, 5 lumbar, and 5 sacral), each named after the corresponding vertebra near which the nerve exits from the vertebral canal. The one exception in the number of spinal pairs not matching the vertebrae is in the cervical segments, where there are eight nerves and only seven vertebrae.

As a refresher, the nerve areas of the spine from top to bottom include the cervical nerves (C1–C8), thoracic nerves (T1–T11), lumbar (L1–L4), sacral (S1–S3), and coccygeal. The vertebral canal is longer than the spinal cord itself; as a result some spinal nerves, particularly at the lower levels, have to travel down a significant distance before leaving the vertebral canal. In particular, the nerve complex *cauda equina* (horse's tail) at the L2 vertebral level must travel inferiorly in the column extending downward to the S5 vertebral level. From the L2 vertebral level downward, therefore, up to eight pairs of spinal nerves occupy this space within the vertebral canal.

The upper half of the cervical level (C1–C5) consists of the *cervical plexus*, while the lower half of the cervical level (C5–C8), as well as a contribution for T1, consists of *the brachial plexus*. The nerves that form the brachial plexus merge in the neck region that form peripheral nerves, each of which has axons from more than one spinal level. The cervical spinal nerves control movement of the upper body such as shoulder and arm muscles and collectively receive sensory information from specialized receptors located within the skin, muscles, bones, and joints.

The thoracic spinal nerves (T1–T11) do not merge into a plexus. The anterior roots of the thoracic spinal nerves innervate peripheral and visceral motor fibers of the muscles of the abdomen and the back, while the posterior roots receive afferent information about the abdominal organs and innervation of the skin, muscles, joints, chest, abdomen, and upper back.

The lumbar (L1–L4) and sacral (S1–S3), however, do merge in the pelvis after leaving the vertebral column and form the *lumbosacral plexus*. This plexus provides sensory and motor innervation to the lower extremity, bladder, and anal sphincter.

Reflexes are an important component of the spinal cord. A reflex is an automatic involuntary response of a body part in response to a stimulus. Reflexes are not consciously processed in the brain and are quick reactions due to interneuron communication. Some reflexes only require a single synapse between an afferent (sensory) and efferent (motor) nerve, which are termed *monosynaptic reflexes*. A common example of such a monosynaptic reflex is a tendon (stretch) reflex or the patellar "knee-jerk" reflex. The stretch of the tendon sends an afferent impulse through a posterior root, which in turn synapses with an anterior horn at the same level in the spinal cord as it entered. This synapse will trigger an efferent impulse in the anterior horn axon to the anterior root of the spinal nerve back to the tendon that was stretched, resulting in muscle contraction. *Polysynaptic reflexes* include several nerves, where synapses are interposed between the afferent and efferent nerves. An example of a polysynaptic nerve is the withdrawal reflex (immediate withdrawal of a hand from a hot stove). Reflexes also exist which govern the action of various body organs such as the heart, blood vessels, and gastrointestinal (GI) tract movement.

Autonomic Nervous System

The autonomic nervous system is intimately connected to the brain and spinal cord. Ultimately, the autonomic nervous system is not under voluntary control, otherwise known as the "automatic" nervous system. Its function is to regulate automatic body functions such as the stomach and intestines, the heart, the smooth muscle around the arteries, the sweat glands, the salivary glands, and the bladder. The autonomic nervous system can be further divided into two subsystems, the *sympathetic* and the *parasympathetic*. These two systems are antagonistic toward each other.

The sympathetic nervous system is also known as the "fight or flight" system when the body needs to quickly react to external stimuli or danger. The sympathetic nervous system begins in the center of the spinal cord and relays signals to the ganglia located close to the spine followed by shorter second neurons. The brain will send immediate signals to the rest of the body such as dilating pupils, inhibiting salivation, dilating airways, increasing heart rate, inhibiting the activity of the stomach and intestines, and stimulating the release of glucose, secreting epinephrine and norepinephrine, and releasing the bladder. All these functions help to elicit fast reactions to a threat. The sympathetic nerve fibers act as a circuit by leaving the spinal cord through the anterior roots of all the thoracic spinal nerves (located below the shoulders around the chest) and the first three lumbar spinal nerves (located within the lower back). Then, these nerve fibers branch off the spinal nerves to join a chain of ganglia lying on either side of the vertebral column where the first synapse will occur. Next, the second sympathetic fiber (*postganglionic*) then returns to the spinal nerve to be distributed throughout the extremities or proceed directly to blood vessels and organs.

The parasympathetic nervous system is also known as the "rest and digest" system and creates contrasting effects on the sympathetic nervous system. The parasympathetic nervous system begins in the brainstem or the bottom of the spine and sends long axons out to ganglion target cells and shorter second neurons. This system is in effect when the body is in a resting state and no threat is available. The brain will send impulses throughout the body to constrict pupils, stimulate saliva, constrict airways, slow heartbeat (controlled by the vagus nerve, cranial nerve X), stimulate the activity of the stomach and intestines, inhibit the release of glucose, and constrict the bladder. The parasympathetic nervous system consists of two parts: the cranial portion, which leaves the CNS with cranial nerves III, VII, IX, and X, and the sacral part (located around the top portion of the gluteus maximus), which exits the spinal cord with sacral spinal nerves 2, 3, and 4. Both subsystems can be influenced by hormones and emotions.

Musculoskeletal System

The musculoskeletal system is an interplay of collaboration between the skeletal system (bones and joints) and the muscle system (voluntary or striated muscles). The human body could not function without the collaboration between these two systems to create accurate, smooth movements. The functions of the musculoskeletal system are:

1. To provide a rigid support framework for the body.
2. To protect vital internal body organs.
3. To manufacture blood cells (hematopoietic function).
4. To store minerals such as calcium and phosphorus for the maintenance of bones.
5. To provide a series of lever arms on which muscles act across joints to produce force and resulting body movements to combat the effects of gravity.

Tissues

The musculoskeletal system is composed of multiple forms of connective tissue such as cartilage, ligament, tendon, bone, and muscle. Connective tissue is further characterized by multiple components: the fibroblast, collagen, elastic fibers, and proteoglycans.

The *fibroblast* is the most common form of connective tissue. Fibroblasts secrete *collagen* which allows for and maintains a structural framework of tissue.

Collagen is the most abundant protein in the body and creates the building blocks for cartilage. It forms long, thin fibrils that intertwine into strong, structural fibers. Due to the strength of collagen proteins, it is utilized in bones, skin, hair, muscles, tendons, and ligaments. Collagen and elastin are known for both their strength and flexibility.

Elastin, elastic fibers, however, oppose collagen proteins by their flexible, stretchy characteristics. Elastic fibers are utilized in areas of the body that need to be stretched, such as arteriole walls.

Finally, all aspects of the connective tissue are found embedded within a matrix, a nonliving, extracellular substance called the ground substance (*proteoglycans*). Proteoglycans consist primarily of carbohydrates and protein.

Cartilage

Cartilage is composed of connective tissue and fats, while also containing a high content of proteoglycans and water, giving it its gel-like flexibility. Cartilage is not innervated, meaning it does not receive nerve cells, and it is also avascular, only receiving its blood supply and nourishment from surrounding capillaries.

Cartilage is separated into three different types: hyaline cartilage, elastic cartilage, and fibrous cartilage. Hyaline cartilage is the most important cartilage, responsible for reducing friction and absorbing shock. Hyaline cartilage serves three major functions: (a) it forms the "original skeleton" in the embryo, from which bone later develops; (b) it is responsible for the growth of long bones; and (c) it lines the opposing surfaces of the most important joints in the body, the synovial joints. Hyaline cartilage is found in the larynx, trachea, throat, and joints. Elastic cartilage is used for shape and support due to a large concentration of elastic fibers. Elastic cartilage is found in the ear and epiglottis. Finally, fibrous cartilage functions for its rigidity and shock absorption between joints with a high concentration of collagen. Fibrous cartilage is found mainly in the intervertebral discs and pelvis.

Ligaments

Ligaments are fibrous tissue that connects bone directly to bone. They are a strong, dense connective tissue structure that is largely composed of collagen and some elastic fibers. They also stabilize joints and determine certain ranges of motion. A well-known example of a ligament is the anterior cruciate ligament (ACL), which connects the thigh to the shin.

Tendons

Tendons are tough cords of tightly packed, thick, parallel fibers that connect the contracting part of the muscle to bone. Tendons are highly composed of collagen fibers and fewer elastic fibers. A primary example of a tendon is the Achilles tendon located in the ankle that connects the calf muscle to the heel bone.

Muscles

Muscles are the contracting unit of the skeletal system, and muscle fibers are long, narrow, mult-inucleated cells attached to tendons on each end. There are three different categories of muscle cells: skeletal muscle, cardiac muscle, and smooth muscle. Cardiac muscles are branched, striated muscle units with one or two nuclei and are only found in the heart. Smooth muscles are non-striated, single-nuclei cells attached to a spindle. Smooth muscles are found in hollow organs such as blood vessels. Both cardiac and smooth muscles are under involuntary control. Finally, skeletal muscles are striated, multinucleated cells under voluntary control. Within each muscle fiber are two essential proteins for muscle contraction, *actin* and *myosin*. The striation of muscle cells is a result of where the actin and myosin fibers overlap. There are two types of muscle-skeletal fibers: type I and type II. Type I muscle fibers appear red in color due to a high concentration of mitochondria present within the muscle cell. The mitochondria is a power-house in the cell that produces the energetic adenosine triphosphate (ATP) molecule responsible for oxidative phosphorylation. Due to type I muscle fibers containing a high number of mito-chondria, type I fibers are used for tasks that include a lot of energy for a long amount of time such as the legs. Type I fibers are fatigue-resistant and have strong power. Conversely, type II muscle fibers appear white due to their lack of mitochondria within the fibers. Type II muscle fibers are responsible for fast-paced, short movements such as flicking a finger. Type II fibers fatigue quickly but contract fast.

During muscle contraction, myosin will attach to actin through a myosin cross-bridge and utilize energy to contract and shorten muscle fibers. This contraction is largely due to the avail-ability of energy, the activation through a motor nerve attached to each muscle fiber, and the release of Ca^{2+} ions into the muscle sarcolemma. Myosin and actin are also controlled and monitored by troponin and tropomyosin that are directly attached to the actin protein. Troponin and tropomyosin act as gatekeepers and prevent the muscle fiber from randomly contracting. The attachment of the motor neuron occurs at the motor endplate, where acetylcholine (Ach) is released at the motor endplate when the electrical impulse reaches the muscle fiber. The location where motor neurons synapse and communicate with muscle fibers is known as the *neuromus-cular junction*. Finally, motor control through the nervous system is due to the motor neuron control located within the cerebrum. The upper motor neurons will send axonal tracts through the brainstem and spinal cord to communicate with the lower motor neurons, which will eventu-ally send a message to the muscle to contract.

Bone

Bone is a specialized form of connective tissue that derives its strength from the production and deposition of calcium crystals on the collagen fiber framework. Bone regulates the varying cal-cium levels within the blood, which are controlled through the endocrine system. The endocrine system monitors calcium levels and secretes varying hormones throughout the bloodstream to control the ratio of bone construction to destruction. The intestines, vitamin D, the kidney, the parathyroid gland, and sex and adrenal hormones also have important roles in this bone bal-ance. The cellular components that make up bone are osteoprogenitor cells, osteoblasts, and osteoclasts. Osteoprogenitor cells are the precursor cells to osteoblasts and provide the growth factors. Osteoblasts synthesize collagen and protein that form osteoid, which will eventually mature into the osteocyte. Osteoblasts are responsible for building up bone, while osteoclasts are responsible for bone reabsorption, which leads to the breakdown of bone.

Bones are identified in two main types: (a) flat bones and (b) the long bones of the extremi-ties. Flat bones are composed of inner spongy or cancellous bone and an outer compact bone shell. Some examples of flat bones include the skull, ribs, and pelvis. Conversely, long bones are composed of spongy medullary cavities and a hard compact outer layer. Examples of long bones include the humerus, femur, and upper leg.

There are two different types of bone marrow: (a) red bone marrow and (b) yellow bone marrow. Red bone marrow is the primary site for hematopoiesis (the production of red blood cells) and is primarily found in the epiphysis of long bones. Most red bone marrow changes to yellow bone marrow in adults, where it will be the primary fat storage center for adipocytes. Yellow bone marrow is predominantly found in the diaphysis of bone.

On each end of the long bone is a structure called the *epiphysis*, and the shaft that runs along and connects them is the *diaphysis*. The point between the epiphysis and diaphysis is called the metaphysis, or *epiphyseal plate* of hyaline cartilage, which is also where the growth plate is located.

The *periosteum* is the outermost layer of bone. It is a tough, connective tissue with cells capable of producing compact bone, which overlies the entire shaft. Flat bones are formed from the periosteum alone.

Loose Connective Tissue

Loose connective tissue includes a network of very loosely arranged fibroblasts, collagen, and elastic fibers in a "ground substance". Loose connective tissue works to hold organs in place and lies between muscles that slide past each other and between bone and muscle (Kamrani et al., 2022).

Joints

Joints are a point where bone articulates with one or more bone(s). There are three different classifications of joints: immovable (fibrous), slightly movable (cartilaginous), and freely movable (synovial).

Immovable (fibrous) joints are found in areas of the skeleton between the skull bones that connect bones by rough collagenous connective tissue. Slightly movable (cartilaginous) joints unite bones by cartilage such as intervertebral discs. Finally, freely movable (synovial) joints unite the extremities of the skeleton through distinct features.

Synovial joints are the main functional joints of the body and consist of four constant features:

1. The *joint capsule* fully surrounds the joint and is composed of connective tissue that is reinforced by ligaments. The capsule extends from the cortex and periosteum in the region of the epiphyseal plates of the two opposing bones.
2. The *synovial membrane*, a continuous sheet of loose connective tissue, lines the inside of the capsule and has a thin layer of specialized synovial cells on its surface.
3. The hyaline *articular cartilage* surfaces at the ends of each of the bones that make up the joint are in constant contact during movement. The joint cavity borders the hyaline cartilages and the synovial membrane, where it receives most of its fluid.
4. The viscous *synovial fluid* is produced by the synovial membrane. It provides a high level of lubrication for the opposing hyaline cartilage surfaces and for the synovial membrane itself during joint movement.

Synovial joints can also be further classified into six categories, which are determined by the type of movements they permit: hinge, saddle, planar, pivot, condyloid, and ball and socket (Juneja et al., 2021).

Skeletal System

The human body is composed of 206 bones, each of which is divided into two subgroups, axial and appendicular skeletons. The axial skeleton can also be referenced due to the "axis of the body", which is composed of the skull, ribcage, vertebral column, lower jaw (*mandible*), and breastbone (*sternum*). The appendicular skeleton is composed of all the extremities outside of the axis of the body such as the pelvis and appendages.

Axial Skeleton

Skull. The main function of the skull is to protect and encase the vulnerable brain tissue from any sort of impact or damage. The skull's 22 total bones consist of two fundamental parts: the bones of the cranium and the bones of the facial skeleton. The upper teeth are embedded within the immovable maxilla, and the lower teeth are embedded in the mandible (jaw), which is the only freely movable skull bone. The facial skeleton supports the muscles of the face and scalp by acting as an attachment point.

Thorax. The thoracic cage consists of the sternum anteriorly, the 12 thoracic vertebrae posteriorly, and the 12 pairs of ribs, which function to protect the thoracic cavity, including the lungs and the heart. The ribs are connected posteriorly to the thoracic vertebrae. Anteriorly, 10 ribs are connected to the sternum by cartilage, and two ribs are "floating".

Vertebral column. The essential function of the vertebral column is to encase and protect the spinal cord. (See Figure 5.5 for vertebral column illustration.) There are 33 total vertebrae, discussed previously in the chapter, and each one essentially has the same basic components, differing in function and structure based on the permitted movements allotted according to the location. The vertebral column is also responsible for transmitting body weight from the head, thorax, and abdomen to the lower extremities.

Appendicular Skeleton

The appendicular skeleton consists of the extremities of the body, the shoulder girdle, and the pelvis (which function as attachment points between the appendicular skeleton and the axial skeleton).

Upper extremity. The *sternoclavicular joint* is the point at which the appendicular skeleton directly articulates with the axial skeleton. The arm is attached to the thorax via the collar bone (*clavicle*), and the upper arm bone (*humerus*) is united to the shoulder bone (*scapula*) at the shoulder joint (*synovial joint*). The scapula is further attached to the thoracic cage by muscles. Following the anatomy of the arm medially to distally starting at the shoulder, the humerus unites the forearm bones (*radius* and *ulna*) and the elbow joint; the forearm bones unite with the bones of the palm (*metacarpals*) through three different sets of joints via the eight *carpal* bones of the wrist; and, finally, the knuckles (*metacarpophalangeal*, or MCP, joints) connect the metacarpals to the proximal *phalanx* of the fingers. Each finger consists of three phalanges—proximal, middle, and distal—except for the thumb, which only consists of two phalanges (Anderson et al., 2021a).

Lower extremity. The sacroiliac joint is another point at which the appendicular skeleton directly articulates with the axial skeleton. The sacroiliac joint is also a synovial joint where the sacrum articulates with the ilium. The pelvis (*innominate bone*) transmits the upper body weight from the sacrum to the legs. Following the anatomy of the leg from medially to distally, the hip bone consists of three fused hipbones (*ilium, ischium*, and *the pubis*), which are united through the pelvic bone to the thigh bone (*femur*). The knee joint, which includes the kneecap (*patella*), unites the femur to the two bones in the lower leg (*tibia and fibula*). The ankle joint is what unites the lower leg bones to the talus, where body weight is distributed

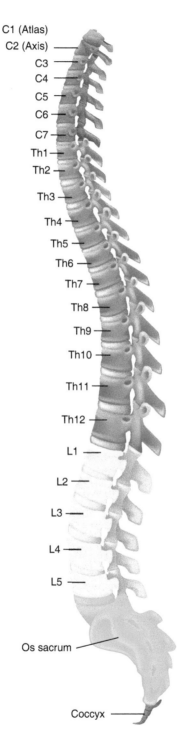

C1 (Atlas)
C2 (Axis)
C3
C4
C5
C6
C7
Th1
Th2
Th3
Th4
Th5
Th6
Th7
Th8
Th9
Th10
Th11
Th12
L1
L2
L3
L4
L5
Os sacrum
Coccyx

Figure 5.5 Spinal Vertebral Column

through the heel (*calcaneus*) and balls of the feet (via the *tarsals* and *metatarsals*—similar to the carpals and metacarpals in hand anatomy). The toes have the same phalangeal structure as the fingers as well (Anderson et al., 2021a).

Skeletal Muscle System

Three different muscle types are within the body: skeletal muscle, cardiac muscle, and smooth muscle. Skeletal muscle is visibly different from the other two muscle types through distinctions of striations and multinucleated cells. The striated appearance of skeletal muscle types is a direct result of the myosin and actin fibers overlapping in the cell, used for their characteristic muscle contractions. Skeletal muscles are under voluntary control, unlike cardiac and smooth muscles, which are under involuntary control. Two ends of a muscle are attached to different bones, meaning muscles cross at least one synovial joint. Thus, when a muscle contracts, or shortens, one bone is moved in relation to the other and the axis of movement is at the joint connecting the two bones. The *origin* of the muscle is the area that is attached closest to the head or body (proximal attachment) and remains stationary during contraction. The distal end of the muscle attachment is termed the *insertion*, which moves during contraction.

All muscles have specific names that are described by the function of the muscle. Muscles or groups of muscles that bend a limb are flexors, while muscles that straighten a limb are called extensors. Muscles that move a limb to the side away from the axis of the body are called abductors, while muscles that move a limb toward the midline are adductors. The other functional groups of muscles are elevators (muscles for biting and chewing), depressors (downward motion), rotators, dorsiflexors (foot and ankle), plantar flexors (stretching the foot), and palmar flexors (flexing in the hand).

Cardiovascular System

The cardiovascular system distributes nutrients, oxygen, and hormones to all living cells through the blood and carries waste products and carbon dioxide away from the cells. Blood cells are the main functional component of the cardiovascular system that travels from the heart to the rest of the body through blood vessels. Blood vessels are composed of smooth muscle that lacks striations and is under involuntary control. The main contributing factor to the circulation of blood throughout the body is the driving force due to the pumping of the heart.

Two distinct circulatory methods are functioning simultaneously in the body. *Pulmonary circulation*, driven by the "right heart", delivers deoxygenated blood (rich in carbon dioxide) to the lungs. *Systemic circulation*, driven by the "left heart", delivers oxygenated blood that had returned from pulmonary circulation out to the tissues.

Blood vessels that transport blood away from the heart are arteries, and the blood vessels that return blood to the heart from the tissues (or lungs) are veins. The largest artery is the aorta, and the largest veins are the superior/inferior vena cava. The flow of blood through blood vessels during systemic circulation is artery, arterioles, capillaries, venules, and veins. During systemic circulation, tissues and vessels exchange oxygen, nutrients, and waste products. Therefore, when the blood returns to the heart through veins, it is predominantly rich in carbon dioxide. Pulmonary circulation includes the flow of carbon dioxide–rich blood pumped through the right heart into the lungs, where the nutrient exchange occurs. In the lungs, the blood becomes rich in oxygen and is pumped back into the left heart after the completion of pulmonary circulation. The oxygen-rich blood is then pumped through the systemic circulation and carried away in arteries.

Blood

Healthy adults have between five and six liters of blood. The hematologic system is composed of three main features: plasma (consisting of mostly water and proteins), white blood cells and platelets, and red blood cells. Plasma comprises 55% of blood, and of the proteins found in plasma, globulins are essential for immunity. There are five types of white blood cells: neutrophils, basophils, eosinophils, lymphocytes, and monocytes. White blood cells play an essential role in innate immunity (the body's natural response to foreign pathogens or bacteria). Platelets make up approximately less than 1% of blood and play a major role in blood clotting after damage to the skin occurs, with albumin and fibrinogen proteins.

Red blood cells (erythrocytes) are the densest component of blood and constitute around 45% of total blood content. Red blood cells consist of hemoglobin, which is an iron-containing heme-protein structure that is directly responsible for the cooperative binding activities of oxygen. Red blood cells are the main oxygen carriers from the heart to the tissues and carbon dioxide from the tissues back to the heart.

Heart

Structure

The heart is approximately the size of one's fist, and it lies to the left of the midline positioned toward the left lung. The right lung has three distinct lobes, while the left lung only has two lobes and a cardiac notch that allows the heart to rest in the lungs. The heart is enclosed by a double-layered loose sac, the *pericardium*. A small amount of fluid between the two layers lubricates the surface, allowing the heart to change its shape without friction as it pumps. The heart is composed of three layers: the innermost layer (*endocardium*), the thick middle layer which is responsible for the heart's ability to pump without stopping (*myocardium*), and the outermost layer (*epicardium*). The myocardium contains the contractile cardiac muscles (not under voluntary control).

Chambers. The heart is composed of four distinct chambers: two atria and two ventricles. The ventricles consist of thicker muscles, and their contractions are responsible for the driving force of blood through the systemic circulation. Blood returning from the systemic circulation will first drain into the right atrium from the superior and inferior *vena cava*. Deoxygenated blood will flow from the right atrium through the *tricuspid valve* into the right ventricle. The right ventricle will then contract and propel blood through the *pulmonary semilunar valve* into the *pulmonary artery* for pulmonary circulation. Once the blood has become oxygenated, it will return from the lungs into the left atrium through the *pulmonary vein*. Once blood collects in the left atrium, it will be pushed through the mitral valve into the left ventricle. Finally, left ventricular contraction forces the blood through the *aortic semilunar valve* into the *aorta* for systemic circulation. The function of valves in the heart is to separate the chambers and to prevent blood backflow from happening and halting the process of circulation. The walls between the two ventricles and the two atria, the interventricular septum and the interatrial septum, block the mixing of the two circulations in the normal condition.

Cardiac Cycle and Heart Sounds

Each cycle of the heart consists of two parts, *diastole* and *systole*. During diastole, the chambers of the heart are relaxed while both atria are receiving and filling with blood from the two circulatory systems. During systole, the cycle first begins with right and left atrial contraction, propelling blood through the mitral and tricuspid valves followed by the strong contraction of the ventricles. Ventricular systole, the main pumping action, forcefully propels blood into the pulmonary artery and aorta through the pulmonary and aortic semilunar valves. During this contraction, the mitral and tricuspid valves snap shut to prevent the backflow of blood into the atria, and the shutting of the valves causes the audible sound of the heartbeat. The first heart sound (S1) is also called "lub". The forcing of blood through arteries from the ventricles causes the pulse beat that can be felt. When ventricular contraction stops, the vessels recoil, and the semilunar valves slam shut to prevent the flow of blood back into the ventricles, and this closure results in the second heart sound. The second heart sound (S2) is also known as "dub". "Lub-dub" is the informal description of the heart sounds heard through a stethoscope.

Murmurs. Murmurs are sounds other than the two normal heart sounds, which can sometimes be heard and signify disease. Murmurs develop due to alteration in blood flow or valve dysfunction. Murmurs can be heard through changes in pitch, volume, or rhythm changes in heartbeats.

Blood pressure. Blood pressure is typically recorded in the arm and records two numbers: *systolic pressure* (ventricular systole) and *diastolic pressure* (diastole). Normal blood pressure is approximately recorded as 120/80, measured in millimeters of mercury (mmHg). The magnitude of the blood pressures is directly proportional to the force produced by the myocardial contraction of the ventricle and the resistance to flow produced by the narrowing peripheral arterial blood vessel diameters. Blood pressure and blood volume are regulated through hormones of the endocrine and excretory system (kidney). Examples of hormones that affect blood pressure are ADH, angiotensin, aldosterone, and atrial natriuretic hormone (ANP) (Evrard et al., 1999).

Cardiac output. Cardiac output is the amount of blood pumped by the heart per minute. It is calculated by multiplying the volume ejected with each ventricular contraction (stroke volume) by the number of beats per minute (heart rate). Stroke volume should vary from 60 to 70 cc, and a regular adult heart rate ranges from 60 to 100 beats per minute. Lower heart rates indicate healthier individuals consisting of more efficient heart functions. Similarly to blood pressure, cardiac output is a highly regulated process as well, since all tissues in the body require nutrient-rich, oxygenated blood to function. Regulation of cardiac output involves the autonomic nervous system (sympathetic versus parasympathetic), the endocrine system (circulating hormones), and the paracrine signaling pathways (denomination of the endocrine system) (King & Lowery, 2021).

Cardiac rhythm. Cardiac muscle cells consist of an inherent capacity to contract rhythmically through specialized cells located within the myocardial heart layer. A typical cycle begins with the signaling of the sinoatrial node (SA node), or the "pacemaker", located on the top left side of the right atrium. This bundle of cells does not require any electrical input, but instead sets regular excitatory intervals. The electrical interval of signals from the SA node causes the walls of the atria to contract, resulting in the stimulation of the *atrioventricular node* (AV node) lying on the bottom right end of the atrium. Electrical signals take a slight pause here until the completion of the atrial systole. Following systole, the AV node sends impulses down cardiovascular fibers (*bundle of His*) on both sides of the interventricular septum. The bundle of His further branches out into *Purkinje fibers* that branch throughout both ventricles, resulting in ventricular contraction. The electrocardiogram (ECG) records the travel time for these impulses, as well as the electrical events associated with atrial and ventricular contractions.

The autonomic nervous system plays a distinct role in the regulation of heart rate. The sympathetic and parasympathetic branches act as antagonists toward one another; therefore, control from the autonomic nervous system controls the SA node's rate of electrical intervals. Certain hormones also regulate heart rates such as epinephrine, norepinephrine, and thyroid hormone.

Vascular System

Arterial System

Once blood leaves the heart, the first direction in which the oxygenated blood travels is through the arterial system. This system allows blood to reach the head, abdomen, and extremities and deliver oxygenated blood to these tissues. Blood travels from the aorta, branching through the arteries and finally the arterioles. In this direction, the arteries become progressively thinner in wall thickness and smaller in vessel diameter. Arterial walls are composed of three distinct layers: (a) the *intima*, a smooth thin layer of endothelial cells; (b) the *media*, a relatively thick middle layer composed of smooth muscle and elastic connective tissue fibers; and (c) the *adventitia*, the outer fibrous layer. Due to the media being composed of smooth muscle, this results from involuntary control of the sympathetic nervous system, allowing for the walls to distend and recoil during systole. Changes in the diameter of the vessels also determine the quantity of blood delivered to the capillaries. Finally, the arterioles are also regulated tightly with the urinary system to control blood pressure, and as diameter changes, resistance to blood flow also changes. ANP is a cardiac hormone released through the endocrine system to decrease blood pressure when it gets too high. ANP inhibits the release of adrenocorticotropic hormone (ACTH) and vasopressin in the kidney (Tucker et al., 2021).

The heart contains a set of right and left *coronary arteries* that supply the heart itself, specifically the myocardium, with gases and nutrients. The right coronary arteries supply the majority of the heart with nutrients, spanning from the right atrium, right ventricle, and bottom of the left ventricle. Conversely, the left coronary artery supplies the left atrium and the remainder of the left ventricle. Both systems, however, have an interconnection (anastomosis) between the two coronary arteries, in which each vessel alone can deliver blood to the myocardium of all four chambers. The blood flow in the coronary arteries occurs during diastole when the heart walls are relaxed and the aortic semilunar valves are closed.

Capillaries

The capillaries are essential for the gas exchange that occurs between the tissues and blood vessels. The capillaries are the middle ground between the arterioles that outflow blood from the heart to the tissues and the venules that return blood from the tissues to the heart. Capillaries are microscopic and branched, with very thin endothelial cell walls that lie in close approximation to the *interstitial* fluid. The capillaries are widely branched to maximize the surface area to allow for efficient diffusion of oxygen to the tissues. The thin walls of the capillary system, consisting only of the intima, permit the exchange of blood plasma containing dissolved nutrients and oxygen into the interstitial fluid with the collection of waste products from the tissues such as carbon dioxide.

Venous System

Once the gas exchange is accomplished through the arteriole system, the capillaries drain the deoxygenated blood with waste products into the venous system. While the arteriole system delivers blood from the heart to the tissues, the venous system will, in turn, deliver blood from the tissues back to the heart. Veins are thin walled with the same three layers as the arteries, except the media is a much thinner layer. Blood pressure drops from the arteriole system to the venous system; thus, blood pressure is the lowest in veins; however, the venous system can hold large volumes of blood. Throughout the lower extremities, veins must work against gravity to return blood to the heart, and this task is accomplished through the use of valves. Valves function in one direction to keep the blood from pooling. All of the blood collected from the lower extremities enters through the inferior vena cava, while the blood from the head and upper extremities enters through the superior vena cava.

Portal System

The liver is an essential organ that conducts a large variety of important physiological functions:

1. Execution of several important steps in the utilization of proteins, fats, and carbohydrates that utilize multiple metabolic pathways to obtain energy
2. Storage of important substances, such as iron, various vitamins, triglycerides, glycogen, and lipoproteins
3. Neutralization of potentially toxic products of digestion

The *portal vein* collects blood from the walls of the GI tract, gallbladder, pancreas, and spleen and delivers it to the liver. Most of the nutrients derived from food come from the digestion within the walls of the intestine and diffusion through these capillaries. The nutrients from the capillaries are then contained in the blood collected by the portal vein. The portal vein enters the liver and branches into venules and then into liver cell capillaries. The capillaries then recombine into more venules followed by the *hepatic vein* eventually draining oxygen-poor blood into the inferior vena cava (Carneiro et al., 2019).

Lymphatic System

The lymphatic system has a few key functions that include:

1. Acting like an immune system defender, sweeping up foreign particles or bacteria and translocating them to a lymph node for immune system interaction
2. Returning and restoring excess molecules such as glucose and fatty acids back into the systemic circulation
3. Restoring excess protein molecules and interstitial fluid into circulation

Lymph fluid is produced due to high blood pressure, where open-ended microscopic lymphatic capillaries are located close to the interstitial fluid bathing all cells. Blood plasma gets forced through these capillary beds where the lymphatic system collects the interstitial fluid (lymph), plasma (lacking red blood cells), and proteins that are too large to fit through the walls of the capillaries. The lymphatic capillaries join to form lymphatic vessels, which will eventually combine back into larger vessels. There are two main vessels: (a) the *thoracic duct*, which enters the left subclavian vein after draining the interstitial fluid for most of the body, and (b) the right *lymphatic duct*, which enters the right subclavian vein after draining the right arm and right upper trunk areas. These lymph vessels utilize valves, similar to the venule system, where smooth muscle contracts with skeletal muscle to prevent the backflow of lymph fluid. All lymphatic fluid is emptied into the left subclavian vein and left internal jugular vein (Null & Agarwal, 2021).

Lymph nodes (glands) are dispersed throughout the body, which manufacture and contain lymphocytes that produce antibodies. Due to the lymphatic system and its immune response, infections are usually caught early and localized so foreign particles cannot enter the bloodstream.

Pulmonary System

The pulmonary system, otherwise known as the lungs, functions through gas diffusion and delivers oxygen to the blood while removing carbon dioxide from the blood. The right lung has three lobes (the right inferior lobe, right middle lobe, and right inferior lobe), while the left lung only has two lobes (the left superior and inferior). The left lung has an indent, called the cardiac notch, where the heart is positioned into. Inspired air contains approximately 21% oxygen and little to no carbon dioxide, while expired air consists of 16% oxygen and 4.5% carbon dioxide. Additionally, the temperature of the air inhaled is close to that of ambient air temperature, while the pulmonary system works to humidify and equilibrate the expired air with body temperature, as well as saturating it with water. Finally, the pulmonary system acts as a filter to essentially eliminate any particles typically referring to smaller items than particulate matter from ambient air (Ochs et al., 2004).

Air enters in through the nose/mouth and passes through to the pharynx, larynx, trachea, into the lungs dispersed into bronchioles, and eventually alveoli. The actual exchange between oxygen and carbon dioxide occurs within the thin walls of the alveoli. Hundreds of millions of alveoli are located deep within the lungs that work to maximize the surface and are needed for gas exchange.

Contraction of the chest cavity is a result of contracting (inhalation) and relaxing (exhalation) of muscles. The main muscle responsible for respiration is the diaphragm, which comprises the floor of the lungs. The rhythmicity of respiration is controlled by respiratory centers in the upper part of the pons and medulla. Respiration primarily relies on chemoreceptors which detect changing levels in oxygen, carbon dioxide, and pH to maintain a steady state of homeostasis (Ochs et al., 2004).

Air distribution. On inspiration, ambient air enters the nose through the nostrils (nares). The nostrils consist of nasal hairs and mucus to collect and filter out any dust or bacterial particles, and the nose also works to warm and humidify the air through the moist lining of the nose (nasal mucosa). Further, the nose and mouth orifices combine and enter the throat, or *pharynx*. The pharynx consists of the *tonsils, adenoids*, and opening of the *auditory (eustachian) tube* that connects to the middle ear. Further warming of the air also occurs within the pharynx.

The end of the pharynx consists of two openings that connect either to the GI tract or to the lungs. One opening is the *esophagus* for the passage of food, and the other is the *larynx* for the continued flow of inspired air. There is a small flap of cartilage, the *epiglottis*, which prevents food from entering the larynx. The larynx also houses the vocal cords, is lined with a mucous membrane, and has a rigid wall of cartilage.

Inspired air flows from the larynx down into the *trachea* ("windpipe"). The trachea begins at the neck and ends in the chest cavity, where it branches into the left and right main *bronchi*. Air finally enters the lungs, where it will continue to flow. Bronchi continue to branch into the smallest unit of branches called the *bronchioles*.

The trachea, bronchi, and most of the bronchioles consist of cells with hair-like projections (cilia), which drive mucus that acts as a final filter of bacteria and particles. Bronchiole walls consist of smooth muscles, similar to the walls of arterioles. At this point, inspired air has reached body temperature, has reached 100% humidity, and has been completely filtered.

The final destination of the inspired air rests in the *alveolar ducts* into *alveolar sacs*. The walls of each sac have many pockets, called *alveoli*. The gas exchange of oxygen and carbon dioxide occurs between the thin walls of the alveoli and the capillary blood.

Thorax

The thorax is the region inferior to the neck and superior to the abdomen. The thoracic wall is formed by 12 ribs, 12 thoracic vertebrae, cartilage, sternum, and five muscles. The main functions of the thorax include movement, respiration, and protection of the thoracic cavity. The diaphragm is the separation point between the abdomen and the chest cavity. The contraction of the diaphragm changes the volume of the thoracic cavity and allows for negative pressure to build for respiration. The intercostal muscles are the muscles between the ribs, which function to tighten and expand the ribcage to allow the lungs to fully expand or help to add pressure to the lungs to deflate during expiration (Kudzinskas & Callahan, 2021).

The thoracic cavity is divided into a right and left chest cavity, consequentially containing the right and left lungs, termed the pleural cavities. The *mediastinum* is central and divides the two pleural cavities and is extended through the entire length of the thoracic cavity. The mediastinum consists of the trachea, esophagus, nerves, lymph nodes, and heart.

Pulmonary Circulation

During systemic regulation of the blood, oxygen-deficient blood returns from the body through the superior (head, neck, and upper extremities) and inferior (trunk and lower extremities) vena cava back into the heart into the right atria. Blood is pumped from the right atria into the right ventricle, where it is sent to the lungs through the main pulmonary artery to be distributed to both lungs for gas exchange to occur. In the lungs, carbon dioxide is diffused out while the blood becomes reoxygenated. The oxygenated blood recombines into venules, veins, and eventually the right and left pulmonary veins to get pumped back into the heart through the left atria. The final step is having the oxygen-rich blood pumped to the rest of the body by the left ventricle.

Gas Exchange

Alveoli and capillaries both consist of a single layer of thin endothelial cell walls that permit the passive diffusion of small non-polar molecules such as dissolved carbon dioxide and oxygen. There are drastic concentration differences between the alveoli and blood capillaries that allow simple diffusion to occur. There is a higher concentration of oxygen within the walls of the alveoli compared to the concentration within the blood in the capillaries; thus, oxygen diffuses from the alveolar walls into the blood. Conversely, the opposite concentration exists between carbon dioxide within the blood capillaries compared to the carbon dioxide concentration of the alveolar cell walls, and the carbon dioxide passively diffuses from the blood to the alveoli. The gaseous-aqueous interphase of the lungs is protected by surfactants, agents that decrease the surface tension of the two in medium (Akella & Deshpande, 2013).

Red blood cells within the blood plasma utilize a multisubunit, heme-protein complex called hemoglobin to maximize its oxygen and carbon dioxide uptake. Hemoglobin has cooperative binding properties that tightly bind four dissolved oxygen molecules, allowing for red blood cells to carry over 70 times more oxygen than they could carry if oxygen were just dissolved in the plasma. The total amount of oxygen that can be taken into the blood each minute depends on (a) the oxygen concentration difference within the alveoli and blood, (b) the total healthy function surface area of the alveoli, and (c) the rate of respiration.

Tissues have a unique property that also monitors the pH levels of blood called the bicarbonate buffer system. The bicarbonate buffer system uses chemoreceptors to maintain homeostatic levels of carbon dioxide found in the blood.

Pleura

The pleura is a membrane that folds back onto itself forming two layers: the visceral and parietal pleura. The thin space located between the pleura membrane is the pleural cavity that contains a small amount of pleural fluid. The parietal pleura is the outer layer of the double-layered membrane, which is connected to the chest wall and faces the lung. The visceral (inner) pleura surrounds the lobes of the lungs via blood vessels, bronchi, and nerves. The surfaces of the parietal and visceral pleura contain cells that secrete a small amount of fluid, which minimizes the friction of the lungs during respiration (Charalampidis et al., 2015).

Mechanics of Respiration

Inspiration

The driving factor that promotes regulatory breathing patterns based on the stimuli on the partial pressure ratio of carbon dioxide to oxygen is located within the brainstem. The medulla oblongata is the structure in the brain that initiates impulses through the nerve (phrenic nerve) that activate the contraction of the diaphragm muscle and the intercostal muscles (spinal nerves T2–T12). The driving force of inspiration is due to the contraction of the diaphragm—this results in an increase in the volume of the thorax. The intercostal muscles between the ribs will also contract, causing the ribcage to expand and furthering the increase of volume. The volume increase triggers an immediate decrease in pressure, or negative pressure, resulting in the pressure of the thorax dropping below atmospheric pressure. The pressure in the bronchi will equilibrate to atmospheric pressure and, in turn, allows for air to rush in through the nose or the mouth.

Expiration

At the height of inspiration, the medulla will cease activation of neural impulses to the phrenic and intercostal nerves. Alveoli are surrounded by elastin proteins that allow them to expand and recoil; as a result, the expanded alveoli simply recoil, and air passively rushes out of the lungs. The pressure of the lungs will increase again as the volume decreases back to its resting state. Activation of the abdominal muscles will also trigger the rise in abdominal pressure, assisting in the expiration of air out of the lungs (Troyer & Boriek, 2011).

Lung Volumes

Lung volumes adapt to different physiological conditions and are flexible in the extent to which they can expand. Lung volumes of importance include the following:

1. *Tidal volume* (TV or V_T) is the volume of gas inhaled or exhaled during a respiratory cycle at rest (about 500 mL) per breath.
2. *Inspiratory reserve volume* (IRV) is the maximum volume of gas that can be inhaled past the tidal volume at maximum inhalation effort (about 3,000 mL). This can occur at peak physical activity.
3. *Expiratory reserve volume* (ERV) is the volume of gas that can be maximally exhaled after standard tidal volume (about 1,000 mL).
4. *Vital capacity* (VC) is the volume change, or the sum of the TV, IRV, and ERV (about 4,500–5,000 mL).

5. *Residual volume* (RV) is the volume of gas remaining in the lungs after ERV (Wanger et al., 2005, p. 12).

Regulation of Respiration

Respiration is tightly regulated by a handful of physiological factors, including (a) the control centers in the brain and (b) chemical and pressure receptors. These respiration centers are located in the brainstem. The medulla works intricately with the pons to regulate the respiration centers and nerves that automatically activate breathing. Central chemoreceptors gather information regarding carbon dioxide levels in the brainstem to tightly regulate blood pH. The blood has a critical bicarbonate buffer system that acts to maintain a homeostatic pH of approximately 7.40. If the levels of carbon dioxide are too high in the blood, the brainstem will trigger rapid and deeper breathing to increase the diffusion of carbon dioxide out of the bloodstream and lower the pH. When carbon dioxide levels are too low, the brainstem will generate the opposite effect and slow breathing down.

Similar to chemoreceptors located in the blood, there are mechanoreceptors located in lung tissue that relay information about pressure, specifically the depth and rhythm of respiration. This pressure signaling is called the Hering-Breuer inspiratory reflex. The vagus nerve (cranial nerve X) controls when the maximum lung expansion is reached and stops the activation of the medulla. Equally, when the minimum lung volume is reached and the lung tissue is collapsed, the vagus nerve stimulates the respiration cycle to start again.

Visual System

The eye is a complex organ that relies on multiple moving systems to relay visual information to the optic nerve into the brain. Cranial nerves I, II, III, IV, and VI innervate to allow visual stimuli to be processed within the occipital lobe of the brain. The eye itself has a multitude of moving parts to allow the eyes to adjust to the afferent light entering to focus and process different stimuli. Light initially enters the eye through the pupil, the dark circle in the center of the eye. The size of the pupil is determined by the iris, the pigmented portion surrounding the pupil. Depending on the amount of light being exposed to the eye, the iris will either constrict the pupil when too much light is trying to enter or dilate the pupil when there are not enough light stimuli to elicit a visual response.

The next structure light will pass through is the lens, which is located directly behind the pupil. The lens reacts to light in a similar way that glasses correct vision. The lens will bend light by assuming a thin or fat shape ("zoom") through the utilization of the ciliary muscle to which it is attached. The lens is essential for focusing images.

The retina is a specific area located on the opposite end of the eyeball situated above the fovea and optic nerve. The retina develops visual stimuli into impulses that will travel through the optic nerve to the occipital lobe for interpretation.

The eyeball is protected by a white, opaque structure called the *sclera* which surrounds the entirety of the eyeball except over the pupil. The *cornea* is the thin, clear layer protecting the pupil. Further protecting the sclera, cornea, and eyelids is a thin, transparent layer called the *conjunctiva*. Eyelashes also serve to keep foreign material out of the eyes.

In the corner of the eye sockets behind the eyelids are *lacrimal glands*, which secrete tears to cleanse the eye when it is irritated or debris passes the eyelashes. The tears enter through holes in the outer aspects of the upper eyelid and drain into the nose through the *nasolacrimal duct*, located in the inner aspect of the lower eyelid. Damage to any of these areas can result in damage to the visual system.

Cornea and Sclera

The cornea is very thin, transparent, and curved. It is the first structure exposed to light rays and is the anterior-most portion of the eye. The curved structure of the cornea bends the light rays before it reaches the lens.

The sclera, however, is fibrous and maintains the shape of the eyeball. The sclera completely encloses and protects the internal contents of the eyeball, except where the optic nerve protrudes in the posterior. No light can pass through the sclera, and it is inelastic. The sclera is supported and internally lined by the choroid, which is predominantly composed of blood vessels that nourish aspects of the eye and are enmeshed in connective tissue and pigmented cells.

Iris and Pupil

The iris is immediately encased by the cornea and is connected directly to the choroid. The iris is composed of colored pigments that control the size of the pupil and the amount of light that enters through the lens, and these reflexes are controlled by cranial nerve III. The pupil is black due to all of the light striking the retina, and no visible light is reflected. In some cases, this is why eyes appear red in a picture that used a flash because the flash of the camera is reflected off of the retina into the image.

Lens and Ciliary Body

The *ciliary body* is a muscular structure that is also attached to the choroid. The ciliary body and the iris work synchronously to control the amount of light that enters the pupil. The *suspensory ligaments* extend from the ciliary body to the lens to maintain their position behind the pupil.

The lens of the eye is similar to the lens of glasses; it is firm and transparent. It consists of an outer cortex and an inner nucleus. When visualizing nearby objects, the ciliary muscle contracts, relaxing the suspensory ligament. The tension on the lens is released, and the lens fattens ("zooms"). This fattening results in the light rays bending more, therefore allowing the eye to focus the image on the retina. The opposite happens for far objects—the ciliary muscles relax, the suspensory ligaments tighten, and the lens thins out.

Hyperopia, or farsightedness, is a condition where light rays focus behind the retina, which results in objects up close appearing out of focus. Conversely, myopia, or nearsightedness, is when light rays bend to focus in front of the retina, which results in objects far away appearing out of focus.

Many other conditions are linked to aging and vision. In presbyopia, the lens is unable to increase its curvature, and near objects cannot be focused on the retina. Also, lens degeneration, which results in the clouding of the lens (cataracts), prevents light rays from reaching the retina. In severe cases of diabetes, patients can develop diabetic retinopathy, where blood vessels in the retina are affected and ultimately can lead to vision loss or blindness.

Anterior and Posterior Cavities

The anterior cavity comprises two different chambers, the anterior and the posterior chambers, separated by the iris. These chambers contain a watery fluid called the *aqueous humor*. The aqueous humor nourishes the cells within these chambers. This fluid passes through the pupil into the anterior chamber, where it is absorbed in the *canal of Schlemm*. The secretion and absorption of the aqueous humor are done in unison to maintain the appropriate pressure in the entire eye.

The posterior cavity behind the lens contains the *vitreous humor*, a transparent, colorless gel, which consists of a mesh of clear liquid and cells but has no blood vessels. The vitreous humor acts as a shock absorber for the retina and becomes less gel-like as age progresses.

Retina

The retina is arguably the most important structure in regard to vision and sensory relay of visual signals. The retina is located on the internal layer in the posterior region of the eyeball, and it is connected to almost all of the choroid. There are two layers to the retina. The inner layer contains light-sensitive cells and blood vessels that are firmly fixed to the choroid. Two main cell types make up the light-sensitive, photoreceptor cell portion of the retina: *rods* and *cones*.

Rods are rod-shaped cells that process dim to dark images (scotopic vision) and have low-resolution acuity. Rods function best in dim or dark light. Rod cells contain a light-sensitive protein called rhodopsin. In the presence of light, the rhodopsin in rod cell discs rapidly breaks down and initiates nerve impulse conduction. Rhodopsin must have a period of darkness for rhodopsin to reform and activate the rod cells again.

Cones are shorter, cone-shaped cells that process color vision and provide higher spatial acuity plus clearer visual details (photopic vision). Cones contain a less sensitive protein, iodopsin, which requires a higher amount of light to break down.

There are far more cones within the area of the retina, except in one particular location. The portion of the retina called the *macula* is responsible for processing color vision and fine visual details. The center of the macula, the *fovea*, only contains cone cells and is the point of clearest vision. When in well-lit conditions, the eye will focus the image directly on the fovea versus in dimly lit conditions, the eye will move to focus the image toward the periphery of the retina where rods are more plentiful.

The conduction of light stimuli through the cells of the retina is a backward process. The photoreceptor cells, the rods, and the cones are closest to the epithelial cells rooted to the choroid on the outermost portion of the retina. Light travels through the cornea, pupil, aqueous humor, and lens and then through the vitreous humor, where light rays excite the photoreceptor cells of the retina. Depending on the amount of light entering the back of the eye, the rods or cones will excite and transduce signals from the photoreceptor cells inward to the bipolar cells of the retina, which act as visual mediators of signals. The final step of the phototransduction cascade concludes at the ganglion cells, which is the final destination where the electrical impulse will be transduced to a chemical one. The axons of the ganglion cells condense together to form the optic nerve.

The optic nerve enters the back of the eye at the *optic disc*, which itself does not contain light-sensitive cells and is therefore sometimes called the *blind spot*. The optic nerve receives signals from the ganglion cells, which will essentially deliver these signals to the occipital lobe of the brain.

Nerve Pathways to the Brain

When both eyes focus on an object, the structures bend the light in an appropriate manner to focus the image on each corresponding retina. Due to the curvature of the eyeball, the image focuses upside-down on the retina, and it is up to the systems of the optic nerve and occipital lobe to correctly interpret the image.

There are four distinct segments to the field of vision. There are left and right fields of vision as a result of two distinct eyes receiving visual input, but there is also the fraction of the retina that is closer to the nose called the *nasal portion*, while the other fraction is called the *temporal portion*. Images located within the right visual field will focus on the left portion of each retina, while images located within the left visual field will focus on the right portion of each retina. If an image is located within the right visual field, the light rays will strike the left nasal portion of the retina in the right eye and the left temporal portion of the retina in the left eye. Inversely, if there was an image located within the left visual field, light rays from the image will strike the right temporal portion of the right eye and the left nasal portion of the left eye.

Similar to how the hemispheres communicate with one another, images located within the right visual field will transpire in the left occipital lobe, and images in the left visual field will end in the right occipital lobe. In total, four fibers are affiliated with the retina. The left temporal and nasal portions constitute the left optic nerve, while the right temporal and nasal portions constitute the right optic nerve. The two optic nerves from both eyes unite at the *optic chiasma*. At the optic chiasma junction, the fibers from the corresponding left nasal portion and the right temporal portion interconnect to form the image (and vice versa). The connection of the fibers forms the *optic tract*, and the left optic tract corresponds to images from the right visual field and the right optic tract corresponds to images from the left visual field. These fibers next synapse within the left and right lateral geniculate bodies of the thalamus, and these fibers continue as *optic radiations* to terminate in the final destination of the right and left occipital cortex. The brain heavily relies on cranial nerves III, IV, and VI (oculomotor, trochlear, and abducens), respectively, for communication and coordination between the two visual systems.

Communication of a three-dimensional image between the two visual fields accounts for highly detailed depth perception. (See Figure 5.6 for eye anatomy illustration.) The same light rays enter each eye at different, unique angles, while fibers and tracts communicate with each other to form a fully comprehensible image. Through one eye, the retina only receives an image from a singular perspective, and the brain relies on monocular cues to form an image. Only using monocular cues results in poor depth perception. The eye utilizes seven monocular clues

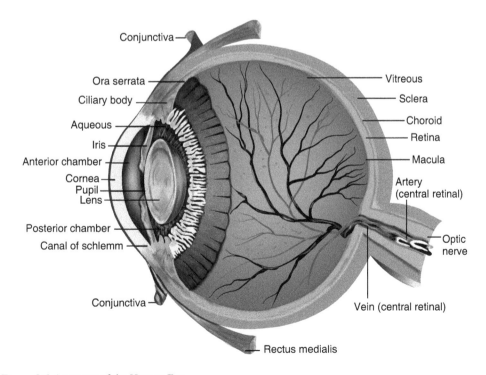

Figure 5.6 Anatomy of the Human Eye

to interpret images: relative size, interposition, linear perspective, aerial perspective, light and shades, and the motion parallax. However, with both eyes, light rays converge and are compared using binocular cues, thus resulting in a three-dimensional image.

Auditory and Vestibular Systems

The vestibular system and the auditory system are structurally linked with one another within the ear. The auditory system relays and encodes sound waves, whereas the vestibular system monitors and controls body equilibrium.

Sound waves do not travel in a vacuum, nor would it be possible to hear any sound within a vacuum. Instead, successions of pressure waves vibrate within a medium, and specialized structures within the ear detect the sound wave to interpret audio. Sound waves travel the slowest through the air at 742 miles (1,197 km) per hour versus 3,424 miles (5,478 km) per hour in water. As a result, structures within the ear evolved to convert the vibrations collected from the air to fluid dispositions to allow the brain to interpret signals gathered from the environment. However, not all sounds can be perceived by the human ear, and the range of frequencies that can be distinguished is between 20 and 20,000 cycles per second (Hz).

The vestibular system actively senses both static position and movements. Specialized nerve cells are signaling the brain nonstop with nerve impulses that allow the rest of the body to interpret where it is in space.

Anatomically the ear is divided into three separate sections: the outer ear, the middle ear, and the inner ear. The outer and middle ear convert the vibrations from the environment into pressure—transverse waves for the ear to interpret. The inner ear consists of two separate systems with their own sets of specialized cells. The inner ear is composed of the physical structures for both the auditory and vestibular systems that interpret the conducted vibrational signals into nerve impulses. These nerve impulses travel to the brain through the *vestibulocochlear nerve* (cranial nerve VIII), which consists of the combination of the *cochlear nerve* for hearing and the *vestibular nerve* for equilibrium.

Auditory Systems

External Ear

The *auricle*, or *pinna*, is the anatomical name for the visible structure of the ear. The shape of the external ear is structurally similar to a satellite dish, essentially collecting sound waves into the opening, the *external acoustic meatus*, and funneling them into the ear canal. These sound waves then travel down the ear canal and meet the entrance of the eardrum (tympanic membrane). The eardrum is a small, sensitive structure that is exposed to the environment; thus, the ear canal utilizes modified sweat glands that secrete *cerumen*, or earwax, for protection.

Middle Ear

The middle ear is the continuation of sound waves through the air. The external ear gathers sound waves from the environment, which then perpetuate forward through the tympanic cavity. The tympanic cavity is contained within the temporal bone behind the cheekbone and connected to the throat by the auditory (eustachian) tube, which is necessary for normal hearing. The eustachian tube allows for the maintenance of air pressure, and thus the eardrum functions efficiently. Typically, the walls of the eustachian tube are closed, except during actions of swallowing or chewing for the equalization of pressure. In high- or low-pressure environments such as flying in an airplane or scuba diving underwater, it is necessary to equalize the pressure within the ears to prevent damage to the eardrum.

The *tympanic membrane* is the thin connective tissue that is exposed to the air-filled cavity of the external/middle ear and a mucous lining inside the eardrum. The tympanic membrane is the connection between the external and middle ear. Directly connected to the tympanic membrane are three small, moveable bones that act as a medium to which air pressure converts into fluid pressure through vibrations. The first bone that is rooted in the tympanic membrane is the *malleus*, and the malleus bone moves whenever the tympanic membrane vibrates. The malleus bone is then connected to the *incus* bone through a joint. The last in the chain is the *stapes* bone, which in turn has a flat expanse (footplate) that fits into a hole, the *oval window*, in the wall of the inner ear. The stapes is the smallest bone in the human body. The ossicles react to vibrations received from the tympanic membrane, and these bones, in turn, transmit and transform these vibrations at the entrance of the inner ear.

Inner Ear

The inner ear is an elaborate, fluid-filled, *bony labyrinth* that serves two specialized functions carved within the temporal bone. The two connected sections are the auditory system's *cochlea* and the vestibular system's *semicircular canals*. The oval window opens into the *vestibule* of the inner ear between the two sections.

It is the responsibility of the inner ear to transmute vibrational frequencies into signals that can be interpreted by the brain. The inner ear is filled with a fluid membranous sac, the *membranous labyrinth* (endolymphatic), and is maintained by cranial nerve VIII (vestibulocochlear). The membranous labyrinth is surrounded by a cushioning fluid called the *perilymph*, and the fluid within the sac is the *endolymph*.

The cochlea contains specialized cells for auditory interpretation and signaling. The cochlea is located on the medial end of the inner ear and has the characteristic coiled shape of a snail. The cochlea has thousands of inner hair cells and thousands of outer hair cells. The inner hair cells detect fluid signals and convert them into electrical signals, whereas outer hair cells are more abundant and amplify low-level sounds. These specialized hearing cells are located within the *organ of the Corti*. The pounding of the stapes onto the oval window creates waves of movement in the perilymph, which will, in turn, transmit through the membranous labyrinth into the endolymph. The movement of the hair cells helps convert fluid waves to electrical signals. The hair cells are located throughout the coiled interior of the cochlea. Different frequencies will trigger different locations of hair cells within the cochlea, and the farther medial inside of the cochlea, the higher the frequencies that can be detected. Once the organ of Corti is activated, the *round window* connecting the middle and inner ears will dissipate the remaining sound to prevent overstimulation of auditory signals. Damage or a nonfunctional cochlea can lead to deafness. Some deaf individuals are born with low to nonfunctional cochlea. Cochlear implants can be surgically inserted into the cochlea using an electrode and a magnetic audio amplifier. Depending on the severity of deafness, some individuals can successfully hear through the use of the artificial firing of the hair cells and activation of the cochlear nerve.

Then the frequency activation of the hair cells relays electrical signals to the fibers of the cochlear nerve. The cochlear nerve enters the skull cavity through a hole in the temporal bone, the *internal acoustic meatus*. The nerve then enters the medulla at the base of the brain before the signals are sent to both auditory cortices of the temporal lobes.

Vestibular System

The organ of the vestibular system is also located within the distal portion of the inner ear called the semicircular canals. The semicircular canals and the central vestibular portion of the bony membranous labyrinths contain different specialized cells that can sense movement and position, which is ultimately responsible for body equilibrium. There are three branches of the semicircular canals, and they are all placed perpendicularly to one another to sense all three directions in space (x, y, and z). At the base of each of the canals lies an enlarged membrane cavity (*ampulla*) that contains hair cells termed the *crista ampullaris*. Depending on the direction or position in space the head is oriented, the endolymph will activate the appropriate specialized hair cells. Within the vestibule, enlargements of the membranous labyrinth, the *utricle* and *saccule*, contain the hair cells that sense static head position. The utricle and saccule are particularly sensitive to motion and acceleration. The utricle is chiefly sensitive to horizontal acceleration, while the saccule is sensitive to vertical acceleration. Depending on what position the head is located in, gravity-activated hair cells shift as a result of the head position with the assistance of small calcium carbonate stones (otoliths). The endolymph fluid located within the vestibular system can be altered during a state of intoxication. Alcohol can be absorbed into the endolymph fluid and result in disequilibrium due to severe intoxication.

The activation of the hair cells as a result of the position of the head due to gravity creates nerve impulses. The nerve impulses collect at the vestibular nerve, which enters the skull cavity through the internal acoustic meatus, similar to the cochlea nerve. The vestibular system has no signaling connection to any area of the cortex. Instead, the impulses from the vestibular nerve are processed through various regions of the brainstem, cerebellum, and spinal cord. There is no higher processing of the vestibular impulses; therefore, it is concluded to be a reflexive response.

References

Akella, A., & Deshpande, S. B. (2013). Pulmonary surfactants and their role in pathophysiology of lung disorders. *Indian Journal of Experimental Biology*, *51*(1), 5–22. https://pubmed.ncbi.nlm.nih.gov/23441475/#:~:text=Surfactant%20is%20an%20agent%20that,II)%20cells%20of%20the%20lungs

Anderson, B. W., Ekblad, J., & Bordoni, B. (2021). Anatomy, appendicular skeleton. In *StatPearls*. StatPearls Publishing. www.ncbi.nlm.nih.gov/books/NBK535397/

Carneiro, C., Brito, J., Bilreiro, C., Barros, M., Bahia, C., Santiago, I., & Caseiro-Alves, F. (2019). All about portal vein: A pictorial display to anatomy, variants, and physiopathology. *Insights into Imaging*, *10*(1), 38. https://doi.org/10.1186/s13244-019-0716-8; www.ncbi.nlm.nih.gov/pmc/articles/PMC6428891/

Charalampidis, C., Youroukou, A., Lazaridis, G., Baka, S., Mpoukovinas, I., Karavasilis, V., Kioumis, I., Pitsiou, G., Papaiwannou, A., Karavergou, A., Tsakiridis, K., Katsikogiannis, N., Sarika, E., Kapanidis, K., Sakkas, L., Korantzis, I., Lampaki, S., Zarogoulidis, K., & Zarogoulidis, P. (2015). Pleura space anatomy. *Journal of Thoracic Disease*, *7*(Suppl 1), S27–S32. https://doi.org/10.3978/j.issn.2072-1439.2015.01.48; www.ncbi.nlm.nih.gov/pmc/articles/PMC4332049/

Daniel, P. M., Prichard, M. M. (1966). Observation of the vascular anatomy of the pituitary gland and its importance in pituitary function. *American Heart Journal*, *72*(2), 147–152. https://doi.org/10.1016/0002-8703(66)90437-6

Evrard, A., Hober, C., Racadot, A., Lefebvre, J., & Vantyghem, M. C. (1999). Hormone natriurétique auriculaire et fonctions endocrines [Atrial natriuretic hormone and endocrine functions]. *Annales de Biologie Clinique*, *57*(2), 149–155.

Herrero, M. T., Barcia, C., & Navarro, J. M. (2002). Functional anatomy of thalamus and basal ganglia. *Child's Nervous System: ChNS: Official Journal of the International Society for Pediatric Neurosurgery*, *18*(8), 386–404. https://doi.org/10.1007/s00381-002-0604-1

Johnson, S. (2019). What are the 12 cranial nerves? *Medical News Today*. Retrieved April 4, 2022, in the public domain from www.medicalnewstoday.com/articles/326621

Juneja, P., Munjal, A., & Hubbard, J. B. (2021). Anatomy, joints. In *StatPearls*. StatPearls Publishing. PMID: 29939670. https://pubmed.ncbi.nlm.nih.gov/29939670/

Kaiser, J. T., & Lugo-Pico, J. G. (2021, July 31). Neuroanatomy, spinal nerves. In *StatPearls*. StatPearls Publishing. Retrieved January 2022, from www.ncbi.nlm.nih.gov/books/NBK542218/

Kamrani, P., Marston, G., & Jan, A. (2022). Anatomy, connective tissue. In *StatPearls*. StatPearls Publishing. Updated January 24, 2022. www.ncbi.nlm.nih.gov/books/NBK538534/

King, J., & Lowery, D. R. (2021). Physiology, cardiac output. In *StatPearls*. StatPearls Publishing. Updated July 23, 2021. Retrieved January 2022, from www.ncbi.nlm.nih.gov/books/NBK470455/

Kudzinskas, A., & Callahan, A. L. (2021). Anatomy, thorax. In *StatPearls*. StatPearls Publishing. www.ncbi.nlm.nih.gov/books/NBK557710/#:~:text=The%20thorax%20is%20the%20region,skin)%20and%20the%20thoracic%20cavity

Null, M., & Agarwal, M. (2021). Anatomy, lymphatic system. In *StatPearls*. StatPearls Publishing. Retrieved January 2022, from www.ncbi.nlm.nih.gov/books/NBK513247/

Ochs, M., Nyengaard, J. R., Jung, A., Knudsen, L., Voigt, M., Wahlers, T., Richter, J., & Gundersen, H. J. (2004). The number of alveoli in the human lung. *American Journal of Respiratory and Critical Care Medicine*, *169*(1), 120–124. https://doi.org/10.1164/rccm.200308-1107OC; https://pubmed.ncbi.nlm.nih.gov/14512270

Porras-Gallo, M., Pena-Melian, A., Viejo, F., Hernandez, T., Puelles, E., Echevarria, D., & Sanudo, J. (2019). Overview of the history of the cranial nerves: From Galen to the 21st century. *Anatomical Record (Hoboken)*, *302*(3), 381–393. http://doi.org/10.1002/ar.23928. Epub November 9, 2018. PMID: 30412363.

Riva, D., Matilde, T., & Bulgheroni, S. (2018). The neuropsychology of basal ganglia. *European Journal of Paediatric Neurology*, *22*(2), 321–326. https://doi.org/10.1016/j.ejpn.2018.01.009; www.sciencedirect.com/science/article/pii/S1090379817318330?via%3Dihub

Trejo, J. (2019). Cranial nerves: Mind your head. *The Anatomical Record*, *302*, 374–377.

Troyer, A. D., & Boriek, A. M. (2011). Mechanics of the respiratory muscles. *American Physiological Society, Comparative Physiology*, *1*(3), 1273–1300. https://doi.org/10.1002/cphy.c100009; https://onlinelibrary.wiley.com/doi/10.1002/cphy.c100009

Tucker, W. D., Arora, Y., & Mahajan, K. (2021). Anatomy, blood vessels. In *StatPearls*. StatPearls Publishing. https://pubmed.ncbi.nlm.nih.gov/29262226/#:~:text=Capillaries%20are%20thin%2Dwalled%20vessels,of%20blood%20through%20the%20capillaries

Wanger, J., Clausen, J., Coates, A., Pedersen, O., Brusasco, V., Burgos, F., Casaburi, R., Crapo, R., Enright, C., van der Grinten, C. P., Gustafsson, P. Hankinson, J., Jensen, R., Johnson, D., MacIntyre, N., McKay, R., Miller, M. R., Navajas, D., Pellegrino, R., & Viegi, G. (2005). Standardization of the measurement of lung volumes. *European Respiratory Journal*, *26*, 511–522. https://doi.org/10.1183/09031936.05.00035005; https://erj.ersjournals.com/content/26/3/511

6 Psychosocial Aspects of Chronic Illness and Disability

Kathleen Acer

Historically, the understanding and conceptualization of chronic illness and disability have been viewed through the lens of a medical model wherein physical conditions were "problems" evidenced by an individual (Smart, 2001). This model emphasized the generation of a diagnosis and the development of a cure, thus returning the individual to a state of "normalcy" (Fowler & Wadsworth, 1991; McCarthy, 1993; Longmore, 1995). This state of "normalcy" was traditionally based upon societal norms and roles. Thus, individuals who proved incurable were subsequently deemed "disabled". Therefore, functional limitations and impairments were judged using the individual's degree of deviation from social norms. This model relied upon the diagnostic assessment procedures of the disease process, failing to place importance on the individual's subjective experience of wellness and functionality (Peterson & Elliot, 2008). This emphasis on diagnostic information alone while devaluing the individual's functionality also ignores the role of environment and societal factors on a person's existence.

In contrast to the rather narrow perspective of the medical model, the social model of disability views societal and environmental barriers as primarily being responsible for the state of disability (Paley, 2002). Rather than effecting a "cure" on the individual, the central focus of the social model is to effect change in society and the environment, which would then provide the individual opportunity and equality (Hurst, 2003). This model, however, does not distinguish who would qualify as a person with a disability or how the disability could even be measured or determined. This failure to generate empirical evidence through research has continued to hamper the development of the social model (Peterson & Elliot, 2008).

Out of the medical and social model's shortcomings grew the biopsychosocial model of disability. Initially proposed by Engel (1977), this model highlights the complex and interconnected effects of an individual's biological, psychological, and social factors that determine functionality. The conceptualization of an individual's health conditions in terms of its functional capacity, rather than as a medical diagnosis, incorporates the specific, individualized, and personal experience of the health issues in the individual's life (Falvo & Holland, 1977).

The natural outgrowth of this progression from a strictly medical, diagnosis-driven perspective was the development of a classification system that assesses illness and disability and is reflective of a continuum of health and functioning (Peterson, 2011). The International Classification of Functioning, Disability, and Health (IFC), (WHO, 2001) emphasized a positive view of health and sought to integrate health conditions (biological factors) with personal, societal, and environmental variables. Health is deemed to be a continuum of disability; a social construct that reflects the individual's interaction with the social and physical environment (Peterson & Kosciulek, 2005). Thus, disability is viewed as a uniquely universal human experience and not limited to a minority of the population. Regarding the determination of the extent of one's disability, the ICF requires that the health condition be placed within the individual's

DOI: 10.4324/b23293-6

unique life context, circumstance, and goals. As such, health conditions which result in a disability for a particular individual may not result in a disability for another individual (i.e. the loss of an index finger, which would be a more significant disability for a professional piano player than for a fork-lift operator).

Models of Psychosocial Adaptation to Illness and Disability

The progression of the conceptualization of disability from a rigid, disease-centric model to a multifaceted model encompassing the individual, society, physical, and functional capacities has facilitated a greater understanding of health and wellness, illness, and disability as a unique, individual experience. Likewise, the progression from a more biologically driven, individually focused perspective of psychosocial adaptation or adjustment to disability toward a more complex paradigm has been evident in the literature and the practice of clinicians working within the rehabilitation field. This paradigm has allowed the inclusion of social, interpersonal, and environmental influences in the individual's adaptation and/or adjustment to the respective disability (Kim et al., 2016; Livneh, 2001, 2019; Martz & Livneh, 2016).

One of the earliest theories on adjustment to chronic illness and disability was presented by Dembo et al. (1956). Dembo asserted that positive adjustment was characterized by successful coping, while the lack of ability to adjust was characterized by a negative "succumbing" to disability. Coping involved an individual recognizing their residual functional capacity. Individuals who emphasized personal accomplishments took control of their lives, successfully negotiated physical and social barriers, expanded social activities that were still achievable, and dealt with negative life experiences effectively had successfully adapted (adjusted) to their disability. Conversely, individuals who "succumbed" to their disability placed an emphasis on their limitations, passively accepted societal roles for persons with disabilities (i.e. vulnerable, pitied, and incompetent), and persisted in dwelling on past abilities rather than focusing on current strengths.

In a later refinement of this theory, Wright (1983) proposed four changes or cognitive reevaluations necessary for successful adaptation. These included a subordination of physique or minimization of self-worth as reflecting one's physical appearance, constraining the "spread" of the negative effect of the disability to other unrelated areas of functioning and activities, an expansion of interests and values consistent with residual functional capacity, and the placement of focus upon remaining abilities and qualities rather than a comparison of oneself to those without challenges and disabilities. This conceptualization increased the importance of the social environment, environmental barriers, and interpersonal interactions.

There are also multiple ecological models of adjustment to disability which involve the interplay of the nature of the disability, the characteristics of the individual, and the influence of the environment upon the individual (Marini, 2018). The nature of the disability includes information regarding the time and type of onset of the disability or illness. Additionally, the severity of the disability, the level of pain involved, how visible the disability is, the type of functions impaired, and the stability of the disability are also considered. Individual characteristics include gender; the nature of the activities affected; the individual's interests, values, and goals; the residual resources retained; and the individual's spiritual and philosophical beliefs. Environmental influences include family, social, and community support and resources; physical settings; and attitudinal barriers or supports. Ecological models posit that the interaction of these variables determines the degree and speed of psychosocial adjustment to disability (Miller Smedema et al., 2009).

An additional ecological model was developed by Bishop (2005). This quality-of-life-based model termed the disability centrality model proposes that the individual's overall quality of life following a disabling event is viewed as a disruption in an individual's life, impacting their psychological well-being and quality of life. This model is composed of four components incorporating the impact of the disabling event on various life domains typically cited in the quality-of-life literature, the importance of the domain to the individual, the perceived control over functioning in that domain, and the overall satisfaction with the domain. These factors interact to produce an overall indication of the individual's adjustment to the disability.

Within many ecological adaptation models, the process is described in discrete stages or phases. The initial or early reactions to a potentially disabling condition include shock, anxiety, and denial. Intermediate reactions may be characterized by depression and internally and externally directed hostility or anger, while later stages of adaptation are described as adjustment, acknowledgment, or acceptance. Thus, psychosocial adaptation consists of a wide range of reactions both adaptive and maladaptive.

A significant evolution in the development of theories of adaptation to chronic illness and disability is the stage model of adjustment. These models differ in their theoretical underpinnings, specificity, and number of phases, with most models describing four to six stages. Livneh (1986) provides a comprehensive summary of more than 40 such stage models. Numerous models describe the psychosocial adjustment process in terms of five fundamental categories.

The first fundamental emergent or initial phase is marked by a period of shock secondary to the individual's reaction to the diagnosis of a disease or condition or the sudden onset of disability, which is an emotionally overwhelming experience. This reaction often results in a numbing of emotions and cognitive disorganization. The individual may also freeze up and demonstrate dramatically decreased speech and movement (Livneh & Antonak, 1997). Anxiety ensues following the initial understanding of the disabling event and is characterized by physical reactivity (increased heart rate and breathing), confused cognition, a sense of being overwhelmed, and possibly repetitive rumination and non-purposeful behavior. This anxiety is deemed a more "state-like" reaction.

Defense mobilization comprises denial and overlaps with bargaining. Denial, or psychological retreat, involves a minimalization or negation of the scope and/or chronicity of the disability or illness (Naugle, 1988). Denial often includes wishful recovery expectations without the component of a restitution agreement inherent in bargaining (Bray, 1978). This stage is highlighted by an inability to accept the nature and extent of the disability. The individual may employ selective attention to reality to mitigate the painful realization of the present and future implications of the trauma.

Following these initial stages, mourning or grief may develop (Marini, 2018). Termed the initial realization period by Livneh (1986), emotional turmoil results from an understanding of the reality of the disabling condition. Typically of briefer duration than depression, the individual grieves both the loss of physical functioning and their way of life. However, decrements in physical capacity and a realization of the potential for resultant physical, emotional, social, and behavioral limitations may ultimately foster the development of depression. Depression in disability research reflects various causal factors including premorbid disposition, biological and chemical changes due to disease and disability, the reaction to a damaged self-image, and a loss of functional roles (Rodin et al., 1991). However, Livneh and Antonak (1997) observed that feelings of hopelessness, intense sadness, withdrawal, despair, and despondency are common during this stage. A gradual acceptance of the losses associated with a disability was noted to occur over 24 months (Livneh & Antonak, 1991).

Anger, characterized as internally generalized and externally directed, has been termed the retaliation or rebellion stage. Feelings of guilt and self-blame for the disability or illness (i.e. viewing one's behavior as responsible for the onset of the illness, the extent of the disability, or the failure to improve) may especially be evident in individuals who recognize the chronic nature of their condition (Levin & Grossman, 1978). Hostility directed outward is viewed as a retaliation against functional limitations. Aggression, other blaming behavior, accusations, and even more passive-aggressive modes of interacting may be present in this phase and tend to be evident as the disability or illness becomes increasingly chronic (Brooks, 1988).

A major step toward a healthy adaptation to chronic disability is acknowledgment. Reintegration or reorganization is the final step of adaptation. In this stage, the individual has demonstrated an initial recognition that the disability is a permanent condition. A state of cognitive reorientation is then initiated. During this critical phase, the individual must accept himself or herself as evidencing a disability. The person must reappraise their life values, seek new achievable goals, and develop a new self-concept as an individual with a disability (Livneh & Antonak, 1997). This final stage of adjustment reflects an emotional acceptance of the functional limitations placed upon the individual and a behavioral acceptance of new life circumstances. The person recognizes newly discovered potentials, actively pursues social and vocational goals, and successfully negotiates obstacles. Reestablishment of positive self-worth is thus achieved through internalization of the functional limitations and subsequent development of self-acceptance and self-approval.

It is important to note that while the literature abounds with a plethora of stage theory models, there are still common assumptions inherent in all phase models of adaptation (Livneh & Antonak, 1997). Adaptation is a dynamic and unfolding shift from an experience of distress (shock, anxiety, depression) to a realignment and integration of the loss. These stages or phases are, in the main, internally driven; however, external events including direct interventions (environment, counseling) can modify the pace and nature of the reactions. The temporal ordering of the stages is influenced by the individual, and the sequences of phases are not universal. Adjustment or adaptation is not a linear progression, and regression to an earlier phase or even skipping of phases is possible. Further, not all individuals reach the theoretical endpoint of the process. The actual stages themselves are non-discrete, and overlapping reactions are possibly resulting in the individual experiencing more than one phase at a time. In this way, quantification of the duration of each phase, or even the whole process of adaptation, is not possible, as many individual factors interact, such as the age of onset, premorbid personality, severity and type of disability, nature of support systems available, available resources, etc., all influencing the process to varying degrees.

References

Bishop, M. (2005). Quality of life and psychosocial adaptation to chronic illness and acquired disability: A conceptual and theoretical synthesis. *Journal of Rehabilitation, 71*(2), 5–13.

Bray, G. P. (1978). Rehabilitation of spinal cord injured: A family approach. *Journal of Applied Rehabilitation Counseling, 9*(3), 70–78.

Brooks, N. (1988). Behavioral abnormalities in head-injured patients. *Scandinavian Journal of Rehabilitation Medicine Supplement, 17*, 41–46.

Dembo, T., Leviton, G. F., & Wright, B. A. (1956). Adjustment to misfortune: A problem of social-psychological rehabilitation. *Artificial Limbs, 3*(2), 4–62.

Engel, G. L. (1977). The need for a new medical model: A challenge for biomedicine. *Science, 196*, 129–136.

Falvo, D., & Holland, B. E. (2017). *Medical and psychosocial aspects of chronic illness and disability* (6th ed.). Jones & Bartlett Learning.

Fowler, C. A., & Wadsworth, J. S. (1991). Individualism and equity: Critical values in North American culture and the impact on disability. *Journal of Applied Rehabilitation Counselling, 22*, 19–23.

Hurst, R. (2003). The International disability rights movement and the ICF. *Disability and Rehabilitation, 25*, 572–576.

Kim, J. H., McMahon, B. T., Hawley, C., Brickham, D., Gonzalez, R., & Lee, D. H. (2016). Psychosocial adaptation to chronic illness and disability: A virtue based model. *Journal of Occupational Rehabilitation, 26*(1), 45–55. https://doi-org.proxy.library.vcu.edu/10.1007/s10926-015-9622-1

Levin, H. S., & Grossman, R. G. (1978). Behavioral sequelae of closed head injury. *Archives of Neurology, 35*, 720–727.

Livneh, H. (1986). A unified approach to existing models of adaptation to disability: Part I-A model adaptation. *Journal of Applied Rehabilitation Counselling, 17*, 5–16.

Livneh, H. (2001). Psychosocial adaptation to chronic illness and disability: A conceptual framework. *Rehabilitation Counseling Bulletin, 44*(3), 151–160.

Livneh, H. (2019). The use of generic avoidant coping scales for psychosocial adaptation to chronic illness and disability: A systematic review. *Health Psychology Open, 6*(2). https://doi-org.proxy.library.vcu.edu/10.1177/2055102919891396

Livneh, H., & Antonak, R. F. (1991). Temporal structure of adaptation to disability. *Rehabilitation Counselling Bulletin, 34*(4), 298–320.

Livneh, H., & Antonak, R. F. (1997). *Psychosocial adaptation to chronic illness and disability*. Aspen Publishers.

Longmore, P. K. (1995). Medical decision making and people with disabilities: A clash of cultures. *Journal of Law, Medicine, and Ethics, 23*, 82–87.

Marini, I. (2018). *The psychological and social impact of illness and disability*. Springer Publishing Company.

Martz, E., & Livneh, H. (2016). Psychosocial adaptation to disability within the context of positive psychology: Findings from the literature. *Journal of Occupational Rehabilitation, 26*(1), 4–12. https://doi-org.proxy.library.vcu.edu/10.1007/s10926-015-9598-x

McCarthy, H. (1993). Learning with Beatrice A. Wright: A breath of fresh air that uncovers the unique virtues and human flaws in us all. *Rehabilitation Education, 10*, 149–166.

Miller Smedema, S., Bajjen-Giien, S. K., & Dalton, J., (2009). Psychosocial adaptation to chronic illness and disability: Models and measurement. In *Understanding psychosocial adjustment to chronic illness and disability: A handbook for evidence-based practitioners in rehabilitation* (F. Chan, Ed.). Springer Publishing Company.

Naugle, R. I. (1988). Denial in rehabilitation: Its genesis, consequences, and clinical management. *Rehabilitation Counselling Bulletin, 31*, 218–231.

Paley, J. (2002). The Cartesian melodrama in nursing. *Nursing Philosophy, 3*(3), 189.

Peterson, D. B. (2011). *Psychological aspects of functioning, disability, and health*. Springer Publishing Company.

Peterson, D. B., & Elliot, T. R. (2008). Advances in conceptualizing and studying disability. In S. Brown & R. Lent (Eds.), *Handbook of counselling psychology* (4th ed.). John Wiley & Sons.

Peterson, D. B., & Kosciulek, J. F. (2005). Introduction to the special issue of rehabilitation education: The international classification of functioning, disability, and health (IFC). *Rehabilitation Education, 19*(2–3), 75–80.

Rodin, G., Craven, J., & Littlefield, C. (1991). *Depression in the medically ill: An integrated approach*. Brunner/Mazel.

Smart, J. F. (2001). *Disability society, and the individual*. Pro-Ed.

WHO. (2001). *ICF: International classification of functioning, disability, and health*. WHO.

Wright, B. A. (1983). *Psychosocial aspects of disability*. Harper & Row.

7 The Pediatric Life Care Plan and Vocational Evaluation

Jennifer Canter[1]

A pediatric life care plan addresses the needs of an individual who has experienced an alleged event leading to medical or developmental outcomes that would not otherwise have occurred. After the age of 21, when an individual reaches the age of majority, the pediatric life care plan will transition into an adult life care plan. This is because the structure of needs such as care and educational support will inherently change with age, although individuals may remain under a pediatrician's care beyond age 21 (Hardin et al., 2017).

Recommendations in the pediatric life care plan, as with adults, should be supported through an evidence-based methodology that ideally includes the integration of epidemiologically strong research with objective clinical judgment. Children and teens require careful consideration regarding the likelihood of developmental progress over time, the utility of therapeutic interventions, and support for families caring for a child with a disability. Medication dosing, durable equipment specifications, and transition to adult care clinicians are further aspects of pediatric care. It is essential to consider the whole child and utilize a family-centered approach when interpreting and synthesizing the materials available for plan generation (Murphy et al., 2011). Vocational aspects may also be included, especially regarding federal, state, and local support services available, to assist in achieving optimal educational and career goals (Laws and Regulations, n.d.).

This chapter will address life care planning assessments and vocational evaluations in children, teens, and young adults. These types of assessments and the analysis processes to create them overlap in many regards. Therefore, the philosophy and development methods discussed for either can often be used interchangeably.

Role of the Pediatrician

There is wide variation in the conditions affecting individuals for whom a life care plan has been requested. Incidents prompting the creation of the assessment and plan include but are not limited to birth injury, trauma, infection, congenital anomalies, and accidents. Pediatrics is the specialty of medical science concerned with the physical, mental, and social health of children from birth to young adulthood. As with adults, the biological, behavioral, physical, and social aspects of a child play a significant role in their health and welfare (Children's Health, the Nation's Wealth, 2004). The field of pediatrics includes preventive health and anticipatory guidance in addition to the diagnosis, treatment, and care of acute and chronic conditions. Pediatricians also consider the impact that genetic, social, and environmental influences have on child development and health, as a growing child differs psychologically, anatomically, and developmentally from an adult (Definition of a Pediatrician, 2015). Fundamental to the field of pediatrics is family-centered care, and the "medical home" philosophy is a well-supported approach to child

DOI: 10.4324/b23293-7

and family welfare. A medical home is not an actual building—it is an extension of the medical practice that "builds partnerships with clinical specialists, families, and community resources." The medical home ensures that the family and community of a constant child's life partner with health care professionals (What Is a Medical Home?, 2021).

Integration of medical specialists, therapists, and educators into the medical home model is a key factor in creating a nurturing environment for any child, and all the more important for a child with a medical or developmental disability (Denboba et al., 2006).

Like the medical home, the pediatric life care plan is founded on the premise that health and wellness extend beyond traditional notions of disease and disability to include myriad factors external to the individual (Children's Health, the Nation's Wealth, 2004). It is essential to be cognizant of the fact that the life care plan is a tool for non-medical individuals to understand effective means of addressing often complex, multidisciplinary needs. These include social factors, specialist coordination, home safety, and durable medical equipment needs. As the life care plan designed in a forensic capacity may be applied clinically in the future as a roadmap to lifetime care, recommendations for the needs of the child and family should be concise and practical. Since life care planners have varied backgrounds that bring different perspectives to the plan, a non-treating pediatrician may be a helpful contributor to the assessment and/or plan.

Person-First Language and Respect

Regardless of the context through which the pediatric life care plan is generated, an approach founded on dignity and respect when interviewing and documenting is paramount. A child should not be defined by the medical diagnoses or disabilities for which their care needs are being evaluated. Certain jurisdictions have laws requiring respectful language when referring to people with disabilities in regulations, rules, and publications (People First Language, 2006). Person-first language conveys respect by recognizing the individual as a person with a medical condition or disability rather than presenting that condition as their defining characteristic.

For example, a "child with epilepsy" is preferred over "an epileptic child." It is similarly respectful to avoid terms such as "suffering" or "victim" when discussing disabilities or mental health challenges. The "child who has limb loss" is preferred over the "amputee." Rather than referring to an individual as "suffering from depression" or "abusing drugs," person-first language principles suggest stating the person "has depression and a substance use disorder." Such language avoids the connotation of negative assumptions about the child's quality of life and family unit and establishes the objectivity of the author. It further conveys a forward-looking outlook on abilities and strengths within the child and family unit.

When meeting the child and their family in the forensic setting, which often involves discussing difficult and emotionally charged topics, it is important to remain respectful and sensitive to the challenges the child and their family have faced and the difficulties the interview or meeting may pose. Conducting a courteous interview is accomplished through using professional and sensitive terminology, maintaining objectivity, focusing on the necessary information, and avoiding unnecessary intrusion. For example, when conducting a social history with a parent, if the child is due for feeding via gastrostomy tube, stop the interview and observe the parent-child interaction. This interaction in the home environment is mutually beneficial for both parties. Observation of a child and family within the home setting additionally allows for assessment of the need for potential adaptations for accessibility. However, a remote interview or evaluation outside the home may also suffice (Cho et al., 2016).

Further inclusive language considerations include race, ethnicity, religion, culture, language, literacy, neurodiversity, sexual orientation, and gender (Advancing Health Equity, 2021). These aspects of a family should be explored and respected during the assessment process.

For example, it is traditional in some cultures to take off one's shoes before entering the home (Advancing Health Equity). The use of an interpreter and how to most effectively integrate this into the assessment must also be considered (Karliner et al., 2007).

Pediatric Life Care Plan Components

The philosophy of and approach to these evaluations focus on abilities rather than disabilities, while at the same time assuring the life care plan is ethical, evidence-based, and provides for a safe living environment. The first step in the process is becoming familiar with the child's over-all condition. This involves using concrete data from professionals who are qualified to render opinions about the child's rehabilitation potential and remaining steadfast in the production of objective work.

The timeline for engagement to create a life care plan in a forensic context varies. The opportunity to interview a child or family may have passed due to the stage of litigation. Materials that afford as comprehensive an approach to the plan as possible should be requested from the referring professional (e.g., attorney). It may be helpful to provide a list of requested materials such as pre- and post-incident medical records, depositions, specialist expert reports, school records, and therapy records.

A pediatric life care plan assignment should be accepted only by a qualified planner who is familiar and comfortable with the subject and able to inform the referring source what input will be necessary from experts. For example, a child with limb loss will have a lifelong requirement for prosthetics that exceeds the adult with limb loss given the child's expected growth. In this instance, it is imperative to have access to a prosthetics expert. A child with a high-level spinal cord injury will not ambulate, yet a child with a lower-level injury may have the potential to do so. In this instance, input from a pediatric neurologist is indicated.

Many planners utilize full life expectancy in costing analysis from a methodological perspective as a blanket approach, regardless of the case specifics. Life expectancy discussions should not take place with families due to the inherent sensitivities. For example, a child in a persistent vegetative state will have a significantly truncated life expectancy with no evidence base to support the potential for developmental progress. However, the family may not yet have come to terms with this or even been informed by treating clinicians of the expected prognosis. An objective, yet sensitive, balance is required during the interview process (Strauss et al., 2000).

Social History

The social environment of the child is a critical component of the pediatric life care plan. Factors such as family and household composition, sibling health and developmental status, the role of extended family, and the family's occupations and work schedules assist in understanding the whole child. The family environment may have a protective or harmful impact on the child's long-term health and welfare. Further, a family may have pre-existing needs that are not related to cost allocations. It is relevant to understand the home size and structure to allocate properly for relevant modifications. Social history is useful not only in identifying risk factors and needs but also in identifying issues that may contribute positively or negatively to a child's medical or developmental issues. Family structure is also important to consider when multiple parties were involved in the event prompting litigation. A healthy parent who sustains a traumatic brain injury may no longer be capable of rendering care to a child who sustained injuries in the same incident, such as in a motor vehicle collision. Various portions of the social history will also be relevant to the vocational analysis, discussed later in this chapter.

Elements to explore in social histories are discussed in the following sections.

Home Setting

1. Where does the child live?
2. Is the living space owned or rented?
3. What is the physical home structure (e.g., bathrooms, stairs, bedrooms)?
4. Have any modifications been made to the living space since the issue prompted life care plan creation?
5. Were there prior residences and, if so, what were the reasons for moving?
6. Is there exposure to smoke?
7. Are there pets in the home?

Family and Household Composition

1. Who lives in the home?
2. Who is considered the primary caregiver and, if more than one, what is the relationship between these individuals (e.g., legally married, common-law marriage)?
3. What is the gender identity of the individuals in the home?
4. What is the legal relationship between the caregivers and child (e.g., biological, adopted, step-parent)?
5. Are there siblings and, if so, are there any health or developmental issues?
6. Are there individuals involved in the child's life who do not live in the home?
7. Are there paramours, close family friends, professional caregivers, babysitters, etc.?
8. What family support (e.g., aunts, uncles, grandparents) is available?
9. If applicable, who (if anyone) has been trained to care for the child if there are special health care needs (e.g., tracheostomy)?
10. What is the immigration status of the family?
11. What are the language preferences and abilities?
12. Is a religion practiced in the home?
13. Are there familial dietary preferences (e.g., vegetarian, kosher)?
14. What is the caregiver's literacy status?

Family Dynamics

1. What stressors have been expressed by caregivers or identified by treating clinicians (e.g., need for mental health support, respite care, support groups)?
2. If the caregivers work outside the home, what are their occupations?
3. Has the incident impacted the family financially?
4. Adverse childhood experiences (ACEs) such as:

   - Abuse or neglect
   - Witnessing violence in the home or community
   - Having a family member attempt or die by suicide
   - Growing up in a household with substance use or mental health conditions
   - Household member incarceration (Preventing Adverse Childhood Experiences, 2021)

Outside Activities

1. Does the child attend school or daycare?
2. If so, what is the family's perception as to the school or daycare's role, successes, and challenges?

3. If therapy is outside the home, how does a child get there?
4. What are the family's transportation needs?

In reviewing all this, it is important to understand how the social history may have changed since the event prompting litigation. In some instances, families with children who have developmental or medical needs may face depression, anxiety, and/or isolation due to the impact on socialization, changes in employment, and discord in familial relationships (Seltzer et al., 2001; Herring et al., 2006). Caring for a child with a disability may impact the caregivers' ability to work outside the home, resulting in adverse financial consequences and further increasing stressors in family dynamics (Kuhlthau & Perrin, 2001). Conversely, with appropriate resources and support, families of children with disabilities may show resilience and adaptation. With the exception of children who sustain the condition at the time of birth, outside activities such as school and sports, among others, may have changed since the event.

Pre-Incident Medical and Developmental Conditions

As many life care plans are generated within a forensic context, documentation of a child's pre-incident medical conditions is essential to differentiate any needs that are attributable to the event leading to ligation. For example, if a child with diabetes sustains a traumatic injury, needs allocation should be related solely to the injury, not pre-existing diabetes. However, the fact that a child had diabetes before the injury may impact elements of post-event care (e.g., a greater risk for infection). In these instances, it is essential to have input from specialist experts to opine on pre -and post-incident needs and how to properly differentiate. A previously active teenage child with a traumatic brain injury requires a wholly different approach than a child with pre-existing disabilities who sustains the same injury.

A child's pre-incident developmental and educational performance and trajectory are additional important factors for the development of a life care plan. For example, if a child sustains an orthopedic injury and has pre-existing speech therapy in place, any costs for the speech therapy would not be allocated in the life care plan. Documents including early intervention records, Individualized Education Plans (IEPs), standardized testing results, teacher commentary, and other academic records are helpful in this regard. However, interpretation of these records should not be undertaken by anyone without the credentials to do so. Children with complex pre-incident developmental or educational trajectories may require input from experts (e.g., pediatrician, pediatric neurologist, neuropsychologist) to determine which changes, if any, can be attributed to the incident.

All children require routine care, including well-child exams, immunizations, dental care, vision screening, and management of routine childhood conditions (e.g., ear infections, respiratory viruses) (2021 Recommendations for Preventive Pediatric Health Care, 2021). These visits are most frequent in the first year of life, with decreasing frequency thereafter. In designing a pediatric life care plan, differentiation of incremental care should be considered. In other words, routine visits that are expected for any child should not be included in the life care plan. Only those visits that are necessary as a result of the inciting event should be included.

Event Prompting Life Care Plan Creation

A general understanding of the event prompting the generation of a life care plan is relevant for determining pre- and post-injury needs, as well as developing an overall understanding of how the event affected the family unit. In a forensic context, for example, a life care plan may be relevant to determine post-incident needs after a motor vehicle crash. Alternatively, a life care plan may be requested by a family engaged in estate planning or the development of a special needs trust. In the forensic realm, documentation of the objective circumstances surrounding the incident prompting litigation should be included in the pediatric life care plan. The purpose of a forensic pediatric life care plan is to establish post-incident needs, and it is not appropriate to comment on causation or standard of care.

Post-Incident Medical and Developmental Conditions

To understand a child's post-incident trajectory, it is useful to establish a timeline from the incident to as close to issuing the plan as feasible. This timeline should include the immediate interventions and medical care after the incident, including the initial hospital course, if applicable. All required medical care, surgical procedures, equipment, and medications to date are paramount to understanding the post-incident trajectory. The timeline should include how the social situation may have changed as well. Importantly, a child's needs may change over time. For example, a child who was initially able to feed by mouth may progress to require enteral nutrition via a feeding tube. On the contrary, a child may improve in some regards, including gaining respiratory independence, mobility improvement, or developmental progress with therapy. Equipment needs may evolve based on the child's ability, growth, or interval changes in health conditions.

At times, proposed interventions are futile in improving certain conditions. If an intervention has been attempted repeatedly without desired results, it is reasonable to consider whether this is appropriate to include in the plan. A healthy child will naturally advance developmentally over time, while a child who sustains a medical or developmental event may reach a static state with little objectively supported improvement. It is important to understand that not all interventions a child has received in the past are appropriate to include for the future. Some equipment, such as a stroller, may need to be replaced with a wheelchair, for example, to allow a child independent mobility if possible. Physical growth may also necessitate adjustment or replacement of equipment. Changes in activity level and physical function over time may also require new equipment allocations or discontinuation of previous equipment, as well as changes in replacement frequency (Marini et al., 2019).

Open-ended questions such as those that follow may help solicit this information from the treating clinician or the family for whom the plan is being prepared. Patience is essential: give the family ample time to respond. Similarly, observing a child in tasks such as eating requires time. It is important to explain this to the referral source to allow sufficient time for the evaluation. Example questions include:

1. Has there been any improvement noted with the use of a particular medication?
2. What impact has there been from a particular therapeutic intervention?
3. Has a particular consumable or durable medical good been helpful? What does the individual and/or caregiver perceive as helpful or not helpful?

Current plans for medical care, diagnostics, and interventions are a further consideration:

1. What do you believe may help with (a certain component of) a child's condition?
2. Who are a child's clinicians, and when were the last appointments?
3. What future plans were made at the last appointment?
4. Are there any upcoming planned diagnostic studies or surgical procedures?

5. Are there upcoming plans that are no longer desired (e.g., a family wishes to forgo a planned procedure because it was not effective in the past or it poses a risk to the individual outweighing the perceived benefit)?

With the extended time frame of the litigation process, it may be years between pediatric life care plan creation and presentation of this information in a forensic setting. As with adults, the pediatric life care plan is an evolving roadmap that may change significantly over time. Education of the plan requestor (e.g., attorney) as to the importance of updating the document if new information becomes available is recommended. At times, a second interview may be warranted to assess the interim developmental status or social changes (e.g., transition from a facility to home).

Future Needs

Projections of future medical care for pediatric patients require consideration of the probable developmental trajectory of a child and recognition of changing medical care and equipment needs as the child ages. It is essential to anchor medical recommendations in a thorough review of the available medical records recommendations of treating clinicians.

Future procedures or interventions planned by treating physicians at the time of plan preparation should be included; when evaluating future interventions, medical necessity should be considered. Medicare considers services medically necessary that are needed to diagnose or treat an illness, injury, condition, disease, or its symptoms and that meet the accepted standards of medicine. Medical necessity is supported by documentation and recommendations from the treating physicians and health care team, as well as accepted treatment practices in the medical literature.

The evidence base available and medical necessity standard must be considered when evaluating complementary or alternative medical treatments. Some medical treatments may not have an established consensus as to their efficacy or safety in the medical literature, making it difficult to evaluate whether they are appropriate for inclusion in a life care plan. It is important to adhere to the medical necessity standard in such circumstances and refrain from recommending treatments outside of the accepted standards of medicine. Planners who are not qualified by licensure or education to integrate such methodology should educate the referral source as such and qualify applicable recommendations.

Medical and Developmental Conditions

Although no two pediatric life care plans are the same, due to the nature of the events that commonly prompt the development of a pediatric life care plan, certain elements of care are frequently addressed. Thus, those who plan to develop pediatric life care plans should have a comprehensive understanding of these regularly encountered issues. Each should be considered separately when determining current and future needs.

Cerebral Palsy and Spasticity

Although the incidence of cerebral palsy has fallen substantially in recent years, most likely due to improved antenatal and neonatal interventions, it is still the most common physical disability in the pediatric population (Novak et al., 2020). Cerebral palsy describes a category of permanent movement disorders that are non-progressive. While patients often have concurrent epilepsy, intellectual disability, or behavior disturbances, among others, this is not always the case. The etiology of cerebral palsy can be related to a wide variety of infectious, developmental, genetic, metabolic, ischemic, and other acquired causes (Johnston, 2019).

Cerebral palsy is classified based on the nature of the motor abnormality and the portion of the body involved. Children with spastic diplegia (the most common classification) are more affected in their lower extremities than their upper extremities. Spastic tetraplegia affects all four extremities and is generally the most severe form of the disease that is most likely to be accompanied by additional comorbidities. Children with spastic hemiplegia are more affected on one side of the body than the other and often show a preference for use of one side early in life. Extrapyramidal cerebral palsy accounts for 15% of cases and is also known as athetoid, choreoathetoid, or dyskinetic, as opposed to spastic (Johnston, 2019).

Spasticity is the condition of an abnormal increase in muscle tone or stiffness of a muscle that might interfere with movement or speech or may be associated with discomfort or pain. It is usually caused by damage to nerve pathways in the brain or spinal cord responsible for muscle movement and is often associated with cerebral palsy, spinal cord injury, multiple sclerosis, stroke, or brain or head trauma (Spasticity Information Page, 2019). Spasticity may be treated through rehabilitation alone (e.g., physical therapy and home-based exercise). Alternatively, treatment can include pharmacological and interventional approaches, and the recommendations of treating physicians and therapists should be examined when assessing the needs of a child. Spasticity may affect a child's quality of life, their ability to function independently, and their caregiver's ability to care for the child and their hygiene needs. Importantly, spasticity management needs can be complex and often change over time as a child grows.

Multiple medical and interventional options are available for spasticity management, and the involvement of a spasticity management specialist (e.g., neurologist, physical medicine and rehabilitation physician) may be required for the integration of a spasticity management plan that is effective and balances risks and benefits.

Seizures

Seizure disorders in children can be idiopathic and occur in children with no other medical or developmental issues. However, seizures are also a common occurrence in infants with birth injury and are often associated with later epilepsy, cerebral palsy, and/or intellectual disability (Glass et al., 2018). In addition, several epilepsy syndromes are associated with genetic mutations. Alternatively, seizure activity in the newborn period may resolve entirely, negating the need for long-term follow-up.

The workup and treatment of seizures can vary depending on a child's presentation, although it often includes brain imaging and laboratory and genetic testing. There is also extensive variation in the ability of a child's seizures to be adequately controlled with available medications, and many children have drug-resistant epilepsy that requires frequent follow-up with specialists and considerations for safety in the child's environment (Mikati & Tchapyjnikov, 2019).

Feeding, Swallowing, and Nutrition Disorders

Children being evaluated for a life care plan will often have needs associated with feeding and nutrition that need to be addressed. Some children with cerebral palsy may have associated dysphagia and require nutrition either fully or in part via a gastrostomy tube. Attention to needs related to dysphagia is critical in this patient population not only to ensure adequate nutrition but also to prevent aspiration and respiratory complications that can arise from dysphagia (Novak et al., 2020).

Chronic Respiratory Conditions

Chronic respiratory conditions that may be encountered when developing a pediatric life care plan include neonatal chronic lung disease, asthma, or the host of respiratory complications associated with cerebral palsy, including aspiration, impaired airway clearance or lung function, recurrent respiratory infections, or pulmonary effects of spinal deformities. It is essential to appreciate the effect of concurrent medical issues such as abnormal tone or gastroesophageal reflux on a child's respiratory status and engage in a holistic approach to a child's respiratory care needs (Boel et al., 2019).

Intellectual Disability

The diagnosis of intellectual disability requires subaverage scores on standardized intelligence testing and difficulties in adaptive behavior, both of which must be present before age 18. In the United States, the prevalence of intellectual disability is about 3%. Importantly, rates of psychiatric disorders are higher in children with intellectual disabilities (Platt et al., 2019). Among children with cerebral palsy, about half have an intellectual disability, and the concurrence of intellectual disability and severe motor impairment is associated with an increased risk of premature death (Novak et al., 2020).

Abuse and Neglect

Children with disabilities are at higher risk for abuse than those without disabilities. Caregiver stress can contribute to this risk, and those children with compromised independence or ability to communicate are particularly vulnerable. While some signs of physical abuse are more obvious, such as bruises, burns, or fractures, other behavioral signs such as a sudden change in behavior may be more nonspecific. Neglect is also a concern among children who are disabled and can manifest in several ways, including poor hygiene or missed medical appointments (Childhood Maltreatment Among Children, 2019).

Limb Loss (Amputation)

Limb loss can be associated with a number of causes in the pediatric population, including trauma, cancer, burns, or congenital malformations (Osoro et al., 2019). Acquired amputations are characterized by the level of limb loss. In the acute phase following limb loss, wound healing and pain are the primary concerns. Following this, special attention should be paid to the choice of prosthetics devices, when desired, matching the individual's needs. Early rehabilitation is also important to optimize independence with limb loss. The majority of individuals with congenital or acquired limb loss go on to live independent lives with vibrant vocational options.

Birth Injuries

Common birth injuries are often temporary in nature, such as subconjunctival hemorrhages, clavicle fractures, or bruising. However, some birth injuries may necessitate rehabilitation and/or medical interventions beyond the postnatal period, particularly brachial plexus injury (Birth Injuries, n.d.).

Categories of Future Needs

Equipment

When allocating for pediatric equipment needs, there are certain factors beyond the nature of a child's medical conditions or disabilities that should be taken into account. For example, a lift may not be necessary for a small child with motor delays, but a larger child who is unable to participate in transfers may require a lift for safety. Similarly, a small child with physical disabilities may be able to use a standard crib, but as they grow a hospital bed may become necessary to accommodate their care needs. An additional consideration for any type of equipment that requires electricity is whether the family has consistent, reliable electricity in their home. When applicable, devices that are not electricity-dependent should be available for backups, such as a manual wheelchair or portable oxygen concentrator. Space for use, movement, and storage of larger pieces of equipment should also be evaluated.

A child who is unable to take food by mouth may have a gastronomy tube for nutrition and medication administration. A nasogastric tube may also be present in some circumstances. It is important to consider not only the costs directly associated with these items but also those of the supplies related to maintaining the tube and site. The need for more frequent replacement or adjustment as a child grows should also be considered in comparison to an adult patient with similar equipment. The necessity of a feeding pump should also be taken into account in these circumstances, along with regular maintenance, service, and replacement of the pump as necessary.

Wheelchairs are an important consideration for mobility and independence depending on a child's age and physical and developmental abilities. Additionally, mobility equipment will require adjustment and replacement as a child develops. It is important to recognize a child's developmental trajectory and level of function in allocating future mobility equipment. A very young child, for example, may make use of a stroller, while they may transition to a wheelchair as they develop. There is considerable variation in available mobility devices, and the plan should outline which device is appropriate for the abilities and developmental stage of the child.

Ankle-foot orthoses and other braces and orthoses will need to be replaced more frequently in pediatric patients than in adults due to rapid growth. Wear and tear in active children may also contribute to more frequent replacement needs during childhood.

Prosthetic replacement needs will also likely be more frequent for the pediatric patient than an adult. Different prosthetic devices will be appropriate at various developmental stages. Input from a prosthetist to allocate appropriate replacement frequencies and prosthetic components for a child with an amputation is essential.

Augmentative and alternative communication (AAC) describes a variety of processes that augment, support, or replace the speech of individuals with communication needs. AAC solutions may be no-tech, low-tech, or high-tech. No-tech solutions include sign language and other gesturing; low-tech solutions may include books, cards, or display boards for common words or phrases; and high-tech typically describes an electronic device used for communication. These high-tech devices may be operated by touch, eye gaze, or microphones, among other options, to meet the specific needs and abilities of the user. Given the great variety of available devices, input from a speech therapist is generally required to match a child with the best method or device for their needs. As with other equipment, maintenance for wear and tear and adaptations as children grow and develop should be considered when developing a life care plan (Elsahar et al., 2019).

Rehabilitation Services

Rehabilitation services for children may include physical, occupational, and/or speech therapy. The Individuals with Disabilities Education Act (IDEA) requires a school district to provide certain "related services" if necessary for an individual to receive a free, appropriate education (Individuals with Disabilities Education Act, 1975). These services are defined to include transportation and such developmental, corrective, and other supportive services as are required to assist a child with a disability to benefit from education. These services may include speech-language pathology and audiology services, interpretation services, psychological services, and physical and occupational therapy, among others. It is important to understand which services will be provided by a child's school district and which will not, to allocate for additional services as needed, and to refrain from providing duplicative services already provided through the district.

Regarding allocation of therapies within a life care plan, the goal is to include differential services (i.e., what the child would not otherwise be entitled to through the school district) to improve or maintain the progress that has already been made. In some cases, it is necessary to allocate additional therapeutic services not directly related to education. These services may include physical and occupational therapy outside of the academic year.

Physical therapists play a role in rehabilitation by addressing gross motor skills, strength building, endurance, and fitness. They may help with mobility through strengthening programs and the use of adaptive equipment and mobility aids. Physical therapists work to minimize activity limitations and address participation restrictions.

Occupational therapists address limitations in activities of daily living such as feeding, eating, dressing, and toileting and instrumental activities of daily living such as cooking or shopping. Occupational therapists also play a role in identifying a child's equipment needs. They may address fine motor skills, upper extremity function, visual-motor skills, and the occupations or tasks that can be expected of a child.

Speech therapists, or speech and language pathologists, address communication and cognition. They work with children to improve expressive language skills verbally or through alternative communication. Speech therapists may also evaluate and treat swallowing problems such as dysphagia (Houtrow et al., 2019).

The optimal frequency of therapies varies by injury or illness and the specific needs of a child, yet generally follows a progression of intensive therapy through childhood to maximize recovery and development followed by tapering of frequency once a maintenance state has been reached. Therapies may be completed in the home (either in person or virtually), at a therapeutic center, or in school. In some cases, a combination of these locations best meets the child's needs.

The three laws most applicable to the rights of students with disabilities in public schools are the IDEA, Section 504 of the Rehabilitation Act, and Title II of the Americans with Disabilities Act (ADA). It is important to understand these and how they apply to allocated resources within a life care plan or vocational evaluation.

Care and Supervision

During days when school is in session, a child will receive care through their school district as a requirement of the legislation previously described. Once the child is of an age that they are no longer entitled to educational services, care needs and associated costs may increase as additional hours are needed. Similarly, needs during periods when school is not in session should be considered, such as summer breaks, and costs allocated accordingly.

Respite care may be allocated for families of children with extensive care needs to benefit caregivers' psychological adjustment, fatigue, and mental health quality of life. The level of care needs and additional care already in place should be considered when determining the appropriate quantity of respite care to allocate. Respite care allocations may also increase over time, as a family would expect reduced care needs with growth and development when a child develops typically, which may not be realized in a child with a disability or injury.

It is imperative to refrain from a broad-stroke recommendation for agency-based care without careful consideration of the needs and preferences of the individual and/or guardian. The level of care and/or supervision required by a child will determine what level of care provider is necessary for their needs and where that care will take place. At times, an extension of what would otherwise be unskilled care (e.g., babysitter, safety chaperone) through the teenage years is appropriate to provide supervision for teens with isolated developmental disabilities (i.e., no medical conditions). When there are medical needs beyond safety/supervision, care may be provided by a home health aide, licensed practical nurse, or registered nurse. The scope of licensure of each of these professions varies and is determined at the state level. Relevant laws and scope of practice should be reviewed where the child resides to determine the appropriate level of in-home care. Facility care may also be appropriate in circumstances where a child's care needs exceed what can be provided in the home due to limitations of space, equipment, and family comfort.

Understanding the distinction between a physical disability, an intellectual disability, and a medical condition is imperative. Avoid broad-stroke labeling and assumptions: not all children with physical disabilities have developmental disabilities. Similarly, not all children with developmental disabilities have medical conditions. Disability does not mean a child is "sick." Although a child may have a need, not all situations require differential care. While some children with physical, intellectual, or medical conditions require care, the care needs and training and licensure of the individual providing the care may vary considerably. Determining the nature of a child's care needs and the appropriate level of training and background of the care provider allocated to address these needs is necessary for life care plan development. Not every child requires skilled and/or unskilled care over what would otherwise be part of the caregiver role, and each situation requires careful consideration.

For allocation of care, family preference for hiring care through a staffing agency or by self-hire should be considered. Self-hire of one or multiple caregivers by a family empowers them to select someone they and their child are comfortable with and gives them control of future staffing decisions. Self-hire may offer more consistency in who is providing care for a child. If the self-hire option is offered in the life care plan, the allocation for additional expenses beyond direct hourly wage, including the employer portion of the Federal Insurance Contributions Act payroll tax and a payroll service, should be included. Hiring care through an agency may alleviate the family of some administrative burdens, including managing payroll, employer taxes, and coordinating time off, but offers limited options in terms of consistency of the caregiver and gives the family limited power to choose the personnel providing care. Statistical data for hourly wages of various levels of caregivers may be accessed on O*NET Online, a database of occupational information sponsored by the U.S. Department of Labor (O*NET OnLine, 2021).

Understanding the family's preferences and a child's needs impacts decisions regarding a live-in or live-out caregiver. A live-in caregiver may offer advantages for a family and child with extensive care needs and may be supplemented with a second caregiver when needed. A live-out caregiver may be more appropriate for a child with care needs that do not necessitate a full-time caregiver if the family's preference is not for an individual to live in the home or if the lack of available living space does not allow for this option.

Family Support and Mental Health

Families caring for a child with a disability or injury may face increased financial, social, and emotional pressures that require additional care. This extends to any other children in the family as well who may face behavioral and social impairment at higher rates than siblings of only typically developing children. The allocation of appropriate supportive mental health resources, such as short-term family or individual counseling, should be considered not only for the child but also for the family and their mental health care needs arising from the child's injury or disability. Support groups catering to specific conditions, including online forums, may be helpful options for some families.

Case Management

Case management is a collaborative process that assesses, plans, implements, coordinates, monitors, and evaluates the options and services required to meet a child's health and human service needs. It is characterized by advocacy, communication, and resource management and promotes quality and cost-effective interventions and outcomes. Case managers may hold a variety of health care qualifications, including registered nurses, physical therapists, occupational therapists, and licensed social workers, among other professions. Several case manager certifications exist, including Certified Case Manager (CCM) and Accredited Case Manager (ACM). A case manager may be allocated as a resource to assist the family and child in navigating the complexities of the health care and education systems and ensure the care plan remains updated and is carried out effectively. Some families choose to coordinate care independent of an outside party. As with other aspects of the life care plan, self-management should be considered.

Vocational Evaluation

At times, a non-vocationally trained clinician "closes the door" for vocational potential by stating the individual will have no chance at meaningful employment merely due to a disability. Instead, it is essential to consider the extensive opportunities for individuals with disabilities to dispel these myths of unemployability. Life care planners, if credentialed to do so, may conduct a vocational evaluation. Alternatively, the planner may be provided with a vocational evaluation from another expert or as part of school records. Vocational considerations are an important component of future needs and thus are important elements of a pediatric life care plan. As such, this component of the whole-child approach is included in this chapter.

Benefits of Employment

Employment is a positive influence on self-efficacy and socialization. It provides structure and a source of income and enables individuals with disabilities to contribute to local businesses and the national economy. The positive effects experienced by individuals with disabilities are most substantial for those who participate in integrated employment (Competitive Integrated Employment, n.d.). Although the planner may not be a vocational evaluator, the vocational analysis may be integrated into the life care plan.

The progress made by the child or adolescent over time is important. Behavioral issues and social skills, for example, may be positively influenced when the individual is employed. Key medical needs, such as seizures, are paramount considerations in a safe work environment. For individuals with physical disabilities, extensive adaptive resources are available, and it is best to start learning about these as early as possible. For example, the individual with upper limb loss may be able to learn to use a one-handed keyboard. With appropriate accommodations, some individuals will be capable of successful employment in a paid work setting.

PEEDS-RAPEL Model

In a forensic context, there are two main components of a vocational analysis: 1) determining what the educational and vocational outcomes would have been absent the issue prompting litigation and 2) devising a plan to assure optimization of vocational potential considering the issue. For a minor with no vocational history of their own, the evidence-based method for evaluating vocational potential is the PEEDS-RAPEL model (Weed & Field, 2002). The analysis seeks to determine the probable vocational trajectory and earnings of an individual. In determining the earnings potential of children, the PEEDS-RAPEL model considers the occupational and educational history of the parents, siblings, and other family members. The educational and income success of children is closely related to the socioeconomic standing of their parents. The following components may be considered in the PEEDS-RAPEL analysis, although it may not be feasible to obtain all of these depending on a child's developmental status or available historical information.

1. Parental/family occupations
2. Educational attainment
3. Evaluation results
4. Developmental state
5. Synthesis
6. Rehabilitation plan
7. Access to the labor market
8. Placeability
9. Earnings capacity
10. Labor force participation

Vocational Rehabilitation and Education

There is extensive federal legislation and funding supporting the integration of vocational rehabilitation into the school setting. The pathway for the continuation of vocational rehabilitation is largely provided through mandated services found in the IDEA, which requires that services be provided at no cost to individuals verified as needing them. The IDEA focuses on teaching and learning and establishes high expectations for children with disabilities to achieve authentic educational and vocational results. Another piece of federal legislation is the Workforce Innovation and Opportunity Act (WIOA), which mandates increased funding and services for individuals with disabilities to help them participate in integrated employment (Workforce Innovation and Opportunity act, n.d.). Further, the ADA and its amendments prohibit discrimination in employment based on disability and require that employers make reasonable accommodations for employees unless this would result in an undue hardship for the business (Americans with Disabilities Act, n.d.).

The school district is required to provide children with vocational transition services. Vocational goals are integrated into the IEP at age 14. Transition planning includes:

1. Transition assessments
2. Involvement of the family and student
3. Interagency collaboration (e.g., school, vocational rehabilitation agency, therapists, employment setting)
4. Community experiences (e.g., job shadowing, visits to postsecondary training institutions, participation in leisure/recreation activities, and/or meeting with agencies that can provide support after high school)
5. The student's goals for:

   • Employment
   • Education/training
   • Practicing self-advocacy
   • Self-determination skills

As the process evolves, the school district typically works with their state division of vocational rehabilitation to transition from school to post–high school employment, education, training, and independence. To qualify, the individual must have a physical, mental, cognitive, or other disability that substantially impedes employment. Once qualified, services include:

1. Job exploration of a variety of workplace settings
2. Paid work experiences with job coaches
3. Soft skills for work and independence
4. Self-advocacy (request and accept support)
5. Counseling on educational and training options
6. Connection to ongoing support options

Another vocational option for some individuals with disabilities is sheltered workshops. These are work centers that exclusively or predominantly employ people with disabilities. They provide greater opportunities for fostering friendships, offer structure during the weekdays, and ensure assistance for life without affecting disability benefits. Activities tend to be adaptable for a variety of skill sets, and responsibilities may involve repetitive tasks such as assembling and packing. Some individuals in sheltered workshops may qualify for transition into supported employment in an integrated setting.

Family-Centered Approach

Understanding a family's wishes as their child progresses toward adulthood and how they would like the child to be cared for once they reach adulthood is critical when developing a life care plan. These goals must be reconciled with the reality of a child's probable developmental trajectory, the probability of the child living longer than any family member's ability to provide care, and changes in a child's care needs over time. Given that there may be multiple possibilities for care as a child ages, it may be appropriate to develop multiple care plans to address all possible scenarios, including the duration of family care and potential placement in a residential facility.

Determination of the family's understanding and expectations of the child's life expectancy should compassionately take place without informing the family of any life expectancy projections. This should be explained to the family and understanding ensured. As in all matters related to the interview, respectful and empathetic communication is essential.

In creating a life care plan, it is important to understand any choices the family has made regarding interventions when a child is not expected to improve, such as a child in a persistent vegetative state or with a terminal illness. In these circumstances, it is important to both understand the decisions already made and those that remain to be made so the life care plan can reflect these choices and provide appropriate support for the child and family.

Interviews and Independent Medical Examinations

The interview and independent medical examination (IME) represent an opportunity to learn more about the day-to-day life of the child and their family. Items covered may include clarification of information in the medical record or collateral sources; discussion of any upcoming procedures; and review of current clinicians, medications, educational plans, and care needs. Family preferences may also be discussed for particular levels of care, interventions, or schooling.

Consider whether an interview will be necessary to gain additional information from the child or family early in the planning process. At times, an interview may not be possible, and the only information available in medical records or collateral sources can be used to create the life care plan.

If other medical experts are also conducting interviews, consider communication where possible to avoid overlap in independent roles and reduce the number of duplicate questions asked of the family and child. Questions regarding planned or potential interventions should be limited to those with a reasonable probability of occurring.

For concurrent interviews or IMEs, details such as family address, current medications, or current clinicians do not need to be asked twice. However, each expert should address the issues relevant to their respective independent evaluations, which may include obtaining additional detail regarding questions previously asked. Coordination of logistical items, including structure and order of the interview, should occur beforehand with any other individuals present.

Respect for the family and child is of the utmost importance, and difficult questions may raise emotions during the interview. Breaks from the interview or IME should be taken as needed, particularly if the child is present. In conducting an interview regarding a child, it may also be appropriate to excuse the child for a portion to allow the family the freedom to discuss sensitive matters they may not wish to discuss in the presence of the child.

Interviews and IMEs may be conducted in person or, at times, remotely via videoconference. In-person interviews present the opportunity for more direct communication and eliminate the possibility of technological difficulties. However, they may be more logistically complex or pose a burden for the family and child. Remote interviews are logistically simpler but are more limited in their possibility for physical examination and observation.

Ethics and Professionalism

Ethical dilemmas related to the age or needs of the child and their family can arise during the process. It is often useful to be aware of the four ethical principles commonly applied to medical decision-making: autonomy, or respecting the decision-making of autonomous persons; nonmaleficence, or avoiding causing harm; beneficence, or providing benefits and balancing risks and costs against benefits; and justice, or fair distribution of the risks, benefits, and costs. It should be the goal to respect these core principles in any ethical dilemmas that occur during the creation of the life care plan.

A common ethical dilemma is the extent to which older children should be involved in medical decision-making, particularly if their wishes do not align with those of their family. In circumstances where a decision has not been reached among the child, their family, and treating clinicians, it may be prudent to present multiple options in the life care plan.

It is essential that the life care plan or vocational evaluation is evidence-based and that the emotions and challenges an ethical dilemma may present do not cause the plan to stray beyond the accepted treatment and practices for a given disease or disability.

The role of the evaluator must be made clear to the child and their family. The goal is to create a plan that will allow the child to achieve optimal outcomes through an appropriate plan of rehabilitation, prevention, and reduction of complications. In this role, a life care planner is not an advocate for a particular "side," but rather tasked with the responsibility to determine evidence-based care needs for the child.

Life care planners must remain aware of their professional scope of practice and any limitations this scope may place on their ability to make projections, diagnoses, or recommendations for treatments. Scope of practice varies by state, and life care professionals are responsible for knowing the limits of their qualifications and including additional experts when necessary. For example, consultation with a physician is necessary for medication recommendations, and appropriate qualification is necessary to determine life expectancy. It is prudent to advise the client early in the process regarding any additional experts needed to make recommendations. For example, consultation with a prosthetist may be necessary for care needs related to amputations, and a neurologist may offer valuable insight into cases involving the management of seizure disorders.

A consistent process should be used for planning and organizing data, creating a narrative report, and projecting costs. It is good practice to be transparent with an individual and their family about the approach to creating the life care plan. This allows for the creation of a repeatable and defensible methodology and an effective life care plan that can evolve with the needs of the child.

Evidence-based costing methodologies should be thoroughly understood and used. Cost establishment can be completed through several methodologies depending on the child's current care and probable future care needs and location. If it is probable that the child will continue to receive care in their current location and with current providers, prior medical bills may be a useful resource. Commercially available usual, customary, and reasonable (UCR) charge databases may also be a useful resource in determining probable care costs. These databases allow searching for a percentile of charges for a specified procedure and geographic area and are useful for estimating outpatient and inpatient care costs. Some knowledge of medical coding is necessary to use these databases. Vendors can also be contacted directly in the child's probable location of care to provide an estimate of costs for a particular item. In this circumstance, it is advisable to survey multiple vendors to establish an average cost and limit the impact of outliers. As in other areas of the life care plan, personal experience alone should not be used to establish the cost. As personal experience may vary considerably by profession, patient population, and geographic area, it is essential to rely on an evidence base of established literature and resources beyond personal experience in drafting a life care plan.

Respectful and professional language should be used at all times in the life care plan, both when referring to the child and their family and when offering comments on other expert reports.

Disclaimer and Acknowledgements

This chapter represents the most up-to-date evidence, literature, and best practices currently available for the evolving field of pediatric life care planning and vocational evaluations. It is intended by the author, who is not associated with other chapters in this textbook, to be a comprehensive and independent resource.

The author wishes to acknowledge the content contributions of Jack Canter (prosthetics), Lucas Canter (adaptive aids), Olivia Canter (person-first language), and Marleigh Canter (family-centered care). The author wishes to acknowledge the contribution of Kyle Otto, BS, Merrie Deitch, BA, and Morgan Leafe, MD, MHA who participated in background research for this publication.

Note

1 I have no known conflict of interest to disclose. This chapter represents the most up-to-date evidence, literature, and best practices currently available for the evolving field of pediatric life care planning and vocational evaluations. It is intended by the author, who is not associated with other chapters in this textbook, to be a comprehensive and independent resource.

References

Advancing Health Equity: A Guide to Language, Narrative, and Concepts. (2021). *American medical association and the association of American medical colleges center for health justice.* www.ama-assn.org/system/files/ama-aamc-equity-guide.pdf

Americans with Disabilities Act, United States Department of Labor. (n.d.). Retrieved June 13, 2022, from www.dol.gov/general/topic/disability/ada

Birth Injuries. (n.d.). *Stanford children's hospital.* Retrieved January 18, 2022, from www.stanfordchildrens.org/en/topic/default?id=birth-injuries-90-P02687

Boel, L., Pernet, K., Toussaint, M., Ides, K., Leemans, G., Haan, J., Van Hoorenbeeck, K., & Verhulst, S. (2019). Respiratory morbidity in children with cerebral palsy: An overview. *Developmental Medicine and Child Neurology, 61*(6), 646–653. https://doi.org/10.1111/dmcn.14060

Childhood Maltreatment Among Children with Disabilities. (2019, September 18). *Centers for disease control and prevention.* Retrieved January 18, 2022, from www.cdc.gov/ncbddd/disabilityandsafety/abuse.html

Children's Health, the Nation's Wealth: Assessing and Improving Child Health. (2004). *National research council and the institute of medicine.* National Academies Press. https://doi.org/10.17226/10886

Cho, H. Y., MacLachlan, M., Clarke, M., & Mannan, H. (2016). Accessible home environments for people with functional limitations: A systematic review. *International Journal of Environmental Research and Public Health, 13*(8), 826. https://doi.org/10.3390/ijerph13080826

Competitive Integrated Employment (CIE). (n.d.). U.S. Department of Labor. Retrieved December 1, 2021, from www.dol.gov/agencies/odep/program-areas/integrated-employment

Definition of a Pediatrician. (2015). Committee on pediatric workforce. *Pediatrics, 135*(4).

Denboba, D., McPherson, M. G., Kenney, M. K., Strickland, B., & Newacheck, P. W. (2006). Achieving family and provider partnerships for children with special health care needs. *Pediatrics, 118*(4), 1607–1615. https://doi.org/10.1542/peds.2006-0383

Elsahar, Y., Hu, S., Bouazza-Marouf, K., Kerr, D., & Mansor, A. (2019). Augmentative and alternative communication (AAC) advances: A review of configurations for individuals with a speech disability. *Sensors (Basel, Switzerland), 19*(8), 1911. https://doi.org/10.3390/s19081911

Glass, H. C., Grinspan, Z. M., & Shellhaas, R. A. (2018). Outcomes after acute symptomatic seizures in neonates. *Seminars in Fetal & Neonatal Medicine, 23*(3), 218–222. https://doi.org/10.1016/j.siny.2018.02.001

Hardin, A. P., Hackell, J. M., & Committee on Practice and Ambulatory Medicine. (2017). Age limit of pediatrics. *Pediatrics, 140*(3), e20172151. https://doi.org/10.1542/peds.2017-2151

Herring, S., Gray, K., Taffe, J., Tonge, B., Sweeney, D., & Einfeld, S. (2006). Behaviour and emotional problems in toddlers with pervasive developmental disorders and developmental delay: Associations with parental mental health and family functioning. *Journal of Intellectual Disability Research, 50*(Pt 12), 874–882. https://doi.org/10.1111/j.1365-2788.2006.00904.x

Houtrow, A., Murphy, N., & Council on Children with Disabilities. (2019). Prescribing physical, occupational, and speech therapy services for children with disabilities. *Pediatrics, 143*(4), e20190285. https://doi.org/10.1542/peds.2019-0285

Individuals with Disabilities Education Act, Publ. L. No. 94–142, Section 300.34 Related Services. (1975). https://sites.ed.gov/idea/regs/b/a/300.34

Johnston, M. V. (2019). Cerebral palsy. In R. M. Kliegman (Ed.), *Nelson textbook of pediatrics* (21st ed.). Elsevier.

Karliner, L. S., Jacobs, E. A., Chen, A. H., & Mutha, S. (2007). Do professional interpreters improve clinical care for patients with limited English proficiency? A systematic review of the literature. *Health Services Research, 42*(2), 727–754. https://doi.org/10.1111/j.1475-6773.2006.00629.x

Kuhlthau, K. A., & Perrin, J. M. (2001). Child health status and parental employment. *Archives of Pediatrics & Adolescent Medicine, 155*(12), 1346–1350. https://doi.org/10.1001/archpedi.155.12.1346

Laws and Regulations. (n.d.). *U.S. department of labor*. Retrieved December 9, 2021, from www.dol.gov/agencies/eta/disability/laws

Marini, I., Chia, V., Antol, D. L., Mora, E. M., Quijano, P., Macarena, P. R., & Cuevas, S. (2019). Redux: Empirical validation of medical equipment replacement schedules in life care plans. *Journal of Life Care Planning, 17*(2), 5–17. www.proquest.com/openview/99ce9ce51059b8bd358456e75392eca6/1?pq-origsite=gscholar&cbl=5107878

Mikati, M. A., & Tchapyjnikov, D. (2019). Seizures in childhood. In R. M. Kliegman (Ed.), *Nelson textbook of pediatrics* (21st ed.). Elsevier.

Murphy, N. A., Carbone, P. S., & Council on Children With Disabilities. (2011). Parent-provider-community partnerships: Optimizing outcomes for children with disabilities. *Pediatrics, 128*(4), 795–802. https://doi.org/10.1542/peds.2011-1467

Novak, I., Morgan, C., Fahey, M., Finch-Edmondson, M., Galea, C., Hines, A., Langdon, K., Namara, M. M., Paton, M. C., Popat, H., Shore, B., Khamis, A., Stanton, E., Finemore, O. P., Tricks, A., Te Velde, A., Dark, L., Morton, N., & Badawi, N. (2020). State of the evidence traffic lights 2019: Systematic review of interventions for preventing and treating children with cerebral palsy. *Current Neurology and Neuroscience Reports, 20*(2), 3. https://doi.org/10.1007/s11910-020-1022-z

O*NET OnLine (CIE). (2021, November 16). *U.S. department of labor*. Retrieved December 1, 2021, from www.onetonline.org

Osoro, M., Tsao, E., & Apkon, S. D. (2019). Ambulation assistance. In R. M. Kliegman (Ed.), *Nelson textbook of pediatrics* (21st ed.). Elsevier.

People First Language. (2006, July). *DC office of disability rights*. Retrieved December 1, 2021, from https://odr.dc.gov/page/people-first-language

Platt, J. M., Keyes, K. M., McLaughlin, K. A., & Kaufman, A. S. (2019). Intellectual disability and mental disorders in a US population-representative sample of adolescents. *Psychological Medicine, 49*(6), 952–961. https://doi.org/10.1017/S0033291718001605

Preventing adverse childhood experiences. (2021, April 6). *Centers for disease control and prevention*. Retrieved December 1, 2021, from www.cdc.gov/violenceprevention/aces/fastfact.html?CDC_AA_refVal=https%3A%2F%2F

Seltzer, M. M., Greenberg, J. S., Floyd, F. J., Pettee, Y., & Hong, J. (2001). Life course impacts of parenting a child with a disability. *American Journal on Intellectual and Developmental Disabilities, 106*(3), 265–286. https://doi.org/10.1352/0895-8017(2001)106<0265:LCIOPA>2.0.CO;2

Spasticity information page. (2019 March 27). *National Institute of neurological disorders and stroke*. Retrieved December 1, 2021, from www.ninds.nih.gov/Disorders/All-Disorders/Spasticity-Information-Page

Strauss, D. J., Ashwal, S., Day, S., & Shavelle, R. M. (2000). Life expectancy of children in vegetative and minimally conscious states. *Pediatric Neurology, 23*(4), 312–319. https://doi.org/10.1016/s0887-8994(00)00194-6

2021 Recommendations for Preventive Pediatric Health Care. (2021). Committee on practice and ambulatory medicine, bright futures periodicity schedule workgroup. *Pediatrics, 147*(3), e2020049776. https://doi.org/10.1542/peds.2020-049776

What is a medical home? (2021, October). *National resource center*. Retrieved December 1, 2021, from https://medicalhomeinfo.aap.org/overview/Pages/Whatisthemedicalhome.aspx

Weed, R. O., & Field, T. F. (2002). *Rehabilitation consultant's handbook*. E &F Publishing, Inc.

Workforce Innovation and Opportunity Act. United States Department of Labor. (n.d.). Retrieved June 13, 2022, from www.dol.gov/agencies/eta/wioa/

8   Disability Sequelae of Immobility

A Systems Perspective

Robert S. Djergaian

Dr. Paul Corcoran, a renowned physiatrist, started his 1991 article, "Use It or Lose It" when discussing the hazards of bed rest and inactivity (Corcoran, 1991). Corcoran noted that post–World War II rehabilitation programs in the Veterans Administration hospitals taught that the avoidable complications of bed rest were often more disabling than the original injury. He noted that before the 1940s, strict bed rest was the rule for four weeks or more after myocardial infarction (Corcoran). The origin of bed rest as treatment goes back to Hippocrates who said, "In every movement of the body whenever one begins to endure pain, it will be relieved by rest" (Hippocrates, 1849).

Studies done by the aerospace industry on the effects of bed rest concluded that long periods of immobility are detrimental to the health of all body systems, and also that inactivity is an important factor in the development of chronic degenerative diseases and is highly prevalent among the elderly (Booth et al., 2012). Besides effects on multiple body systems, mobility difficulties are associated with higher rates of depression, fear, anxiety, confusion, obesity, dizziness, imbalance, and increased risks of falls (Iezzoni et al., 2001). Deconditioning can be a separate diagnosis, and the importance of early mobilization for those with illness or injury has been demonstrated (Convertino, 1997; Convertino et al., 1997).

Immobility can occur from multiple causes including enforced bed rest (illness or convalescence), paralysis, immobilization of body parts with braces or casts, joint stiffness or pain with protective limitations of motion, mental disorders, and loss of sensation (discomfort does not dictate a change of position) (Dittmer & Teasell, 1993). The normal aging process is associated with mobility limitations affecting the physical, psychological, and social aspects of an older adult's life (Brown & Flood, 2013). These issues become even more problematic with a preexisting disability (Rantanen, 2013).

Complications of immobility are much easier to prevent than to treat and can negatively impact recovery from illness or trauma. Paradigm shifts have occurred in intensive care unit (ICU) care with more emphasis being placed on early mobilization. It has been demonstrated that physical and occupational therapy commencing within the first 48 hours of ICU admission leads to improved functional recovery at hospital discharge, reduced delirium duration, and increased discharge to home (Schweickert et al., 2009). Ongoing monitoring for increasing immobility during the aging process with potential interventions such as physical activity, counseling, or further therapy and training may prevent or reduce mobility decline (Rantanen, 2013).

DOI: 10.4324/b23293-8

Effects of Immobility on Specific Body Systems

Neurological System

Lipshutz and Gropper (2013) state that 25–50% of critically ill patients develop neuromuscular weakness and give an excellent review of the multifactorial causes and pathophysiology. Bed rest is considered one of the factors leading to critical illness neuromyopathy (CINM), leading them to advocate for early mobilization in the ICU setting. Other causative factors may include critical illness, cytokine production, possible drugs such as neuromuscular blockers and steroids, protein malnutrition, electrolyte imbalances, and glutamine deficiency (Lipshutz & Gropper). Additionally, compression mononeuropathies, particularly of the peroneal nerve at the fibular head and ulnar at the elbow, can occur. Corcoran (1991) notes there is a substantial decrease in the central nervous system content of the neurotransmitters dopamine, norepinephrine, and serotonin after inactivity. Serotonin plays a key role in mood, cognition, and appetite, so reduced serotonin levels associated with immobility may be linked to the depressed mood, reduced cognitive skills, and loss of appetite commonly seen in patients confined to bed (Knight et al., 2018c; Lipshutz & Gropper). Sleep appears to be affected by prolonged time in bed, and chronic insomnia can be perpetuated by prolonged bed rest (Spielman et al., 1987). Yuan et al. (2018) found that prolonged bed rest is associated with sensorimotor dysfunction leading to postural instability and a dysregulated sense of balance. Negative effects on balance and coordination are not due mostly to disuse weakness, but to problems with neural control, leading to increased fall risk (Halar & Bell, 1988). Finally, immobilized patients, especially those who are cognitively impaired (stroke and brain-injured patients), are prone to complications of sensory deprivation. These may include intellectual regression, depression, reduced attention, and poor motivation. Social isolation in combination with physical inactivity can result in intellectual deterioration. Sensory deprivation may manifest itself as restlessness, increased aggression, insomnia, and reduced pain threshold (Knight et al., 2018c).

As stated previously, prevention is the best management strategy to combat weakness associated with immobility. Early mobilization has been recommended to minimize the weakness and deconditioning associated with a critical illness. Studies and reviews have shown that early mobilization is feasible and effective in the ICU population (Schweickert et al., 2009; Lipshutz & Gropper, 2013; Needham et al., 2010; Pohlman et al., 2010; Bailey et al., 2007; Morris et al., 2008). Efforts at minimizing or reducing sedating medications can potentially help encourage early mobilization. Attention should be focused on avoiding pressure at the elbows and fibular heads as well as maintaining continued monitoring for early compression neuropathy. Watching how patients are positioned in bed or sitting in a wheelchair is critical. Disabled persons who either become ill or suffer a new trauma later in life should be remobilized as quickly as possible.

Musculoskeletal System

Immobility can have profound effects on muscles, bones, and joints and can occur quite rapidly. Muscle strength and endurance will decline significantly, as a muscle at complete rest will lose 10–15% of its strength each week and nearly half of normal strength within 3–5 weeks of immobilization (Dittmer & Teasell, 1993). Muscle weakness can negatively affect performing activities of daily living, transfers, locomotion, work, and leisure activities. Muscle atrophy or loss of muscle mass associated with immobility can be superimposed on the atrophy that occurs with peripheral nerve injuries or spinal injuries, causing flaccid paralysis. After 2 months, normal muscles at rest lose half their bulk (Muller, 1970). It has been shown that 72 hours of limb immobilization can cause the atrophy of slow- and fast-twitch muscle fibers by 14% and 17%, respectively (Lindboe & Platou, 1984). With paralysis associated with spasticity (cerebrovascular accident [CVA], traumatic brain injury [TBI], spinal cord injury [SCI]) or with limb immobilization with splints or casts, muscle atrophy is less (Dittmer & Teasell, 1993). It should be noted that weight-bearing muscles of the lower limb are affected to a greater degree than the muscles of the arm (LeBlanc et al., 1992). Prolonged bed rest can also cause selective atrophy in lumbar musculature (Belavy et al., 2011). Backache and fatigue during recovery are often due to disuse atrophy of the underlying core muscle groups than the initial condition (Knight et al., 2019c).

Catabolism also plays a role, marked by a significant increase in urinary excretion of nitrogen by the fifth day of bed rest, reflecting protein degradation and an early sign of muscle atrophy (Deitrick et al., 1948). It has also been noted that prolonged bed rest increases the long-term stress hormone cortisol, which is known to stimulate the catabolic breakdown of muscle (Knight et al., 2019b).

Reduced muscle strength with bed rest may also be affected by metabolic changes within muscle fibers. Glucose, stored in muscle fibers as glycogen, is critical for muscle contraction. Immobility has been linked with decreased glycogen stores along with the reduced activity of oxidative capacity of mitochondrion, which contributes to muscles tiring more easily (Knight et al., 2019b; Bloomfield, 1997).

Finally, there is evidence for reduced motor neuron activation after immobilization and the resultant need for increased neuronal activation that can contribute to loss of strength (Sale et al., 1982). Fatigue may also be caused partially by changes in electrical activity within muscles and a loss of integrity of the neuromuscular junction following immobility (Blottner & Salanova, 2015).

It has been shown the rate of recovery from disease weakness is slower than the rate of loss. Disuse weakness is reversed at a rate of only 6% per week using submaximal exercise (65–75% of maximum) (Muller, 1970). Besides limiting the extent and duration of immobility, this underscores the importance of focusing on muscle strengthening and conditioning as patients become more active.

The primary function of bones is the mechanical support for the tissues of the body and the maintenance of mineral homeostasis promoting the reserves of calcium, phosphorus, and magnesium salt (Nigam et al., 2009). Wolff's law states that the relationship between bone formation and resorption is influenced by stress on the bone and that bone density is directly proportional to the stress placed on it. Maintaining normal bone mass requires a balance between osteoblasts (bone formation) and osteoclasts (bone resorption) (Convertino et al., 1997). Removal of normal weight-bearing activity during bed rest disrupts the balance and resorption is increased, altering calcium balance and resulting in bone loss (Krasnoff & Painter, 1999). After bed confinement, calcium loss begins immediately, and increased urinary clearance of calcium is detectable within a few days. Calcium clearance is four to six times normal within 3 weeks of total immobilization (Deitrick et al., 1948). This process can lead to urolithiasis and heterotopic ossification (Corcoran, 1991).

Loss of bone mass and density may lead to osteoporosis, which renders bones increasingly fragile and susceptible to fractures (Knight et al., 2019c). The National Osteoporosis Foundation lists reduced mobility along with age, smoking, being female, diet low in vitamin D or calcium, family history, and low body weight as risk factors for osteoporosis.

People with disabilities who may be at increased risk of falling will be at higher risk of fractures. Non-spastic paralyzed or paretic limbs will be more at risk for osteopenia or bone loss. Nearly all fractures after falls occur on the hemiparetic side in stroke survivors (Chiu et al., 1992). Bone density loss is significant in the limbs following SCI (Biering-Sørensen et al., 1990; Lazo et al., 2001). Disuse and immobility play a role in the pathogenesis of osteoporosis, but other non-mechanical factors appear to play a role such as altered nutrition, disordered vasoregulation, hypercortisolism (therapeutic or stress-related), and endocrine dysfunction (Winslow & Rozovsky, 2003). The degree of bone loss may also be affected by the level of lesion in SCI, the extent of functional impairment, duration of injury, and age. It is also thought the loss may be more severe in patients with complete injury than with incomplete SCI (Jiang et al., 2006). Reports suggest that over 50% of patients with complete SCI develop osteoporosis by 1 year post-injury (Szollar et al., 1998). An unfortunate consequence of this process can be fragility or spontaneous fractures, which can occur in up to 50% of patients with complete SCI during their lifetime (Battaglino et al., 2012).

Calcium and vitamin D supplementation have been recommended after SCI, but caution should be used after stroke if hypercalcemia occurs (Bell & Shenouda, 2012; Varacallo et al., 2022). Bisphosphonates have been used for osteoporosis following SCI, but efficacy seems more for preventing further bone loss compared to increasing bone density. This is in contrast to improvements in bone density treating postmenopausal women with osteoporosis. Standing, walking, and functional electric stimulation have been advocated. Standing and orthotopically aided walking appear to have a positive effect during acute stages of SCI (Jiang et al., 2006).

The other aspects of the musculoskeletal system that are adversely affected by immobility are connective tissue and joints. A decrease in the normal range of motion of a joint is a contracture that, depending on the joint involved and the degree of range of motion loss, can lead to significant functional loss.

Contractures can begin forming within 8 hours after immobility. Tendons and ligaments that surround joints are largely composed of collagen, as is periarticular connective tissue. With immobility, the normally loose connective tissue/collagen fibers will become more densely packed and shortened (Dittmer & Teasell, 1993). Besides affecting tendons and ligaments, immobility negatively affects articular cartilage (Knight et al., 2019b). Additionally, muscle shortening, muscle spasticity, and muscle imbalance that occur with various neurologic conditions or trauma can accelerate the formation of contractures.

Many fractures can contribute to or complicate the clinical picture. Besides paralysis and spasticity noted earlier, edema, bleeding, infections, burns, or other healing of surgical or traumatic wounds pose challenges (Corcoran, 1991). Also, joints often need to be immobilized in casts or splints. Other issues can include poor bed or wheelchair positioning or inappropriate use of slings.

Joints crossed by muscles that span two joints are at higher risk of contractures such as the hip, knee, or ankle. The functional limitations that result can become quite significant, leading to problems with bed positioning, transfers, ambulation, and self-care.

Prevention needs to be the initial focus in the management of contractures, and multiple disciplines (physicians, advanced practice providers, therapists, and nursing staff) bear responsibility, and it must begin in ICU settings. Proper bed and wheelchair positioning and appropriate and judicious use of slings and splints with regular passive and active range-of-motion (ROM) exercises are key. Consistent monitoring for early development of ROM loss with early and frequent mobilization will help.

It is imperative to respond quickly if contractures are noted with more intensive and aggressive ROM. Family education and participation in ROM exercises will be essential, especially when patients are at home or alternative settings. Early and expert management of spasticity is essential with certain conditions (CVA, TBI, SCI, multiple sclerosis [MS], etc.) and can include therapy, antispasmodic medication, and Botox. Monitoring for heterotopic ossification, especially in the TBI and SCI population, is important. Initially, this includes serial ROM examinations looking for a loss of motion followed by consideration of plain radiographs, computed tomography (CT) scans, or bone scans.

Often, despite optimal efforts, contractures will occur. Depending upon whether it is thought the contracture may be more dynamic or fixed, inhibitive or serial casting may be indicated. This strategy is most commonly used for contractures identified at ankles, knees, wrists, fingers, and elbows. Evaluation and management of contractures should be guided by what functional limitations are present. Self-feeding can be impacted by contractures of the hands and wrist, as well as dressing with shoulder contractures. Standing can be limited by hip and knee contractures, and ambulation is often impaired by plantar flexion contractures. It is critical to have at-risk patients monitored over a long period post-illness or trauma, and at times, this monitoring may be required over the patient's remaining life span. Increasing disability may occur within the normal aging process due to falls (orthopaedic fracture[s], acquired brain injury, etc), or loss or change in caregiver of skilled nursing. With a negative change in function observed with contractures, surgical referral should be considered. Periarticular connective tissue release, muscle-tendon lengthening, or even manipulation under anesthesia can lead to improvement in self-care or mobility function (Fahmy & Seffinger, 2018; Kraal et al., 2019; Fitoussi & Bachy, 2015).

Of significant note is the fact that the prevalence of contractures in nursing home residents is estimated at 55% with significant functional and medical consequences (Offenbächer et al., 2014). Dementia, especially with disease progression, has been connected with reduced physical activity, increasing immobility, and leading to contractures and functional decline (Brach et al., 2003). Additionally, Miller (1975) identified poor patient motivation, depression, fear of falling, and disordered family relationships as major determinants of immobility in the elderly, along with overuse of restraints or sedating medications.

Renal and Urologic Systems

Immobile patients are at increased risk for urinary retention, urinary tract infections, and kidney stones (Petruccio et al., 2018; Knight et al., 2019a; Hwang et al., 1988). Recumbency is associated with a reduced urinary flow rate. Drainage of urine from renal calyces is assisted by gravity while the body is upright. The urinary stasis that occurs, coupled with the hypercalcemia/hypercalciuria previously discussed, predisposes the immobilized patient to renal calculi (Petruccio et al.; Bell & Shenouda, 2012; Knight et al., 2019a; Hwang et al.). Bladder emptying is also more challenging for supine patients, especially if coupled with neurologic conditions that affect bladder function (CVA, TBI, SCI, MS) and certain medications that impact bladder emptying (anticholinergics) or males with prostate issues.

Urinary stasis, bladder retention, and renal calculi all increase the risk of urinary tract infections. This risk would be magnified by the use of indwelling catheters or intermittent catheterization, especially in the presence of bowel incontinence.

Mobilizing patients as quickly as possible is important. Patients should be encouraged to get out of bed to void, either to the bathroom or bedside commode. Staff and family should strive to promote adequate hydration. Excellent bladder management is critical, especially with patients who have a neurogenic bladder, to avoid long periods of high bladder volumes. With the presence of recurrent urinary tract infections in immobile patients, clinicians should consider and evaluate for bladder or renal calculi serving as a nidus for recalcitrant infections. It is also prudent to minimize or eliminate the use of anticholinergic agents when possible.

Gastrointestinal System

Immobility has been linked to reduced appetite, fluid intake, and a reduced sense of taste and smell (Corcoran, 1991; Knight et al., 2018c; Bortz, 1984). Swallowing is more difficult with recumbent patients, and gastric transit time may be reduced by up to 66% (Corcoran; Thomas et al., 2002). Therefore, they are more susceptible to gastroesophageal reflux. Many patients with central nervous system (CNS) injury (i.e., TBI and CVA) are already at risk for dysphagia.

The other major issue seen with long-term immobility or bed rest is constipation. The risks of constipation result from reduced motility in the gut, increased transit times, increased water reabsorption, increased hardening of stools, and reduced urge to defecate due to stool not reaching the rectum (Knight et al., 2018c). The problem is worsened with the concurrent use of certain medications such as opiates or anticholinergics. Performing bowel programs in bed is not helpful unless the program may be unsafe given the patient's condition or not practical for the patient to get up. Also, patients with CNS injuries and/or neurogenic bowel are at a higher risk for system complications (Bell & Shenouda, 2012; Sezer, 2015).

Awareness of the problem is critical to avoid bowel impactions or obstruction. Promoting adequate nutrition with a higher fiber diet and good fluid intake is key. Early use of stool softeners, laxatives, and the patient engaging in a regular out-of-bed bowel routine is important. Minimizing medication that can affect bowel function is helpful. Early use of proton pump inhibitors should be considered, especially for patients on steroids. Having patients eat out of bed and early mobilization will also minimize these complications. Patients who present with infrequent bowel movements, abdominal discomfort, or bloating should be evaluated for constipation or impaction.

Cardiovascular System

The most common significant cardiovascular complications of immobility include tachycardia, decreased cardiac reserve (reduced exercise tolerance), orthostatic hypertension, and venous thromboembolism (Dittmer & Teasell, 1993).

Initially, with bed rest, there is a shift of fluids away from the legs to the abdomen, thorax, and head. This redistribution of fluid has shown to be up to 1 liter from the legs to the chest, temporarily increasing venous return to the heart and increasing intracardiac pressure (Perhonen et al., 2001). Increased venous return stretches the right atrium, causing a hormonal response that causes diuresis, leading to increased urine output and reduced blood volume (Knight et al., 2018a). Maximal oxygen uptake (VO_2 max) is reduced with immobilization (Convertino, 1997; Convertino et al., 1997). Increased heart rate occurs due to hypovolemia and altered sympathetic activity. Cardiac muscle atrophy, similar to skeletal muscle atrophy, may occur (Corcoran, 1991; Levine et al., 1997). These pathophysiologic changes result in the heart being less capable of responding to metabolic demands above the basal level (Dittmer & Teasell, 1993). Cardiac deconditioning occurs that can become magnified in patients with pre-existing heart disease (precipitation of angina or congestive heart failure [CHF]) as well as anemic patients. Of importance is the fact that Corcoran noted exercise tolerance did not return to normal again until after 5–10 weeks of vigorous reconditioning.

Orthostatic hypotension (a postural drop in systolic blood pressure accompanied by an increase in heart rate) can be both common and cause troublesome symptoms. It can occur within 20 hours of bed rest in the elderly and within 3 weeks of bed rest for healthy individuals (Petruccio et al., 2018; Dittmer & Teasell, 1993). This issue is even more prevalent in patients with SCIs, especially with high thoracic and cervical injuries, and has been reported to be as high as 21% (Sezer et al., 2015). Symptoms that occur with the change in the position include dizziness, headache, pallor, fatigue, and sometimes syncope, which can increase fall risk.

The risk and causes of thromboembolic disease in the immobilized patient have been well described (Petruccio et al., 2018; Dittmer & Teasell, 1993; Bell & Shenouda, 2012;

Knight et al., 2018b). The factors of the Virchow triad (venous stasis, hypercoagulability, and endothelial damage) are seen in many patients who face immobility, especially with neurologic disability resulting in paretic or plegic limbs. The incidence of deep vein thrombosis (DVT) associated with prolonged bed rest is up to 13% (Kierkegaard et al., 1987). Clots are seen more frequently in the paralyzed limb of hemiparetic patients (Turpie, 1997). Both limb weakness and bed rest contribute to venous stasis. Traumatic injury, especially if accompanied by bleeding, can promote a hypercoagulable state (Bell & Shenouda, 2012). Prolonged bed rest has also been shown to lead to endothelial damage (Knight et al., 2018b). Therefore, all aspects of the Virchow triad become potential risk factors.

The most serious consequence of DVT is embolization, especially pulmonary emboli (PE), which can be fatal. PE are still one of the most common causes of unexpected deaths in hospitalized patients (Knight et al., 2018b).

Rapid and continued mobilization is still the optimal plan to limit cardiovascular complications of immobility. Quickly getting and keeping patients out of bed and starting an exercise program as soon as possible should be encouraged. It is important to monitor fluid and electrolyte balance, keep patients well hydrated, and attempt to reverse anemia if present. Patients who are having difficulty being mobilized should be evaluated for orthostatic hypotension. Appropriately sized compression stocking, ACE wraps, and tilt tables may be helpful. Preventing DVT involves lower extremity exercise, early ambulation, compression stockings, mechanical compression, and pharmacologic agents such as low-dose heparin, Lovenox, antiplatelet agents, or anticoagulants. The latter may be precluded with neurotrauma or CVA associated with bleeding. While immobile, patients should be regularly monitored for signs and symptoms of either DVT or PE.

Respiratory System

There are significant negative effects on the respiratory system with prolonged immobility. When supine, body weight restricts movement of the rib cage, which reduces tidal volume. Normally, 78% of tidal volume is due to the motion of the rib cage, but when supine, this is reduced to 32% (Petruccio et al., 2018; Knight et al., 2018b). Normal residual lung volumes are reduced due to blood being shunted from lower limbs to the thorax, causing an increase in pulmonary blood volume and abdominal organs shifting toward the thorax and compressing the lungs (Petruccio et al.; Manning et al., 1999). The mucous film that lines smaller air passages tends to pool when supine due to gravity, leading to local atelectasis (Corcoran, 1991). Diffusing capacity can become reduced by 4–5% (Bell & Shenouda, 2012). The diameter of the airways, particularly bronchioles, decreases with prolonged periods of being supine (Knight et al., 2018b). These pathophysiologic changes become more problematic with smokers, history of chronic obstructive pulmonary disease (COPD), obesity, sedated patients, obstructive sleep apnea, dysphagia, and patients with neurologic injuries causing weakness of respiratory muscles. All these changes put patients at higher risk for atelectasis, hypoxia, and pneumonia.

Pneumonia can cause a two- to threefold increase in death in the stroke population (Katzan et al., 2003; Halar, 1994). It has been stated that TBI patients are four times more likely to die of respiratory complications compared to the general population (Harrison-Felix et al., 2009). Respiratory complications associated with SCI are the most significant cause of morbidity and mortality in both acute and chronic stages (Tollefsen & Fonderes, 2012; Garshick et al., 2005). Patients with complete tetraplegia are at the highest risk (Chen et al., 1999). Pneumonia is the primary cause of death during chronic SCI (McKinley et al., 2002). Elderly patients, either with a new disability or those aging with a disability, already have an increased risk of respiratory complications due to normal respiratory system changes that occur with age (Mobily & Skemp Kelley, 1991).

Preventative and management measures include frequent turning, early mobilization, breathing techniques, cough assistance, suctioning, respiratory therapy, and incentive spirometry. Adequate hydration is essential. Sedating medications should be minimized. Patients should be kept current on influenza and pneumococcal vaccines (will need to monitor for ultimate recommendations for COVID-19 vaccines). Keeping patients isolated from sick friends and family would be prudent. Appropriate screening for dysphagia should be considered and treated when necessary. Early identification and treatment of respiratory tract infections, especially pneumonia, is critical. Finally, modifiable risk factors such as obesity and smoking should be addressed.

Integumentary System

Immobility is the factor most likely to put an individual at risk of altered skin integrity (Knight et al., 2019c). The major issues that result are pressure sores or decubitus ulcers, which are localized areas of cellular necrosis from lack of adequate circulation. The most common areas are over bony prominences, where skin tissue is subjected to external pressure greater than capillary pressure (32 mm Hg) for prolonged periods. Microscopic tissue changes secondary to ischemia have been observed with pressures of 70 mm Hg after only 2 hours. Regarding skin breakdown, 95% of decubitus ulcers occur at five major sites: the sacrum, ischial tuberosities, greater trochanters, heels, and ankles (Teasell & Dittmer, 1993). They can occur in both the supine patient as well as patients confined to a wheelchair. Generally, in response to discomfort, people regularly or automatically shift their weight to relieve pressure. Weak patients, either from immobility or underlying pathology, may not be able to move frequently. Altered sensations seen with diabetes, neuropathies, or SCI may inhibit discomfort associated with pressure. Cognitive dysfunction causes a lack of awareness either from traumatic or nontraumatic brain injuries or dementia, and sedating medication may be a significant factor. Lying or sitting on a hard surface such as an inadequate mattress or wheelchair cushion adds to the risks. Tissue shearing occurring with changing bed positions or transfers can be a cause of skin breakdown or inhibit skin ulcer healing. The longer the duration and the greater degree of pressure, the higher the risk of developing decubitus ulcers, so obesity is also a risk factor. Pressure ulcers most frequently occur in elderly immobilized patients, critical care patients, and spinal injured patients (Knight et al., 2019c).

Unfortunately, once a patient develops a pressure sore, this often is followed by further immobilization, leading to an increased risk of other decubitus ulcers and further/increased sequelae of immobility (Mobily & Skemp Kelley, 1991). Multiple complications can result from decubitus ulcers like osteomyelitis, sinus tracts, septic joints, septicemia, amyloidosis, protein and water loss, and localized damage to muscles, tendons, and nerves as well as be a trigger for increased spasticity (Teasell & Dittmer, 1993). Infection becomes the most common problem, as decubitus ulcers can lead to deep, significant infections that can become life-threatening (Teasell & Dittmer). Incontinence, especially bowel or infected urine, can be an additive factor, depending on the location of the ulcer. Smoking and poor nutrition (leading to loss of soft tissue padding) can contribute to ulcer formation. In one large study, around 6.2% of patients over the age of 65 developed pressure sores within 2 days of hospital admission (Knight et al., 2019c). Patients older than 70 have been shown to have 70% of all pressure sores. This issue becomes one of the most significant areas of management and education for SCI patients and their caregivers. The risk starts at the time of injury and becomes a lifelong commitment for those living with SCI (Regan et al., 2009). Management of decubitus ulcers has been reported to be the second most common etiology for rehospitalization after SCI during a 20-year follow-up (Cardenas et al., 2004). The development of pressure sores in the nursing home population has been a known source of concern.

Prevention is the mainstay of the "management" of decubitus ulcers. Maintaining adequate nutrition and hydration is critical. Risk assessment should begin at the time of hospitalization and any subsequent change of condition or living environment. Patients should be turned every 2 hours, and skin inspections looking for areas of redness or skin loss should occur frequently, especially those assessed to be at high risk for skin breakdown Patients should be lifted when repositioned or transferred to minimize shearing. Spasticity should be adequately treated, and attempts should be made to minimize incontinence through a scheduled, facilitated bowel program. Appropriate mattresses or cushions should be utilized for high-risk patients. Facilitating getting patients out of bed and ambulatory as quickly as possible is important. Responding early to skin breakdown and the use of specialized wound care teams can prevent the worsening of ulcers and promote more rapid healing. It should be remembered that healing from deep decubitus ulcers can be a risk factor for later ulcers due to the fragility of the scar or healed skin. The cost of care for a significant decubitus ulcer cannot be overemphasized. The cost of treating one decubitus ulcer has been conservatively estimated to be between $15,000 and $20,000 (Teasell & Dittmer, 1993).

Psychological Sequelae

National Aeronautics and Space Administration (NASA) studies of normal young men who were kept in bed for 5 weeks showed significant increases in anxiety, hostility, and depression, together with altered sleep patterns (Ryback et al., 1971). Corcoran (1991) stated that bed rest appears to be a subtle form of sensory deprivation. Teasell and Dittmer (1993) maintained that immobilized patients, especially those who are cognitively impaired (stroke, head injury, dementia), and the elderly are prone to complications of sensory deprivation. These complications include intellectual regression, depression, a short attention span, and poor motivation. Social isolation in combination with physical inactivity can result in intellectual deterioration (Halar & Bell, 1990; Haythorn, 1973).

Knight et al. (2019c) discussed how immobility can affect self-concept and self-worth. Self-concept is described as a set of beliefs about one's qualities and attributes, and self-esteem is the feeling of self-worth and a central component of psychological well-being (Marks et al., 2018; Walker et al., 2007). Self-concept and self-esteem are directly related to an individual's body image, achievement, social functioning, and self-identification. Knight et al. (2019c) maintained that acute or chronic illness along with prolonged bed rest can affect both function and self-concept. The prolonged ability to work or engage in hobbies can become a positive factor. Overall, the reduced opportunity to interact with friends or family negatively impacts a patient's support system.

With the decline in function also comes a sense of dependency, loss of independence, and stress of imposing on others. Corcoran (1991) talked about "learned helplessness" as a negative consequence of prolonged hospitalization or bed rest. He suggested patients confined to bed are expected to play a sick role, be compliant without questions, and that care providers whether in a hospital, long-term care, or at home often reinforce this. Bedbound patients lose control over all aspects of their lives, and Corcoran concluded that regaining a sense of independence and an ability for decision-making after prolonged bed rest is challenging.

Regarding management, the recurring theme is to limit bed rest and encourage activity and to improve function. Patients should be encouraged to perform all functions of which they are capable. For example, feeding or dressing a patient just because it is faster should be discouraged when realistic to do so. Effective pain management also helps encourage mobilization. Patients, especially those with chronic diseases, should be given choices to facilitate active decision-making and reduce passivity and dependence. Educating patients and families about the harmful effects of dependency and immobility is useful (Teasell & Dittmer, 1993). Expectations for improving function and increasing mobilization should be set before and after transfer to new environments and especially upon return home. Practitioners who manage patients as they age, with or without disability, should monitor them for progressive immobility and offer guidance as indicated. Much concern has been expressed about the negative psychological consequences of isolation on the elderly, especially in various long-term residential care facilities during the current COVID-19 pandemic, which significantly reduced visitation. Finally, it should be noted that the issues affecting the mental health and sense of well-being of immobilized patients are additive to the psychological consequences of disease-specific illness and trauma as well as those that can occur with normal aging.

Life Expectancy

The target audience for this text is life care planners, medical-legal experts, nurse case managers, physiatrists, and various other rehabilitation professionals. Gonzales (2017) wrote the basic questions of life care planning that include: 1) What is a subject's condition? 2) What medically related goods and services does a subject's condition require? and 3) How much will the goods and services cost over time? These are applied to the overarching issue affecting potential future medical costs throughout care. Duration of care is directly connected to projected life expectancy and is often not easy to accurately or objectively determine. Life expectancy for various disability groups is beyond the scope of this chapter. The Life Expectancy Project found at www.lifeexpectancy.com is an excellent resource. Life expectancy adjustments should be individualized and are impacted by various factors including disabilities, pre-existing comorbidities, adverse lifestyle behaviors, mental health issues, new complications, and family history (Gonzales). Potential other factors that could play a role include economic status and availability of state-of-the-art health care (resources are different for traumatic injury in a no-fault state or workers' compensation case than patients on Medicaid). Availability of caregiver assistance, along with the presence of a strong family or friend advocate, is critical. Finally, the locus of control is applied to a person with a disability, moderate or severe, and includes such factors as self-educating, self-advocating, and avoiding a victim mentality, but these factors require further study to confirm. Social inequities leading to health care disparities potentially affecting life expectancy need further investigation and will not be discussed here.

For this chapter, there is little doubt that functional status and immobility play major roles in reductions in life expectancy and have been discussed in multiple publications related particularly to survival after stroke, brain injury, and SCI. Dr. Robert Shavelle, a leading researcher and contributor to the Life Expectancy Project, along with colleagues, has analyzed much of the available data. Shavelle et al. (2019) stated that functional ability has long been recognized as a key prognostic factor for survival at older ages and in persons with disabilities due to either congenital or acquired brain injury. They further stated that it was not surprising that persons with Rankin Grade 0 or 1 have a modest reduction in life expectancy, while persons with Rankin 5 (severe disability—bedridden, incontinent, requiring constant care) have very low life expectancies, similar to those in persistent vegetative states, due to both groups being confined to bed and unlikely to improve in function.

Baguley et al. (2000) speculated that inactivity-related morbidity may have been a factor in the increased death rate in TBI patients, predominantly from cardiorespiratory arrest and bronchopneumonia/sepsis. Wannamethee et al. (1998) stated that a permanently sedentary lifestyle is known to lead to an increased risk of heart disease and other conditions and can be shown to lead to a reduction of about 4 years. Shavelle and Strauss (2000) found an increase in mortality rates after TBI, particularly among non-ambulatory patients. Ratcliff et al. (2005) demonstrated that there is more than a twofold increase in long-term mortality for individuals with moderate or severe brain injury compared to the general population, and the risk is more pronounced in the most disabled groups as indicated by the level of independence in basic activities of daily living (ADLs). Finally, Harrison-Felix et al. (2009) studied data from the Brain Injury Model Systems and found the strongest risk factors for reduced survival after 1 year post–brain injury were older age, not being employed as a result of injury, and greater disability at rehabilitation discharge. Disability was the only risk factor that is potentially "modifiable" from a rehabilitation perspective. The authors suggest that rehabilitation efforts focusing on reducing disability may be important to long-term survival (Harrison-Felix et al., 2004). Finally, Shavelle et al. (2000) found that mobility is the most powerful predictor of long-term survival after TBI. The risk of death for persons with no mobility was approximately four times higher than for those with fair or good mobility (Shavelle et al., 2007). Additionally, the key factor in life expectancy is the severity of a disability, especially motor dysfunction, measured by simple functional tasks such as the ability to walk, use hands, and self-feed.

Realizing these are overlapping issues with TBI patients, Slot et al. (2008) concluded that the functional status of patients 6 months after the onset of an ischemic stroke had a significant effect on their long-term survival. Kammersgaard's (2010) data determined that the two most prominent factors affecting both short- and long-term survival after stroke are age and stroke severity at the onset.

Survival after SCI has been another area of study. Mobility and function have been shown to play significant roles in survival rates. Yeo et al. (1998) analyzed a large cohort of spinal injured patients in Australia and found the projected mean life expectancy compared to the general population was estimated to approach 70% of normal for patients with complete tetraplegia and 84% of normal for complete paraplegia. Patients with incomplete lesions and motor function capabilities are projected to have a life expectancy of at least 92% of the normal population. McColl et al. (1997) also found that quadriplegic patients had a risk of death one to seven times greater than paraplegics, resulting in a median survival time for paraplegics of about 9 years greater than quadriplegics. Finally, Shavelle et al. (2015) maintained that life expectancy for spinal injured patients is greater in those who can walk independently than in those who use support, which in turn is greater in those who are wheelchair-bound. Survival after ASIA Impairment Scale (AIS) D SCI seems to be more related to the severity of functional disability than the nominal level or grade of injury (Shavelle et al.). The common thread in all of the references cited in this section is that reduction in life expectancy is directly related to the degree of functional loss and the resultant immobility.

Conclusions

The intention behind this chapter has been to highlight the multiple negative sequelae of immobility that can occur following illness or trauma that can lead to worsening complications and reduced function and potentially shorten an individual's life. Essentially all major body systems can be negatively impacted by immobility. A focus on rapid and continuous mobilization should begin in the ICU and should remain an important issue throughout life. Efforts to maximize function are critical, as it has been demonstrated that higher-level function leads to greater mobility. This principle speaks to the importance of early and intensive rehabilitation. Post-acute follow-up is necessary to monitor for decreasing mobility or function as well as the multiple complications that can result from immobility. Rapid intervention is critical. Education of patients, families, and caregivers about the importance of maximizing mobility should occur and be regularly reinforced. Education of primary care providers, who often are the ones providing follow-up, and third-party payors (if justification is needed for late intervention or complications) should be facilitated.

Not enough emphasis has been placed on aging with a disability, as both can contribute to reduced function and increasing immobility. Minkler and Fadem (2002) offered an excellent perspective on successful aging from a disability perspective. They cite Kahn and Rowe's (1998) successful aging paradigm and its three components: low probability of disease and disease-related disability, high cognitive and physical functioning, and active engagement with life. They identified physical fitness and exercise as the crux of successful aging and are dependent upon individual choices, behaviors, and efforts. The value of active engagement with life facilitated by maximal mobility and function speaks to the importance of vocational rehabilitation, addressing avocational interests and goals, as well as volunteerism and community involvement, which can help improve and maintain mobility through motivating to maximize function and engagement.

This focus on combating the multiple negative aspects of immobility must be an evolving interdisciplinary effort between primary care practitioners; acute, post-acute, and long-term care staff; physiatrists; other rehabilitation professionals; and potentially multiple physician specialists. New medical illnesses or trauma, changes in the environment, or new social situations should trigger red flags for reevaluation and intervention if indicated. Nurse case managers, life care planners, and medical-legal experts also play a role in providing for some of the complications noted in this chapter when developing long-term care plans or pointing them out when doing evaluations, which often occur years after trauma or illness.

Finally, there is a role for advocacy by all rehabilitation professionals to help combat unsuccessful aging with a disability. Health and social policy that can potentially impact systemic barriers to community living, active engagement with life, and ultimately an improved quality of life can make a true difference. Issues here include accessibility, transportation, and caregiver assistance, as well as other social or health care inequities. It is without a doubt that the ADA has helped those with physical disabilities become more involved and connected in their communities and ultimately more mobile.

It seems most appropriate to end this chapter with how Corcoran ended his important 1991 article. He cited Asher (1947), who had composed a prayer for physicians:

Teach us to live that we may dread
unnecessary time in bed.
Get people up and we may save
our patients from an early grave. (p. 967)

References

Asher, R. (1947). The dangers of going to bed. *British Columbia Medical Journal, 2*, 967–968.

Baguley, I., Slewa-Younan, S., Lazarus, R., & Green, A. (2000). Long-term mortality trends in patients with traumatic brain injury. *Brain Injury, 14*(6), 505–512. https://doi.org/10.1080/026990500120420

Bailey, P., Thomsen, G. E., Spuhler, V. J., Blair, R., Jewkes, J., Bezdjian, L., Veale, K., Rodriquez, L., & Hopkins, R. O. (2007). Early activity is feasible and safe in respiratory failure patients. *Critical Care Medicine*, *35*(1), 139–145. https://doi-org.proxy.library.vcu.edu/10.1097/01.CCM.0000251130.69568.87

Battaglino, R. A., Lazzari, A. A., Garshick, E., & Morse, L. R. (2012). Spinal cord injury-induced osteoporosis: Pathogenesis and emerging therapies. *Current Osteoporosis Reports*, *10*(4), 278–285. https://doi-org.proxy.library.vcu.edu/10.1007/s11914-012-0117-0

Belavy, D. L., Armbrecht, G., Richardson, C. A., Felsenberg, D., & Hides, J. A. (2011). Muscle atrophy and changes in spinal morphology: Is the lumbar spine vulnerable after prolonged bed-rest? *Spine*, *36*(2), 137–145. https://doi-org.proxy.library.vcu.edu/10.1097/BRS.0b013e3181cc93e8

Bell, K., & Shenouda, C. (2012). Complications associated with immobility. In N. Zasler, D. Katz, R. Zafonte, D. Arciniegas, M. Bullock, & J. Kreutzer (Eds.), *Brain injury medicine* (2nd ed., pp. 809–820). Springer Publishing Company. https://doi.org/10.1891/9781617050572.0049; https://connect.springer-pub.com/content/book/978-1-6170-5057-2/part/part10/chapter/ch49

Biering-Sørensen, F., Bohr, H. H., & Schaadt, O. P. (1990). Longitudinal study of bone mineral content in the lumbar spine, the forearm, and the lower extremities after spinal cord injury. *European Journal of Clinical Investigation*, *20*(3), 330–335. https://doi-org.proxy.library.vcu.edu/10.1111/j.1365-2362.1990.tb01865.x

Bloomfield, S. A. (1997). Changes in musculoskeletal structure and function with prolonged bed rest. *Medical and Science in Sports and Exercise*, *29*(2), 197–206.

Blottner, D., & Salanova, M. (2015). *The neuromuscular system: From earth to space life science: Neuromuscular cell signaling in disuse and exercise*. Springer. https://doi.org/10.1007/978-3-319-12298-4

Booth, F. W., Roberts, C. K., & Laye, M. J. (2012). Lack of exercise is a major cause of chronic diseases. *Comprehensive Physiology*, *2*(2), 1143–1211. https://doi-org.proxy.library.vcu.edu/10.1002/cphy.c11002514

Bortz, W. M., II. (1984). The disuse syndrome. *The Western Journal of Medicine*, *141*(5), 691–694.

Brach, J. S., FitzGerald, S., Newman, A. B., Kelsey, S., Kuller, L., VanSwearingen, J. M., & Kriska, A. M. (2003). Physical activity and functional status in community-dwelling older women: A 14-year prospective study. *Archives of Internal Medicine*, *163*(21), 2565–2571. https://doi-org.proxy.library.vcu.edu/10.1001/archinte.163.21.2565

Brown, C., & Flood, K. (2013). Mobility limitations in the older patient a clinical review. *Journal of the American Medical Association*, *310*(11), 1168–1177.

Cardenas, D. D., Hoffman, J. M., Kirshblum, S., & McKinley, W. (2004). Etiology and incidence of rehospitalization after traumatic spinal cord injury: A multicenter analysis. *Archives of Physical Medicine and Rehabilitation*, *85*(11), 1757–1763. https://doi.org/10.1016/j.apmr.2004.03.016. PMID: 15520970

Chen, D., Apple, D. F., Jr., Hudson, L. M., & Bode, R. (1999). Medical complications during acute rehabilitation following spinal cord injury—current experience of the model systems. *Archives of Physical Medicine and Rehabilitation*, *80*(11), 1397–1401. https://doi-org.proxy.library.vcu.edu/10.1016/s0003-9993(99)90250-2

Chiu, K. Y., Pun, W. K., Luk, K. D., & Chow, S. P. (1992). A prospective study on hip fractures in patients with previous cerebrovascular accidents. *Injury*, *23*(5), 297–299. https://doi-org.proxy.library.vcu.edu/10.1016/0020-1383(92)90171-n

Convertino, V. A. (1997). Cardiovascular consequences of bed rest: Effect on maximum oxygen uptake. *Medicine & Science in Sports and Exercise*, *29*(2), 191–196.

Convertino, V. A., Bloomfield, S. A., & Greenleaf, J. E. (1997). An overview of the issues: Physiological effects of bed rest and restricted physical activity. *Medicine and Science in Sports and Exercise*, *29*(2), 187–190. https://doi-org.proxy.library.vcu.edu/10.1097/00005768-199702000-00004

Corcoran, P. (1991). Use it or lose it: The hazards of bed rest and inactivity. *Western Journal of Medicine*, *4*, 536–538.

Deitrick, J. E., Whedon, G. D., & Shorr, E. (1948). Effects of immobilization upon various metabolic and physiologic functions of normal men. *The American Journal of Medicine*, *4*(1), 3–36. https://doi-org.proxy.library.vcu.edu/10.1016/0002-9343(48)90370-2

Dittmer, D. K., & Teasell, R. (1993). Complications of immobilization and bed rest. Part 1: Musculoskeletal and cardiovascular complications. *Canadian Family Physician*, *39*, 1428–1432, 1435–1437.

Fahmy, K., & Seffinger, M. (2018). Manipulation under anesthesia thaws frozen shoulder. *The Journal of the American Osteopathic Association*, *118*, 485–486.

Fitoussi, F., & Bachy, M. (2015). Tendon lengthening and transfer. *Orthopaedics & Traumatology, Surgery & Research, OTSR*, *101*(Suppl 1), S149–S157. https://doi.org/10.1016/j.otsr.2014.07.033

Garshick, E., Kelley, A., Cohen, S. A., Garrison, A., Tun, C. G., Gagnon, D., & Brown, R. (2005). A prospective assessment of mortality in chronic spinal cord injury. *Spinal Cord, 43*(7), 408–416. https://doi-org.proxy.library.vcu.edu/10.1038/sj.sc.3101729

Gonzales, J. (Ed.). (2017). *A physician's guide to life care planning: Tenets, methods, and best practices for physician life care planners.* American Academy of Physician Life Care Planners.

Halar, E. M. (1994). Disuse syndrome: Recognition and prevention. In R. M. Hays, G. Kraft, & W. Stolov (Eds.), *Chronic disease and disability: A contemporary rehabilitation approach to the practice of medicine.* Demos Medical.

Halar, E. M., & Bell, K. R. (1988). Contracture and other deleterious effects of immobility. In J. A. Delisa (Ed.), *Rehabilitation medicine, principles and practices* (pp. 448–462). JB Lippincott Co.

Halar, E. M., & Bell, K. R. (1990). Rehabilitation's relationship to activity. In F. J. Kottke & F. Lehmann (Eds.), *Krusen's handbook of physical medicine and rehabilitation* (4th ed., pp. 1113–11133). WB Saunders Co.

Harrison-Felix, C., Whiteneck, G., DeVivo, M., Hammond, F. M., & Jha, A. (2004). Mortality following rehabilitation in the traumatic brain injury model systems of care. *Neuro Rehabilitation, 19*(1), 45–54.

Harrison-Felix, C. L., Whiteneck, G. G., Jha, A., DeVivo, M. J., Hammond, F. M., & Hart, D. M. (2009). Mortality over four decades after traumatic brain injury rehabilitation: A retrospective cohort study. *Archives of Physical Medicine and Rehabilitation, 90*(9), 1506–1513. https://doi-org.proxy.library.vcu.edu/10.1016/j.apmr.2009.03.015

Haythorn, W. W. (1973). The miniworld of isolation: Laboratory studies. In J. Rasmussen (Ed.), *Man in isolation and confinement* (pp. 218–239). Aldine Publishing.

Hippocrates. (1849). *The genuine works of Hippocrates., Francis Adams, the Milwaukee academy of medicine.* Book Collection, The Sydenham Society.

Hwang, T. I., Hill, K., Schneider, V., & Pak, C. Y. (1988). Effect of prolonged bed rest on the propensity for renal stone formation. *The Journal of Clinical Endocrinology and Metabolism, 66*(1), 109–112. https://doi-org.proxy.library.vcu.edu/10.1210/jcem-66-1-109.

Iezzoni, L. I., McCarthy, E. P., Davis, R. B., & Siebens, H. (2001). Mobility difficulties are not only a problem of old age. *Journal of General Internal Medicine, 16*(4), 235–243. https://doi-org.proxy.library.vcu.edu/10.1046/j.1525-1497.2001.016004235.x

Jiang, S. D., Dai, L. Y., & Jiang, L. S. (2006). Osteoporosis after spinal cord injury. *Osteoporosis International: A Journal Established as Result of Cooperation Between the European Foundation for Osteoporosis and the National Osteoporosis Foundation of the USA, 17*(2), 180–192. https://doi-org.proxy.library.vcu.edu/10.1007/s00198-005-2028-8

Kahn, R. L., & Rowe, J. W. (1998). *Successful aging.* Pantheon Books.

Kammersgaard, L. P. (2010). Survival after stroke: Risk factors and determinants in the Copenhagen stroke study. *Danish Medical Bulletin, 57*, B4189.

Katzan, I. L., Cebul, R. D., Husak, S. H., Dawson, N. V., & Baker, D. W. (2003). The effect of pneumonia on mortality among patients hospitalized for acute stroke. *Neurology, 60*(4), 620–625. https://doi-org.proxy.library.vcu.edu/10.1212/01.wnl.0000046586.38284.60

Kierkegaard, A., Norgren, L., Olsson, C. G., Castenfors, J., Persson, G., & Persson, S. (1987). Incidence of deep vein thrombosis in bedridden non-surgical patients. *Acta Medica Scandinavica, 222*(5), 409–414. https://doi-org.proxy.library.vcu.edu/10.1111/j.0954-6820.1987.tb10957.x

Knight, J., Nigam, Y., & Jones, A. (2018a). Effect of bed rest 1: Introduction and the cardiovascular system. *Nursing Times (Online), 114*(12), 54–57.

Knight, J., Nigam, Y., & Jones, A. (2018b). Effects of bed rest 2: Respiratory and hematological systems. *Nursing Times (Online), 115*(1), 44–47.

Knight, J., Nigam, Y., & Jones, A. (2018c). Effects of bed rest 3: Gastrointestinal, endocrine and nervous systems. *Nursing Times (Online), 115*(2), 50–53.

Knight, J., Nigam, Y., & Jones, A. (2019a). Effects of bed rest 4: Renal, reproductive, and immune systems. *Nursing Times (Online), 115*(3), 51–54.

Knight, J., Nigam, Y., & Jones, A. (2019b). Effects of bed rest 5: The muscles, joints, and mobility. *Nursing Times (Online), 115*(4), 54–57.

Knight, J., Nigam, Y., & Jones, A. (2019c). Effects of bed rest 6: Bones, skin, self-concept, and self-esteem. *Nursing Times (Online), 115*(5), 58–61.

Kraal, T., Beimers, L., The, B., Sierevelt, I., van den Bekerom, M., & Eygendaal, D. (2019). Manipulation under anaesthesia for frozen shoulders: Outdated technique or well-established quick fix? *EFORT Open Reviews, 4*(3), 98–109. https://doi-org.proxy.library.vcu.edu/10.1302/2058-5241.4.180044

Krasnoff, J., & Painter, P. (1999). The physiological consequences of bed rest and inactivity. *Advanced Renal Replacement Therapy*, 6, 124–132.

Lazo, M. G., Shirazi, P., Sam, M., Giobbie-Hurder, A., Blacconiere, M. J., & Muppidi, M. (2001). Osteoporosis and risk of fracture in men with spinal cord injury. *Spinal Cord*, 39(4), 208–214. https://doi-org.proxy.library.vcu.edu/10.1038/sj.sc.3101139

LeBlanc, A. D., Schneider, V. S., Evans, H. J., Pientok, C., Rowe, R., & Spector, E. (1992). Regional changes in muscle mass following 17 weeks of bed rest. *Journal of Applied Physiology (Bethesda, Md.:1985)*, 73(5), 2172–2178. https://doi-org.proxy.library.vcu.edu/10.1152/jappl.1992.73.5.2172

Levine, B. D., Zuckerman, J. H., & Pawelczyk, J. A. (1997). Cardiac atrophy after bed-rest deconditioning: A nonneural mechanism for orthostatic intolerance. *Circulation*, 96(2), 517–525. https://doi-org.proxy.library.vcu.edu/10.1161/01.cir.96.2.517

Lindboe, C. F., & Platou, C. S. (1984). Effect of immobilization of short duration on the muscle fiber size. *Clinical Psychology*, 4(2), 183–188.

Lipshutz, A., & Gropper, M. (2013). Acquired neuromuscular weakness and early mobilization in the intensive care unit. *Anesthesiology*, 118, 202–215.

Manning, F., Dean, E., Ross, J., & Abboud, R. T. (1999). Effects of side-lying on lung function in older individuals. *Physical Therapy*, 79(5), 456–466.

Marks, D. F., Murray, M., & Estacio, E. (2018). *Health psychology: Theory research and practice*. Sage.

McColl, M. A., Walker, J., Stirling, P., Wilkins, R., & Corey, P. (1997). Expectations of life and health among spinal cord injured adults. *Spinal Cord*, 35(12), 818–828. https://doi.org/10.1038/sj.sc.3100546

McKinley, W. O., Gittler, M. S., Kirshblum, S. C., Stiens, S. A., & Groah, S. L. (2002). Spinal cord injury medicine. 2. Medical complications after spinal cord injury: Identification and management. *Archives of Physical Medicine and Rehabilitation*, 83(3 Suppl 1), S58–S98. https://doi-org.proxy.library.vcu.edu/10.1053/apmr.2002.32159.

Miller, M. B. (1975). Iatrogenic and nursigenic effects of prolonged immobilization of the ill aged. *Journal of American Geriatric Society*, 23, 360–369.

Minkler, M., & Fadem, P. (2002). "Successful aging": A disability perspective. *Journal of Disability Policy Studies*, 12(4), 229–235. https://doi.org/10.1177/104420730201200402

Mobily, P. R., & Skemp Kelley, L. S. (1991). Iatrogenesis in the elderly: Factors of immobility. *Journal of Gerontological Nursing*, 17(9), 5–11. https://doi-org.proxy.library.vcu.edu/10.3928/0098-9134-19910901-04

Morris, P. E., Goad, A., Thompson, C., Taylor, K., Harry, B., Passmore, L., Ross, A., Anderson, L., Baker, S., Sanchez, M., Penley, L., Howard, A., Dixon, L., Leach, S., Small, R., Hite, R. D., & Haponik, E. (2008). Early intensive care unit mobility therapy in the treatment of acute respiratory failure. *Critical Care Medicine*, 36(8), 2238–2243. https://doi-org.proxy.library.vcu.edu/10.1097/CCM.0b013e318180b90e

Muller, E. A. (1970). Influence of training and of inactivity on muscle strength. *Archives of Physical Medicine and Rehabilitation*, 51, 449–462.

Needham, D. M., Korupolu, R., Zanni, J. M., Pradhan, P., Colantuoni, E., Palmer, J. B., Brower, R. G., & Fan, E. (2010). Early physical medicine and rehabilitation for patients with acute respiratory failure: A quality improvement project. *Archives of Physical Medicine and Rehabilitation*, 91(4), 536–542. https://doi-org.proxy.library.vcu.edu/10.1016/j.apmr.2010.01.002

Nigam, Y., Knight, J., & Jones, A. (2009). Effects of bed rest 3: Musculoskeletal and immune systems, skin, and self-perception. *Nursing Times*, 105(23), 18–23.

Offenbächer, M., Sauer, S., Rieß, J., Müller, M., Grill, E., Daubner, A., Randzio, O., Kohls, N., & Herold-Majumdar, A. (2014). Contractures with special reference in elderly: Definition and risk factors—a systematic review with practical implications. *Disability and Rehabilitation*, 36(7), 529–538. https://doi.org/10.3109/09638288.2013.800596. Epub June 17, 2013. PMID: 23772994.

Petruccio, L., Cunha de Oliveira, M., & Carvalho, G. (2018). Deleterious effects of prolonged bed rest on the elderly—a review. *Brazilian Journal of Geriatrics and Gerontology*, 21(4), 499–506. https://doi.org/10.1590/1981-22562018021.170167

Perhonen, M. A., Zuckerman, J. H., & Levine, B. D. (2001). Deterioration of left ventricular chamber performance after bed rest: "Cardiovascular deconditioning" or hypovolemia? *Circulation*, 103(14), 1851–1857. https://doi-org.proxy.library.vcu.edu/10.1161/01.cir.103.14.1851

Pohlman, M. C., Schweickert, W. D., Pohlman, A. S., Nigos, C., Pawlik, A. J., Esbrook, C. L., Spears, L., Miller, M., Franczyk, M., Deprizio, D., Schmidt, G. A., Bowman, A., Barr, R., McCallister, K., Hall, J. B., & Kress, J. P. (2010). Feasibility of physical and occupational therapy beginning from initiation of mechanical ventilation. *Critical Care Medicine*, 38(11), 2089–2094. https://doi-org.proxy.library.vcu.edu/10.1097/CCM.0b013e3181f270c3

Rantanen, T. (2013). Promoting mobility in older people. *Journal of Preventive Medicine and Public Health*, *46*(Suppl 1), 550–554.

Ratcliff, G., Colantonio, A., Escobar, M., Chase, S., & Vernich, L. (2005). Long-term survival following traumatic brain injury. *Disability and Rehabilitation*, *27*(6), 305–314. https://doi.org/10.1080/09638280400018338

Regan, M. A., Teasell, R. W., Wolfe, D. L., Keast, D., Mortenson, W. B., Aubut, J. A., & Spinal Cord Injury Rehabilitation Evidence Research Team (2009). A systematic review of therapeutic interventions for pressure ulcers after spinal cord injury. *Archives of Physical Medicine and Rehabilitation*, *90*(2), 213–231. https://doi-org.proxy.library.vcu.edu/10.1016/j.apmr.2008.08.212

Ryback, R. S., Trimble, R. W., Lewis, O. F., & Jennings, C. L. (1971). Psychobiologic effects of prolonged weightlessness (bed rest) in young healthy volunteers. *Aerospace Medicine*, *42*(4), 408–415.

Sale, D. G., McComas, A. J., MacDougall, J. D., & Upton, A. R. (1982). Neuromuscular adaptation in human thenar muscles following strength training and immobilization. *Journal of Applied Physiology: Respiratory, Environmental and Exercise Physiology*, *53*(2), 419–424. https://doi-org.proxy.library.vcu.edu/10.1152/jappl.1982.53.2.419

Schweickert, W. D., Pohlman, M. C., Pohlman, A. S., Nigos, C., Pawlik, A. J., Esbrook, C. L., Spears, L., Miller, M., Franczyk, M., Deprizio, D., Schmidt, G. A., Bowman, A., Barr, R., McCallister, K. E., Hall, J. B., & Kress, J. P. (2009). Early physical and occupational therapy in mechanically ventilated, critically ill patients: A randomized controlled trial. *Lancet (London, England)*, *373*(9678), 1874–1882. https://doi-org.proxy.library.vcu.edu/10.1016/S0140-6736(09)60658-9

Sezer, N., Akkuş, S., & Uğurlu, F. G. (2015). Chronic complications of spinal cord injury. *World Journal of Orthopedics*, *6*(1), 24–33. https://doi-org.proxy.library.vcu.edu/10.5312/wjo.v6.i1.24

Spielman, A. J., Saskin, P., & Thorpy, M. J. (1987). Treatment of chronic insomnia by restriction of time in bed. *Sleep*, *10*(1), 45–56.

Szollar, S. M., Martin, E. M., Sartoris, D. J., Parthemore, J. G., & Deftos, L. J. (1998). Bone mineral density and indexes of bone metabolism in spinal cord injury. *American Journal of Physical Medicine & Rehabilitation*, *77*(1), 28–35. https://doi-org.proxy.library.vcu.edu/10.1097/00002060-199801000-00005

Shavelle, R. M., Brooks, J. C., Strauss, D. J., & Turner-Stokes, L. (2019). Life expectancy after stroke based on age, sex, and ranking grade of disability: A synthesis. *Journal of Stroke and Cerebrovascular Diseases: The Official Journal of the National Stroke Association*, *28*(12), 1–7, 104450. https://doi-org.proxy.library.vcu.edu/10.1016/j.jstrokecerebrovasdis.2019.104450

Shavelle, R. M., Paculdo, D. R., Tran, L. M., Strauss, D. J., Brooks, J. C., & DeVivo, M. J. (2015). Mobility, continence, and life expectancy in persons with Asia impairment scale grade D spinal cord injuries. *American Journal of Physical Medicine & Rehabilitation*, *94*(3), 180–191. https://doi.org/10.1097/PHM.0000000000000140

Shavelle, R. M., & Strauss, D. (2000). Comparative mortality of adults with traumatic brain injury in California, 1988–97. *Journal of Insurance Medicine*, *32*, 163–166.

Shavelle, R. M., Strauss, D., Day, S., & Ojdana, K. (2007). Life expectancy. In N. Zasler, D. Katz, & R. Zafante (Eds.), *Brain injury: Principles and practice*. Demos Medical Publishing.

Slot, K. B., Berge, E., Dorman, P., Lewis, S., Dennis, M., Sandercock, P., Oxfordshire Community Stroke Project, the International Stroke Trial (UK), & Lothian Stroke Register. (2008). Impact of functional status at six months on long term survival in patients with ischaemic stroke: Prospective cohort studies. *British Medical Journal (Clinical Research Ed.)*, *336*(7640), 376–379. https://doi.org/10.1136/bmj.39456.688333.BE

Teasell, R., & Dittmer, D. (1993). Complications of immobilization and bed rest. Part 2: Other complications. *Canadian Family Physician*, *39*, 1440–1446.

Thomas, D. C., Kreizman, I. J., Melchiorre, P., & Ragnarsson, K. T. (2002). Rehabilitation of the patient with chronic critical illness. *Critical Care Clinics*, *18*(3), 695–715. https://doi-org.proxy.library.vcu.edu/10.1016/s0749-0704(02)00011-8

Tollefsen, E., & Fonderes, O. (2012). Respiratory complications associated with spinal cord injury. *Tidsskr Nor Laegeforen*, *132*, 1111–1114.

Turpie, A. G. (1997). Prophylaxis of venous thromboembolism in stroke patients. *Seminars in Thrombosis and Hemostasis*, *23*(2), 155–157. https://doi-org.proxy.library.vcu.edu/10.1055/s-2007-996084

Varacallo, M., Davis, D. D., & Pizzutillo, P. (2022). Osteoporosis in spinal cord injuries. In *StatPearls*. StatPearls Publishing.

Walker, J., Payne, S., Smith, P., & Jarrett, N. (2007). *Psychology for nurses and the caring professions*. McGraw Hill, Open University Press.

..

Wannamethee, S. G., Shaper, A. G., & Walker, M. (1998). Changes in physical activity, mortality, and incidence of coronary heart disease in older men. *Lancet (London, England)*, *351*(9116), 1603–1608. https://doi-org.proxy.library.vcu.edu/10.1016/S0140-6736(97)12355-8

Winslow, C., & Rozovsky, J. (2003). Effect of spinal cord injury on the respiratory system. *American Journal of Physical Medicine & Rehabilitation*, *82*, 803–814.

Yeo, J. D., Walsh, J., Rutkowski, S., Soden, R., Craven, M., & Middleton, J. (1998). Mortality following spinal cord injury. *Spinal Cord*, *36*(5), 329–336. https://doi.org/10.1038/sj.sc.3100628

Yuan, P., Koppelmans, V., Reuter-Lorenz, P., De Dios, Y., Gadd, N., Wood, S., Riascos, R., Kofman, I., Bloomberg, J., Mulavara, A., & Seidler, R. (2018). Vestibular brain changes within 70 days of head-down bed rest. *Human Brain Mapping*, *39*(7), 2753–2763. https://doi-org.proxy.library.vcu.edu/10.1002/hbm.24037

9 Acquired Brain Injury

Huma Haider

Background

Traumatic brain injuries (TBIs) significantly impact the daily lives of those who have suffered from one, as well as their family members, friends, and caregivers. Often referred to as the "silent epidemic", TBIs are defined by the Centers for Disease Control (2015) as "a disruption in the normal function of the brain that can be caused by a bump, blow, or jolt to the head or a penetrating head injury" (Marr & Coronado, 2004; Wright, 2013, p. 549). Coronado et al. (2012) added acceleration/deceleration forces in a revised definition and noted that such forces were associated with decreased level of consciousness, amnesia, objective neurologic or neuropsychological abnormality(ies), skull fracture(s), diagnosed intracranial lesion(s), or head injury listed as a cause of death in the death certificate. Explosive blasts can also cause TBI, particularly among those who serve in the U.S. military (Centers for Disease Control, National Center for Injury Prevention and Control, n.d., 2022; The CDC et al., 2013). A person who is suffering from a TBI may appear to have no physical or mental deficits to the general population; however, with proper testing and diagnosis, these deficits can be identified and treated. There are approximately 2.8–2.9 million reported TBI-related emergency department visits, hospitalizations, and deaths of all ages every year (Lo et al., 2021). However, this number is grossly underreported primarily with mild TBI (Putnam et al., 2019). The annual estimated global burden of disease (GBD) on health care is estimated for annual direct costs to be $27.2 billion for TBI-related admissions and $8.2 billion for discharge/transports (Lo et al.). The annual indirect costs total $75.6 billion, resulting in an annual cost of $93.0 billion for TBI for all ages (Lo et al.).

Advancements in modern medicine are improving the outcomes and livelihoods of those with traumatic and moderate to severe brain injuries, many of whom would have died ten years ago without the treatment options of the present. TBIs can be clinically classified as either mild, moderate, or severe. Those with severe TBIs typically have visible external impairments, for example, quadriplegic, paraplegic, spasticity, amputations, etc. With a mild TBI, the person may appear to be physically fit without impairments; however, there has been significant long-term damage to the brain. It is well documented that TBI increases long-term mortality regardless of severity level and is associated with increased incidences of neurodegenerative and psychiatric diseases (Chen et al., 2021). Mild TBIs are often undiagnosed, underdiagnosed, untreated, and misunderstood. Many times, the cognitive, behavioral, and physical impairments of a mild TBI are as severe as those seen with a severe TBI (Chen et al.). Out of the 3 million TBIs reported each year, approximately 75% of them are classified as mild (National Center for Injury Prevention and Control, 2003). This missed diagnosis of a mild TBI has become an epidemic in industrialized countries resulting in undertreatment and

DOI: 10.4324/b23293-9

fatalities. Regarding children in the United States, an estimated 475,000 children aged 0–14 suffer a TBI each year. TBI results in more than 7000 deaths, 60,000 hospitalizations, and 600,000 emergency department (ED) visits annually among American children (Dewan et al., 2016). This trauma travels the world over, as statistics for brain injury are documented annually in all countries (Hyder et al., 2007). TBI studies have revealed that this trauma contributes to more than half of pediatric injuries in Iran, around 20% of trauma ED admissions in India, and about 30% of pediatric injuries in Korea (Dewan et al.). Australia has approximately 486 adolescents per 100,000 people per year with a TBI and approximately 280 children out of 100,000 people in the United Kingdom (Dewan et al.). TBI is not a single diagnosis, but it is a symptom of a complex biopsychosocial interaction of physical, cognitive, and emotional symptoms in all countries.

The three most common causes of TBIs are falls, motor vehicle accidents, and head strikes, or hitting of the head on an external object. Other causes of a TBI include blast injuries, penetrating injuries, and inhalation injuries. TBIs are categorized as primary and secondary (Andriessen et al., 2010). Primary injuries are those with mechanical forces that affect the cerebral tissues. Secondary injures are those that affect the cascade of the cellular and molecular processes resulting from the head strike (Andriessen et al.). There are also secondary causes of brain injuries that consist of brain tissue damage, including hypoxic or ischemic injuries, hypoglycemia, hypotensive events, and increased intracranial pressure. A TBI is caused by "a sudden impact or acceleration/deceleration trauma of the head" (Vos et al., 2012). This impact or acceleration/deceleration causes damage to the brain tissue and structures, which leads to cognitive, physical, and/or emotional impairments in the patient.

Pathophysiology

There are four main causes of TBIs: focal injuries, diffuse axonal injuries, hypoxic-ischemic injuries, and increased intracranial pressure. Focal injuries directly impact the area of the brain associated with the location of external impact. For example, a blow to the head may incite brain injury at the site of the blow, but also brain injury may result directly opposite the site of impact (O'Sullivan et al., 2007). Common sites of focal brain injury are the anterior-inferior temporal lobes and prefrontal lobes. Symptoms after a focal brain injury are directly correlated with the area of the brain that is impacted. Focal injuries can be caused by a coup/contrecoup injury, where the brain strikes the inside of the skull after the head has an impact with a fixed object. An injury directly related to trauma at the site of impact is called a coup injury. On impact, the brain can travel back and strike the back of the skull. This is called a contrecoup injury (see Figure 9.1).

Diffuse axonal injuries occur when the brain rapidly shifts inside the skull as the injury is occurring with acceleration, deceleration, and rotational forces impacting the brain. These types of injuries are characterized by widespread shearing and retraction of damaged axons (O'Sullivan et al., 2007). The significance of these axonal changes is that they eventually separate from the soma. Thus, multiple areas of the brain are involved in addition to the cortical white matter and include the corpus callosum, basal ganglia, brainstem, and cerebellum (O'Sullivan et al.). Diffuse axonal injuries can occur in high-speed motor vehicle collisions, causing the rapid acceleration/deceleration of the brain within the skull. Andriessen et al. (2010) noted that characteristically diffuse brain injury involves the widely distributed damage of axons in addition to diffuse vascular injury, hypoxic-ischemic injury, and brain swelling (edema). Andriessen et al. also noted that due to the structure of the brain being heterogeneous regarding the degree of fixation to other parts of the brain and skull, it is a very consistent-structured complex organ, such that during the movement of the head, some segments of the brain move slower than others

Coup injury   Contrecoup
                                 injury

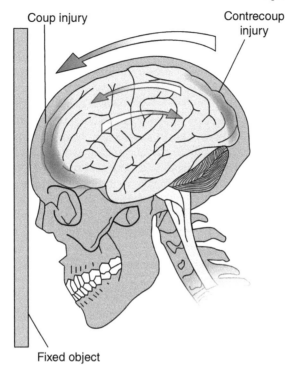

Fixed object

Figure 9.1 Contrecoup Injury

causing "shear, tensile, and compressive forces within the brain tissue" (p. 2383). When the damage is significant, it can be seen on a head computed tomography (CT) scan as an intracranial hemorrhage.

Park et al. (2009) identified diffuse axonal injury as being recognized as severe post-traumatic brain injury, Park et al. noted that this diffuse axonal injury is characterized as having a post-traumatic coma following injury, with an intracranial mass lesion. Hypoxic/ischemic injuries occur when there is a lack of oxygenated blood flow to the brain tissue for an extended period. There are many causes of this type of injury including systemic, hypotension, anoxia, and near-drowning. O'Sullivan et al. (2007) added that a hypoxic-ischemic event that is associated with poorer cognitive function and lower expected outcomes can lead to global damage.

Neuromembrane Events Associated With Traumatic Brain Injury

Increased intracranial pressure (ICP) can also damage the brain tissue and result in a TBI. Increased ICP is an important cause of secondary brain injury. Smith (2008) noted that intracranial mass lesions, contusional injuries, vascular engorgement, and brain edema can lead to increased ICP. Increased ICP typically leads to poorer outcomes and higher mortality rates after a TBI. O'Sullivan et al. (2007) reported that a variety of cellular events that follow tissue damage can cause secondary cell death, such as glutamate neurotoxicity, the influx of calcium and other ions, free radical release, and cytokines.

Function of the Brain Lobes and Associated Impairments

The frontal lobes of the brain are involved in tracking and a sense of self as well as arousal and initiations, the consciousness of the environment, reaction to self and environment, executive functioning, judgment, emotional response, stability, language usage, personality, word associations and meaning, and memory for motor activity habits. When there is damage to the frontal lobe, the person may demonstrate difficulties with planning and carrying out complex tasks in the correct order. They may also perseverate on something, meaning they will repeat their words or actions over and over again without consciously knowing they are doing it. These people may also have decreased attention and concentration and can be easily distracted. They may demonstrate mental rigidity, or an inability to think flexibly, as well as diminished abstract reasoning or imagination. Emotionally they may have difficulty controlling their emotions and demonstrate mood swings frequently. Family and friends may notice changes in the person's personality and social behavior. Frontal lobe damage may also result in difficulty with problem-solving, expressive language, and word-finding difficulties, as well as loss of simple movements of various body parts.

The temporal lobes of the brain are involved in auditory processing, long-term memory, object categorization, visual perception, and intellect. When there is damage to the temporal lobe, the person may have difficulty understanding spoken language, an inability to categorize objects, and difficulty identifying and verbalizing about objects. They can have difficulty with concentration and short-term memory loss. Behaviorally they may demonstrate extreme aggression or demonstrate aggressive behavior overall. Some of their long-term memories may be lost. If the damage is to the right temporal lobe, they may demonstrate persistent talking. They may have difficulty locating objects within their environment. Temporal lobe damage may also cause seizure disorders, changes in sexual interest, and auras.

The parietal lobes of the brain are involved in visual perception, tactile or touch perception, object manipulation, integration of sensory information, and goal-directed voluntary movements. When there is damage to the parietal lobe, a person may demonstrate difficulty with naming objects, writing words, performing math calculations, and/or drawing. They may demonstrate an inability to attend to more than one object at a time or focus their visual attention, which leads to difficulty reading. Damage to the parietal lobe may also lead to poor hand-eye coordination, confusion between right/left orientation, and/or lack of awareness of certain body parts and where they are in space.

The occipital lobes are responsible for visual perception. Many of the visual impairments are related to damage to the occipital lobe. These impairments include visual field cuts, hallucinations, visual illusions, word blindness, and difficulty perceiving movement. Other limitations may include difficulty recognizing drawn objects and a loss of academic skills such as reading and writing (see Figure 9.2).

Cognitive Characteristics

TBIs present with many different characteristics depending on the areas of the brain that were affected by the injury. Cognitive impairments are frequently seen in both mild and severe TBIs. Many of the cognitive impairments are not initially obvious to the general public and can pose a significant impact on the lives of those with TBIs. The sequelae of TBI and its associated functional deficits are not consistent across patients with this diagnosis. Impairments from TBI are referred to as post-concussion symptoms and include cognitive (e.g., difficulty concentrating and taking longer to think), word-finding difficulties, short-term and long-term memory loss, difficulty understanding written or spoken words, and difficulty communicating (Theadom et al., 2018). Cognitive deficits can evolve into behaviors that impair one's productivity in the

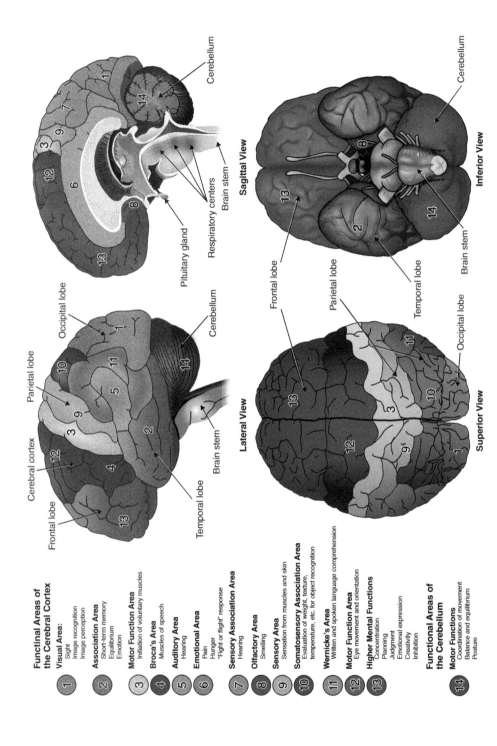

Functinal Areas of the Cerebral Cortex

(1) Visual Area:
Sight
Image recognition
Image perception

(2) Association Area
Short-term memory
Equilibrium
Emotion

(3) Motor Function Area
Initiation of voluntary muscles

(4) Broca's Area
Muscles of speech

(5) Auditory Area
Hearing

(6) Emotional Area
Pain
Hunger
"Fight or flight" response

(7) Sensory Association Area
Hearing

(8) Olfactory Area
Smelling

(9) Sensory Area
Sensation from muscles and skin

(10) Somatosensory Association Area
Evaluation of weight, texture,
temperature, etc. for object recognition

(11) Wernicke's Area
Written and spoken language comprehension

(12) Motor Function Area
Eye movement and orientation

(13) Higher Mental Functions
Concentration
Planning
Judgment
Emotional expression
Creativity
Inhibition

Functional Areas of the Cerebellum

(14) Motor Functions
Coordination of movement
Balance and equilibrium
Posture

Figure 9.2 Functional Areas of the Brain

workplace, create a need for higher health service delivery, and cause the development of anti-social behaviors. Often, cognitive symptoms go unnoticed in polytrauma cases, as the more severe trauma is addressed at the time of hospitalization at which time acquired brain injury sequelae have not evolved, are not noticeable, or are not identified (Theadom et al., 2018).

Cognitive symptoms can have a significant impact on a person's daily life and activities of daily living. If the cognitive symptoms persist longer than the acute period after injury, persons with mild TBIs may have difficulty maintaining or obtaining employment. Theadom et al. found in their study that people with mild TBIs have an increased occurrence of self-reported cognitive symptoms and reduced community participation. "The persistence of cognitive symptoms four years post-injury, suggests that cognitive symptoms which fail to resolve in the acute phase post-injury are likely to become chronic, and impact participation without intervention" (Theadom et al., p. 7).

Physical Characteristics

Physical characteristics of TBIs can have as much as or more of an impact on a person's daily life; the typical and inclusive complaints include headaches, balance problems, dizziness, and fatigue (The CDC et al., 2013). These physical impairments can greatly impact the daily living of a person with a TBI. A person with post-traumatic brain injury headaches may experience headaches for several hours to days at a time, making working and daily activities extremely difficult or impossible. With severe TBIs, the person may develop abnormal tone in their muscles and they may demonstrate primitive postures as a result. Impaired sensation is another physical characteristic that occurs after a TBI. The person may experience numbness or tingling in their arms or legs. O'Sullivan et al. (2007) noted that sensation modifications following TBI may include impairments in light touch, pain, deep pressure, and temperature, as well as sensory trait factors such as proprioception and kinesthesia. Decreased sensation poses a safety risk to these people while they complete activities of daily living. They may not be able to determine the proper water temperature for a shower or the temperature of the cooked food. They may also not be able to feel when they nick their finger while chopping vegetables.

Cerebellar injuries are common in TBIs, and the cerebellum plays a vital role in balance. Balance problems pose a high safety risk for overall mobility in persons with mild TBIs. Vestibular and physical therapy play a vital role in providing these patients with compensatory strategies and balance-strengthening to improve their overall quality of life. At times a person may require a cane or walker to assist them in walking due to significant balance impairments. Balance impairments may decrease the person's ability to have gainful employment, depending on what their occupation was before the TBI.

Behavioral Characteristics

Behavioral characteristics may not initially be seen in persons with TBIs. As time progresses post-injury, certain behavioral characteristics may evolve that interfere with the patient's daily life activities as well as social interactions. Such behavioral characteristics may include undesirable behavioral patterns that can vary from apathy, disinhibition, and agitation, to aggression and violent behavior, and these behavioral traits may frequently exist simultaneously (Timmer et al., 2020). These characteristics can have a significant impact on the relationship between the person with a TBI and their family, friends, and co-workers. It is noteworthy that such undesirable behavioral trait factors can negatively affect familial relationships. Timmer et al. documented in their study of 226 patients, of which 107 were diagnosed with having mild TBI and 119 were diagnosed as having moderate to severe TBI. Regarding the mild TBI patients, 24% of them showed serious behavioral disturbances and 76% showed mild behavioral disturbances. In comparison to the severe TBI patients, the data showed serious behavioral disturbances almost three times more present in severe TBI patients (35%) when compared to mild TBI patients (13%).

Behavioral characteristics can lead to difficulty reintegrating into society. Additional behavioral characteristics include sexual disinhibition, low frustration tolerance, and depression.

Diagnostic Imaging

TBIs can be difficult to diagnose initially. Traditionally, a head CT scan will be done in the emergency room to look for acute bleeding. There can still be brain damage even if it is not seen on the CT scan. A head CT will show a subdural hematoma, an epidural hematoma, a subarachnoid hemorrhage, and a diffuse axonal injury. A negative CT scan will not show the damage and disruption of the axons and dendrites on a microscopic level. These disruptions have a significant impact on the functioning of the brain. Magnetic resonance imaging (MRI) of the brain can also be used to diagnose a TBI; however, it may still not show the damage at the microscopic level (see Figures 9.3 and 9.4).

Diffusion tensor imaging (DTI) is another diagnostic imaging technique that can show brain tissue damage and damage to the white matter tracts. Alexander et al. (2007) stated that "Diffusion tensor imaging is a promising method for characterizing microstructural changes or differences with neuropathology and treatment. The diffusion tensor may be used to characterize the magnitude, the degree of anisotropy, and the orientation of directional diffusion" (p. 316). DTI provides valuable information to providers regarding the areas of the brain that are affected by TBIs and greatly assists providers in determining the best course of treatment. The DTI provides three segments of information: tractography from the DTI, fractional anisotropy analysis from the DTI, and general brain imaging with susceptibility-weighted imaging. DTI provides objective evidence that a mild brain injury ceases to be mild and becomes a permanent brain injury. It will allow more precise discovery into the areas damaged at a level unable to be viewed with traditional MRI or CT; these techniques are not sensitive to detecting diffuse axonal injuries/traumatic axonal injuries (DAIs/TAIs)—the major brain injuries observed in mild TBI (Shenton et al., 2012). Symptoms in this patient group are the result of alterations undetectable by traditional CT and/or MRI machinery. Information garnered from DTI reveals microscopic damage and is very helpful for the targeted neurocognitive rehabilitation and prognostication (see Figure 9.5).

Electromyography (EMG) measures muscle response or electrical activity in response to a nerve's stimulation of the muscle. The EMG is a diagnostic procedure that assesses the health of the muscles and the motor neurons that control them. Electroencephalography (EEG) is a test that is used to detect the electrical activity of the brain and help providers identify abnormalities.

Treatment

Treatment for persons with TBIs varies greatly across the population based on the area of the brain impacted by the injury. Ninety-five percent of TBI sufferers will have headaches. One treatment option for headaches is medication. Providers must be sure to monitor the person's response to the medication and adjust or alter it as necessary. Nerve blocks and nerve stimulation are other options for treating headaches. Memory loss, decreased attention, and brain fog are common symptoms as well. In the acute phase after a TBI, the person will benefit from inpatient rehabilitation services for up to three months. If these symptoms are noticed in the acute phase, the person will benefit from outpatient therapy and at-home exercises to improve their overall memory and attention and decrease the brain fog. Also important is community reintegration and getting the person back to work if physically able. People with balance disorders

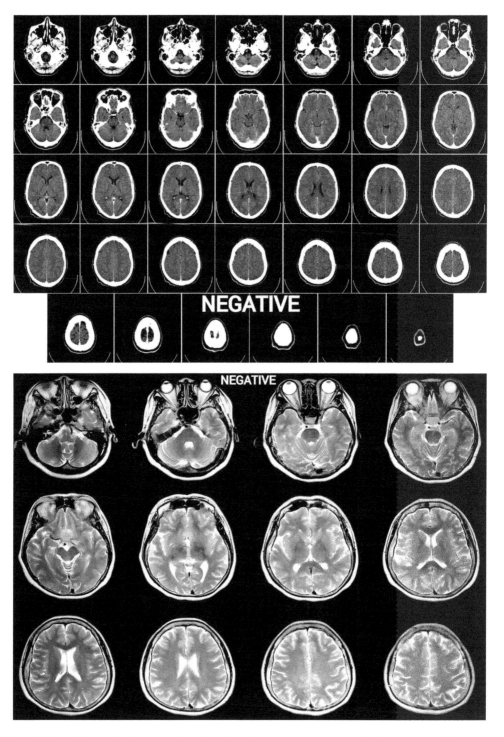

Figure 9.3 and Figure 9.4 Negative Brain Imaging. These Images are Negative for Any Acute Trauma or Brain Tissue Damage, Even Though the Patient did Suffer a TBI

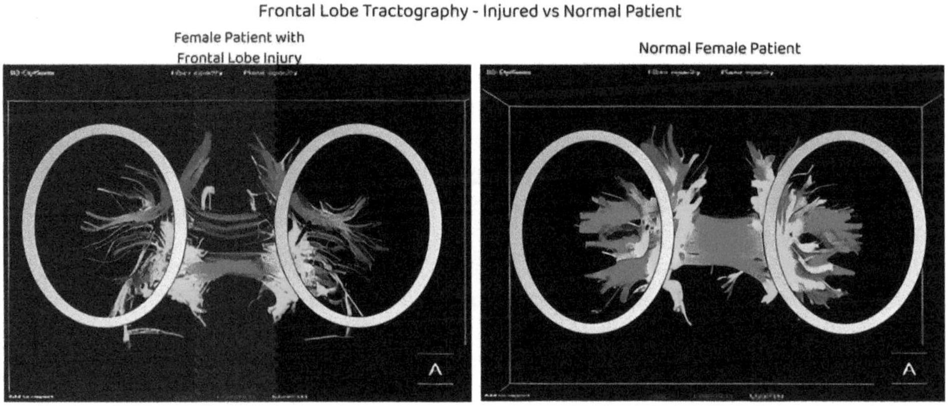

Figure 9.5 Brain Injury vs. Normal Brain

will benefit greatly from vestibular therapy to improve their overall balance and teach them compensation strategies to ensure safety with their activities of daily living.

Depression is common after TBI, affecting half of sufferers in the first year and two-thirds within seven years of injury. Of those suffering depression, half will present with newly onset concomitant anxiety (Delmonico et al., 2021; Depression After Traumatic Brain Injury, n.d.). Proactive treatment of these psychiatric symptoms following a brain injury has been shown to improve mental health outcomes, cognition, somatic symptoms, and daily functioning. (Silverberg & Panenka, 2019). Mood swings, depression, and anxiety are commonly treated with antidepressant/anxiety medications as well as therapy and counseling. Transcranial magnetic stimulation is another treatment method used to treat depression. It is a non-invasive procedure that uses magnetic fields to stimulate nerve cells in the brain to improve symptoms of depression. TBI increases the risk of developing psychiatric disorders by nearly three-fold. Mild TBI increases the risk of subsequent or comorbid post-traumatic stress disorder (PTSD) (Bryant, 2011). Signs and symptoms of PTSD include unwanted and repeated memories of the incident, flashbacks with a loss of reality in which the incident is relived, intentional avoidance of reminders (places, items, sounds, etc.), detachment from loved ones and/or depersonalization, shame surrounding the incident, survivor guilt, hypervigilance, irritability absent discernible cause, intense and/or unwarranted arousability, and/or paranoia.

Sleep disturbances such as difficulty falling asleep and staying asleep, as well as suffering from fatigue unabated by rest, and hypersomnia (sleeping more than normal amounts) though fatigue persists unabated by rest are common and affect up to 70% of TBI sufferers, while up to 53% endorse enduring fatigue (Viola-Saltzman & Watson, 2012). Treatment for insomnia and sleep disturbances includes sleep aids, sleep studies, and proper sleep hygiene.

Ringing in the ears, also known as tinnitus, is another common symptom persons with TBIs experience. Up to 53% of those who have suffered a TBI develop tinnitus. Causes include mechanical trauma, pressure-related injury, noise-associated trauma, and neck injury or emotional trauma (Kreuzer et al., 2014). Treatment considerations for ringing in the ears include an audiological evaluation, prescription ear drops, and devices such as white noise makers or soft background music to distract the person from concentrating on the noise.

Vision is the most important source of sensory information. Consisting of a sophisticated complex of subsystems, the visual process involves the flow and processing of information to the brain. The visual system is really a relationship of sensory-motor functions, which are controlled and organized in the brain. After TBI, there is frequently a shifting of the visual midline, vitreous hemorrhaging, and macular or retinal abnormalities. Common visual changes following an injury include blurred vision, double vision, and decreased peripheral vision. Others suffer photophobia, accommodation, eye movement, convergence, pupillary function, and/or visual field impairments or changes. Studies indicate that up to 60% of TBI patients suffer from some visual dysfunction in at least one eye (Armstrong, 2018). Treatment considerations for vision changes include a neuro-optometrist evaluation, anti-inflammatory eye drops, and ocular rehabilitation.

Brain damage, such as that imparted by trauma, is a major cause of adult-onset communication disorders, specifically aphasia, apraxia, and dysarthria. Diffuse brain injury is known to cause difficulties in comprehension and expression. Damage to the left hemisphere often manifests as aphasiac conditions and dysarthria, while right hemisphere damage accounts for confrontational naming, word fluency, reading, writing, and related impairments (Bobba et al., 2019). Professional intervention for those suffering from communication impairments following brain injury has been proven effective for the majority of patients. With tailored treatment plans, studies show that between 67% and 82.5% of patients showed improvement in language-based capabilities (Coelho et al., 1996). Treatment for communication disorders is a formal evaluation and treatment by a speech-language pathologist.

The Life Care Plan

A life care plan (LCP) is a document that outlines a comprehensive plan for medical requirements for people with long-term treatment needs. People with TBIs that suffer from multiple chronic conditions as a result will require ongoing and perhaps lifelong care and will benefit from an LCP. An LCP is a document that is based upon the current published standards for practice, comprehensive assessment, data analysis, and research. The LCP document is created with the patient at the center and is aptly named person-centered planning (PCP). PCP supports personal independence to the extent possible based upon comprehensive assessments by trained and credentialed providers. Moreover, this plan also endeavors to provide for personal freedom of movement within the community in a supported and safe manner, as well as aims to account for appropriate services and support based upon individual needs. Also integral to personal well-being, and as determined by legal mandates, this plan addresses the needs of a safe, accessible home in a residential setting with adequate privacy. Holistic supports discussed within this document also delve into vocational and meaningful activity to provide community integration and a sense of self-efficacy. LCPs are vital for the long-term, lifelong care of a person with a TBI.

The remaining part of this chapter focuses on preparing an LCP for a brain-injured patient. The LCP for brain-injured patients is a highly structured document with multiple sections, the first being that of the clinical interview.

Clinical Interview

In this section, the history of the patient's present illness is written out in a narrative paragraph. Then the medical and surgical history before injury are listed, followed by the medical and surgical history after the injury. This demonstrates the changes in medical conditions from before the injury to after the injury and is vital for the proper long-term cost analysis. The current medications and allergies are included in this section and are important in the proper long-term cost analysis. The next three subsections are the educational, social, and family history. The educational history plays an important role in identifying any potential jobs or careers the person might be able to do post-injury, depending on their impairments. Family history identifies any potential of having common disorders such as high blood pressure, heart disease, etc. The social history identifies any potential lifestyle habits that may contribute to a shorter lifespan or habits that may need to be stopped or altered for the best health of the patient. The background information section is vital in developing proper future needs and costs associated with the needs and in identifying the support system that the patient has as well as any traumatic events they may have experienced prior to their injury. The remaining subsection is the review of systems. This is completed to obtain a subjective report on the patient's body systems and any current issues or complaints from the patient.

Physical Examination

The second section of the LCP is the physical examination. This allows the medical practitioner to assess the patient formally by looking at all body systems, range of motion of the joints, and the patient's mental status, mood, and speech, as well as specialized assessments to determine areas of impairment in sensation and vision. A cranial nerve exam, motor strength exam, deep tendon reflexes, sensory light touch, and pinprick are also completed. Coordination, gait, and adventitious movements are also assessed to identify any potential safety issues with functional mobility.

Neuropsychological Testing

The third section in an LCP for brain injuries is the ImPACT Testing section. ImPACT testing is a computer-delivered assessment to quantify the neurocognitive capacity and facility of those who have suffered a brain injury. Following a simple point-and-click style exam and taking into account previous injury, medical history, age, and related pertinent information, scores are given across multiple domains. Subtest scores and summaries are provided, as are the composite scores. These scores not only identify cognitive strengths and weaknesses but are a useful indicator of domains requiring further evaluation and prognostication. The next section of the LCP is the summarized medical records and sources. This section provides a chronological record of what the patient has experienced since their injury. This section tends to be very extensive and long, depending on the amount of records the patient has provided.

Impact of the Injury

The fifth section of the LCP is the impact of injury section. This section is completed during a process called the LCP interview, where the patient is assessed by a medical professional and specific assessments are completed.

Impact of Injuries on Activities of Daily Living and Instrumental Activities of Daily Living

The first subsection is the impact of injuries on activities of daily living (ADLs) and instrumental activities of daily living (IADLs). This section is important in identifying how the patient's life has been impacted from the injury/injuries and identifies specific areas of ADLs they are no longer able to independently complete. The medical assistant and provider will collect this information from the patient during their LCP interview. Once the information is collected, a summary statement is completed and placed at the bottom of the table. Sample tables are found in Appendix 9A.

Impact on Complex Tasks

The second subsection of the report is the impact on complex tasks. This section takes information obtained through a neuropsychological evaluation and identifies the level of impairments in a variety of categories such as response inhibition, working memory, emotional control, task initiation, sustained attention, planning/prioritization, organization, time management, flexibility (cognitive), metacognition, goal-directed persistence, and stress tolerance. At the end of these charts the patient's strongest skills and weakest skills are identified. The next two subsections are the impact on psychosocial well-being and the impact on family well-being. The impact on psychosocial well-being looks at how the injury has impacted the patient's self-esteem, autonomy, ability/opportunities to make choices/decisions, and adaptive behavior and related skills. The impact on family well-being looks at how the injuries of the patient have impacted their relationships and roles within the family. It identifies if a strain has been placed on their relationships and what they no longer can do with or for the family. Familial observations are also collected in this section to gain more insight into the impact on the family's well-being.

Personalized Brain Injury Map

The next section is the personalized brain injury map, which is modified for each and every patient. Figure 9.6 is an example of the map that identifies impairments based on the lobes impacted by injury and a general description of the general functions of each lobe (see Figure 9.6).

Long-Term Complications of TBI

The next subsection is the long-term complications of a TBI. This section identifies the potential complications a person may develop due to the severity of their injuries. These complications can require additional treatments and therapies that are above and beyond those listed within the LCP.

Leading Impressions

The sixth section is discusses the leading impressions of the LCP. This includes the diagnoses, disabilities post-injury, and life expectancy. The diagnoses include all diagnoses that have been identified by all providers for the patient. Many times during the medical record review these diagnoses can be identified and captured here. The disabilities post-injury section identifies what the patient can no longer do that they were able to prior to the injury as well as any activities that were affected and identified in the ADL/IADL chart in the impact section. The life expectancy section is important to identify how many anticipated years the patient has in their life. This information is vital and used to calculate the costs in the future medical requirements section. That section will calculate treatment according to the potential years left of life remaining, as elucidated from both the most recent National Vital Statistics reports in combination with the Social Security Administration's Life Expectancy Calculator. The National Vital Statistics report accounts for the patient's race in determining their life expectancy. The Social Security Administration's Life Expectancy Calculator accounts for gender and exact age of the patient.

Future Medical Requirements

The seventh section is the future medical requirements section. This section identifies all services, equipment, physician appointments, laboratory work, and future diagnostics that the

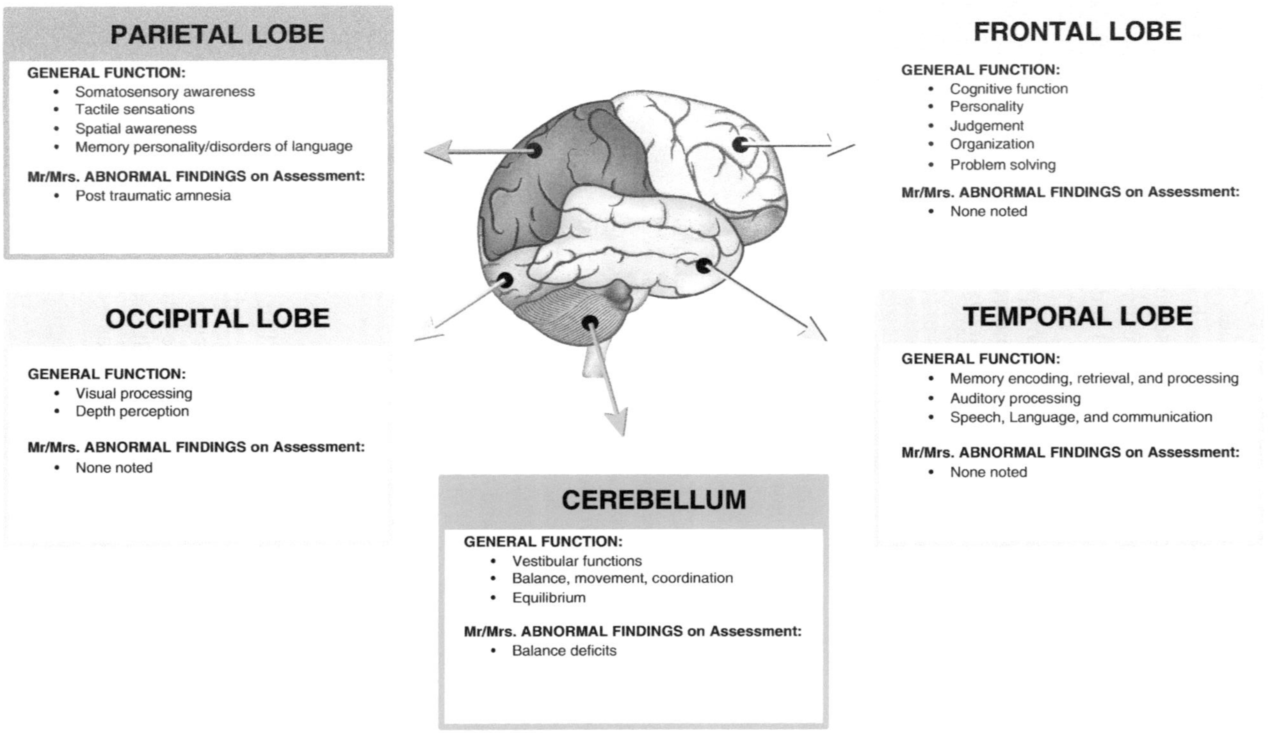

FRONTAL LOBE

GENERAL FUNCTION:
- Cognitive function
- Personality
- Judgement
- Organization
- Problem solving

Mr/Mrs. ABNORMAL FINDINGS on Assessment:
- None noted

TEMPORAL LOBE

GENERAL FUNCTION:
- Memory encoding, retrieval, and processing
- Auditory processing
- Speech, Language, and communication

Mr/Mrs. ABNORMAL FINDINGS on Assessment:
- None noted

CEREBELLUM

GENERAL FUNCTION:
- Vestibular functions
- Balance, movement, coordination
- Equilibrium

Mr/Mrs. ABNORMAL FINDINGS on Assessment:
- Balance deficits

PARIETAL LOBE

GENERAL FUNCTION:
- Somatosensory awareness
- Tactile sensations
- Spatial awareness
- Memory personality/disorders of language

Mr/Mrs. ABNORMAL FINDINGS on Assessment:
- Post traumatic amnesia

OCCIPITAL LOBE

GENERAL FUNCTION:
- Visual processing
- Depth perception

Mr/Mrs. ABNORMAL FINDINGS on Assessment:
- None noted

Figure 9.6 Personalized Brain Injury Map: Brain Lobes and Their Functions

patient will need for the remainder of their life expectancy. This section is tailored to each person individually. Following this section is the cost data/vendor source section that identifies the costs from three different resources and the average cost of each. Three sources are used to determine the average cost, and the patient's ZIP code is used to find the most accurate cost. When completing the costing for the LCP, it is industry standard to create them with self-pay prices to provide optimal care to the patients at all times. This section directly correlates with the future medical requirement section and prices out each service, piece of equipment, physician appointment, laboratory test, and future diagnostic service. Within this section several subsections are typically used for the patients. Following are the main subsections used with associated services and Current Procedural Terminology (CPT) codes. Each of these sections are customized for the patient and their specific needs; there are services not captured in the charts that can and are added as necessary. These charts are found in Appendix 9B.

Additional tables are used to factor in the future medical requirements and costs that are specific to each patient's needs. Once the services and needs are determined and identified, costing is then completed.

Cost Analysis

The next section is the cost analysis section, and it contains tables and pie charts demonstrating the costs of associated needs. This cost analysis exhibits the future medical requirements for the patient and their associated monetary value. The information in the sections titled Future Medical Requirements and Cost Data/Vendor Sources were used to calculate these total costs. The average costs associated with the CPT code/service are determined by four main resources that include Context4Healthcare, FAIR Health, 2021 Medical Fees, and Veterans Administration (VA) reasonable costs. These sources take into account the patient's ZIP code and age. Within the cost analysis, the following variables are considered to calculate the number of visits, items, and services the patient will require for the remainder of their life: 1) age at which recommendations are pursued; 2) quantity of visits, items, and services; 3) duration of treatment and use in years; and 4) cost per visit, items, and services. The patient's age, sex, race, and life expectancy are references and used as a basis to calculate the total costs. A restatement of the patient's diagnoses and disabilities is placed before the tables and graphs to support the necessity of the future medical requirements.

Recommendations

The tenth section is the recommendations section. This section contains all recommendations the provider has for the care of the patient currently and in the future. These recommendations are captured within the Future Medical Requirements, Cost Data/Vendor Sources, and Cost Analysis sections. The final section of the LCP is the summary section, where the entire LCP is summarized. There is a summary table containing all costs mentioned in the previous costs that provides a total for all future medical requirements as well as a pie chart.

Rehabilitation Potential

The rehabilitation potential for patients with TBIs varies greatly depending on the severity of the brain injury and other injuries sustained during the damaging event as well as the patient's comorbidities. It is noteworthy that when a patient is discharged from a rehabilitative or medical treatment facility, it does not suggest that the individual has attained maximum medication improvement (MMI) or maximum rehabilitative achievement (MRa) (Marini et al., 2009). It is essential that the discharged patient continue with follow-up therapy to continue to progress toward their maximum level of independence (Marini et al.). Patients with TBIs may require physical, occupational, speech, vestibular, and/or cognitive therapies to recover from their injuries. Cognitive impairments influence rehabilitation outcomes significantly given their common sequelae in acquired brain injury (Whyte et al., 2011). Research evidence suggests that pharmacologic and nonpharmacologic interventions can improve rehabilitation outcomes, as these treatment methodologies have been shown to manipulate impairments in cognitive functions (Whyte et al.). The rehabilitation process for patients with TBIs is often seen as a lifelong process. It is necessary to maintain their highest level of independence and ensure the highest quality of life. Almost all patients with a TBI will require services from multiple therapists. O'Sullivan et al. (2007) noted that the TBI patient receives treatment across a continuum of care in a variety of settings, and therefore it is essential that an interdisciplinary team is involved in the rehabilitation process of the respective patient.

Medical Treatment and Follow-Up Care

The treatment for a patient with a TBI starts at the scene of the accident. The goal is to stabilize the patient's cardiovascular and respiratory systems so they can be transported to a medical facility. Continuous monitoring of the patient's blood pressure, oxygen saturation, and Glasgow Coma Scale should be performed throughout transport to the emergency room. In the emergency room, the patient will be assessed by the emergency room physician, and a variety of tests and imaging will be performed. Lab work can include chemistry, complete blood count (CBC), prothrombin time/partial thromboplastin time (PT/PTT), toxicology, alcohol level, and pregnancy test on females. Imaging can include a head CT, cervical spine x-ray, chest x-ray, abdomen and pelvis x-ray, and other imaging as indicated by any other injuries sustained during the accident. Once the patient is stabilized, the physician will determine if they require hospitalization in the intensive care unit (ICU) or other unit within the hospital. If the patient presents with a mild TBI or the brain injury is not detected or diagnosed in the emergency room, the patient may be treated for their other injuries and released home. If the patient is transferred to the ICU or other unit within the hospital, they will have constant neurological assessments, vital signs monitoring, and potentially the initiation of therapy. If the patient presents with difficulty swallowing, a speech language pathologist (SLP) will be consulted to perform a swallowing assessment and, if indicated, a swallow study to determine the swallowing abilities of the patient and make recommendations on food and liquid consistency. The SLP will also determine if it is safe for the patient to eat and drink or if they require alternative routes for nutrition such as a percutaneous endoscopic gastrostomy (PEG) tube. When the physician determines the patient is stable to participate, early mobilization with physical therapy and occupational therapy will be initiated to begin determining the functional abilities of the patient and what equipment, modifications, and assistance they may require when they return home.

Once the patient returns home, follow-up care is necessary. The patient will need to follow up with their primary care physician or establish a primary care physician if they did not have one prior to the injury. The patient should also follow up with any physicians the hospital recommended upon their discharge such as a neurologist, orthopedic surgeon, ear/nose/throat (ENT) doctor, etc. The primary physician can make referrals to the appropriate specialists as needed and will order outpatient or home health therapy services based on the patient's needs. In a study by Marini et al. (2009) 63 physical therapists were surveyed to obtain their opinions on the long-term therapy needs of six diagnoses, one of which was TBIs. Marini et al. concluded that ongoing therapy was indicated and extremely important given the patients' losses or impairments in motor skills, ambulation skills, and self-care skills. Patients with TBIs benefit from ongoing and lifelong therapy interventions, including physical, occupational, speech, cognitive, and psychotherapy. Marini et al. also noted that to better achieve one's maximum level of independence and function as well as prevent secondary complications, it is necessary to administer periodic evaluations followed by treatment based on the respective evaluation outcome. Long-term complications associated with brain injuries include post-traumatic headaches, movement disorders, psychiatric illnesses, PTSD, depression, anxiety, chronic pain, insomnia, and emotional dysregulation. These long-term complications may lead to long-term disability of the patient and the patient's inability to return to their normal day-to-day activities and lifestyles.

Evaluation Standards

Comprehensive neurological evaluations are designed to assist in the quantification of the patient's symptom severity as related to their brain injury, and neuropsychological assessment battery evaluations are used to determine suspected cognitive decline secondary to TBIs. Neuropsychological assessment battery evaluations are completed by a licensed clinical psychologist or neuropsychologist. Comprehensive neurological evaluations are completed by physicians who are treating the patient with a TBI. The information garnered from the neuropsychological assessment battery facilitates diagnostic decision making, management, and treatment planning for the long-term needs of the patient. "Cognitive assessment and rehabilitation should be tailored to the patient's neuropsychological profile, premorbid cognitive characteristics, and goals for life activities and participation" (Bayley et al., 2014, p. 1). The patient will need an interdisciplinary team to address all impairments, and each discipline will follow specific evaluation processes (O'Sullivan et al., 2007).

Appendix 9A

Impact of Injuries on Activities of Daily Living (ADLs) and Instrumental Activities of Daily Living (IADLs)

Table 9.1.1 Feeding ADLs

Activity	Reduced Ability Since Injury	Before Incident	After Incident	Comments
Feeding		☐ Feeds self completely independently, including food movement to the mouth, swallowing, and related tasks	☐ Feeds self completely independently, including food movement to the mouth, swallowing, and related tasks	**Is it taking you longer than your pre-injury status to complete this task?** Yes/No
		☐ Needs assistance with cutting, chopping, and/or related tasks	☐ Needs assistance with cutting, chopping, and/or related tasks	**Do you perform this task by taking multiple breaks to alleviate the pain?** Yes/No
		☐ Needs assistance spooning or moving food/drinks to mouth.	☐ Needs assistance spooning or moving food/drinks to mouth.	**Is any pain experienced while completing this task?** Yes/No
		☐ Difficulty swallowing and/or moving food from mouth to stomach.	☐ Difficulty swallowing and/or moving food from mouth to stomach.	
		☐ Tube feeding or other completely dependent food intake.	☐ Tube feeding or other completely dependent food intake.	

Notes:

Table 9.1.2 Bathing ADLs

Activity	Reduced Ability Since Injury?	Before Incident	After Incident	Comments
Bathing		☐ Takes a shower or bath completely independently with an adequate level of cleanliness achieved. Includes drying off and safely entering/departing shower or tub.	☐ Takes a shower or bath completely independently with an adequate level of cleanliness achieved. Includes drying off and safely entering/departing shower or tub.	**Is it taking you longer than your pre-injury status to complete this task?** Yes/No
		☐ Needs assistance with entering/ departing shower or tub, but can wash self without aid.	☐ Needs assistance with entering/ departing shower or tub, but can wash self without aid.	**Do you perform this task by taking multiple breaks to alleviate the pain?** Yes/No
		☐ Needs assistance to wash hard-to-reach spots, such as back or feet.	☐ Needs assistance to wash hard-to-reach spots, such as back or feet.	**Is any pain experienced while completing this task?** Yes/No
		☐ Difficulty washing resulting in inadequate levels of cleanliness and safety issues without moderate aid. Unable to perform most tasks of bathing, such as hair washing, use of soap, drying with a towel, etc.	☐ Difficulty washing resulting in inadequate levels of cleanliness and safety issues without moderate aid. Unable to perform most tasks of bathing, such as hair washing, use of soap, drying with a towel, etc.	
		☐ Requires total assistance to bathe, such as in-shower/ tub help, sponge baths, etc.	☐ Requires total assistance to bathe, such as in-shower/ tub help, sponge baths, etc.	
Notes:				

Table 9.1.3 Grooming ADLs

Activity	Reduced Ability Since Injury?	Before Incident	After Incident	Comments
		☐ Is completely independent in self-presentation and hygiene tasks including brushing teeth, combing hair, shaving, make-up application, etc.	☐ Is completely independent in self-presentation and hygiene tasks including brushing teeth, combing hair, shaving, make-up application, etc.	**Is it taking you longer than your pre-injury status to complete this task?** Yes/No
Grooming		☐ Needs assistance with gathering items or reminders to complete certain tasks, but otherwise independent.	☐ Needs assistance with gathering items or reminders to complete certain tasks, but otherwise independent.	**Do you perform this task by taking multiple breaks to alleviate the pain?** Yes/No
		☐ Needs assistance with physical tasks, such as reaching to brush long hair or holding a razor steady (mechanical/physical).	☐ Needs assistance with physical tasks, such as reaching to brush long hair or holding a razor steady (mechanical/physical).	**Is any pain experienced while completing this task?** Yes/No
		☐ Needs assistance with cognitive-based tasks such as reminders of what toothpaste is for or frequency required for toothbrushing (planning/steps/memory).	☐ Needs assistance with cognitive-based tasks such as reminders of what toothpaste is for or frequency required for toothbrushing (planning/steps/memory).	
		☐ Unable to groom to a level of satisfactory standards absent complete or nearly complete assistance.	☐ Unable to groom to a level of satisfactory standards absent complete or nearly complete assistance.	

Notes:

Table 9.1.4 Dressing ADLs

Activity	Reduced Ability Since Injury?	Before Incident	After Incident	Comments
Dressing		☐ Is completely independent in clothes and shoes dressing, including zippers, buttons, and shoe tying.	☐ Is completely independent in clothes and shoes dressing, including zippers, buttons, and shoe tying.	**Is it taking you longer than your pre-injury status to complete this task?** Yes/No
		☐ Needs assistance with fine motor movements and/or coordinated movements such as buttons, zippers, and/or shoe tying.	☐ Needs assistance with fine motor movements and/or coordinated movements such as buttons, zippers, and/or shoe tying.	**Do you perform this task by taking multiple breaks to alleviate the pain?** Yes/No
		☐ Needs assistance with smaller items, such as socks, ties, suspenders, and/or belts.	☐ Needs assistance with smaller items, such as socks, ties, suspenders, and/or belts.	**Is any pain experienced while completing this task?** Yes/No
		☐ Needs assistance with taking off/putting on shirt, pants, and/or sweaters.	☐ Needs assistance with taking off/putting on shirt, pants, and/or sweaters.	
		☐ Needs assistance with appropriate attire reminders, such as a coat in the snow or a swimsuit for the pool.	☐ Needs assistance with appropriate attire reminders, such as a coat in the snow or a swimsuit for the pool.	
		☐ Unable to groom to dress self absent major help to include complete or nearly complete dressing.	☐ Unable to groom to dress self absent major help to include complete or nearly complete dressing.	

Notes:

Table 9.1.5 Bathroom/Toileting

Activity	Reduced Ability Since Injury	Before Incident	After Incident	Comments
		☐ Is completely independent in toileting and experiences no incontinence. Can remove and rearrange clothing before and after toileting independently.	☐ Is completely independent in toileting and experiences no incontinence. Can remove and rearrange clothing before and after toileting independently.	

Activity	Reduced Ability Since Injury	Before Incident	After Incident	Comments
		☐ Needs assistance with clothing removal and/or rearrangement for toileting, but experiences no incontinence.	☐ Needs assistance with clothing removal and/or rearrangement for toileting, but experiences no incontinence.	
Bathroom/Toileting		☐ Needs physical help on/off the toilet, but otherwise independent.	☐ Needs physical help on/off the toilet, but otherwise independent.	
		☐ Experiences increased urinary frequency, but has not experienced incontinence.	☐ Experiences increased urinary frequency, but has not experienced incontinence.	
		☐ Experiences increased bowel frequency, but has not experienced incontinence.	☐ Experiences increased bowel frequency, but has not experienced incontinence.	
		☐ Experiences increased constipation.	☐ Experiences increased constipation.	
		☐ Experiences occasional incontinence of bowels (1–4 × per month).	☐ Experiences occasional incontinence of bowels (1–4 × per month).	
		☐ Experiences occasional incontinence of bladder (1–4 × per month).	☐ Experiences occasional incontinence of bladder (1–4 × per month).	
		☐ Experiences frequent incontinence of bowels (5+ × per month).	☐ Experiences frequent incontinence of bowels (5+ × per month).	
		☐ Experiences frequent incontinence of bladder (5+ × per month).	☐ Experiences frequent incontinence of bladder (5+ × per month).	
		☐ Unable to control bowels and/or bladder or has assistive device (catheter or other) to aid in function.	☐ Unable to control bowels and/or bladder or has assistive device (catheter or other) to aid in function.	

Notes:

Table 9.1.6 Transfers

Activity	Reduced Ability Since Injury	Before Incident	After Incident	Comments
		☐ Is completely independent in transferring from one area to another safely.	☐ Is completely independent in transferring from one area to another safely.	**Is it taking you longer than your pre-injury status to complete this task?** Yes/No
		☐ Needs verbal reminders/assistance to transfer safely, but can physically do so independently.	☐ Needs verbal reminders/assistance to transfer safely, but can physically do so independently.	**Do you perform this task by taking multiple breaks to alleviate the pain?** Yes/No
Transfers		☐ Needs minimal physical assistance to do so safely or without pain (hold an arm to stand up, steadying hand, etc.).	☐ Needs minimal physical assistance to do so safely or without pain (hold an arm to stand up, steadying hand, etc.).	**Is any pain experienced while completing this task?** Yes/No
		☐ Needs moderate physical assistance to do so safely or without pain (supporting more than half of person's weight, or responsible for more than half of the task involved).	☐ Needs moderate physical assistance to do so safely or without pain (supporting more than half of person's weight, or responsible for more than half of the task involved).	
		☐ Requires transfer benches, hand-hold pegs or slots, or other self-dependent devices for aid.	☐ Requires transfer benches, hand-hold pegs or slots, or other self-dependent devices for aid.	
		☐ Requires assistive devices, such as belts, halters, or slings to move from one surface to another.	☐ Requires assistive devices, such as belts, halters, or slings to move from one surface to another.	
		☐ Is unable to sit or stand independently due to lack of balance; safety issues. Requires complete assistance for transfers.	☐ Is unable to sit or stand independently due to lack of balance; safety issues. Requires complete assistance for transfers.	
Notes:				

Table 9.1.7 Mobility

Activity	Reduced Ability Since Injury	Before Incident	After Incident	Comments
Mobility		☐ Is completely independent in moving through the community on reasonably level surfaces.	☐ Is completely independent in moving through the community on reasonably level surfaces.	**Is it taking you longer than your pre-injury status to complete this task?** Yes/No
		☐ Independently moves in the community on reasonably level surfaces with the use of cane, walking stick, or related device.	☐ Independently moves in the community on reasonably level surfaces with the use of cane, walking stick, or related device.	**Do you perform this task by taking multiple breaks to alleviate the pain?** Yes/No
		☐ Independently moves through the community with the aid of assistive device such as rollator walker, wheelchair, or related device.	☐ Independently moves through the community with the aid of assistive device such as rollator walker, wheelchair, or related device.	**Is any pain experienced while completing this task?** Yes/No
		☐ Mobile only with the aid of another person's direct physical assistance, such as holding waist or shoulder for support. Unable to walk more than 50 yds. unaided.	☐ Mobile only with the aid of another person's direct physical assistance, such as holding waist or shoulder for support. Unable to walk more than 50 yds. unaided.	
		☐ Unable to walk more than 50 yds. absent pain.	☐ Unable to walk more than 50 yds. absent pain.	
		☐ Uses an assistive device, but is not independent. Requires verbal or physical reminders for safe use.	☐ Uses an assistive device, but is not independent. Requires verbal or physical reminders for safe use.	
		☐ Completely immobile in the community. Requires total movement assistance.	☐ Completely immobile in the community. Requires total movement assistance.	

Notes:

Table 9.1.8 Hearing

Activity	Reduced Ability Since Injury	Before Incident	After Incident	Comments
		☐ Hearing is not a source of worry and seems to be within normal limits.	☐ Hearing is not a source of worry and seems to be within normal limits.	**Is it taking you longer than your pre-injury status to complete this task?** Yes/No
		☐ Hearing of some frequencies or levels is reduced, but overall not a source of concern.	☐ Hearing of some frequencies or levels is reduced, but overall not a source of concern.	**Do you perform this task by taking multiple breaks to alleviate the pain?** Yes/No
Hearing		☐ Hearing is moderately difficult, with repetition of words at times and an increased need for higher volumes for understanding.	☐ Hearing is moderately difficult, with repetition of words at times and an increased need for higher volumes for understanding.	**Is any pain experienced while completing this task?** Yes/No
		☐ Hearing is difficult due to tinnitus but remains overall within normal limits.	☐ Hearing is difficult due to tinnitus but remains overall within normal limits.	
		☐ Hearing loss has been diagnosed laterally.	☐ Hearing loss has been diagnosed laterally.	
		☐ Hearing loss has been clinically diagnosed bilaterally.	☐ Hearing loss has been clinically diagnosed bilaterally.	
		☐ Hearing is aided by an assistive device laterally.	☐ Hearing is aided by an assistive device laterally.	
		☐ Complete loss of functional hearing and/or deafness is experienced and/or has been diagnosed.	☐ Complete loss of functional hearing and/or deafness is experienced and/or has been diagnosed.	

Notes:

Table 9.1.9 Seeing

Activity	Reduced Ability Since Injury	Before Incident	After Incident	Comments
Seeing		☐ Sight and visual function are seemingly within normal limits and are not an area of concern.	☐ Sight and visual function are seemingly within normal limits and are not an area of concern.	**Is it taking you longer than your pre-injury status to complete this task?** Yes/No
		☐ Sight is aided by glasses/contacts to a reasonably functional level and is not a source of concern.	☐ Sight is aided by glasses/contacts to a reasonably functional level and is not a source of concern.	**Do you perform this task by taking multiple breaks to alleviate the pain?** Yes/No
		☐ Vision is reduced and difficulty seeing due to blurriness exists.	☐ Vision is reduced and difficulty seeing due to blurriness exists.	**Is any pain experienced while completing this task?** Yes/No
		☐ Floaters, flashes of lights, or similar issues impede vision.	☐ Floaters, flashes of lights, or similar issues impede vision.	
		☐ Prescription lenses no longer provide a level of visual function adequate for daily life.	☐ Prescription lenses no longer provide a level of visual function adequate for daily life.	
		☐ Monocular vision loss is experienced and/or has been clinically diagnosed.	☐ Monocular vision loss is experienced and/or has been clinically diagnosed.	

Notes:

Table 9.1.10 Speech/Communication

Activity	Reduced Ability Since Injury	Before Incident	After Incident	Comments
		☐ Speaks, reads, and understands spoken words adequately and within seemingly normal limits. No concern was experienced regarding communication.	☐ Speaks, reads, and understands spoken words adequately and within seemingly normal limits. No concern was experienced regarding communication.	**Is it taking you longer than your pre-injury status to complete this task?** Yes/No
		☐ Difficulty with oral production and/or changes in speech patterns experienced (stuttering, slowness, misused words).	☐ Difficulty with oral production and/or changes in speech patterns experienced (stuttering, slowness, misused words).	**Do you perform this task by taking multiple breaks to alleviate the pain?** Yes/No
Speech Communication		☐ Difficulty with understanding spoken or heard words.	☐ Difficulty with understanding spoken or heard words.	**Is any pain experienced while completing this task?** Yes/No
		☐ Difficulty with written words or communications.	☐ Difficulty with written words or communications.	
		☐ Struggles with communication due to anxiety and social changes.	☐ Struggles with communication due to anxiety and social changes.	
		☐ Completely or nearly unable to communicate orally.	☐ Completely or nearly unable to communicate orally.	
Notes:				

Table 9.1.11 Tactile Feeling and Grasping

Activity	Reduced Ability Since Injury	Before Incident	After Incident	Comments
		☐ Sensation and grip are adequate for daily life and are not a source of worry.	☐ Sensation and grip are adequate for daily life and are not a source of worry.	**Is it taking you longer than your pre-injury status to complete this task?** Yes/No
Tactile Feeling and Grasping		☐ Some changes in the ability to recognize temperature, vibration, light touch, and/or pain are experienced.	☐ Some changes in the ability to recognize temperature, vibration, light touch, and/or pain are experienced.	**Do you perform this task by taking multiple breaks to alleviate the pain?** Yes/No
		☐ Some loss of grip or the ability to securely grasp desired large items is experienced (cup, book, ball).	☐ Some loss of grip or the ability to securely grasp desired large items is experienced (cup, book, ball).	**Is any pain experienced while completing this task?** Yes/No
		☐ Some loss of grip or the ability to securely grasp desired small items is experienced (pen, pill, key).	☐ Some loss of grip or the ability to securely grasp desired small items is experienced (pen, pill, key).	
		☐ Total or nearly total loss of the ability to grasp large items meaningfully (hold a ball, open a door with the handle, etc.) is experienced.	☐ Total or nearly total loss of the ability to grasp large items meaningfully (hold a ball, open a door with the handle, etc.) is experienced.	
		☐ Total or nearly total loss of the ability to grasp small items meaningfully (use forks, write with pencils, etc.) is experienced.	☐ Total or nearly total loss of the ability to grasp small items meaningfully (use forks, write with pencils, etc.) is experienced.	

Notes:

196   *Huma Haider*

Table 9.1.12 Sleep

Activity	Reduced Ability Since Injury	Before Incident	After Incident	Comments
		☐ Sleeping is restful and adequate for daily life most times. Refreshment is experienced upon waking and fatigue is not present on most days.	☐ Sleeping is restful and adequate for daily life most times. Refreshment is experienced upon waking and fatigue is not present on most days.	**Is it taking you longer than your pre-injury status to complete this task?** Yes/No
Sleep		☐ Sleep is restless and refreshment is not experienced with waking. Fatigue is present as a result.	☐ Sleep is restless and refreshment is not experienced with waking. Fatigue is present as a result.	**Do you perform this task by taking multiple breaks to alleviate the pain?** Yes/No
		☐ Sleep is plentiful and in sufficient amounts, but refreshment is not experienced and/or fatigue is common.	☐ Sleep is plentiful and in sufficient amounts, but refreshment is not experienced and/or fatigue is common.	**Is any pain experienced while completing this task?** Yes/No
		☐ Sleep is pervaded by pain.	☐ Sleep is pervaded by pain.	
		☐ Sleep is pervaded by a racing mind or inability to relax.	☐ Sleep is pervaded by a racing mind or inability to relax.	
		☐ Use of medication or aids allows for restful sleep and refreshed feeling.	☐ Use of medication or aids allows for restful sleep and refreshed feeling.	
		☐ Medication is ineffective and sleep remains deficient.	☐ Medication is ineffective and sleep remains deficient.	
		☐ Sleep is experienced in excess.	☐ Sleep is experienced in excess.	

Notes:

Table 9.1.13 Ability to Handle Finances

Activity	Reduced Ability Since Injury	Before Incident	After Incident	Comments
Ability to Handle Finances		☐ Is completely independent in money matters. Can adequately budget, pay bills, perform banking activities, understand financial documents, etc.	☐ Is completely independent in money matters. Can adequately budget, pay bills, perform banking activities, understand financial documents, etc.	**Is it taking you longer than your pre-injury status to complete this task?** Yes/No
		☐ Needs minor assistance, such as bill pay reminders or digital/app aids for banking.	☐ Needs minor assistance, such as bill pay reminders or digital/app aids for banking.	**Do you perform this task by taking multiple breaks to alleviate the pain?** Yes/No
		☐ Independent in everyday money matters, but requires assistance for major purchases or to understand financial documents, such as with a mortgage, loan, or bank statement.	☐ Independent in everyday money matters, but requires assistance for major purchases or to understand financial documents, such as with a mortgage, loan, or bank statement.	**Is any pain experienced while completing this task?** Yes/No
		☐ Needs moderate assistance, without which rent would not be paid, finances would be at risk, and income management would not be done.	☐ Needs moderate assistance, without which rent would not be paid, finances would be at risk, and income management would not be done.	
		☐ Depends upon a third party to handle financial matters.	☐ Depends upon a third party to handle financial matters.	
		☐ Completely unable to handle financial matters and has experienced repercussions as a result.	☐ Completely unable to handle financial matters and has experienced repercussions as a result.	

Notes:

Table 9.1.14 Food Preparation

Activity	Reduced Ability Since Injury	Before Incident	After Incident	Comments
		☐ Is completely independent in planning, preparing, and serving adequate meals.	☐ Is completely independent in planning, preparing, and serving adequate meals.	**Is it taking you longer than your pre-injury status to complete this task?** Yes/No
Food Preparation		☐ Independently prepares and serves meals with planning assistance and provided ingredients.	☐ Independently prepares and serves meals with planning assistance and provided ingredients.	**Do you perform this task by taking multiple breaks to alleviate the pain?** Yes/No
		☐ Experiences difficulty with physically intense food preparation tasks, such as chopping, slicing, or pouring.	☐ Experiences difficulty with physically intense food preparation tasks, such as chopping, slicing, or pouring.	**Is any pain experienced while completing this task?** Yes/No
		☐ Experiences difficulty with following recipes.	☐ Experiences difficulty with following recipes.	
		☐ Can heat, reheat, and/or order food independently, but is unable to independently prepare meals.	☐ Can heat, reheat, and/or order food independently, but is unable to independently prepare meals.	
		☐ Unable to order and/or prepare meals sufficient for nutritional intake.	☐ Unable to order and/or prepare meals sufficient for nutritional intake.	
		☐ Is completely dependent upon assistance for alimentation, including tube feedings.	☐ Is completely dependent upon assistance for alimentation, including tube feedings.	

Notes:

Table 9.1.15 Housekeeping

Activity	Reduced Ability Since Injury	Before Incident	After Incident	Comments
Housekeeping		☐ Independently handles all tasks related to household care. Included tasks: vacuuming, lawn care, dusting, sweeping, etc.	☐ Independently handles all tasks related to household care. Included tasks: vacuuming, lawn care, dusting, sweeping, etc.	**Is it taking you longer than your pre-injury status to complete this task?** Yes/No
		☐ Needs minor assistance with heavy items such as refuse removal or furniture moving for vacuuming, but otherwise independent.	☐ Needs minor assistance with heavy items such as refuse removal or furniture moving for vacuuming, but otherwise independent.	**Do you perform this task by taking multiple breaks to alleviate the pain?** Yes/No
		☐ Needs assistance with physically intensive tasks such as lawn care or deep cleaning, but can independently perform light or daily cleaning tasks.	☐ Needs assistance with physically intensive tasks such as lawn care or deep cleaning, but can independently perform light or daily cleaning tasks.	**Is any pain experienced while completing this task?** Yes/No
		☐ Is responsible for small tasks, such as throwing own trash away or picking up discarded items, but otherwise unable to perform housekeeping tasks.	☐ Is responsible for small tasks, such as throwing own trash away or picking up discarded items, but otherwise unable to perform housekeeping tasks.	
		☐ Employs household services.	☐ Employs household services.	
		☐ Completely or nearly completely unable to perform household tasks at an adequate level of cleanliness.	☐ Completely or nearly completely unable to perform household tasks at an adequate level of cleanliness.	

Notes:

Table 9.1.16 Laundry

Activity	Reduced Ability Since Injury	Before Incident	After Incident	Comments
		☐ Can independently carry, insert/ remove, and handle all aspects of laundering.	☐ Can independently carry, insert/ remove, and handle all aspects of laundering.	**Is it taking you longer than your pre-injury status to complete this task?** Yes/No
Laundry		☐ Needs assistance carrying, but can handle all other tasks of laundering.	☐ Needs assistance carrying, but can handle all other tasks of laundering.	**Do you perform this task by taking multiple breaks to allevi- ate the pain?** Yes/No
		☐ Needs assistance for most physical tasks of laundry.	☐ Needs assistance for most physical tasks of laundry.	**Is any pain expe- rienced while completing this task?** Yes/No
		☐ Requires verbal or other reminders about laundry- related tasks such as moving loads, adding soap, etc.	☐ Requires verbal or other reminders about laundry- related tasks such as moving loads, adding soap, etc.	
		☐ Completely unable to launder independently.	☐ Completely unable to launder independently.	
Notes:				

Table 9.1.17 Transportation

Activity	Reduced Ability Since Injury	Before Incident	After Incident	Comments
Transportation		☐ Travels within the community completely independently via self-driven vehicle or public transportation.	☐ Travels within the community completely independently via self-driven vehicle or public transportation.	**Is it taking you longer than your pre-injury status to complete this task?** Yes/No
		☐ Can independently arrange travel via paid taxi or related service, but is unable to travel otherwise.	☐ Can independently arrange travel via paid taxi or related service, but is unable to travel otherwise.	**Do you perform this task by taking multiple breaks to alleviate the pain?** Yes/No
		☐ Travels with another person accompanying on public transportation.	☐ Travels with another person accompanying on public transportation.	**Is any pain experienced while completing this task?** Yes/No
		☐ Travels as a passenger only with a trusted person operating the vehicle.	☐ Travels as a passenger only with a trusted person operating the vehicle.	
		☐ Can travel via public transportation with reminders or cues such as provided funds, maps, or other aids.	☐ Can travel via public transportation with reminders or cues such as provided funds, maps, or other aids.	
		☐ Is completely or nearly unable to travel in the community.	☐ Is completely or nearly unable to travel in the community.	
Notes:				

Table 9.1.18 Medication Management

Activity	Reduced Ability Since Injury	Before Incident	After Incident	Comments
Medication		☐ Medication is independently managed, to include taking the right doses of the right medication at the right times/ intervals.	☐ Medication is independently managed, to include taking the right doses of the right medication at the right times/ intervals.	**Is it taking you longer than your pre-injury status to complete this task?** Yes/No
		☐ Digital or other reminders are used to assure medication is taken correctly but can be done absent other assistance.	☐ Digital or other reminders are used to assure medication is taken correctly but can be done absent other assistance.	**Do you perform this task by taking multiple breaks to alleviate the pain?** Yes/No
		☐ Medication must be prepared by another, but can then be taken independently.	☐ Medication must be prepared by another, but can then be taken independently.	**Is any pain experienced while completing this task?** Yes/No
		☐ Assistance is required in the form of verbal reminders to take medications as directed.	☐ Assistance is required in the form of verbal reminders to take medications as directed.	
		☐ Medication is frequently forgotten, and non-compliance may be an issue due to cognitive process changes.	☐ Medication is frequently forgotten, and non-compliance may be an issue due to cognitive process changes.	
		☐ Medication must be delivered directly at the exact time and in the correct dose required to ensure medication compliance.	☐ Medication must be delivered directly at the exact time and in the correct dose required to ensure medication compliance.	

Notes:

Table 9.1.19 Provisions/Shopping

Activity	Reduced Ability Since Injury	Before Incident	After Incident	Comments
Provision/Shopping		☐ Shopping and/or the provision of needed goods is done independently and without pain.	☐ Shopping and/or the provision of needed goods is done independently and without pain.	**Is it taking you longer than your pre-injury status to complete this task?** Yes/No
		☐ Shopping and/or the provision of needed goods is done independently, though pain creates some difficulty.	☐ Shopping and/or the provision of needed goods is done independently, though pain creates some difficulty.	**Do you perform this task by taking multiple breaks to alleviate the pain?** Yes/No
		☐ Shopping and/or the provision of needed goods is done independently, though items are frequently forgotten or incorrectly purchased (products bought without a need, or those not typically purchased, etc.).	☐ Shopping and/or the provision of needed goods is done independently, though items are frequently forgotten or incorrectly purchased (products bought without a need, or those not typically purchased, etc.).	**Is any pain experienced while completing this task?** Yes/No
		☐ Shopping trips require accompaniment to provide oversight and aid in supply acquisition.	☐ Shopping trips require accompaniment to provide oversight and aid in supply acquisition.	
		☐ Shopping trips require accompaniment to provide physical support, such as lifting, carrying, and/or ambulation assistance.	☐ Shopping trips require accompaniment to provide physical support, such as lifting, carrying, and,/ or ambulation assistance.	
		☐ Completely unable to shop or adequately provide supplies for daily life.	☐ Completely unable to shop or adequately provide supplies for daily life.	

Notes:

Table 9.1.20 Sexual Health

Activity	Reduced Ability Since Injury	Before Incident	After Incident	Comments
Sexual Health		☐ Sexual health (stamina, drive, arousability, etc.) is seemingly within normal limits and is not a cause of concern.	☐ Sexual health (stamina, drive, arousability, etc.) is seemingly within normal limits and is not a cause of concern.	**Is it taking you longer than your pre-injury status to complete this task?** Yes/No
		☐ Reductions in sexual wellness and/or performance are experienced.	☐ Reductions in sexual wellness and/or performance are experienced.	**Do you perform this task by taking multiple breaks to alleviate the pain?** Yes/No
		☐ Reductions in sexual stamina and/or arousability are experienced.	☐ Reductions in sexual stamina and/or arousability are experienced.	**Is any pain experienced while completing this task?** Yes/No
		☐ Hyper or increased sexual impulses, arousal, desires, and/or related changes are experienced.	☐ Hyper or increased sexual impulses, arousal, desires, and/or related changes are experienced.	
		☐ Sexual dysfunction has been clinically diagnosed.	☐ Sexual dysfunction has been clinically diagnosed.	

Notes:

Appendix 9B

Life Care Plan Subsection Charts

Table 9.2.1 Evaluations

Service	CPT Code
Audiology	92620
Dentistry	D0150
Internal Medicine	99214
Neurology	99214
Neuropsychology	99214
Pain Specialist/Management	99214
Orthopedic Provider/Surgeon	99214

Table 9.2.2 Treatments and Therapies

Treatment/Therapy	CPT
33-Point Botox Injections	64615
Epidural Steroid Injection: Cervical Spine	62321
Epidural Steroid Injection: Thoracic Spine	62321
Epidural Steroid Injection: Lumbar Spine	62323
Greater Occipital Nerve Block	64405
Lesser Occipital Nerve Block	64450
Neurocognitive Rehabilitation	97130
Neuropsychological Evaluation	96132, 96133
Trigger Point Injection 3+ Muscles	20553

Table 9.2.3 Future Diagnostics

Service	CPT
CT of the Brain	70450
Diffusion Tensor Imaging	70554
MRI of the Brain Without Contrast	70551
MRI of the Cervical Spine	72141
MRI of the Lumbar Spine	72148
Computerized Dynamic Posturography	92548

Table 9.2.4 Medications

Medication	Type
Acetaminophen-Codeine 300–30 mg	Pain reliever
Gabapentin 300 mg	Neuroleptic
Alpha Lipoic Acid (ALA) 100 mg daily	Supplement
Coenzyme Q10 100 mg daily	Antioxidant
Fish Oil/Omega-3 Supplements 2–3 grams daily	Supplement
Glucoraphanin 15 mg	Supplement
Magnesium L Threonate 1–2 grams daily	Supplement
N-Acetyl Cysteine 150 mg daily	Antioxidant
Phosphatidylserine (PS) 100 mg daily	Supplement
Probiotics	Probiotic
Super B Complex	Supplement
Zinc 20 mg daily	Supplement

Table 9.2.5 Laboratory Studies

Service	CPT
Complete Blood Count (CBC)	85025
Comprehensive Metabolic Panel	80053
Urinalysis	81001

Table 9.2.6 Rehabilitation Services

Service	CPT
Cognitive/Behavioral Therapy	90832
Gym Membership	n/a
Occupational Therapy	97530
Pain Management Program	99214
Physical Therapy	97110
Psychotherapy	90834
Speech/Language Therapy	92507
Vestibular Therapy	97112
Gait Training	97116
Auditory Rehabilitation	92633

Table 9.2.7 Medical Equipment and Supplies

Equipment/Supply	CPT/HCPCS
Bedside Toilet	E0163
Cervical Pillow	E0190
Heating Pad	E0210
Ice Pack	A9273
Lumbar Support Pillow	E0190
Lumbar Support Brace	L0625
Reacher	A9281
Rollator Walker With Seat	E0143, E0156

Equipment/Supply	CPT/HCPCS
TENS Unit	E0730
TENS Unit Supplies	A4595
Transfer Bench	E0247
Bed Handrails	E0310
Rose-Tinted Glasses	N/A
White Noise Machine/Tinnitus Maskers	N/A
Pillbox; Digital With Reminder Function	N/A
Notebooks, Calendar, Post-Its, etc.; Annual Allotment	N/A
Balance Footwear	N/A

Table 9.2.8 Home Alterations and Furnishings

Equipment/Furnishing	CPT/HCPCS
Bathtub Safety Rail	E0241
Handheld Showerhead	E1399
Shower Chair	E0240
Shower Hose	E1399
Toilet Safety Rail	E0243
Traction Strips	n/a
Padded Carpeting, Installed, 1,200 ft.	n/a

Table 9.2.9 Personal Care and Home Services

Service	CPT/HCPCS
Home Health Aide, living tasks; 2 hours daily	S9122
Home Health Aide, living tasks; 4 hours daily	S9122
Home Health Aide, living tasks; 6 hours daily	S9122
Direct Care in-home by LVN/LPN; once weekly visit	G0300
Direct Care in-home by LVN/LPN; once weekly visit	G0300
Housekeeping	n/a
Direct nursing care, in the home, by an RN	G0299

References

Alexander, A. L., Lee, J. E., Lazar, M., & Field, A. S. (2007). Diffusion tensor imaging of the brain. *Neurotherapeutics: The Journal of the American Society for Experimental NeuroTherapeutics, 4*(3), 316–329. https://doi.org/10.1016/j.nurt.2007.05.011

Andriessen, T. M., Jacobs, B., & Vos, P. E. (2010). Clinical characteristics and pathophysiological mechanisms of focal and diffuse traumatic brain injury. *Journal of Cellular and Molecular Medicine, 14*(10)2381–2392. https://doi.org/10.1111/j.1582-4934.2010.01164.x

Armstrong, R. A. (2018). Visual problems associated with traumatic brain injury. *Clinical and Experimental Optometry, 101*(6), 716–726. https://doi.org/10.1111/cxo.12670

Bayley, M. T., Tate, R., Douglas, J. M., Turkstra, L. S., Ponsford, J., Stergiou-Kita, M., Kua, A., Bragge, P. (2014, July–August). INCOG guidelines for cognitive rehabilitation following traumatic brain injury. *Journal of Head Trauma Rehabilitation, 29*(4), 290–306. https://doi.org/10.1097/HTR.0000000000000070

Bobba, U., Munivenkatappa, A., Agrawal, A. (2019). Speech and language dysfunctions in patients with cerebrocortical disorders admitted in a neurosurgical unit. *Asian Journal of Neurosurgery, 14*(1), 87–89. https://doi.org/10.4103/ajns.AJNS_240_17

Bryant, R. (2011). Post-traumatic stress disorder vs traumatic brain injury. *Dialogues in Clinical Neuroscience, 13*(3), 251–262.

The CDC, NIH, DoD, & VA Leadership Panel. (2013). *Report to congress on traumatic brain injury in the United States: Understanding the public health problem among current and former military personnel.* Centers for Disease Control and Prevention (CDC), the National Institutes of Health (NIH), the Department of Defense (DoD), and the Department of Veterans Affairs (VA).

Centers for Disease Control and Prevention. (2015). *Report to congress on traumatic brain injury in the United States: Epidemiology and rehabilitation.* National Center for Injury Prevention and Control, Division of Unintentional Injury Prevention. Retrieved February 6, 2022, from www.cdc.gov/traumaticbraininjury/pdf/tbi_report_to_congress_epi_and_rehab-a.pdf

Center for Disease Control and Prevention. (2022). *Traumatic brain injury and concussion: Get the facts: TBI data.* www.cdc.gov/traumaticbraininjury/data/index.html

Centers for Disease Control, National Center for Injury Prevention and Control. (n.d.). *Report to congress traumatic brain injury in the United States.* CDC.

Chen, H., Li, Y., Jiang, B., Zhu, G., Rezaii, P. G., Lu, G., & Wintermark, M. (2021). Demographics and clinical characteristics of acute traumatic brain injury patients in the different neuroimaging radiological interpretation system (NIRIS) categories. *Journal of Neuroradiology – Journal de Neuroradiologie, 48*(2), 104–111. https://doi-org.proxy.library.vcu.edu/10.1016/j.neurad.2019.07.002

Coelho, C., Deruyter, F., & Stein, M. (1996). Treatment efficacy. *Journal of Speech, Language, and Hearing Research, 39*(5). https://doi.org/10.1044/jshr.3905.s5

Coronado, V. G., McGuire, L. C., Sarmiento, K., Bell, J., Lionbarger, M. R., Jones, C. D., Geller, A. I., Khoury, N., & Xu, L. (2012). Trends in traumatic brain injury in the U.S. and the public health response: 1995–2009. *Journal of Safety Research, 43*(4), 299–307. https://doi-org.proxy.library.vcu.edu/10.1016/j.jsr.2012.08.011

Delmonico, R. L., Theodore, B. R., Sandel, M. E., Armstrong, M. A., & Camicia, M. (2021). Prevalence of depression and anxiety disorders following mild traumatic brain injury. *PM & R: The Journal of Injury, Function, and Rehabilitation, 14.* Advance online publication. https://doi-org.proxy.library.vcu.edu/10.1002/pmrj.12657

Depression After Traumatic Brain Injury. (n.d.). *Depression after traumatic brain injury.* Model Systems Knowledge Translation Center (MSKTC).

Dewan, M., Mummareddy, N., Wellons, J., III, & Bonfield, C. (2016). Epidemiology of global pediatric traumatic brain injury: Quantitative review. *World Neurosurgery, 91,* 497–509.

Hyder, A. A., Wunderlich, C. A., Puvanachandra, P., Gururaj, G., & Kobusingye, O. C. (2007). The impact of traumatic brain injuries: A global perspective. *NeuroRehabilitation, 22*(5), 341–353.

Kreuzer, P. M., Landgrebe, M., Vielsmeier, V., Kleinjung, T., Ridder, D. D., & Langguth, B. (2014). Trauma-associated tinnitus. *Journal of Head Trauma Rehabilitation, 29*(5), 432–442. https://doi.org/10.1097/htr.0b013e31829d3129

Lo, J., Chan, L., & Flynn, S. (2021). A systematic review of the incidence, prevalence, costs, and activity and work limitations of amputation, osteoarthritis, rheumatoid arthritis, back pain, multiple sclerosis, spinal cord injury, stroke, and traumatic brain injury in the United States: A 2019 update. *Archives of Physical Medicine and Rehabilitation, 102*(1), 115–131. https://doi-org.proxy.library.vcu.edu/10.1016/j.apmr.2020.04.001

Marini, I., Luckett, K., Miller, E., & Blanco, E. L. (2009). A Survey of physical therapists: Long term needs for persons with severe disabilities. *Journal of Life Care Planning, 8*(3), 107–123.

Marr, A. L., & Coronado, V. G. (Eds.). (2004). *Central nervous system injury surveillance data submission standards-2002.* US Department of Health and Human Services, CDC. www.dshs.state.tx.us/injury/registry/coronadoandmarrcnsdefinitions.doc

National Center for Injury Prevention and Control. (2003). *Report to congress on mild traumatic brain injury in the United States: Steps to prevent a serious public health problem.* Centers for Disease Control and Prevention.

O'Sullivan, S. B., Schmitz, T. J., & Fulk, G. D. (2007). Traumatic brain injury. In *Physical rehabilitation* (pp. 895–928). Davis.

Park, S. J., Hur, J. W., Kwon, K. Y., Rhee, J. J., Lee, J. W., & Lee, H. K. (2009). Time to recover consciousness in patients with diffuse axonal injury: Assessment with reference to magnetic resonance grading. *Journal of Korean Neurosurgical Society*, *46*(3), 205–209. https://doi-org.proxy.library.vcu.edu/10.3340/jkns.2009.46.3.205

Putnam, L. J., Willes, A. M., Kalata, B. E., Disher, N. D., & Brusich, D. J. (2019). Expansion of a fly TBI model to four levels of injury severity reveals synergistic effects of repetitive injury for moderate injury conditions. *Fly*, *13*(1–4), 1–11. https://doi-org.proxy.library.vcu.edu/10.1080/19336934.2019.1664363

Shenton, M. E., Hamoda, H. M., Schneiderman, J. S., Bouix, S., Pasternak, O., Rathi, Y., Vu, M. A., Purohit, M. P., Helmer, K., Koerte, I., Lin, A. P., Westin, C. F., Kikinis, R., Kubicki, M., Stern, R. A., & Zafonte, R. (2012). A review of magnetic resonance imaging and diffusion tensor imaging findings in mild traumatic brain injury. *Brain Imaging and Behavior*, *6*(2), 137–192. https://doi-org.proxy.library.vcu.edu/10.1007/s11682-012-9156-5

Silverberg, N. D., & Panenka, W. J. (2019). Antidepressants for depression after concussion and traumatic brain injury are still best practice. *BioMed Central (BMC) Psychiatry*, *19*(1). https://doi.org/10.1186/s12888-019-2076-9

Smith, M. (2008). Monitoring intracranial pressure in traumatic brain injury. *Anesthesia and Analgesia*, *106*(1), 240–248. https://doi-org.proxy.library.vcu.edu/10.1213/01.ane.0000297296.52006.8e

Theadom, A., Starkey, N., Barker-Collo, S., Jones, K., Ameratunga, S., Feigin, V., & BIONIC4you Research Group (2018). Population-based cohort study of the impacts of mild traumatic brain injury in adults four years post-injury. *PLOS One*, *13*(1), e0191655. https://doi-org.proxy.library.vcu.edu/10.1371/journal.pone.0191655

Timmer, M. L., Jacobs, B., Schonherr, M. C., Spikman, J. M., & van der Naalt, J. (2020). The spectrum of long-term behavioral disturbances and provided care after traumatic brain injury. *Frontiers in Neurology*, *11*, 246. https://doi-org.proxy.library.vcu.edu/10.3389/fneur.2020.00246

Viola-Saltzman, M., & Watson, N. F. (2012). Traumatic brain injury and sleep disorders. *Neurologic Clinics*, *30*(4), 1299–1312. https://doi.org/10.1016/j.ncl.2012.08.008

Vos, P. E., Alekseenko, Y., Battistin, L., Ehler, E., Gerstenbrand, F., Muresanu, D. F., Potapov, A., Stepan, C. A., Traubner, P., Vecsei, L., & von Wild, K. (2012). Mild traumatic brain injury. *European Journal of Neurology*, *19*, 191–198. https://doi.org/10.1111/j.1468-1331.2011.03581.x

Whyte, E., Skidmore, E., Aizenstein, H., Ricker, J., & Butters, M. (2011). Cognitive impairment in acquired brain injury: A predictor of rehabilitation outcomes and an opportunity for novel interventions. *PM&R*, *3*, S45–S51. https://doi.org/10.1016/j.pmrj.2011.05.007

Wright, D. W., Kellermann, A., McGuire, L., Chen, B., & Popovic, T. (2013). CDC grand rounds: Reducing severe traumatic brain injury in the United States. *Morbidity and Mortality Weekly Report (MMWR)*, *62*(27), 549–552.

10 Traumatic Brain Injury

A Neurosurgeon's Perspective

Gary E. Kraus

The human brain, which is who we in essence are, is at the core of our existence and awareness as we know it. Understanding the human brain and its impact on our daily existence has challenged society since the dawn of civilization. As a neurosurgeon, I have had the privilege of treating patients who have suffered from disorders of the brain. In addition, my experience as a life care planner, along with experiences in neuroanatomy, physics, and electrical engineering, have helped me take an analytical approach to understanding the brain, with the hope of helping individuals who have suffered a traumatic brain injury.

The almost unfathomable coalescence of neurons, glial cells, blood vessels, and much more, all coordinating in a most incredibly harmonious and synergistic manner to create the brain, means that although much has been learned, there is still an enormous amount to be learned. In the relentless quest of physicians, psychologists, and medical scientists to understand the human body, the brain remains the most elusive of structures. With advances in science and technology, significant progress has been made in unraveling the mysteries of the brain, yet only the surface has been scratched. Understanding the brain requires expertise from a variety of fields, including medicine, anatomy, histology, psychology, psychiatry, physics, mathematics, biochemistry, computer science, big data, and philosophy.

Ultimately, our quest to understand the brain and do our best to help treat patients depends not only on merging data from these diverse fields but also on our ability to constantly shift our analysis and questions from the microscopic to the macroscopic and to each level in between, grasping both the big and the small picture. Analogously, the earth appears very differently from 60,000 feet of altitude than it does when one is standing on the ground, but the ability to see the earth from both vantage points, and at intervening levels, provides insights not apparent at only one level. Similarly, the ability to evaluate a patient's neurological status, study advanced imaging of the brain, and review critical and pertinent anatomic features, while correlating function with structure, will ultimately serve to further our understanding of the brain and to better evaluate and treat patients.

People are often extremely capable of recognizing even subtle changes in human behavior, as may be exhibited by an individual who has suffered a traumatic brain injury. With advances in science and technology applied to imaging and studying the anatomy of the brain, as well as improving methods of evaluating cognition and psychological functioning of the brain in a person who has suffered a traumatic brain injury, the goal of matching the form or structure of the brain with the function of the brain is constantly improving and evolving. The intersection of the medical specialties which evaluate structure with those which evaluate function is allowing for anatomical and chemical biomarkers which are greatly improving our ability to recognize, diagnose, and treat traumatic brain injury, as well as predict future needs and likely required care

DOI: 10.4324/b23293-10

of a person who has suffered a traumatic brain injury. Traumatic brain injury is not an isolated event, but rather a chronic disease, and potentially the beginning of life-altering changes for the patient and all those around them.

Experience as a Neurosurgeon

As a neurosurgeon, I have on many occasions had the experience of being called into the emergency department of a hospital at all hours of the day and night to take care of patients who have suffered a traumatic brain injury and multiple traumas to their body. I have pushed my way through a barrage of medical personnel surrounding a patient who had suffered a major trauma and who had just been transported by a helicopter or ambulance and was still strapped to a spine board with a hard collar on the neck and an endotracheal tube protecting the lungs. Surrounding the patient were doctors, nurses, respiratory therapists, and x-ray technicians trying to assess and stabilize the patient's condition, looking for better intravenous access, compressing an Ambu bag to deliver air into the patient's lungs, getting a "stat" lateral "C" (cervical spine) x-ray to rule out a fracture, monitoring vital signs, and getting a Foley catheter into the bladder, yet I pushed my way through this multitude of people who were trying to save the patient's life, so that I could perform my role as a neurosurgeon. I made my way to the patient's head and tried to start my neurological assessment, often beginning in the emergency department, but sometimes continuing as I was running with the patient who was traveling on a gurney en route to the computed tomography (CT) scanner for a view of the brain. Frequently we would go straight from the CT room to the operating room, where I might perform an emergency craniotomy to evacuate a hematoma in an attempt to save the patient's life. The goal was to have the elapsed time from when the patient first arrived at the emergency room to when I actually made an incision in the skin on the scalp, and subsequently opened the skull and decompressed the brain, be as brief as possible. Time is of the essence, as an expanding hematoma around or in the brain, resulting in a shift of the brain from one side to the other, is a severe insult to and is extremely poorly tolerated by the brain for more than a short while before a deteriorating cascade of events occurs, with increasing intracranial pressure building, increasing brain shift worsening, and subsequent death or otherwise extreme neurological damage imminent. Despite such swift measures, the outcome is often very poor, and even if the patient survives, they are often left with severe impairment and permanent deficits for life.

In the operating room, I have rushed to first open the scalp with a large flap, cut open a large bone flap, then widely open the dura mater to expose a very swollen and tense brain. If the patient suffered a subdural hematoma, I would immediately see a large amount of mixed clotted and fresh blood pouring out of the brain, and I would use copious amounts of irrigation to try to wash out any clot which remained beneath the far reaches of the skull. If there were a severely contused frontal or temporal lobe, I may have had to remove a portion of brain tissue and try to stop all active bleeding. After adequately decompressing the brain and achieving hemostasis, I would repair the dura, replace and secure the bone flap, close the scalp, insert an intracranial pressure (ICP) monitor in the brain, apply the wound dressing, and reevaluate the patient shortly thereafter in the neuro-intensive care unit. The patient would have an ICP monitor, and often a ventricular catheter in the brain, which allowed for the drainage of cerebrospinal fluid (CSF) to help to manage ICP.

Meeting with the family after the surgery was difficult, as I had to explain to them what happened and what measures we were taking to try to save the patient's life, as well as possible and probable future outcomes. It was at this point that we would offer a prognosis with conditions.

From the time a brain-injured patient arrives in the emergency department, whether or not they undergo a craniotomy, and throughout their stay in the neuro-intensive care unit, I have on many occasions gone through the neurological assessments and tests to confirm brain death if the patient's neurological condition had severely deteriorated.

As a neurosurgeon, my role in the treatment of patients has been to assess traumatic brain injury in the acute, subacute, and chronic setting and treat patients for their traumatic brain injury to the best of my ability. In the acute phase, this often involves assessing patients in a hospital emergency department, making rapid assessments to save a patient's life, and helping in the management of their postoperative care. In the subacute phase and chronic phase, this requires taking care of issues which had arisen after the patient was stabilized from their initial injury, as well as issues which may have arisen weeks or months after the injury. My interactions would frequently require the input of and coordination with other medical specialists such as intensive care physicians, anesthesiologists, neurologists, radiologists, physiatrists, and ortho-pedic surgeons, as well as occupational and physical therapists, respiratory therapists, nutrition-ists, orthotists, and other medical experts.

Responsibilities of a Life Care Planner

As a life care planner, my role is to assess what has occurred with respect to traumatic brain injury and attempt to determine likely future care that will be needed for the individual, as well as its associated costs. This may include likely future medical treatments, anticipated compli-cations, future therapy, medications, and other adaptive changes to their surroundings such as modifications to living arrangements, attendant care, day-to-day environmental needs (eating utensils, raised toilet seats, etc.), and modification to the architecture of their abode (widened doorways, bathrooms, ramps, etc.).

Evaluating Traumatic Brain Injury

Much of the assessment, whether as a treating physician or as a life care planner, involves trying, as much as possible, to determine the condition of an individual who has suffered a traumatic brain injury, on both a qualitative and quantitative basis, for current and future care. In order to accomplish this, we must do our best to understand the functioning of the injured brain and determine what types of deficits an individual with a traumatic brain injury has. As we attempt to understand the functioning of the brain in an individual who has suffered a traumatic brain injury, we must try to understand both the "structure," or anatomy, and the "function" of the injured brain, which are extremely interrelated, as structure may impact function, and func-tion may reflect structure.

Brain Structure and Function

The structure may be evaluated through advanced imaging studies of the brain, which look at anatomy. Despite the most modern imaging techniques, the level of resolution in a patient is not sufficient to see down to the level of the neuron (as opposed to histologic examination under the microscope in the laboratory). As technology improves, significant insight is being gained into the evaluation of structures and their relationships to function. Among these advances, diffusion tensor imaging (DTI), segmental volume analysis of the brain, positron emission tomography (PET), functional magnetic resonance imaging (fMRI), magneto-encephalography, and other technologies may provide information about both structure and function of the brain.

In addition to clinical evaluation (history, physical examination) of a patient who has suffered a brain injury, much information about functioning ability will be gleaned by talking with the patient's family, friends, etc., about performance at work, in the family setting, in social settings, and in various other environments. Information about performance in various settings will help to provide an understanding as to a patient's ability to function in different environments and under different levels of stress. There may be deficiencies in their functioning which might not be elucidated in evaluation, but which may only be revealed in certain situations that have not been tested. An analogy that comes to mind is a window leak that I had repaired 6 weeks ago. Since then, there has been no leaking, but there has also been minimal rain. It won't be until there is a severe storm, with winds blowing the rain sideways, that the adequacy of the repair will be properly tested. My conclusion could be that there is no leaking when it doesn't rain, but the real test will come when there is a severe rain. Similarly, the real test of a patient who has suffered a traumatic brain injury is how they function under certain conditions, which may test their capacity.

In order to gain an understanding of how a person is affected when there is damage to the brain, it is important to understand the functioning of the brain when everything is working properly. The splendor of the brain can start to be appreciated by recognizing its anatomy and function, its capability of memory across our five senses and more, its processing speed, its higher executive functioning, memory, learning, social cognition, language skills, its intricate pathways interconnecting structure and function of different parts of the brain, the redundancy of the pathways of the brain that attempt to compensate for neurological damage, and much more.

Through the Operating Microscope: A Neurosurgeon's View

To attempt to appreciate the almost unimaginable complexity and delicacy of the brain, it is helpful to look at the surface of the brain. A textbook that I co-authored, *Microsurgical Anatomy of the Brain: A Stereo Atlas* (Kraus & Bailey, 1994), contains three-dimensional (3-D) photographs (the textbook comes with 32 View-Master Reels and a 3-D Viewer) of the neurosurgical approaches to the brain that a neurosurgeon typically encounters. Shown in Figure 10.1 is a two-dimensional (2-D) photograph of the undersurface of the right side of the brain (in a cadaver specimen in which the arteries have been injected with a red latex dye and the veins with blue latex) in an approach known as the pterional approach (Kraus & Bailey, 1994). In Figure 10.2 is seen a 2-D photograph showing the back of the brain, with the cerebellum being lifted, exposing the dorsal aspect of the brainstem with the cervical spinal cord entering it (Kraus & Bailey, 1994).

In Figure 10.1, the undersurface of the right side of the brain is seen after dissecting open the sylvian fissure with the frontal lobe on the left and the temporal lobe on the right, through what is known as the pterional approach. Among the important structures we see are the right internal carotid artery (supplying blood to a large portion of the right cerebral hemisphere), the right optic nerve (sending visual information from the right eye to the brain), the right cranial nerve III (oculomotor nerve controlling a portion of the movement of the right eye), the pituitary stalk (connecting the pituitary gland with the hypothalamus), the posterior cerebral artery (supplying blood to the posterior portion of the cerebral hemispheres), the region anterior to the brainstem, and the tentorium (a dural membrane separating the upper and lower portions of the brain, medial to which the uncal portion of the temporal lobe can herniate, pressing on the third cranial nerve and causing the ipsilateral pupil to dilate). The delicate and dense interweaving of critical structures at the base of the brain is evident, as are the small perforating arteries that are visualized, supplying blood to the thalamus. While thalamoperforating arteries such as those

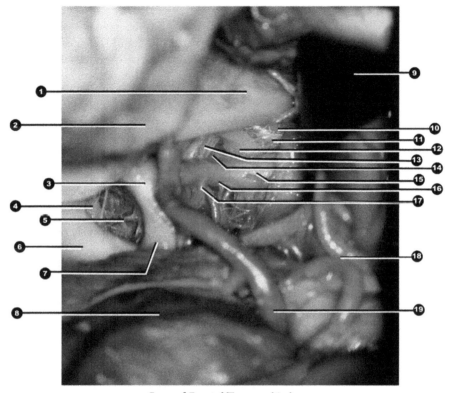

Base of Frontal/Temporal Lobes
Anterior incisural space; right pterional approach

1. Tentorium
2. Lesser wing of sphenoid
3. Right internal carotid artery
4. Pituitary stalk
5. Superior hypophyseal artery
6. Right optic nerve
7. A1 portion of right anterior cerebral artery
8. Right frontal lobe
9. Retractor on temporal lobe
10. Superior cerebellar artery
11. Interpeduncular cistern
12. Third cranial nerve
13. Liliequist's membrane
14. P1 portion of right posterior cerebral artery
15. P2 portion of right posterior cerebral artery
16. Right posterior communicating artery
17. Anterior thalamoperforating arteries
18. M3 branch of middle cerebral artery
19. Superficial sylvian vein

Figure 10.1 Base of Frontal/Temporal Lobes

From Kraus and Bailey (1994) *Microsurgical Anatomy of the Brain* with permission from Wolters Kluwer

seen in Figure 10.1 can be 0.41 to 4.71 mm in diameter, the arteriole diameters progressively decrease as the vasculature bifurcates to eventually reach neurons, the size of which are measured in terms of microns (roughly 1/25,000th of an inch) (Park et al., 2010).

Figure 10.2 shows a photograph after a midline suboccipital approach (portion of skull over posterior fossa removed) and cervical laminectomy has been performed and the is cerebellum

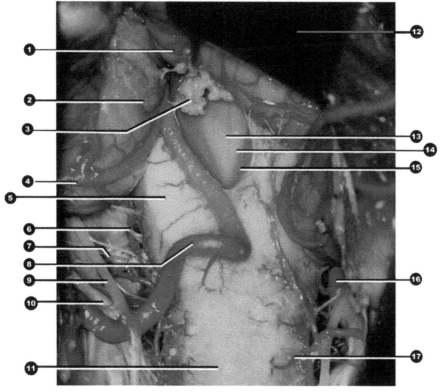

Brainstem
Foramen of Magendie; midline suboccipital approach

1. Uvula
2. Tonsil
3. Choroid plexus of fourth ventricle protruding through foramen of Magendie
4. Tonsillar artery
5. Medulla
6. Medullary rootlet of cranial nerve eleven
7. Cranial nerve twelve entering hypoglossal canal
8. Left posterior inferior cerebellar artery
9. Left cranial nerve eleven (spinal portion)
10. Dentate ligament
11. Spinal Cord
12. Retractor under right tonsil
13. Median sulcus
14. Hypoglossal triangle
15. Vagal triangle
16. Right vertebral artery
17. Posterior spinal artery

Figure 10.2 Brainstem

From Kraus and Bailey (1994). *Microsurgical Anatomy of the Brain: A Stereo Atlas* with permission from Wolters Kluwer

elevated to show the dorsal aspect of the brainstem as the cervical spinal cord ascends through the foramen magnum to merge with it. Again, extremely small arteries are seen, which enter and supply the upper cervical spinal cord and brainstem. The fine and delicate spinal portion of the left cranial nerve XI (spinal portion of the accessory nerve controlling the sternocleidomastoid and trapezius muscles) and left cranial nerve XII (hypoglossal nerve controlling ipsilateral tongue movement) are visualized. Seen on the dorsal surface of the medulla oblongata, the lowest portion of the brainstem, are the vagal trigone (region of vagal nuclei which control cardiac and other vital functions) and the hypoglossal trigone (region of nucleus of cranial nerve XII). Deep within the brainstem are critical structures which, among serving many other vital life-sustaining functions, keep an individual awake instead of being in a coma. Also, the vital and life-sustaining pathways connecting the brain with the body pass through this narrow but critical region.

The importance of the brain may be well recognized and emphasized by the fact that even though its weight (~1400 grams) represents about 2% of a person's body weight, it still receives roughly 20% of the blood that is pumped out of the heart, with the other 80% going to the remainder of the body. While there is debate about the actual number, it has been estimated that there are about 86 billion to 100 billion neurons within the human brain, about 1 trillion glial cells, 164 trillion to 200 trillion connections or synapses, and an estimated processing speed of roughly 52 quadrillion (52 thousand trillion) bits per second. The glial cells (astrocytes and oligodendrocytes) insulate the axons and significantly increase the speed of transmission of nerve impulses, and because they contain a fatty substance called myelin, the tissue is known as white matter, which lies deep to the gray matter (von Bartheld et al., 2016; Zimmer, 2011; Fields, 2020; Tang, 2001; Martins et al., 2019, 2012).

Forces of Brain Injury and Consequences of TBI

During a head injury, the brain may sustain force vectors of translation, rotation, acceleration and deceleration, compression, tension, and shearing, as well as blast-induced forces, coup (trauma to the brain under the location of impact on the skull) and contra coup (trauma to the brain in a location remote to or on the opposite side of the head from the region of impact to the skull) injuries. Many factors play a role in the functional outcome an injured patient may experience, including the severity (force of impact) and location of the injury (which side of the head was struck and with what vector of force), the type of force (blunt or penetrating injury, blast injury), and the patient's age and pre-injury health. These may result in cortical contusions, intracerebral hematomas, subdural hematomas, and epidural hematomas, as well as diffuse axonal injury (DAI)/traumatic axonal injury (TAI). Non-depressed and depressed skull fractures may occur.

Every traumatic brain injury is unique. While an acute epidural hematoma may be life-threatening, its prompt removal may result in the patient having an excellent outcome. On the other hand, a DAI in the brain may not show hemorrhage on an initial CT scan of the brain, but the lifelong consequences and disability might be significant. A brain injury can instantly change a person's life and their ability to care for themselves and interact with others. It can also instantly change the lives of all those around the patient who interact with them on a personal or professional level. The consequences of a brain injury may be temporary or permanent. Traumatic brain injury is one of the largest causes of disability and death. On many occasions, the sequelae that a patient may experience after suffering a traumatic brain injury are significant, with very severe and obvious physical and cognitive findings. As an example, a patient may experience varying degrees of paresis or paralysis, difficulty speaking and understanding (Broca's and Wernicke's aphasia), significant cognitive and psychiatric concerns, and many other issues. Awareness of the consequences of a mild traumatic brain injury may be low, possibly because changes may at times be subtle and may chronically evolve, which may not be apparent to observers. In addition, many individuals who have suffered a mild traumatic brain injury may not seek medical care.

Patients who have suffered moderate and severe traumatic brain injuries will show more obvious clinical findings than those who have suffered a mild traumatic brain injury, in whom objective findings might not be seen. Most likely, many of those patients who are felt to be "normal" may in fact have unrecognized and undiagnosed pathology, both in structure and in function. If a patient sustains a traumatic brain injury and their relatives state that since the injury, the individual is "just not right," or "there is something different about them, but I just can't put my finger on it," and despite this all objective imaging studies, neuropsychological tests, and other evaluations are normal, it may be more likely that medicine and science have not properly evaluated and diagnosed what is wrong, rather than there actually being nothing wrong.

Complications and Comorbidities of TBI

Eventual traumatic brain injury comorbidities may include neurological disorders, sleep disorders, neurodegenerative diseases, Alzheimer's disease, Parkinson's disease, epilepsy, depression, amyotrophic lateral sclerosis (ALS), dementia, endocrine disorders, spasticity, psychiatric disorders, chronic traumatic encephalopathy, sexual dysfunction, incontinence, musculoskeletal disorders, metabolic dysfunction, and many others, as well as an acceleration of the aging process. For these reasons, TBI may be considered a silent epidemic as well as a chronic disease and is a risk factor for future neurological and psychiatric illness, epilepsy, neurodegenerative disease, and a cascade of other negative events, which may act synergistically with each other. TBI has dramatic consequences and impact on injured patients, as well as their families, caretakers, and society as a whole (LoBue et al., 2019; Javaid et al., 2021; Armstrong, 2019; Riggio & Wong, 2009; Masel & DeWitt, 2010).

Neurosurgical Procedures: Avoiding Iatrogenic Brain Injury

The subject of brain injury is close to the heart of every neurosurgeon. Not only does a neurosurgeon treat patients who have a traumatic brain injury as being the reason for their hospital admission, but also every neurosurgical procedure performed has the potential to cause iatrogenic trauma or injury to the brain. Opening the skull to resect a brain tumor or clip an aneurysm that is located within the deep recesses of the brain necessarily exposes the surrounding brain tissue to potential harm. One of the most important tenets of operating on the brain, which is paramount during every brain operation, is to at all times take every possible measure to protect normal brain, which may inadvertently be subject to trauma due to its proximity to the target pathology or which may be harmed during circumnavigation of that tissue during the neurosurgical approach to a deeper region of the brain. Techniques to minimize injury to normal brain include the use of the stereo operating microscope, proper handling of brain tissue with appropriate techniques and use of microsurgical instruments, detailed knowledge of the cisterns (subarachnoid pockets of CSF) which are external to brain parenchyma and provide passage corridors to deep portions of the brain, intraoperative drainage of CSF to "relax" the brain, opening fissures of the brain widely to let the lobes and gyri of the brain separate easily (thus providing deeper exposure while minimizing the peril of retraction), and strategically positioning the patient properly to let gravity assist with the gentle and progressive separation of the more superficial regions of the brain in order to access the deep ones. In addition, medications, anesthetic techniques, and electrical monitoring of brain activity and function are critical.

Despite taking all possible measures to protect normal brain, it is frequently necessary to enter normal brain parenchyma in order to access the target pathology. Although every measure is made to minimize harm to the patient, using the most sophisticated intraoperative navigation techniques, and possibly adding functional mapping, normal brain tissue will be impacted. Neurosurgeons have for decades strived to avoid "eloquent" (such as motor strip or speech area) portions of the brain, and instead go through or, if necessary, remove relatively "silent" areas of the brain. In order to save or vastly improve a patient's life and treat the offending pathology, this entry into normal brain is often necessary, as the anticipated benefits of this surgery outweigh the risks.

"Silent" Areas of the Brain

Insights into the human connectome (discussed later in this chapter) may have importance in the attempt to preserve neurological function in a patient undergoing supratentorial surgery on the brain, as connectomics has contributed to the understanding of human language and other brain functions (Poologaindran et al., 2020). The question as to whether truly "silent" areas of the brain exist is an important one (Baker, 2018). It is possible that all areas of the brain have a significant role, but injury to some regions may be more noticeable in day-to-day life than is injury to other regions of the brain. As an example, disorders of emotional regulation have been seen commonly after injury to the right prefrontal cortex (Salas et al., 2016).

Instead of thinking of regions of the brain as "silent," these areas may instead be portions which are redundant in function. If so, this changes the concept of eloquent versus non-eloquent areas of the brain, and rather suggests these are areas of the brain that, if injured, may have obvious or more subtle changes in the functioning of a patient (Baker et al., 2018).

Another way of asking this important question is to ponder whether it is likely that a portion of the brain can be damaged and remain "silent" to the functioning of an individual, or whether it is more likely that we do not yet have the proper tools, or are not correctly using the tools that we have, in order to assess the damage. Much of the brain's higher executive function may not be easily recognized if there is a small amount of damage, but does our inability to recognize the effect of brain injury mean that the brain is functioning normally?

Cerebral Architecture, Neural Networks, and Assemblies

Theories about brain functioning are evolving. Traditionally, it has been felt that a particular function of the brain resides within a focal region of the brain and that this neural hub provides executive function or cognitive control, with perception, cognition, and action being discrete functions of the human brain. The growing body of data suggests that instead of having a single neural apex to act as an executive, the brain is organized into modules, themselves functioning in parallel rather than in a simple progression. This represents an organizational and functional structure of the brain which is an interaction of neuronal assemblies without the need for a central controller. This is consistent with the understanding that many functions of the brain defy the simple classification as perception, cognition, or action (Gazzaniga et al., 2009).

The growing volume of big data in neuroscience emphasizes the need for theoretical ideas that can unify the understanding of brain structure and function. Network neuroscience may provide a common conceptual framework and toolset with which to do so, connecting theoretical approaches such as dynamic systems, neural coding, and statistical physics (Bassett & Sporns, 2017). The concept of a networking approach of cerebral function has been described as a result of additional knowledge and insight of the brain connectome gained by combining multimodal data from anatomic dissections, lesion studies, neuroimaging, electrophysiological mapping methods, and computational modeling. This networking theory may provide for interindividual anatomo-functional variations and neuroplastic phenomena that go beyond apparent limitations of the white matter connectivity, possibly explaining how the brain can adapt to the environment, with potential implications for traumatic brain injury (Herbet & Duffau, 2020). Concepts of small world networks, local connectivity, long-distance connectivity, hierarchical modularity, interconnected hubs, rich clubs, connectivity backbones, and centrality have been used in analyzing neurological disorders (Hoffman, 2016; Stam, 2014).

The Brain Is the Person: The Person Is the Brain

In two medical novels that I co-authored, *Body Trade* and *Unexpected*, the concepts and ramifications of brain injury and brain transplantation are explored and emphasized, stressing the point that the brain is the person (socially, emotionally, intellectually, occupationally, etc.), with the remainder of the body providing the vital and necessary functions to support the brain (Kraus & Popp, 2014, 2016). To put into context the ramifications to a person's function after suffering an injury to the brain, let us consider the impact of the injury on other body parts and organs and for a moment give thought as to what actually constitutes a person. If an individual suffers an injury to their hand, they are the same person, but they have an injured hand. If they fracture a leg, they are the same person with a fractured leg. However, if they injure the brain, they may be, in essence, a mildly or dramatically different person, because the thoughts, language, memory, perception, awareness, concentration, ambition, attention, emotions, skills, dreams, intelligence, aptitude, hopes, and interpersonal interactions, which for the most part reside within the brain, are the actual person. When these functions are altered through injury, the person is no longer the same. In addition, since the brain controls the functioning of the remainder of the body, the remainder of somatic functions may also be impaired and changed.

Symptom Progression, Comorbidities, Family Impact, and Awareness of TBI

Inability to recognize or measure functional changes does not equate to the conclusion that those changes have not occurred. Some damage may also be progressive and worsen with time (as with chronic traumatic encephalopathy [CCTE]) before it becomes "noticeable." While damage may not be outwardly observable at times, based upon behavior or objective testing, there may come a time at which it will be. Reasons for this delay may include the following: 1) the decline may be progressive, either from natural progression or from further insults to the brain, causing it to exceed the "tipping point" at which symptoms are apparent; 2) the environmental factors and stresses, which may not have elicited symptoms initially, may have changed, placing new stresses or requirements upon an individual that were not existent previously, again crossing the threshold of a "tipping point" for symptoms to appear; and 3) our behavioral and cognitive testing abilities (including neuropsychological, neurological, psychiatric, vocational, and social assessments) and technological testing (imaging modalities of the brain, serum and CSF biomarkers, etc.) will likely continue to improve in the future. It is important to recognize that just because we have not recognized or measured a deficit does not mean that the deficit does not exist, but rather that our measurement and assessment tools may have not been thorough enough, advanced enough, or detailed enough or that not enough time has elapsed for the possible progression of symptoms to become apparent.

The study of the brain is ever evolving and advancing. As we learn more, new tools that result in new discoveries will be retrospectively applied to past clinical data and findings. As this occurs, previous classification methods and scales may become obsolete because they fail to consider new understandings of the intricate workings of the brain. While this may make comparison to historical studies and data difficult, it is inevitable as the field advances. As we answer new questions about the brain, many more questions are created. One would expect nothing less when trying to study the world's most sophisticated and complicated "machine," the human brain.

Subtle But Important Ramifications of TBI

The cases of mild traumatic brain injury, which may represent 75–90% of all cases of traumatic brain injury, may be difficult to understand and detect. Much of the CT and MRI imaging may appear to be normal, although more advanced neuroimaging may at times detect abnormalities. The neuropsychological evaluation may return to relatively normal status. The designs of different tests and scales vary significantly, and the resulting conclusion of a test is only as good as the design of the test and the specificity of the test's conclusions. While imaging and testing may appear to be quite normal, the real test for these patients is determined by how their subsequent functioning in life is affected and how well they integrate into the family, work, and social roles in which they were previously engaged. Are they independent in daily living, or has that been affected, even in a subtle way? What has happened to their job? Are they able to perform the same skills that they used to perform? If they are an accountant, can they process information as proficiently, accurately, and rapidly as they used to? Can they still work with four spreadsheets on a computer simultaneously? If they are a carpenter, is their spatial perception altered, resulting in difficulty visualizing where shelves, cabinets, and doorways will be built? Is their depth perception or ability to see in stereo altered, affecting a pilot's ability to land a plane? Is their hearing or voice altered, affecting a musician's ability to perform on an instrument or sing or recognize music properly? Is their comprehension of verbal or written language impaired, affecting their ability to learn new tasks? If they are a student, is their ability to learn affected? In patients who have suffered injury to the frontal lobes of the brain, have their drive, ambition, and mood been altered? Are social relationships with family and friends changed? Are they angry, depressed, or anxious? Do they have difficulty sleeping or have nightmares? Were there any preexisting cognitive or psychological impairments that might have been aggravated or worsened by the traumatic brain injury? Are there new physical and emotional stressors in life that have occurred as a result of the traumatic brain injury, such as relationship, financial, job, and other, that might interact with each other to worsen any underlying or newly caused traumatic brain injury–related functioning neuropsychological pathology?

Epidemiology

Traumatic brain injury is a global problem and is recognized as one of the most common, disabling, and costly medical problems facing the world. Traumatic brain injury is generally broken down into mild (also sometimes referred to as a concussion), moderate, and severe categories, depending upon the clinical presentation. It causes include falls (~49% of hospital admissions); motor vehicle collisions (~25% of hospital admissions); and gunshot wounds, explosive blasts, sports injuries, and interpersonal violence. Approximately 42–74 million cases of mild traumatic brain injury occur worldwide annually, and mild traumatic brain injury occurs with a tenfold higher frequency than moderate and severe injury (Frieden et al., 2015; Gardner & Yaffe, 2015; Dewan et al., 2018).

During a blast injury, as seen in the military as well as occupational and civilian settings, there is a significant instantaneous rise in atmospheric pressure. This blast overpressure (BOP) or high energy noise may result in damage to solid organs such as the brain, heart, and spleen, as well as hollow organs such as the ears, lungs, and gastrointestinal tract. There may be four aspects to the injury, which include the primary (caused by the BOP wave), secondary (resulting from mechanical and penetrating trauma from airborne debris), tertiary (from transportation of the entire body as a result of structural collapse or blast wind), and quaternary (resulting from exposure to toxic inhalants, burns, asphyxia, etc.) (Elsayed, 1997; Kocsis & Tessler, 2009; Kovacs et al., 2014; Elder & Cristian, 2009; Kennedy et al., 2010; Mathews & Koyfman, 2015).

Traumatic Brain Injury Classification, Scales, and Definitions

By implementing broadly accepted scales for the assessment of traumatic brain injury and outcomes, a standardization is developed that is very helpful for comparing research studies, evaluating the literature, and formulating guidelines and recommendations.

After suffering a mild traumatic brain injury or concussion, a patient may experience confusion and disorientation for less than 24 hours, loss of consciousness for up to 30 minutes, or memory loss lasting less than 24 hours. A CT scan of the brain is typically normal. Those suffering a moderate traumatic brain injury may have confusion or disorientation lasting more than 24 hours, loss of consciousness for over 30 minutes but less than 24 hours, or memory loss for over 24 hours but less than 7 days. Patients suffering from a severe traumatic brain injury may have confusion or disorientation for over 24 hours, loss of consciousness for over 24 hours, or memory loss for over 7 days. A CT scan of the brain is usually abnormal (Defense Medical Surveillance System, 2021).

The Glasgow Coma Scale (GCS) is a widely accepted method of evaluating patients who have suffered a head injury and have associated impaired consciousness. The three components of the scale are ocular, verbal, and motor function, with total scores ranging from 3 to 15, with an alert patient having a score of 15 (Campbell, 2013; Teasdale & Jennett, 1974).

Other scales used to assess patients who have suffered a traumatic brain injury in both the acute, subacute, and chronic setting include the following (it is beyond the scope of this chapter to go into more detail than that given here).

For assessing disability due to physical and cognitive impairment: Glasgow Outcome Scale (GOS) with or without extended scores (GOS-E); Disability Rating Scale (DRS); Rancho Los Amigos Scale (RLOS); Functional Independence Measure (FIM); Functional Assessment Measure (FAM); Community Integration Questionnaire (CIQ); Functional Status Examination (FSE); Supervision Rating Scale (SRS); Sensory Modality Assessment and Rehabilitation Technique (SMART); Sensory Stimulation Assessment Measure (SSAM); and Western Neuro Sensory Stimulation Profile (WNSSP).

For assessing neuropsychological and cognitive outcome assessment: Controlled Oral Word Association for verbal fluency; Rey Complex Figure for visuo-construction and memory; Grooved Pegboard for fine motor dexterity; and Symbol Digit Modalities (verbal) for sustained attention.

For assessing patient's subjective view of their disease: Health-Related Quality of Life (HRQoL); SF-36 (short form 36 health questionnaire); SF-12 (a shorter version); WHOQOL; SIP; EQ-5D; Neurobehavioral Symptom Inventory (NSI); and Quality of Life in Brain Injury (QUOLIBRI) (Nichol et al., 2011; Shukla et al., 2011; Hall et al., 2001).

Brain Neuroanatomy, Function, and Cognition

The anatomy and function of the brain are covered in another chapter in this textbook; therefore, this discussion will be limited to a few pertinent topics. Classically, different regions of the brain were thought to correspond with specific functions. Understanding of the anatomy and function of the brain is significantly improving with the advent of advanced imaging capabilities.

In 1909, K. Brodmann (1909), a pioneer in the field of brain mapping through his studies of the cytoarchitectonic parcellation of the human cerebral cortex, published a seminal textbook *Brodmann's Localization in the Cerebral Cortex* (translated by Laurence Garey) that described

> a topographic analysis of the human cerebral cortex based on its cellular structure . . . the emphasis would be not only on gross divisions of the brain, such as lobes and gyral complexes, but also on the smallest gyri and parts of gyri . . . to describe topographical parcellation and localization in the cortex that would also be of value for clinicians.
>
> (Brodmann, 1909)

Over a century later, this classic work remains important in advancement of the field and has been cited over 170,000 times (as of July 2018) (Zilles, 2018). As neuroimaging studies have advanced, so has the understanding that traditional neuroanatomical maps do not provide the precision to match some aspects of functional segregation (Nieuwenhuys, 2013). Using multimodal MRIs from the Human Connectome Project (HCP), 180 areas per hemisphere were delineated with the use of an objective semi-automated neuroanatomical approach (localizing sharp and reproducible parcellated brain images), of which 97 areas are new and 83 areas were previously reported using postmortem microscopy (Glasser et al., 2016). Functional anatomy is not necessarily constrained by anatomic distinctions, and even within one sulcus, the upper bank may be functionally distinct from the opposite side (Baker et al., 2018). Transcranial magnetic stimulation has also been used for diagnosis and treatment and has been used to perform functional mapping of the motor cortex (Lefaucheur, 2019).

Traditionally, knowledge of the neuroanatomy of the brain has been essential to understanding which regions of the brain are related to various aspects of functioning of the brain. Despite additional concepts regarding neural networks, which may help to understand cerebral and cognitive processing, this knowledge is a prerequisite to evaluating compromise of function in an injured brain and how the changes in anatomy of the brain relate to changes in function. In putting together the complexities of evaluation of traumatic brain injury and how it affects an individual, it is essential to have an understanding of the 1) anatomy of the normal brain, 2) functioning of the normal brain, 3) correlations between normal anatomy and normal functioning, 4) changes in anatomy of the injured brain when compared with the normal brain, 5) changes in functioning of the injured brain compared to the normal brain, and 6) correlations between anatomy and functioning of the injured brain.

To gain an understanding of brain anatomy in a patient, we can use the best imaging technology that is available. To gain an understanding of functioning of the brain, we use clinical input from physicians (neurosurgeons, neurologists, psychiatrists), neuropsychologists, nurses, therapists (physical therapists, occupational therapists, vocational rehabilitation specialists), social workers, and other medical personnel.

DTI is an excellent imaging tool that evaluates the white matter structure of the brain. The brain has white matter tracts which can be classified into three groups (projection, association, and commissural fibers), depending upon which regions of the brain they are connecting:

- **Projection fibers**: connect the cortex with the brainstem, cerebellum and spinal cord, and can be seen on DTI (corticospinal, corticobulbar, and corticopontine fibers; thalamic radiations, geniculocalcarine fibers [optic radiations])
- **Association fibers**: connect cortical regions within the same hemisphere (cingulum, superior occipitofrontal fasciculus, inferior occipitofrontal fasciculus, uncinate fasciculus, superior longitudinal fasciculus, arcuate fasciculus, inferior longitudinal fasciculus)

- **Commissural fibers**: connect analogous cortical regions of the two hemispheres (corpus callosum, anterior commissure, posterior commissure)
- **Additional tracts**: fornix, cerebellar peduncles (inferior, middle, superior), stria terminalis, frontal aslant tract, central tegmental tract, decussation of the superior cerebellar peduncle, medial lemniscus (Wycoco et al., 2013; Mori et al., 2008; Aggarwal et al., 2013)

The understanding of the structure of the brain helps to assess and correlate abnormalities and deficits in the event of injury. Although it is beyond the scope of this chapter to cover the multitude of cortical, brainstem, and white matter tract injuries; their resultant imaging (DTI, etc.) changes; and the correlating impact on the psychological, cognitive, and functional outcomes of a patient who has suffered a traumatic brain injury, several examples will be given.

The uncinate fasciculus, which connects the orbitofrontal and temporal lobes, may be an early biomarker for identification of behavioral problems, as seen in a study using probabilistic diffusion tensor tractography in a group of pediatric patients who suffered moderate to severe traumatic brain injury (Johnson et al., 2011). Using diffusion MRI in another pediatric sample of over 500 patients suffering mild/severe traumatic brain injury, the uncinate fasciculus was particularly vulnerable to white matter disruption, and as it is a frontolimbic tract connecting the ventral prefrontal cortex with the amygdala, it may create an increased risk for behavioral or emotional difficulties after injury. It was found that female patients had a lower uncinate fasciculus fractional anisotropy and higher radial diffusivity compared to controls, whereas this effect of traumatic brain injury was not significant in male patients (Dennis et al., 2021).

It is beyond the scope of this chapter to discuss many of the disorders that may occur after a traumatic brain injury or the intricacies behind each syndrome or deficit. The following review of a number of dysfunctions that may occur with injury to various regions of the brain provides for an appreciation of how complex, intricate, and interdependent the various regions of the brain are and how higher executive functioning of the brain may be impacted.

Vision Deficits Related to the Primary Occipital Cortical Regions

- Hemianopsias, scotomas
- Simple hallucinations, phosphenes, photopsias (perception of light in the absence of light stimulus)
- Visual agnosia
- Cortical blindness (loss of vision without ophthalmological causes)
- Anton's syndrome (denial of visual loss with confabulation in a setting of cortical blindness) (Das & Naqvi, 2022)
- Astereopsis (Hoffman, 2016)

Vision Deficits Related to Ventral Stream Disorders

The three standard ventral tracts are the uncinate fasciculus, inferior frontooccipital fasciculus, and temporofrontal extreme capsule fascicle (the ventral occipitotemporal pathway subserves object perception) (Weiller et al., 2021; Freud et al., 2016).

- Achromatopsia (inability to see colors)
- Color anomia
- Color agnosia
- Prosopagnosia (inability to recognize faces)

- Object agnosia
- Object anomia
- Synesthesia (stimulation of one sensory modality causes experiences in another (colored grapheme: viewing letters and numbers induces perception of color) (Hubbard & Ramachandran, 2005)
- Pareidolia (image of faces and objects seen in patterns such as clouds or plants)

Vision Deficits Related to Dorsal Stream Disorders

Dorsal occipitoparietal pathway (subserves object localization and visually guided action) (Hoffman, 2016)
- Simultanagnosia
- Oculomotor apraxia
- Inverted vision
- Visual perseveration (persistence or reappearance of image)

(Hoffman, 2016)

Temporal Lobe–Related Disorders

- Right or left temporal lobe

  - Vertigo, olfactory hallucinations, gustatory (taste) abnormalities
  - Neuropsychiatric: Kluver-Bucy syndrome, anxiety, agitation, paranoia
  - Cognitive: memory (Korsakoff), cortical deafness, auditory agnosia and hallucinations, difficulty with time perception

- Left temporal lobe

  - Wernicke's aphasia, verbal amnesia, visual agnosia, lexical amusia (difficulty reading music), synesthesia

- Right temporal lobe

  - Visuospatial amnesia, prosopagnosia, auditory agnosia, amusia (receptive and expressive), delusional misidentification syndromes (Hoffman, 2016)

Deficits Related to Right or Left Parietal Lesion Syndromes

- **Cortical sensory impairment**: tactile agnosia; astereognosis (loss of depth perception); impairment of two-point discrimination; agraphesthesia (impairment of palm number tracing); ahylognosia (difficulty recognizing density of material such as liquid, metal, wood)
- **Visuospatial disturbances**: Balint's syndrome (simultagnosia: inability to perceive more than one object at a time; visual apraxia and ataxia); optokinetic reflex and nystagmus; smooth pursuit/saccadic eye movement disorders
- **Precuneus and claustrum**: attention and consciousness hubs, which if injured, may result in minimally conscious or transcendental states
- **Temporo-occipito-parietal junction and other cross-modal abnormalities**: autoscopy (seeing one's double from an out-of-body experience); acquired synesthesia (sensory stimulus in one modality triggers sensations in another modality); autokinesis (impression of movement of objects in the dark) (Hoffman, 2016)

Impairment of the left parietal lobe: anomias; apraxias; Gerstman's syndrome (acalculia, agraphia, finger anomia, difficulty with right/left orientation) (Hoffman, 2016)

Impairment of the right parietal lobe: aprosodia (difficulty comprehending or expressing changes in tone of voice); neglect syndromes; visuospatial impairment; anosognosia (inability of brain to recognize illness of itself or the individual's own body); geographic disorientation (inability to orient oneself in their surroundings); allesthesia (perception of one receiving a stimulus on the body that is remote to where it was actually applied); impairment of three-dimensional sense appreciation; aphonognosia (inability to recognize familiar voices); dressing apraxia (Hoffman, 2016)

Left hemisphere disorders: apraxia

Right hemisphere disorders (right hemisphere is important for attention attributes in both hemispheres; left hemisphere is responsible for attention only contralaterally and emotion): difficulty with attention, prosody, neglect, anosognosia for hemiparesis, visuospatial function) (Hoffman, 2016)

Frontal lobe disorders: cognitive (memory, attention, executive problems), neurological symptoms (dizziness, headaches, vertigo, imbalance), neuropsychiatric impairment (depression, anxiety, irritability, mania, impulsivity, disinhibition), Broca's aphasia (typically left hemisphere)

Injury to Papez's circuit (mammillothalamic tract, medial mammillary nucleus, anterior nucleus of the thalamus, cingulate gyrus, cingulum, entorhinal cortex, subiculum, hippocampus), fornix: affects consolidation of short- and intermediate-term memory into long-term memory (Hoffman, 2016)

Biomarkers of TBI (Imaging and Chemical)

Biomarkers can help to quantify the assessment of traumatic brain injury. They may be chemical, radiological, or other.

Imaging Biomarkers

Imaging of the brain is commonly performed after a patient has suffered a traumatic brain injury. In the acute setting, a CT scan of the brain is usually performed, especially if there is a moderate or severe traumatic brain injury. While the CT scan is often negative when a patient has suffered a mild traumatic brain injury, other advanced imaging studies may detect abnormalities. MRI is frequently performed to obtain more detail. Advanced imaging techniques, such as DTI, may be used to evaluate the white matter fiber tracts of the brain. Segmentation protocols may be incorporated with MRI images in order to evaluate volumes of various regions of the brain, compare right and left sides of the brain, make comparisons to normal controls, and assess a patient on a longitudinal basis, looking for changes that may occur over time. Additional MRI sequences that may help in evaluating traumatic brain injury include fluid attenuated inversion recovery (FLAIR), susceptibility weighted imaging (SWI), high angular resolution diffusion imaging (HARDI), diffusion spectrum imaging (DSI), and fMRI (Irimia et al., 2012a; Ledig et al., 2015).

Advanced imaging of the brain using DTI relies on the tissue diffusion rate of water. Water molecules, which diffuse equally in all directions due to Brownian motion, as they might in a glass of water, do so in a uniform fashion. If the water molecules are constrained in their movement, such as by obstruction from the wall of a cell located within a white matter tract, their diffusion becomes directional, and the diffusion is known as anisotropic. When a volume element of the brain (voxel) is evaluated on an MRI using DTI, the addition of a vector element gives direction to the diffusion, thus yielding information about location, orientation, and anisotropy to the voxel on a DTI scan of the brain. Fractional anisotropy (FA) gives insight into the health of an axons within the white matter tracts and may show information that is not available from CT or other MRI imaging modalities. Quantitative parameters of the diffusion tensor that are commonly used are apparent diffusion coefficient (ADC), which is also known as mean diffusivity (MD); axial diffusivity (AD); radial diffusivity (RD); and FA (Ranzenberger & Snyder, 2021).

Hulkower et al. (2013), in a review entitled "A Decade of DTI in Traumatic Brain Injury: 10 Years and 100 Articles Later," states "despite significant variability in sample characteristics, technical aspects of imaging, and analysis approaches, the consensus is that DTI effectively differentiates patients with TBI and controls, regardless of the severity and timeframe following injury" (p. 2071). Hulkower et al. (2013) felt that diffusion tensor imaging was an extremely important tool that could benefit the neurosurgeon in better diagnosing induced trauma brain abnormalities. He summarized his conclusions in his quoted summary:

> a unifying theme can be deduced from this large body of research: DTI is an extremely useful and robust tool for the detection of TBI-related brain abnormalities. The overwhelming consensus of these studies is that low white matter FA is characteristic of TBI. This finding is consistent across almost all the articles we reviewed, despite significant variability in patient demographics, modest differences in data acquisition parameters, and a multiplicity of data analysis techniques. This consistency across studies attests to the robustness of DTI as a measure of brain injury in TBI.
>
> (Hulkower et al., p. 2071)

Hulkower et al. found the following areas of abnormality in the brain using DTI after a TBI. When evaluating DTI by evaluating abnormal FA and MD, the most common areas of abnormality were the corpus callosum, frontal lobe, white matter, and thalamus. Using tractography analysis, the areas were the corpus callosum, frontooccipital fasciculus, inferior longitudinal fasciculus, uncinate fasciculus, and cingulum bundle. Using whole-brain analysis, the areas were the cingulum bundle, corpus callosum, superior longitudinal fasciculus, posterior limb of the internal capsule, frontooccipital fasciculus, and frontal lobe. White matter lesions and changes in white matter microarchitecture may be the basis of cognitive impairment, as was seen in an evaluation of 50 patients with white matter lesions, in addition to healthy controls, who underwent cognitive evaluation (Hu et al., 2022).

White matter fiber tracking using diffusion MRI provides the ability to map brain connections. In order to create tracks (also known as streamlines), which represent the white matter tracts within the brain (tractography), several processing steps are taken: 1) the diffusion-weighted images are pre-processed (eddy current, motion, and phase distortion correction); 2) fiber resolving is performed (fiber orientation); 3) fiber tracking is achieved (deterministic or probabilistic method, etc.); and 4) post-tracking processing is performed (Yeh et al., 2021). Traumatic brain injury connectomics (mapping of neural connections in the nervous system to create a connectome) allows for evaluation of cortical regions and connectivity as a patient's recovery evolves, allows comparison to populations, and may be used to create a personalized atrophy profile for a patient, which may help with personalized rehabilitation treatments by informing the medical team about recovery prospects and guiding evaluation and need for long-term care (Irimia et al., 2012b).

Tracts that can be analyzed using advanced imaging techniques (in this study, utilizing constrained spherical deconvolusion [CSD] of diffusion MRI) include the following: arcuate fasciculus; cingulum; fornix; frontal aslant tract; inferior frontooccipital fasciculus; inferior longitudinal fasciculus; middle longitudinal fasciculus; superior longitudinal fasciculus (I, II, and III); uncinate fasciculus; vertical occipital fasciculus; anterior commissure; corpus callosum; mediallemniscus; optic radiation; optic tract; pyramidal tract; corticospinal tract; thalamic radiations; and cerebellar bundles (Radwan et al., 2022). It is important to recognize that tractography and connectomes are maps of a macroscale, focusing on large white matter bundles. Many axons in the cerebrum are local, terminating in the same gyrus from which they originated, and may not be visualized using currently available technology (Baker et al., 2018).

Other imaging modalities that may be used to assess traumatic brain injury include magnetic resonance spectroscopy (MRS) (Croall et al., 2015; Gardner et al., 2014), magnetoencephalography (MEG) (Huang et al., 2009, 2012), PET scanning (Byrnes et al., 2014; Kraus et al., 1995; Padma et al., 2004b, 2004a, 2003; Selwyn et al., 2013; Nakayama et al., 2006), and single photon emission computed tomography (SPECT) (Raji et al., 2014).

Chemical Biomarkers

As a result of a brain injury, the blood-brain barrier may be broken down, and neurons as well as glial cells may release proteins, nucleic acids, and metabolites into the extracellular space, which may then enter the bloodstream (Huibregtse et al., 2021).

In an effort to evaluate traumatic brain injury in an analytical method and stratify its outcomes, biomarkers in the blood serum, CSF through a ventriculostomy or spinal tap, brain extracellular fluid, and brain tissue may be examined. Biomarkers are evaluated in clinical research, but generally not in the daily clinical practice of medicine. As summarized by Khellaf et al., 2019, regarding works of Depreitere and Donnelly,

> noteworthy biomarkers in TBI include glia-related biomarkers (GFAP, S100B), neuron/axon-related biomarkers (neuron-specific enolase [NSE], neurofilament light polypeptide [NFL], ubiquitin carboxy-terminal hydrolase [UCH-L1], tau, amyloid β, αII-Spectrin breakdown products among others) and other inflammation-related biomarkers (high mobility group box protein 1 [HMGB1], various cytokines and autoantibodies).
>
> (Khellaf et al., p. 2882)

Acute Neurosurgical Management of Brain Injury

When a patient who has suffered an acute traumatic brain injury arrives in an emergency room, they will be immediately assessed, and depending upon the severity of the injury as determined by a physical examination and imaging studies, their treatment course may vary significantly. When the patient has suffered a mild traumatic brain injury, they may be discharged home, while those suffering from a severe traumatic brain injury may undergo emergent surgery on the brain.

Acute hemorrhages within the head may occur in the epidural space (outside of the dura), subdural space (deep to the dura), intraparenchymal region (in the substance of the brain), subarachnoid space (under the arachnoid membrane), and intraventricular region (within the ventricle). Mass effect, causing shift of the brain from one side to another or from the supratentorial to the infratentorial compartment, may be present.

Whether or not patients undergo a craniotomy for hemorrhage within the brain, they may have an ICP monitor placed to give the medical team the ability to determine how much pressure is present within the skull, and thus determine cerebral perfusion pressure (defined as the difference between mean arterial pressure and ICP). After the initial traumatic insult to the brain, secondary brain injury may set in with edema and ischemia, resulting in a downward cascade of events for the brain. To try to prevent this, measures must be taken to attempt to minimize the consequences of this secondary insult and maintain proper cerebral perfusion. Part of a potential downward cycle of events may include cell death and microvascular occlusion, leading to raised ICP and additional cerebral ischemia and ultimately resulting in a worsening deteriorating spiral of secondary events.

In order to remove an offending hematoma that may be causing mass effect and shift of the brain, a craniotomy may be performed. At times, a decompressive craniectomy may be performed, in which a large bone flap is removed, to allow the swollen brain additional room in which to expand.

Other treatments that may be used to help with the acute management of a traumatic brain injury patient include hyperosmolar therapy (to reduce raised ICP), prophylactic hypothermia, CSF drainage, ventilation therapies to decrease carbon dioxide within the blood, anesthetics/analgesics/sedatives, steroids, nutrition, infection prophylaxis, deep venous thrombosis prevention, seizure prophylaxis, brain tissue oxygen monitoring, and transcranial Doppler (Bullock et al., 2006a, 2006b, 2006c; Sahuquillo & Dennis, 2019; Shahlaie et al., 2017; Carney et al., 2016; Aisiku et al., 2017; Zusman ct al., 2020).

Neuropsychological Testing/Assessment

Neuropsychological testing may be able to not only quantify deficits but also be a predictor of current and future outcomes with respect to real-world measures and help neuropsychologists to guide recommendations regarding life and treatment planning for post– traumatic brain injury patients. Domains tested include cognition, neurobehavior, psychological health, life participation, and physical function (Casaletto & Heaton, 2017; Silverberg et al., 2017).

Although many neuropsychological tests are available, the design of the test may impact the outcomes and which conclusions are drawn. Testing should meet several criteria, in that they should be sensitive (not miss a disorder if a patient has one), specific (only show a positive result if a patient has specific pathology), reliable (tests should be repeatable), and valid (actually test what it is intended to test for) (Gardner et al., 2020; Randolph et al., 2005). Neuropsychological testing has been implemented with pencil and paper tests as well as with computerized tests. Testing is routinely performed for a baseline evaluation on all U.S. military service members before deployment (Meyers & Vincent, 2020) and in professional sports (Echemendia et al., 2020).

Traditional pencil and paper neurocognitive tests include:

- Hopkins Verbal Learning Test
- Brief Visuospatial Memory Test
- WAIS-3 Digit Symbol subtest
- Symbol Digit Modalities Test
- Trail Making Test
- Controlled Oral Word Association Test
- Stroop Color Word Test
- WAIS-III Digit Span Test
- WAIS-III Letter-Number Sequencing Test
- Paced Auditory Serial Addition Test
- Repeatable Battery for the Assessment of Neuropsychological Status

Computerized neurocognitive tests include:

- ANAM (Automated Neuropsychological Assessment Metrics)
- CNS VS (CNS Vital Signs)
- CogSport

- HeadMinder CRI (HeadMinder Concussion Resolution Index)
- ImPACT (Immediate Post-Concussion and Cognitive Testing) (Randolph et al., 2005; Arrieux et al., 2017)

Recovery and Rehabilitation

This topic is covered in another chapter in this textbook, and a detailed review is beyond the scope of this chapter.

The path to recovery after a patient has suffered a traumatic brain injury may be a long one, and many patients may suffer lifelong deficits. After discharge from a hospital, depending upon the severity of the traumatic brain injury, patients may be cared for at inpatient rehabilitation facilities, long-term hospitals, or skilled nursing facilities.

Depending upon the severity of a traumatic brain injury, some of the long-lasting consequences may include difficulties not only for the patients but for their families and caregivers as well. Patients may experience difficulties with neuropsychological, psychiatric, and physical difficulties, and they may experience cognitive, behavioral, emotional, medical, interpersonal, and financial challenges. Activities such as grocery shopping, balancing a checkbook, dialing a phone number, and preparing a meal may be difficult or impossible to perform.

The team of health care providers caring for patients who have suffered a traumatic brain injury may include physicians, nurses, neuropsychologists, psychiatrists, physical therapists, nutritionists, respiratory therapists, occupational therapists, vocational counselors, speech pathologists, social workers, psychotherapists, case managers, and marriage counselors.

Short- and Long-Term Effects and Complications of TBI

This topic is covered in another chapter in this textbook, and therefore coverage here will be brief.

Patients who have suffered a traumatic brain injury may experience the following sequelae and complications:

- Post-concussive symptoms and syndrome
- Cognitive changes
- Psychiatric disorders
- Post-traumatic stress disorder (PTSD)
- Headache
- Somatic disorders associated with brain injury (hemiplegia, aphasia, etc.)
- Chronic pain
- Balance difficulties
- Susceptibility to repeated traumatic brain injury and consequential increased deficits
- Chronic traumatic encephalopathy (CTE)
- Post-traumatic seizures/epilepsy
- Neuroendocrine dysfunction
- Visual changes
- Sleep disturbances
- Movement disorders/Parkinson's disease
- Spasticity
- Swallowing difficulties

Outcome, Disability, and Return to Work

Traumatic brain injury is a major cause of morbidity and mortality in the United States. Despite existing statistics on the incidence of traumatic brain injury and its outcomes, many individuals suffering a traumatic brain injury may not seek medical attention, and many may have suffered cognitive and functional impairments without recognizing it. The moderate and severe cases of traumatic brain injury are easily detected, as these patients usually arrive at an emergency department of a hospital in serious or severe condition. Many of these patients may suffer life-long disabilities, requiring various levels of assistive care. Some may never achieve independent living. Some may not be able to walk, comprehend written or verbal language, eat, or talk, and some may require ventilator support to assist with breathing and an implanted feeding tube to provide nutrition. The patient who was previously functioning well and who is consciously awake enough to recognize that their life as they knew it has been taken from them will be devasted, which will have with it its own associated psychological, neurological, and psychiatric sequelae.

In a review of 13,700 traumatic brain injury patients who were treated with inpatient rehabilitation, at five years after the injury, one in five patients had died. Of the survivors, 12% were institutionalized, one-third did not gain independence in daily activities, 57% were moderately or severely disabled, 29% were dissatisfied with life, and 55% of those previously employed were no longer employed (Corrigan et al., 2014).

Depending upon the severity, traumatic brain injury may adversely affect a patient's ability to return to independent living and work. In the United States, roughly 3.2–5.3 million people live with a disability related to traumatic brain injury, and approximately 43% of those hospitalized for TBI have residual disability a year after discharge (Corrigan et al., 2010; Langlois et al., 2006). Higher severity of head injuries was associated with greater dependence on others, worse GOS ratings, dependent living, and unemployment (Dikmen et al., 1995). In one group of 113 patients studied who had suffered moderate to severe traumatic brain injury, although the employment rate pre-injury was 80%, it was 15% at 3 months post-injury and 55% after 3 years post-injury (Grauwmeijer et al., 2012).

In a prospective cohort of mild traumatic brain injury patients in a TRACK-TBI study at 6 and 12 months after the injury, 82% of patients reported at least one post-concussion syndrome symptom, with approximately 40% having significantly reduced satisfaction with life scores at 12 months post-injury, and 22.4% of patients at 1 year post-injury were below full functional status. It was felt that recovery from a mild traumatic brain injury is a nonlinear process, and the time to full recovery may for some patients be protracted (McMahon et al., 2014).

TBI has significant ramifications on patients and those around them. As medicine and technology improve, so does our understanding of traumatic brain injury and the ability to treat patients who have suffered a traumatic brain injury in the acute, subacute, and chronic setting.

References

Aggarwal, M., Zhang, J., Pletnikova, O., Crain, B., Troncoso, J., & Mori, S. (2013). Feasibility of creating a high-resolution 3D diffusion tensor imaging-based atlas of the human brainstem: A case study at 11.7 T. *NeuroImage, 74,* 117–127. https://doi.org/10.1016/j.neuroimage.2013.01.061
Aisiku, I. P., Silvestri, D. M., Robertson, C. S. (2017). Critical care management of traumatic brain injury. In H. R. Winn (Ed.), *Youmans and Winn neurological surgery* (7th ed., pp. 2876–2897). Elsevier.
Armstrong, R. A. (2019). Risk factors for Alzheimer's disease. *Folia Neuropathologica, 57*(2), 87–105. https://doi.org/10.5114/fn.2019.85929
Arrieux, J. P., Cole, W. R., & Ahrens, A. P. (2017). A review of the validity of computerized neurocognitive assessment tools in mild traumatic brain injury assessment. *Concussion (London, England), 2*(1), CNC31. https://doi.org/10.2217/cnc-2016-0021
Baker, C., Burks, J., Briggs, R., Conner, A., Glenn, C., Sali, G., Mccoy, T., Battiste, J., O'Donoghue, D., & Sughrue, M. (2018). A connection Atlas of the human cerebrum – Chapter 1: Introduction, methods, and significance. *Operative Neurosurgery, 15*(6), 51–59.

Bassett, D. S., & Sporns, O. (2017). Network neuroscience. *Nature Neuroscience, 20*(3), 353–364. https://doi.org/10.1038/nn.4502

Brodmann, K. (1909). *VergleichendeLokalisationslehre der Grosshirnrinde in ihrenPrinzipiendargestellt auf Grund des Zellenbaues.* Verlag von Johann Ambrosius Barth (Garey, L. J. (Trans.). (2006). *Brodmann's localization in the cerebral cortex.* Springer).

Bullock, M. R., Chesnut, R., Ghajar, J., Gordon, D., Hartl, R., Newell, D. W., Servadei, F., Walters, B. C., Wilberger, J. E., & Surgical Management of Traumatic Brain Injury Author Group. (2006a). Surgical management of acute epidural hematomas. *Neurosurgery, 58*(Suppl 3), S7–iv.

Bullock, M. R., Chesnut, R., Ghajar, J., Gordon, D., Hartl, R., Newell, D. W., Servadei, F., Walters, B. C., Wilberger, J., & Surgical management of traumatic brain injury author group. (2006b). Surgical management of traumatic parenchymal lesions. *Neurosurgery, 58*(Suppl 3), S25–iv. https://doi.org/10.1227/01.NEU.0000210365.36914.E3

Bullock, M. R., Chesnut, R., Ghajar, J., Gordon, D., Hartl, R., Newell, D. W., Servadei, F., Walters, B. C., Wilberger, J. E., & Surgical Management of Traumatic Brain Injury Author Group. (2006c). Surgical management of acute subdural hematomas. *Neurosurgery, 58*(Suppl 3), S16–iv.

Byrnes, K. R., Wilson, C. M., Brabazon, F., von Leden, R., Jurgens, J. S., Oakes, T. R., & Selwyn, R. G. (2014). FDG-PET imaging in mild traumatic brain injury: A critical review. *Frontiers in Neuroenergetics, 5,* 13. https://doi.org/10.3389/fnene.2013.00013

Campbell, W. W. (2013). The Examination in coma. In *DeJong's the neurologic examination* (7th ed., pp. 745–762). Wolters Kluwer, Lippincott Williams & Wilkins.

Carney, N., Totten, A. M., O'Reilly, C., Hawryluk, G. W. J., Bell, M. J., Bratton, S. L., Chesnut, R., Harris, O. A., Kissoon, N., Rubiano, A. M., Shutter, L., Tasker, R. C., Vavilala, M. S., Wilberger, J., Wright, D. W., & Ghajar, J. (2016, September). *Guidelines for the management of severe traumatic brain injury* (4th ed.) Brain Trauma Foundation. https://braintrauma.org/uploads/03/12/Guidelines_for_Management_of_Severe_TBI_4th_Edition.pdf

Casaletto, K. B., & Heaton, R. K. (2017). Neuropsychological assessment: Past and future. *Journal of the International Neuropsychological Society: JINS, 23*(9–10), 778–790. https://doi.org/10.1017/S1355617717001060

Corrigan, J. D., Cuthbert, J. P., Harrison-Felix, C., Whiteneck, G. G., Bell, J. M., Miller, A. C., Coronado, V. G., & Pretz, C. R. (2014). US population estimates of health and social outcomes 5 years after rehabilitation for traumatic brain injury. *The Journal of Head Trauma Rehabilitation, 29*(6), E1–E9. https://doi.org/10.1097/HTR.0000000000000020

Corrigan, J. D., Selassie, A. W., & Orman, J. A. (2010). The epidemiology of traumatic brain injury. *The Journal of Head Trauma Rehabilitation, 25*(2), 72–80. https://doi.org/10.1097/HTR.0b013e3181ccc8b4

Croall, I., Smith, F. E., & Blamire, A. M. (2015). Magnetic resonance spectroscopy for traumatic brain injury. *Topics in Magnetic Resonance Imaging: TMRI, 24*(5), 267–274. https://doi.org/10.1097/RMR.0000000000000063

Das, J. M., & Naqvi, I. A. (2022, May 8). *Anton syndrome.* Stat Pearls Publishing.

Defense Medical Surveillance System (DMSS), Theater Medical Data Store (TMDS) provided by the Armed Forces Health Surveillance Division (AFHSD). (2021, November 10). *DOD numbers for traumatic brain injury worldwide—totals.* https://health.mil/Reference-Center/Publications/2022/01/20/2000-Q3-2021-DOD-Worldwide-Numbers-for-TBI

Dennis, E. L., Caeyenberghs, K., Hoskinson, K. R., Merkley, T. L., Suskauer, S. J., Asarnow, R. F., Babikian, T., Bartnik-Olson, B., Bickart, K., Bigler, E. D., Ewing-Cobbs, L., Figaji, A., Giza, C. C., Goodrich-Hunsaker, N. J., Hodges, C. B., Hovenden Aa, E. S., Irimia, A., Königs, M., Levin, H. S., Lindsey, H. M., . . . Wilde, E. A. (2021). White matter disruption in pediatric traumatic brain injury: Results from ENIGMA pediatric moderate to severe traumatic brain injury. *Neurology, 97*(3), e298–e309. Advance online publication. https://doi.org/10.1212/WNL.0000000000012222

Dewan, M. C., Rattani, A., Gupta, S., Baticulon, R. E., Hung, Y. C., Punchak, M., Agrawal, A., Adeleye, A. O., Shrime, M. G., Rubiano, A. M., Rosenfeld, J. V., & Park, K. B. (2018). Estimating the global incidence of traumatic brain injury. *Journal of Neurosurgery,* 1–18. Advance online publication. https://doi.org/10.3171/2017.10.JNS17352Ref 12

Dikmen, S. S., Ross, B. L., Machamer, J. E., & Temkin, N. R. (1995). One-year psychosocial outcome in head injury. *Journal of the International Neuropsychological Society: JINS, 1*(1), 67–77. https://doi.org/10.1017/s1355617700000126

Echemendia, R. J., Thelen, J., Meeuwisse, W., Hutchison, M. G., Rizos, J., Comper, P., & Bruce, J. M. (2020). Neuropsychological assessment of professional ice hockey players: A cross-cultural examination of baseline data across language groups. *Archives of Clinical Neuropsychology: The Official Journal of the National Academy of Neuropsychologists, 35*(3), 240–256. https://doi.org/10.1093/arclin/acz077

Elder, G. A., & Cristian, A. (2009). Blast-related mild traumatic brain injury: Mechanisms of injury and impact on clinical care. *The Mount Sinai Journal of Medicine, New York, 76*(2), 111–118. https://doi.org/10.1002/msj.20098

Elsayed, N. M. (1997). Toxicology of blast overpressure. *Toxicology, 121*(1), 1–15. https://doi.org/10.1016/s0300-483x(97)03651-2

Fields, R. D. (2020). The brain learns in unexpected ways: Neuroscientists have discovered a set of unfamiliar cellular mechanisms for making fresh memories. *Scientific American, 322*(3), 74–79.

Freud, E., Plaut, D. C., & Behrmann, M. (2016). "What" is happening in the dorsal visual pathway. *Trends in Cognitive Sciences, 20*(10), 773–784. https://doi.org/10.1016/j.tics.2016.08.003

Frieden, T. R., Houry, D., & Baldwin, G. (2015). *Report to congress: Traumatic brain injury in the United States: Epidemiology and rehabilitation.* Centers of Disease Control and Prevention, National Center for Injury Prevention and Control: Division of Unintentional Injury Prevention.

Gardner, A. J., Iverson, G. L., & Stanwell, P. (2014). A systematic review of proton magnetic resonance spectroscopy findings in sport-related concussion. *Journal of Neurotrauma, 31*(1), 1–18. https://doi.org/10.1089/neu.2013.3079

Gardner, A. J., Tonks, J., Potter, S., Yates, P. J., Reuben, A., Ryland, H., & Williams, H. (2020). Neuropsychological assessment of mTBI in adults. In J. W. Tsao (Ed.), *Traumatic brain injury: A clinician's guide to diagnosis, management, and rehabilitation* (2nd ed., pp. 57–74). Springer.

Gardner, R. C., & Yaffe, K. (2015). Epidemiology of mild traumatic brain injury and neurodegenerative disease. *Molecular and Cellular Neurosciences, 66*(Pt B), 75–80. https://doi.org/10.1016/j.mcn.2015.03.001

Gazzaniga, M. S., Doron, K. W., & Funk, C. M. (2009). Looking toward the future: Perspectives on examining the architecture and function of the human brain as a complex system. In M. S. Gazzaniga, E. Bizzi, A. Caramazza, L. M. Chalupa, S. T. Grafton, T. F. Heatherton, C. Koch, J. E. LeDoux, S. J. Luck, J. A. Movshon, H. Neville, E. A. Phelps, P. Rakic, D. L. Schacter, M. Sur, & B. A. Wandell (Eds.), *The cognitive neurosciences* (4th ed.). MIT Press.

Glasser, M. F., Coalson, T. S., Robinson, E. C., Hacker, C. D., Harwell, J., Yacoub, E., Ugurbil, K., Andersson, J., Beckmann, C. F., Jenkinson, M., Smith, S. M., & Van Essen, D. C. (2016). A multi-modal parcellation of human cerebral cortex. *Nature, 536*(7615), 171–178. https://doi.org/10.1038/nature18933

Grauwmeijer, E., Heijenbrok-Kal, M. H., Haitsma, I. K., & Ribbers, G. M. (2012). A prospective study on employment outcome 3 years after moderate to severe traumatic brain injury. *Archives of Physical Medicine and Rehabilitation, 93*(6), 993–999. https://doi.org/10.1016/j.apmr.2012.01.018

Hall, K. M., Bushnik, T., Lakisic-Kazazic, B., Wright, J., & Cantagallo, A. (2001). Assessing traumatic brain injury outcome measures for long-term follow-up of community-based individuals. *Archives of Physical Medicine and Rehabilitation, 82*(3), 367–374. https://doi.org/10.1053/apmr.2001.21525

Herbet, G., & Duffau, H. (2020). Revisiting the functional anatomy of the human brain: Toward a meta-networking theory of cerebral functions. *Physiological Reviews, 100*(3), 1181–1228. https://doi.org/10.1152/physrev.00033.2019

Hoffman, M. (2016). *Cognitive, conative and behavioral neurology: An evolutional perspective.* Springer.

Hu, A. M., Ma, Y. L., Li, Y. X., Han, Z. Z., Yan, N., & Zhang, Y. M. (2022). Association between changes in white matter microstructure and cognitive impairment in white matter lesions. *Brain Sciences, 12*(4), 482. https://doi.org/10.3390/brainsci12040482

Huang, M. X., Nichols, S., Robb, A., Angeles, A., Drake, A., Holland, M., Asmussen, S., D'Andrea, J., Chun, W., Levy, M., Cui, L., Song, T., Baker, D. G., Hammer, P., McLay, R., Theilmann, R. J., Coimbra, R., Diwakar, M., Boyd, C., . . . Lee, R. R. (2012). An automatic MEG low-frequency source imaging approach for detecting injuries in mild and moderate TBI patients with blast and non-blast causes. *NeuroImage, 61*(4), 1067–1082. https://doi.org/10.1016/j.neuroimage.2012.04.029

Huang, M. X., Theilmann, R. J., Robb, A., Angeles, A., Nichols, S., Drake, A., D'Andrea, J., Levy, M., Holland, M., Song, T., Ge, S., Hwang, E., Yoo, K., Cui, L., Baker, D. G., Trauner, D., Coimbra, R., & Lee, R. R. (2009). Integrated imaging approach with MEG and DTI to detect mild traumatic brain injury in military and civilian patients. *Journal of Neurotrauma, 26*(8), 1213–1226. https://doi.org/10.1089/neu.2008.0672

Hubbard, E. M., & Ramachandran, V. S. (2005). Neurocognitive mechanisms of synesthesia. *Neuron, 48*(3), 509–520. https://doi.org/10.1016/j.neuron.2005.10.012

Huibregtse, M. E., Bazarian, J. J., Shultz, S. R., & Kawata, K. (2021). The biological significance and clinical utility of emerging blood biomarkers for traumatic brain injury. *Neuroscience and Biobehavioral Reviews*, *130*, 433–447. https://doi.org/10.1016/j.neubiorev.2021.08.029

Hulkower, M. B., Poliak, D. B., Rosenbaum, S. B., Zimmerman, M. E., & Lipton, M. L. (2013). A decade of DTI in traumatic brain injury: 10 years and 100 articles later. *AJNR, American Journal of Neuroradiology*, *34*(11), 2064–2074. https://doi.org/10.3174/ajnr.A3395

Irimia, A., Chambers, M. C., Torgerson, C. M., Filippou, M., Hovda, D. A., Alger, J. R., Gerig, G., Toga, A. W., Vespa, P. M., Kikinis, R., & Van Horn, J. D. (2012a). Patient-tailored connectomics visualization for the assessment of white matter atrophy in traumatic brain injury. *Frontiers in Neurology*, *3*, 10. https://doi.org/10.3389/fneur.2012.00010

Irimia, A., Wang, B., Aylward, S. R., Prastawa, M. W., Pace, D. F., Gerig, G., Hovda, D. A., Kikinis, R., Vespa, P. M., & Van Horn, J. D. (2012b). Neuroimaging of structural pathology and connectomics in traumatic brain injury: Toward personalized outcome prediction. *NeuroImage: Clinical*, *1*(1), 1–17. https://doi.org/10.1016/j.nicl.2012.08.002

Javaid, S., Farooq, T., Rehman, Z., Afzal, A., Ashraf, W., Rasool, M. F., Alqahtani, F., Alsanea, S., Alasmari, F., Alanazi, M. M., Alharbi, M., & Imran, I. (2021). Dynamics of choline-containing phospholipids in traumatic brain injury and associated comorbidities. *International Journal of Molecular Sciences*, *22*(21), 11313. https://doi.org/10.3390/ijms222111313

Johnson, C. P., Juranek, J., Kramer, L. A., Prasad, M. R., Swank, P. R., & Ewing-Cobbs, L. (2011). Predicting behavioral deficits in pediatric traumatic brain injury through uncinate fasciculus integrity. *Journal of the International Neuropsychological Society: JINS*, *17*(4), 663–673. https://doi.org/10.1017/S1355617711000464

Kennedy, J. E., Leal, F. O., Lewis, J. D., Cullen, M. A., & Amador, R. R. (2010). Posttraumatic stress symptoms in OIF/OEF service members with blast-related and non-blast-related mild TBI. *NeuroRehabilitation*, *26*(3), 223–231. https://doi.org/10.3233/NRE-2010-0558

Khellaf, A., Khan, D. Z., & Helmy, A. (2019). Recent advances in traumatic brain injury. *Journal of Neurology*, *266*(11), 2878–2889. https://doi.org/10.1007/s00415-019-09541-4

Kocsis, J. D., & Tessler, A. (2009). Pathology of blast-related brain injury. *Journal of Rehabilitation Research and Development*, *46*(6), 667–672. https://doi.org/10.1682/jrrd.2008.08.0100

Kovacs, S. K., Leonessa, F., & Ling, G. S. (2014). Blast TBI models, neuropathology, and implications for seizure risk. *Frontiers in Neurology*, *5*, 47. https://doi.org/10.3389/fneur.2014.00047

Kraus, G. E., & Bailey, G. J. (1994). *Microsurgical anatomy of the brain: A stereo atlas*. Williams & Wilkins.

Kraus, G. E., Bernstein, T. W., Satter, M., Ezzeddine, B., Hwang, D. R., & Mantil, J. (1995). A technique utilizing positron emission tomography and magnetic resonance/computed tomography image fusion to aid in surgical navigation and tumor volume determination. *Journal of Image Guided Surgery*, *1*(6), 300–307. https://doi.org/10.1002/(SICI)1522-712X(1995)1:6<300::AID-IGS2>3.0.CO;2-E

Kraus, G., & Popp, P. (2014). *Body trade*. TouchPoint Press.

Kraus, G., & Popp, P. (2016). *Unexpected: Body trade 2*. TouchPoint Press.

Langlois, J. A., Rutland-Brown, W., & Wald, M. M. (2006). The epidemiology and impact of traumatic brain injury: A brief overview. *The Journal of Head Trauma Rehabilitation*, *21*(5), 375–378. https://doi.org/10.1097/00001199-200609000-00001

Ledig, C., Heckemann, R. A., Hammers, A., Lopez, J. C., Newcombe, V. F., Makropoulos, A., Lötjönen, J., Menon, D. K., & Rueckert, D. (2015). Robust whole-brain segmentation: Application to traumatic brain injury. *Medical Image Analysis*, *21*(1), 40–58. https://doi.org/10.1016/j.media.2014.12.003

Lefaucheur, J. P. (2019). Transcranial magnetic stimulation. *Handbook of Clinical Neurology*, *160*, 559–580. https://doi.org/10.1016/B978-0-444-64032-1.00037-0

LoBue, C., Munro, C., Schaffert, J., Didehbani, N., Hart, J., Batjer, H., & Cullum, C. M. (2019). Traumatic brain injury and risk of long-term brain changes, accumulation of pathological markers, and developing dementia: A review. *Journal of Alzheimer's Disease: JAD*, *70*(3), 629–654. https://doi.org/10.3233/JAD-190028

Martins, N. R. B., Angelica, A., Chakravarthy, K., Svidinenko, Y., Boehm, F. J., Opris, I., Lebedev, M. A., Swan, M., Garan, S. A., Rosenfeld, J. V., Hogg, T., & Freitas, R. A., Jr. (2019). Human brain/cloud interface. *Frontiers in Neuroscience*, *13*, 112. https://doi.org/10.3389/fnins.2019.00112

Martins, N. R. B., Erlhagen, W., & Freitas, R. A. (2012, June). Non-destructive whole-brain monitoring using nanorobots: Neural electrical data rate requirements. *International Journal of Machine Consciousness*, *4*(1). https://doi.org/10.1142/S1793843012400069

Masel, B. E., & DeWitt, D. S. (2010). Traumatic brain injury: A disease process, not an event. *Journal of Neurotrauma, 27*(8), 1529–1540. https://doi.org/10.1089/neu.2010.1358

Mathews, Z. R., & Koyfman, A. (2015). Blast injuries. *The Journal of Emergency Medicine, 49*(4), 573–587. https://doi.org/10.1016/j.jemermed.2015.03.013

McMahon, P., Hricik, A., Yue, J. K., Puccio, A. M., Inoue, T., Lingsma, H. F., Beers, S. R., Gordon, W. A., Valadka, A. B., Manley, G. T., Okonkwo, D. O., & TRACK-TBI Investigators. (2014). Symptomatology and functional outcome in mild traumatic brain injury: Results from the prospective TRACK-TBI study. *Journal of Neurotrauma, 31*(1), 26–33. https://doi.org/10.1089/neu.2013.2984

Meyers, J. E., & Vincent, A. S. (2020). Automated neuropsychological assessment metrics (v4) military battery: Military normative data. *Military Medicine, 185*(9–10), e1706–e1721. https://doi.org/10.1093/milmed/usaa066

Mori, S., Oishi, K., Jiang, H., Jiang, L., Li, X., Akhter, K., Hua, K., Faria, A. V., Mahmood, A., Woods, R., Toga, A. W., Pike, G. B., Neto, P. R., Evans, A., Zhang, J., Huang, H., Miller, M. I., van Zijl, P., & Mazziotta, J. (2008). Stereotaxic white matter atlas based on diffusion tensor imaging in an ICBM template. *NeuroImage, 40*(2), 570–582. https://doi.org/10.1016/j.neuroimage.2007.12.035

Nakayama, N., Okumura, A., Shinoda, J., Nakashima, T., & Iwama, T. (2006). Relationship between regional cerebral metabolism and consciousness disturbance in traumatic diffuse brain injury without large focal lesions: An FDG-PET study with statistical parametric mapping analysis. *Journal of Neurology, Neurosurgery, and Psychiatry, 77*(7), 856–862. https://doi.org/10.1136/jnnp.2005.080523

Nieuwenhuys, R. (2013). The myeloarchitectonic studies on the human cerebral cortex of the Vogt-Vogt school, and their significance for the interpretation of functional neuroimaging data. *Brain Structure & Function, 218*(2), 303–352. https://doi.org/10.1007/s00429-012-0460-z

Nichol, A. D., Higgins, A. M., Gabbe, B. J., Murray, L. J., Cooper, D. J., & Cameron, P. A. (2011). Measuring functional and quality of life outcomes following major head injury: Common scales and checklists. *Injury, 42*(3), 281–287. https://doi.org/10.1016/j.injury.2010.11.047

Padma, M. V., Jacobs, M., Kraus, G., McDowell, P., Satter, M., Adineh, M., & Mantil, J. (2004a). Radiation-induced medulloblastoma in an adult: A functional imaging study. *Neurology India, 52*(1), 91–93.

Padma, M. V., Jacobs, M., Sequeira, P., Adineh, M., Satter, M., Kraus, G., & Mantil, J. C. (2004b). Functional imaging in Lhermitte-Duclose disease. *Molecular Imaging and Biology, 6*(5), 319–323. https://doi.org/10.1016/j.mibio.2004.06.005

Padma, M. V., Said, S., Jacobs, M., Hwang, D. R., Dunigan, K., Satter, M., Christian, B., Ruppert, J., Bernstein, T., Kraus, G., & Mantil, J. C. (2003). Prediction of pathology and survival by FDG PET in gliomas. *Journal of Neuro-Oncology, 64*(3), 227–237. https://doi.org/10.1023/a:1025665820001

Park, S. Q., Bae, H. G., Yoon, S. M., Shim, J. J., Yun, I. G., & Choi, S. K. (2010). Morphological characteristics of the thalamoperforating arteries. *Journal of Korean Neurosurgical Society, 47*(1), 36–41. https://doi.org/10.3340/jkns.2010.47.1.36

Poologaindran, A., Lowe, S. R., & Sughrue, M. E. (2020). The cortical organization of language: Distilling human connectome insights for supratentorial neurosurgery. *Journal of Neurosurgery, 134*(6), 1959–1966. https://doi.org/10.3171/2020.5.JNS191281

Radwan, A. M., Sunaert, S., Schilling, K., Descoteaux, M., Landman, B. A., Vandenbulcke, M., Theys, T., Dupont, P., & Emsell, L. (2022). An atlas of white matter anatomy, its variability, and reproducibility based on constrained spherical deconvolution of diffusion MRI. *NeuroImage, 254*, 119029. https://doi.org/10.1016/j.neuroimage.2022.119029

Raji, C. A., Tarzwell, R., Pavel, D., Schneider, H., Uszler, M., Thornton, J., van Lierop, M., Cohen, P., Amen, D. G., & Henderson, T. (2014). Clinical utility of SPECT neuroimaging in the diagnosis and treatment of traumatic brain injury: A systematic review. *PLOS One, 9*(3), e91088. https://doi.org/10.1371/journal.pone.0091088Ref 130

Randolph, C., McCrea, M., & Barr, W. B. (2005). Is neuropsychological testing useful in the management of sport-related concussion? *Journal of Athletic Training, 40*(3), 139–152, 149.

Ranzenberger, L. R., & Snyder, T. (2021). Diffusion sensor imaging. In *StatPearls*. StatPearls Publishing.

Riggio, S., & Wong, M. (2009). Neurobehavioral sequelae of traumatic brain injury. *The Mount Sinai Journal of Medicine, New York, 76*(2), 163–172. https://doi.org/10.1002/msj.20097

Sahuquillo, J., & Dennis, J. A. (2019). Decompressive craniectomy for the treatment of high intracranial pressure in closed traumatic brain injury. *The Cochrane Database of Systematic Reviews, 12*(12), CD003983. https://doi.org/10.1002/14651858.CD003983.pub3

Salas, C. E., Castro, O., Yuen, K. S., Radovic, D., d'Avossa, G., & Turnbull, O. H. (2016). "Just can't hide it": A behavioral and lesion study on emotional response modulation after right prefrontal damage. *Social Cognitive and Affective Neuroscience, 11*(10), 1528–1540. https://doi.org/10.1093/scan/nsw075

Selwyn, R., Hockenbury, N., Jaiswal, S., Mathur, S., Armstrong, R. C., & Byrnes, K. R. (2013). Mild traumatic brain injury results in depressed cerebral glucose uptake: An (18)FDGPET study. *Journal of Neurotrauma, 30*(23), 1943–1953. https://doi.org/10.1089/neu.2013.2928

Shahlaie, K., Zwienenberg-Lee, M., & Muizelaar, J. P. (2017). Neuropathology of traumatic brain injury. In H. R. Winn (Ed.), *Youmans and Winn neurological surgery* (7th ed., pp. 2843–2859). Elsevier.

Shukla, D., Devi, B. I., & Agrawal, A. (2011). Outcome measures for traumatic brain injury. *Clinical Neurology and Neurosurgery, 113*(6), 435–441. https://doi.org/10.1016/j.clineuro.2011.02.013

Silverberg, N. D., Crane, P. K., Dams-O'Connor, K., Holdnack, J., Ivins, B. J., Lange, R. T., Manley, G. T., McCrea, M., & Iverson, G. L. (2017). Developing a cognition endpoint for traumatic brain injury clinical trials. *Journal of Neurotrauma, 34*(2), 363–371. https://doi.org/10.1089/neu.2016.4443

Stam, C. J. (2014). Modern network science of neurological disorders. *Nature Reviews: Neuroscience, 15*(10), 683–695. https://doi.org/10.1038/nrn3801

Tang, Y., Nyengaard, J. R., De Groot, D. M., & Gundersen, H. J. (2001). Total regional and global number of synapses in the human brain neocortex. *Synapse (New York, N.Y.), 41*(3), 258–273. https://doi.org/10.1002/syn.1083

Teasdale, G., & Jennett, B. (1974). Assessment of coma and impaired consciousness: A practical scale. *Lancet (London, England), 2*(7872), 81–84. https://doi.org/10.1016/s0140-6736(74)91639-0

von Bartheld, C. S., Bahney, J., & Herculano-Houzel, S. (2016). The search for true numbers of neurons and glial cells in the human brain: A review of 150 years of cell counting. *The Journal of Comparative Neurology, 524*(18), 3865–3895. https://doi.org/10.1002/cne.24040

Weiller, C., Reisert, M., Peto, I., Hennig, J., Makris, N., Petrides, M., Rijntjes, M., & Egger, K. (2021). The ventral pathway of the human brain: A continuous association tract system. *NeuroImage, 234*, 117977. https://doi.org/10.1016/j.neuroimage.2021.117977

Wycoco, V., Shroff, M., Sudhakar, S., & Lee, W. (2013). White matter anatomy: What the radiologist needs to know. *Neuroimaging Clinics of North America, 23*(2), 197–216. https://doi.org/10.1016/j.nic.2012.12.002

Yeh, F. C., Irimia, A., Bastos, D., & Golby, A. J. (2021). Tractography methods and findings in brain tumors and traumatic brain injury. *NeuroImage, 245*, 118651. https://doi.org/10.1016/j.neuroimage.2021.118651

Zilles, K. (2018). Brodmann: A pioneer of human brain mapping-his impact on concepts of cortical organization. *Brain: A Journal of Neurology, 141*(11), 3262–3278. https://doi.org/10.1093/brain/awy273

Zimmer, C. (2011). 100 trillion connections. *Scientific American, 304*(1), 58–63. https://doi.org/10.1038/scientificamerican0111-58

Zusman, B. E., Kochanek, P. M., & Jha, R. M. (2020). Cerebral edema in traumatic brain injury: Ahistorical framework for current therapy. *Current Treatment Options in Neurology, 22*(3), 9. https://doi.org/10.1007/s11940-020-0614-x

11 Post-Traumatic Headaches

Huma Haider

Background

Post-traumatic headaches are a common occurrence in patients with traumatic brain injuries. Ninety-five percent of traumatic brain injury sufferers will have headaches. A post-traumatic headache is defined as one that develops or onsets within the seven days to several weeks following an injury or after regaining consciousness (Defrin, 2014). There is a temporal relationship between an injury causing a traumatic brain injury and the onset of post-traumatic headaches. Post-traumatic headaches are the most frequent complaint following a traumatic brain injury, with a prevalence rate of up to 95%. Even at 12 months post-incident, the cumulative incidence rate remains above 70%. Most of those suffering experience daily or weekly onset, with the temple, forehead, neck, back of the head, eyes, and vertex the most-cited pain locations (Headache Classification Committee, 2018; The International Headache Society, 2021). As per Labastida-Ramírez et al. (2020), "Acute post-traumatic headache[s] resolve after 3 months, but persistent post-traumatic headache[s] usually last much longer and account much longer and account for 4% of all secondary headache disorders" (p. 2). The causes of post-traumatic headaches vary based on the injuries and the areas of the brain impacted.

Etiology

Ashina et al. (2019) noted that post-traumatic headaches are identified as secondary headaches, and the onset of such headaches can occur within seven days of a post-traumatic event. Additionally, traumatic headaches can evolve within seven days of gaining consciousness or recovering the ability to sense and report pain. There have been some patients that do not report the onset of new headaches immediately after a traumatic brain injury and may not report these symptoms until almost a year post-injury. There is a significant increase in developing post-traumatic stress disorder with the presence of post-traumatic headaches. These headaches can present in different forms and require a unique approach to treatment depending on the associated symptoms.

Pathophysiology

The true pathophysiology of a post-traumatic headache is still unknown; however, there are several proposed ideas regarding the underlying cause. Labastida-Ramírez et al. (2020) noted there are three main ideas of the causes, including impaired descending modulation, where there are structural differences in cortical thickness and cerebral volumes. Some people with mild traumatic brain injuries typically have diffuse axonal injuries that can result in the structural remodeling in the somatosensory and insular cortex areas of the brain "leading to impaired neuromodulation of descending pain-modulating pathways." Another potential cause of

DOI: 10.4324/b23293-11

post-traumatic headaches is neurometabolic changes (Labastida-Ramírez et al., p. 14). Physical trauma to the brain causes damage to the tissues and white matter tracts within the brain and leads to cellular injury. After traumatic brain injuries, regardless of the severity, an inflammatory process occurs. This inflammatory process can cause neuroinflammation that may affect the trigeminal sensory system (Labastida-Ramírez et al.). Regardless of the cause of post-traumatic headaches, it is imperative that the treating provider evaluates the patient and quantifies the severity and type of post-traumatic headache. Table 11.1 and Table 11.2 are examples of assessments that assist providers in quantifying post-traumatic headaches.

This scale should only be used if the traumatic brain injury is greater than three months old. Additional evaluations used to diagnose post-traumatic headaches include computed

Table 11.1 Migraine Disability Assessment Tool (MIDAS)

Not Experienced	No More of a	A Mild Problem	A Moderate Problem	A Severe Problem
1	Problem	3	4	5
	2			

On how many days in the last 3 months did you miss work and/or school because of your headaches?
(Select zero if you did not have the activity in the last 3 months, such as you were completely unable to go to work.)
How many days in the last 3 months was your productivity at work and/or school reduced by half or more because of your headaches?
(Select zero if you did not have the activity in the last 3 months. You were able to go but unable to perform your best; do not include missed days.)
On how many days in the last 3 months did you not do household work (cleaning, shopping, child/relative care, cooking, repairs, yard work, etc.) because of your headaches?
(Select zero if you did not have the activity in the last 3 months. You were completely unable to perform the task.)
On how many days in the past 3 months was your productivity in household work reduced by half or more because of your headaches?
(Do not include days you counted in question 3 where you did not do household work. You were able to perform the tasks but unable to perform at your best; do not include missed days.)
On how many days in the past 3 months did you miss family, social, and/or leisure activities because of your headaches?
TOTAL

Table 11.2 MIDAS Scale

MIDAS Grade	Definition	MIDAS Score
I	**Little or No Disability** = Unlikely to affect daily activities and/or independence.	**0–5**
II	**Mild Disability** = Some activities and/or areas of independence are being affected.	**6–10**
III	**Moderate Disability** = More activities and/or areas of independence are being affected significantly.	**11–20**
VI	**Severe Disability** = Activities and/or areas of independence are profoundly affected.	**21+**

tomography (CT) and magnetic resonance imaging (MRI) of the head to rule out other potential causes of the headache.

Types of Post-Traumatic Headaches

There are four main types of post-traumatic headaches after a traumatic brain injury. The presentation of these headaches and the symptoms associated with the impact on the person with a traumatic brain injury appear in different ways.

Tension-Type Headaches

The most common type of headache is tension-type headaches. They are not limited to the head, but can cause pain around the face and neck as well. "These headaches often cause mild-to-moderate pain around the head, face, or neck. They usually don't cause other symptoms (like nausea or vomiting)" (Tension Headaches, n.d.). These types of headaches can frequently be perceived by the person as minimally annoying or moderately disabling. The headache can last as little as 30 minutes and as long as several months, although this is not as common.

Migraine-Type Headaches

Migraine-type headaches are more intense in terms of pain and have frequent secondary symptoms including nausea, vomiting, photophobia, and phonophobia. The pain associated with these headaches is typically described as moderate to severe with a unilateral localization, constant throbbing, and pain exacerbated by physical activity. Traumatic migraine headaches are disabling events that can cause significant lost time from an individual's work schedule as well as loss of family participation and interactions. These painful conditions are considered a common cause of disability resulting from complex brain events that may revolve from hours to days in a recurrent manner (Ruschel & De Jesus, 2022). The most common type of migraine is without aura (Ruschel & De Jesus).

Occipital Neuralgias–Type Headaches

The International Headache Society defines occipital neuralgias as "paroxysmal shooting or stabbing pain in the dermatomes of the greater or lesser occipital nerve" (Choi & Jeon, 2016, p. 479). The characteristic of this disorder is that its locus of pain is in the suboccipital region and spreads through the vertex, commonly affecting the upper neck, back of the head, and behind the eyes (Choi & Jeon). It is believed the pain is caused by compression of the greater and/or lesser occipital nerve, producing an intractable pain that requires a variety of interventions to treat. Another cause can be irritation/inflammation around the peripheral nerve structures. These headaches can be treated with interventional medicine using medication and a variety of modalities.

Cervicogenic-Type Headaches

The common trait factor of cervicogenic headaches is that pain is unilateral and begins in the neck and usually evolves following neck movement. This headache is a common and recurrent pain process that can inhibit the neck's range of motion (Al Khalili et al., 2022). These headaches can last many months if not treated, however, and they seem to resolve after around three months of successful treatment. These headaches typically occur at cervical levels 1, 2, and 3.

A cervicogenic headache is considered an unusual headache impacting "1% to 4%" of the post-traumatic headache population (Al Khalili et al.).

Diagnosis

The diagnosis of post-traumatic headaches varies greatly based on the symptoms that the person presents with as well as the areas of the brain that are impacted by the traumatic brain injury. Various imaging studies can be useful in diagnosing the presence of post-traumatic headaches including an MRI, CT scan, and diffuse tensor imaging (DTI). The DTI is useful in identifying areas of the white matter tracts that are impacted by traumatic brain injury. Electroencephalography (EEG) evaluations are "sparse and the few available often show marked early abnormalities, this includes focal slowing, absence of fast activity and amplitude asymmetries" (Labastida-Ramírez et al., 2020, p. 16).

Treatment

The treatment for each type of headache varies slightly from over-the-counter medication, to prescription medication, to physical modalities and physical therapy interventions. Occipital neuralgia presents as recurring pain most frequently described as 'shooting', 'burning', or 'stabbing'. It commonly results from head trauma, such as that experienced with a collision, fall, or other blow to the head that is associated with a concussion or whiplash-type injury (Zaremski et al., 2015). One medical treatment modality for occipital neuralgia is a nerve block with injection sites located on a line that connects the middle of the ears, 3.19 cm from the midline. Injection points are illustrated in Figure 11.1 (Choi & Jeon, 2016).

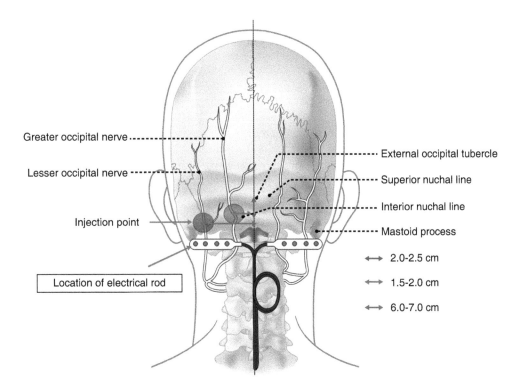

Figure 11.1 Landmarks for Injection of the Occipital Nerves and Electrical Stimulation

Occipital Neuralgia Management

Clinical signs and/or symptoms of occipital neuralgia are present and warrant treatment. Treatment includes gabapentin 100 mg TID. The cost for this medication, absent insurance use, ranges from $800 to $5,500 per year, depending on dosage and formulation. Should relief fail to be actualized with pharmacotherapy alone, nerve blocks, as detailed earlier, will be considered.

Additional headache treatments include prophylaxis: topiramate BID. Preventative therapy such as this is used when the frequency of onset is high; it helps to reduce the severity and duration of post-traumatic headaches, as well as improve the efficacy of abortive treatments (see later).

Vitamin and Herbal Supplementation

Use the following as directed to naturally prevent and/or treat post-traumatic headaches:

- **Riboflavin (vitamin B$_2$) 25–400 mg daily:** Helps to reduce frequency after one month of use with a continued reduction over the following two months. Increases energy and may cause a flushed or warm feeling, which passes. Urine may be bright yellow. Costs for this vitamin supplement range from $13 to $30 per month.
- **Coenzyme Q10 (CoQ10 or ubiquinol) 150–200 mg twice daily:** Reduces frequency by more than 50% in some people by increasing cell energy in the brain. Commonly used to improve memory and cognition. May increase energy levels. Costs for this supplement range from $27 to $55 per month.
- **Magnesium oil topical spray 400–600 md daily/4–5 sprays:** Stimulates blood flow and eases the nervous system for relief from pain. Use close to bedtime, as it induces calmness and restfulness. Apply to areas where the skin is thin, such as the tops of the feet, to aid in rapid absorption. May cause skin irritation at site that resolves after 10–15 minutes. Avoid oral formulation to avoid gastrointestinal side effects. Taking a bath with Epsom salt may also be of benefit for pain relief throughout the body. Costs for this supplement range from $15 to $21 per bottle, with one bottle lasting 2–3 months with prescribed use.
- **Butterbur root extract/blatterdock (*Petasites hybridus*) 50 mg 2–3 times daily:** Works to alleviate spasms and decrease swelling from inflammation in the brain to prevent the onset of pain. May cause indigestion, burping, and some mild gastrointestinal issues that often ease with continued use. Costs for this herbal supplement range from $19.99 to $41.50 per month; using inferior brands is advised against.
- **Medication overuse headaches:** Research also shows "chronic NSAID use increases the risk of peptic ulcer disease, acute renal failure, and stroke/myocardial infarction" (Marcum & Hanlon, 2010, p. 5).
- **PRN (as-needed) therapy:** Another option is diclofenac potassium 50 mg for oral solution. This medication can be taken twice daily as an acute rescue therapy for use when the person suffers from post-traumatic headaches. In conjunction with the diclofenac, the patient is also prescribed promethazine 25 mg as acute abortive medicine. The patient should be counseled to use this medication for ten days or less per month to avoid developing medication overuse headaches, as well as the potential gastrointestinal side effects of the medicine. The requirement for PRN migraine medications will significantly decrease with prophylactic therapy. The cost for this medication, absent insurance and at prescribed use, ranges from $40 to $150 per month for promethazine suppositories and $18 to $500 per three months for the diclofenac potassium, depending upon formulation.
- **Acute abortive medication:** To provide expeditious relief from post-traumatic headaches, a prescription for rizatriptan benzoate 10 mg every 2 hours as needed will benefit the patient.

The requirement for acute abortive medications will significantly decrease with prophylactic therapy. The cost for this medication, absent insurance and at a moderate use, ranges from $400 to $3,900 per year, depending upon dosage and formulation.

- **Neuromodulation device:** The use of a non-invasive neuromodulation device is warranted at times for the patient depending on the post-traumatic headache's impact on the person's life. This device works to alter brain activity and provide both acute relief and aid in onset prevention without the potential side effects of pharmaceutical therapies.
- **Interventional headache/migraine management:** If the medical management does not provide relief as anticipated or fails to provide relief of an adequate nature, escalation will be warranted. An alternative would be onabotulinum toxin A injections to reduce the frequency and intensity of the person's post-traumatic headaches. Additionally, bilateral greater and lesser occipital nerve block under ultrasound guidance, as well as bilateral third occipital nerve block under fluoroscopy will greatly benefit patients with no relief from other alternative therapy options.

  - **33-point Botox injections:** Botox inhibits local neurogenic inflammation and inhibits central sensitization, thus relieving and therefore improving sharp and/or shooting pains in up to 88.9% of sufferers (Choi and Jeon, 2016, p. 7). Costs for this series of injections, absent insurance use, range from $2,000 to $9,000 per treatment.
  - **Greater/lesser occipital nerve block(s):** Nerve blocks, both greater and lesser, are well-accepted, long-utilized treatments for headaches of various types. When adhering to a standard protocol, studies have shown that relief is significant; the number of headaches reduced by 10.48–11.21 days, severity reduced by 3.1 on a ten-point scale, and duration more than halved (Inan et al., 2016). Costs for these procedures, absent insurance use, range from $5,000 to $10,000 per treatment.
  - **Surgical intervention:** If the occipital nerve blocks fail to provide adequate relief, then the person with post-traumatic headaches will be a candidate for the following for the treatment of occipital neuralgia:

    i. **Occipital nerve stimulation:** This surgical treatment involves the placement of electrodes under the skin near the occipital nerves. Costs for this procedure, inclusive of the pulse generator and requisite equipment, absent insurance, may vary widely, though a common range is from $120,000 to $200,000. Facility fees, recovery-related costs, and other miscellaneous charges are not included and should be accounted for separately.

- **Occipital nerve decompression/release:** During this surgical procedure, nerves from six compression points are released from entrapment or entanglement and freed to allow for decompression. This procedure has an 89.5% headache resolution rate (Cedars-Sinai, n.d.), with an additional 6.5% having significant enough relief that care was no longer warranted. Costs for this procedure for self-pay persons, excluding ancillary and facility costs, range from $7,500 to $14,000.

Summary

Post-traumatic headaches can be a major cause of disabilities for people with traumatic brain injuries. Tessler and Horn (2022) noted that of 452 acute consecutive patients admitted to inpatient rehabilitation services with traumatic brain injury, 71% of these patients reported headaches within the first year after moderate or severe traumatic brain injury, 46% of patients reported headaches at initial evaluation, and 44% of patients reported new or persistent headaches at one-year follow-up. Many patients after a traumatic brain injury experience post-traumatic headaches. These headaches can deter patients from a psychosocial perspective by withdrawing from social interaction as they return to their baseline activity in their rehabilitation programs. Up to 35% of post-traumatic headache patients do not return to work after three months (Tessler & Horn, 2022).

References

Al Khalili, Y., Ly, N., & Murphy, P. B. (2022). Cervicogenic headache. In *StatPearls*. StatPearls Publishing. Updated March 9, 2022. Retrieved January 2022, from www.ncbi.nlm.nih.gov/books/NBK507862/

Ashina, H., Porreca, F., Anderson, T., Amin, F. M., Ashina, M., Schytz, H. W., & Dodick, D. W. (2019, October 15). Post-traumatic headache: Epidemiology and pathophysiological insights. *Nature Reviews Neurology*, *10*, 607–617.

Cedars-Sinai. (n.d.). www.cedars-sinai.org/programs/occipital-neuralgia.html

Choi, I., & Jeon, S. R. (2016). Neuralgias of the head: Occipital neuralgia. *Journal of Korean Medical Science*, *31*(4), 479–488. https://doi.org/10.3346/jkms.2016.31.4.479

Defrin, R. (2014). Chronic post-traumatic headache: Clinical findings and possible mechanisms. *Journal of Manual & Manipulative Therapy*, *22*(1), 36–44. https://doi.org/10.1179/2042618613Y.0000000053

Headache Classification Committee of the International Headache Society (IHS). (2018). The international classification of headache disorders, 3rd edition. *Cephalalgia: An International Journal of Headache*, *38*(1), 1–211. https://doi-org.proxy.library.vcu.edu/10.1177/0333102417738202

Inan, N., Inan, L. E., Coşkun, Ö., Tunç, T., & Ilhan, M. (2016). Effectiveness of greater occipital nerve blocks in migraine prophylaxis. *Noro Psikiyatri Arsivi*, *53*(1), 45–48. https://doi.org/10.5152/npa.2015.10003

The International Headache Society. (2021). www.ichd-3.org/other-primary-headache-disorders/4-10-new-daily-persistent-headache-ndph/

Labastida-Ramírez, A., Benemei, S., Albanese, M., D'Amico, A., Grillo, G., Grosu, O., Ertem, D. H., Mecklenburg, J., Fedorova, E. P., Řehulka, P., di Cola, F. S., Lopez, J. T., Vashchenko, N., Maassen Van DenB rink, A., Martelletti, P., & European Headache Federation School of Advanced Studies (EHF-SAS). (2020). Persistent post-traumatic headache: A migrainous loop or not? The clinical evidence. *The Journal of Headache and Pain*, *21*(1), 55. https://doi-org.proxy.library.vcu.edu/10.1186/s10194-020-01122-5

Marcum, Z., & Hanlon, J. (2010). Recognizing the risks of chronic nonsteroidal anti-inflammatory drug use in older adults. *The Annals of Long-Term Care*, *18*(9), 24–27.

Ruschel, M. A. P., & De Jesus, O. (2022, January). Migraine headache. In *StatPearls*. StatPearls Publishing. Updated April 14, 2022. www.ncbi.nlm.nih.gov/books/NBK560787/

Tension Headaches: Symptoms, Causes, & Treatments. (n.d.). *Cleveland clinic*. Retrieved June 6, 2022, from https://my.clevelandclinic.org/health/diseases/8257-tension-type-headaches

Tessler, J., & Horn, L. J. (2022). Post-traumatic headache. In *StatPearls*. StatPearls Publishing. Updated January 14, 2022. Retrieved January 2022, from www.ncbi.nlm.nih.gov/books/NBK556134/

Zaremski, J. L., Herman, D. C., Clugston, J. R., Hurley, R. W., & Ahn, A. H. (2015). Occipital neuralgia as a sequela of sports concussion: A case series and review of the literature. *Current Sports Medicine Reports*, *14*(1), 16–19. https://doi.org/10.1249/JSR.0000000000000121

12 Traumatic Spinal Cord Injury

Stuart Kahn, Rachel Santiago, Michael Chiou, and Sofia Barchuk

Disorder (Disease) Description

Traumatic spinal cord injury (SCI) is a life-changing neurological condition with substantial socioeconomic implications for patients and their caregivers. It is considered to be a permanent condition, with very few people experiencing significant long-term recovery from disability (Winkler & Weed, 2004). There are more than 17,000 new cases of spinal cord injury each year in the United States, with an estimated prevalence of over 290,000 cases. The overall incidence varies from state to state given the population demographics, the definition of SCI, and data collection methodology (Kim et al., 2012). Research studies have reported as low as 29 cases per million to 60 cases per million. To note, this does not include those who died before hospital admission (Kim et al.).

Age of injury is also difficult to accurately estimate due to a lack of uniformity in categorizing reported age ranges (Kim et al., 2012). However, several trends can be deduced from current data. SCI seems to be the least prevalent in the pediatric population. It is the highest for individuals in their late teens and early twenties but declines with age (Kim et al.). The average age at injury has increased from 29 years during the 1970s to 43 years. There is a predilection toward the male gender with a male to female ratio of 4:1, which has stayed consistent over the years (Kim et al.). Though males experience SCI at higher rates, gender-specific annual incidence rates still vary from state to state (Kim et al.).

The etiology of injury is also state-specific and influenced by several important factors including gender, race, and ethnicity (Kim et al., 2012). Motor vehicle collisions remain the leading cause of SCI, but falls, acts of violence, and sports-related injuries tend to change in proportion depending on the patient demographics and location (Kim et al.). Other common causes include violence, primarily gunshot wounds, and recreational activities. Incomplete tetraplegia is the most common neurological category.

The total economic impact of SCI has been estimated to be $9.7 billion annually (Berkowitz, 1998). For individuals, the estimated average lifetime expense, including health care costs and living expenses, depends on the level of injury. In high tetraplegia (C1–C4) the average expense for the first year is estimated to be $1.1 million and an additional $190,000 with each subsequent year. In low tetraplegia (C5–C8) the average expense for the first year is estimated at $800,000 and an additional $120,000 each subsequent year. In paraplegic patients, the average expense for the first year is estimated at $500,000 and $72,000 each subsequent year (DeVivo et al., 2011).

DOI: 10.4324/b23293-12

Spinal Cord Anatomy

The vertebral column includes 7 cervical vertebrae, 12 thoracic vertebrae, and 5 lumbar vertebrae, followed by the sacrum and coccyx. The spinal cord is located behind the vertebral body. The spinal cord is an inner core of gray matter surrounded by white matter. The terminal portion of the spinal cord is the conus medullaris, which becomes the cauda equina at approximately the L2 vertebrae.

There are several important long tracts in the spinal cord:

- The dorsal columns (fasciculus gracilis/cuneatus) are responsible for proprioception, light touch, and vibration sense.
- The spinocerebellar tract conveys proprioceptive data from the spinal cord to the cerebellum.
- The lateral spinothalamic tract is responsible for pain and temperature sensation.
- The ventral spinothalamic tract is responsible for transmitting coarse touch and firm pressure.
- The lateral corticospinal tract is responsible for the control of voluntary movement.
- The anterior corticospinal tract is responsible for neck and trunk movements.

The dedicated blood supply to the spinal cord is as follows. Posterior spinal arteries provide blood to the posterior one-third of the spinal cord. Anterior spinal arteries supply blood flow to the anterior two-thirds of the spinal cord. Posterior and anterior spinal arteries arise directly or indirectly from the vertebral arteries. Radicular arteries, which are branches of local arteries, reinforce the posterior and anterior spinal arteries. The artery of Adamkiewicz is the lumbar radicular artery responsible for the lower anterior two-thirds of the spinal cord. It arises from an intersegmental branch of the descending aorta and joins with the anterior spinal artery in the lower thoracic region. The veins of the spinal cord drain to the internal venous plexus (see Figure 12.1).

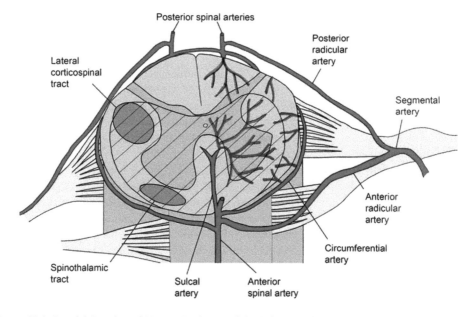

Figure 12.1 Arterial Supply and Venous Drainage of the Spinal Cord

Scales

ASIA Impairment Scale

The American Spinal Injury Association (ASIA)/International Standards for the Neurological Classification of Spinal Cord Injury (ISNCSCI) is a standard neurological examination incorporating sensory and motor components. It is used to determine the neurological level of injury and to qualify the completeness or incompleteness of the injury as measured by the ASIA Impairment Scale (AIS). Key sensory points of the dermatomes C2–S5 are tested bilaterally using a cotton tip applicator for light touch and either a neuro-tip or safety pin for pinprick. The patient's cheek is used as a normal frame of reference. Key motor functions of the myotomes C5–T1 and L2–S1 are tested bilaterally in a standardized fashion to grade muscle strength. The most recent revision of this scale was published in 2019. Figure 12.2 shows the most up-to-date version of the ASIA classification scale (see Figure 12.2).

Frankel Grade Classification

The Frankel Grade Classification provides an assessment of spinal cord function after traumatic SCI. A person's Frankel Grade can range from A (complete neurological injury) to E (normal motor function). The Frankel Grade Classification was introduced in 1969 and was replaced by the ASIA Impairment Scale in 1992.

Glasgow Coma Scale

The Glasgow Coma Scale (GCS) was developed in 1974 and is currently used to assess the level of consciousness in those with an acute traumatic brain injury (TBI) (www.glasgowcomascale.org/what-is-gcs/). It is based on the structured approach to evaluating motor functions, verbal responsiveness, and eye movements. A person's GCS score can range from 3 (unresponsive, coma, or death) to 15 (responsive), and is used to guide immediate medical care after a TBI as well as monitor the level of consciousness throughout hospitalization. It is important to note that GCS is not used for SCI assessment, but there are a number of patients with traumatic SCI that have co-occurring TBI, making it a valuable tool to evaluate for additional injuries (https://pubmed.ncbi.nlm.nih.gov/18586138/).

Modified Ashworth Scale

The modified Ashworth scale is a standardized measure for the evaluation of spasticity and is described as follows:

0: No increase in muscle tone
1: Slight increase in muscle tone with minimal resistance at the end range of motion
1+: Slight increase in muscle tone with minimal resistance throughout less than half the range of motion
2: Increase in muscle tone throughout most of the range of motion but the limb is easily moved
3: Increase in passive muscle tone with difficulty moving the limb
4: Affected limb is rigid in flexion or extension

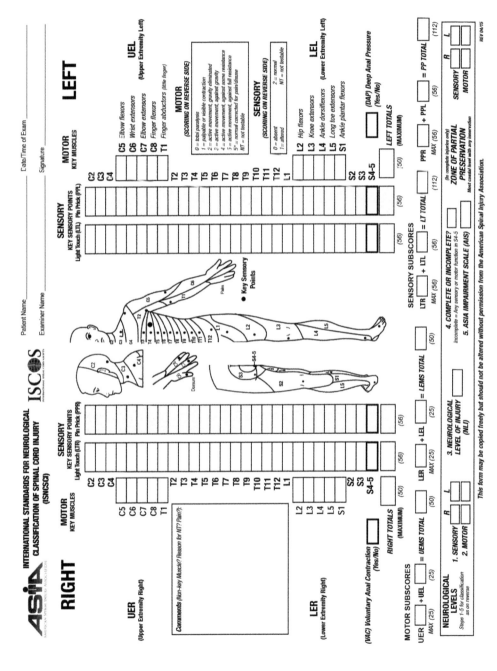

Figure 12.2 International Standards for Neurological Classification of Spinal Cord Injury

Acute and Potential Complications

Acute and potential complications of traumatic SCI can occur during the primary or secondary phase of injury (Vaikuntam et al., 2019), with acute decompensation being most common within the first 72 hours, requiring careful monitoring (Bonner & Smith, 2013). Primary injury takes place during the initial traumatic impact on the spine, which often causes fractures or dislocations of the corresponding vertebrae (Vaikuntam et al.). Secondary mechanisms of injury occur immediately after primary injury and can continue for weeks to months (Vaikuntam et al.). There are several different ways to classify the progression of SCI, but most commonly they can be divided into three phases: acute, sub-acute, and chronic (Vaikuntam et al.).

This section will focus on acute and sub-acute complications that arise after injury and include sequelae that develop as a result of vascular damage, ionic imbalances, inflammation, and ultimately cell death (Merritt et al., 2019). This time period also encompasses the acute hospitalization and acute rehabilitation period as well as long-term acute care and nursing home management. In what follows the sections are divided by organ system to better encompass the global impact that SCI has on the affected individual. This topic is very complex and goes beyond the scope of this chapter, but an overview is useful to understand the implications for life care planning. The average cost for the acute care to recovery phase is approximately $142,366, with the majority of charges covered by the patient's primary medical insurance (Merritt et al.).

Cardiovascular System

Spinal Shock

The cardiovascular system is impacted by traumatic SCI at the level of injury and below. The proportion of the spinal cord that directly affects the cardiac system spans from T1 to T7. Injuries at or above this level result in altered cardiovascular physiology (Winkler & Weed, 2004). It is important to note that altered blood pressure control tends to change over time following injury and can cause long-term morbidity in this patient population (Claydon et al., 2006). According to the National Spinal Cord Injury Statistical Center (NSCISC) hypertension, ischemic heart disease, and other heart diseases were included in the top five leading causes of death in the SCI population.

Shortly after injury, there is a state of hypoexcitability (Claydon et al., 2006). This is commonly known in the medical community as "spinal shock" in which patients present with flaccid paralysis, decreased or absent deep tendon reflexes (DTRs), and impairment of autonomic function (Claydon et al.). SCI leading to severely disrupted blood pressure control with resultant hypotension can cause "neurogenic shock" which often requires management in the intensive care unit (ICU) setting and can last anywhere from 24 hours to several weeks (Claydon et al.; Bonner & Smith, 2013). Acute care costs have been steadily increasing despite decreased lengths of stay in the hospital and are ultimately affected by the need for surgery, secondary medical complications, and in-hospital transfers, among other important variables (Vaikuntam et al., 2019).

Orthostatic Hypotension

After spinal shock resolves, which is commonly days to weeks post-injury, the patient can start to experience sudden drops in blood pressure during postural changes (Claydon et al., 2006). This phenomenon is called orthostatic hypotension and generally affects those with injuries at the T6 level or above (Winkler & Weed, 2004). During these episodes, the patient will experience dizziness, lightheadedness, or even syncopal events, which can interfere with physical and occupational therapies, thereby limiting participation in rehabilitation (Claydon et al.). Orthostatic hypotension can affect the acute phase of recovery, but it also has a profound impact on quality of life. Several studies also show low resting blood pressure in chronic SCI patients can even have an impact on overall cognitive performance (Claydon et al.; Jegede et al., 2010).

Conservative management for orthostatic hypotension usually includes a combination of different techniques to mitigate symptoms. Some common treatments include compression stockings, abdominal binders, reclining chairs, and elevated leg rests (Winkler & Weed, 2004). Physical therapy is geared toward progressive tilt table tolerance (Winkler & Weed). If conservative management fails, pharmaceutical agents can be added to the regimen including midodrine, Florinef, and/or salt tabs (Winkler & Weed). It is important to remember to review a patient's current medications and eliminate any that may be contributing to profound blood pressure drops.

Arrhythmias

SCI has the potential to affect the autonomic nervous system given the level of injury and completeness. Many different complications can develop in the cardiovascular system, and identifying at-risk individuals is extremely important to mitigate medical complications (Hector et al., 2013). Cardiac arrhythmias have the potential to develop due to unopposed parasympathetic control, leading to marked bradycardia and in severe cases asystole (Hector et al.; Winkler & Weed, 2004). If patients at risk for cardiac arrhythmias are identified early, then the need for aggressive pharmacological therapy and potential pacemaker placement can be considered to decrease morbidity and mortality in this unique subset of patients (Hector et al.; Winkler & Weed).

Autonomic Dysreflexia

Autonomic dysreflexia (AD) is a syndrome in which there is a sudden onset of excessively high blood pressure caused by a noxious stimulus below the level of injury (Winkler & Weed, 2004). This includes any painful, irritating, or strong stimulus (AAPMR). AD has an incidence of 48%–98% and it carries a mortality rate of 22% (Winkler & Weed; Chan et al., 2020; AAMPR; Murray & Knikou, 2019). This devastating and debilitating medical complication usually first occurs between 6 months and 1-year post-injury (AAPMR) and is most common in lesions T6 and above (Winkler & Weed, 2004). Although rare, some individuals with injuries at the T7 or T8 level develop AD as well (Winkler & Weed).

Common manifestations of AD include but are not limited to flushing/redness above the level of injury, general malaise, severe headache, elevated blood pressure, and increased/decreased heart rate (Winkler & Weed, 2004, AAMPR). It is important to keep in mind that patients with SCI usually have a lower resting blood pressure, so what is normotensive in fact may be hypertensive for the SCI patient (Winkler & Weed). If overlooked and improperly managed, AD can lead to life-threatening medical complications such as myocardial infarction, stroke, intracranial hemorrhage, hypertensive encephalopathy, seizure, and even death (Winkler & Weed).

Rehabilitation management focuses on lowering blood pressure and eliminating any noxious stimuli, but educating patients and staff on prevention is the ultimate goal (AAPMR). Common causes that are crucial to be addressed during an AD episode are distended bowel or bladder, occult fractures, decubitus ulcers, infections, gastric ulcers, cholelithiasis, improper positioning in a chair, or tight clothing (Winkler & Weed, 2004; PMR). AD also has the potential to greatly impact the well-being of the individual as well as their active participation in therapy programs during the rehabilitation period (Winkler & Weed).

Deep Venous Thrombosis

Deep venous thrombosis (DVT) and pulmonary embolism (PE) are severe complications that lead to prolonged hospitalizations, increased morbidity, and increased mortality in the SCI population (Mackiewicz-Milewska et al., 2016). The pathogenesis of DVT includes thrombogenesis due to activation of Virchow's triad, including blood stasis, hypercoagulability, and endothelial damage (Nanclares et al., 2019). It can also occur from immobilization after SCI leading to increased venous stasis as well as a decrease in antithrombin III and fibrinolysis in trauma patients (Nanclares et al.). Administering the correct DVT prophylaxis in the acute phase of injury is crucial when it comes to helping prevent clot formation.

The incidence of DVT ranges from 5.3% to 64% when correct prophylaxis is given and anywhere between 47% and 100% if prophylaxis is not given (Mackiewicz-Milewska et al., 2016). If a patient develops a DVT, hospital costs can rise as much as 35% (Winkler & Weed, 2004; Mackiewicz-Milewska et al.). The greatest risk for developing a DVT is within the acute phase of SCI, especially the first 3 months of injury. Of those who develop a DVT, recurrence is twice as likely compared with those who do not have a history of a DVT (Geerts et al., 2002). If an individual did not develop a DVT during the acute phase of injury, they have a 14%–20% risk of DVT at some point in time in their life.

Among major trauma patients, those with SCI have been shown to have the highest risk for the development of DVT (Geerts et al., 2002; Gould et al., 2012). Those at increased risk include paraplegia, motor complete, concomitant fractures of the lower extremities and pelvis, previous DVT, and absent or delayed thromboprophylaxis (Consortium Guidelines, third edition). Mechanical prophylaxis is recommended in the initial t2wo weeks post-injury, and thromboprophylaxis with low-molecular-weight heparin (LMWH) should be given up to 8 weeks post-injury if no active bleed is present (Consortium Guidelines, third edition). Once a DVT has developed, medical management changes and patients may require anticoagulation for up to 6 months to 1 year (Winkler & Weed, 2004). For a certain subset of individuals, lifetime anticoagulation may be recommended (Winkler & Weed).

Pulmonary System

Respiratory Failure

The development of respiratory complications is directly related to the level of injury and degree of motor completeness (Cardozo, 2007). It remains the leading cause of death in this vulnerable patient population (Cardozo). The greatest risk of pulmonary complications occurs within the first 2 years post-injury and includes pneumonia, respiratory failure, pulmonary edema, and thromboembolism (Schilero et al., 2018). There are a multitude of different reasons why the SCI population is at a greater risk for developing respiratory issues. Some of these include changes that occur as a direct result of injury and others as secondary complications.

SCI lesions at T12 and below virtually have no problems with the respiratory system, but as SCI injury rises, there is a progressive loss of respiratory mechanics and function. Lesions from

T12 to T5 alter abdominal motor and chest wall function that impairs cough. Individuals are also more prone to hypoxia because lung bases are less aerated (Winkler & Weed, 2004, Demos). SCI ranging from T5 to T1 affects the intercostal muscles, which impacts both inspiration and expiration (Winkler & Weed, 2004). The most detrimental lesions causing severe respiratory compromise include those affecting C3, C4, and C5 leading to diaphragm impairment, where individuals with C3-level injury virtually are all ventilator dependent (Winkler & Weed). Individuals with respiratory issues caused by SCI require a higher level of attendant care and frequent physician follow-ups (Winkler & Weed).

As mentioned previously there are temporal changes in pulmonary function following SCI (Schilero et al., 2018). Immediately after an injury to the cervical region, there is a decrease in vital capacity and expiratory flows (Schilero et al.). This can lead to the development of respiratory failure requiring ventilatory support (Schilero et al.). Improvement in respiratory function can be seen in the years post-injury, but based on level, SCI patients are still at an increased risk for respiratory issues later in life (Schilero et al.). Neuromuscular weakness exhibited in SCI is classically associated with spirometry testing demonstrating restrictive lung disease (Schilero et al.). Tetraplegic patients also show increased hyperactivity of the airways, which has been hypothesized to increase the risk of developing asthma and chronic obstructive pulmonary disease (COPD) (Schilero et al.). Other complications of the respiratory system include but are not limited to sleep apnea, mucus plugging, pneumonia, bronchiectasis, atelectasis, and an overall gradual increase in respiratory fatigue over time (Whiteneck & Jawad, 1993).

Respiratory failure and aspiration are the most common early respiratory compilations seen in the SCI population (Cardozo, 2007). It is most commonly seen in C1–C4 tetraplegic patients (Winkler & Weed, 2004; Cardozo). Studies have hypothesized that respiratory failure may be increased due to copious sputum during the first 6 days of injury and pneumonia (Cardozo). There are several mechanisms unique to the SCI population that can occur leading to increased risk for respiratory failure. Swelling of the spinal cord during high cervical SCI can compromise innervation to the diaphragm leading to altered function and weakness (Cardozo). There is also a decrease in lung compliance and surfactant production leading to an accumulation of secretions superimposed by a poor cough (Cardozo). These alterations can also lead to atelectasis causing impaired aeration and infection (7). Close care must be taken with those who have a vital capacity of less than 15 mL/kg of ideal body weight when attempting to wean from the ventilator (Winkler & Weed; Cardozo). A thorough workup must be done before extubation attempts to eliminate any secondary complications that could affect successful ventilator liberation.

Upper Respiratory Tract Infections and Pneumonia

Upper respiratory tract infections (URIs) and pneumonia are expected to occur at a greater frequency in the SCI population (Winkler & Weed, 2004). It has been documented that 80% of deaths in patients hospitalized from cervical spinal injury are due to pulmonary dysfunction, with pneumonia being the cause in 50% of the cases (Cardozo, 2007). The number of respiratory infections is directly related to the acute care hospital length of stay and overall cost of hospitalization (Cardozo). The prevention of respiratory complications needs to be the immediate priority, with the implementation of a high level of attendant care and frequent physician visits depending on the level of injury and risk for the development of secondary complications (Winkler & Weed; Cardozo).

Many tools can be implemented to prevent and treat respiratory complications associated with SCI. Tetraplegic patients should receive annual influenza vaccinations as well as pneumococcal (Winkler & Weed, 2004). Depending on the level of injury, a variety of equipment may be needed to help sustain life. This includes ventilators, respiratory monitors, suctioning equipment, and pulse oximetry (Winkler & Weed). Emergency equipment may also be a necessity such as backup ventilators, a home generator system, and an Ambu bag (Winkler & Weed). Additional resources include abdominal binders, mechanical insufflation-exsufflation, high chest wall oscillation, incentive spirometry, and abdominal weights (Winkler & Weed).

Urogenital and Renal System

Neurogenic Bladder

In SCI, there is impairment of the normal bladder mechanism that prevents vesicoureteral reflux. If vesicoureteral reflux occurs, increased bladder pressure may result in subsequent hydronephrosis of the kidneys. Thus, routine urodynamic studies and annual renal ultrasounds are used to assess bladder function and screen for hydronephrosis, respectively.

Integumentary System

Pressure Injury

Pressure ulcers are the most common skin complication in SCI and are a significant cause of immobility in this patient population (Whiteneck & Jawad, 1993). It has been reported that most SCI patients will have at least one decubitus ulcer (Winkler & Weed, 2004). According to the 2019 NSCISC, among post-injury year 1 participants, 25% reported the occurrence of pressure ulcers since discharge from rehabilitation. The prevalence has also increased over the post-injury years from 36.2% to 40% (DeVivo et al., 2002). The exact mechanism of pressure ulcer formation is not completely understood, but it is speculated that they develop due to compression and shearing forces leading to tissue breakdown.

Research has shown after SCI an increased collagen metabolism, a higher ratio of weaker type III collagen to type I collagen, a decrease in adrenergic receptor density, atrophy of protective muscles, and reduced cutaneous blood flow below the level of injury all contribute to pressure injury formation. Classification of pressure injuries according to the National Pressure Ulcer Advisory Panel are as follows. Stage I includes diagnosis of non-blanchable erythema. Stage II is described as a shallow, open ulcer with a red-pink wound bed. Stage III is full-thickness tissue loss with visible subcutaneous fat, and stage IV is full-thickness tissue loss with exposed muscle or bone.

Those who develop pressure sores require a higher level of attendant care and increased physician follow-up. The focus is on prevention. Pressure release techniques should be taught to the patient and home attendant (Whiteneck & Jawad, 1993). Cushions can be used to help prevent ulcer formation but should be highly customized to fit the individual's specific needs (Whiteneck & Jawad). SCI patients at risk for pressure ulcers may also need a specialty bed such as a minimal air-loss bed or air fluidized bed (Whiteneck & Jawad). Acute management for decubitus ulcers can include additional hospitalizations with antibiotic therapy treatment, wound debridement, and/or surgical management.

Chronic Phase Complications

Over the years, a model of how aging may affect the total function of individuals with SCI has developed (Whiteneck & Jawad, 1993). There are three phases following SCI, which include the acute restoration phase, maintenance phase, and decline. The maintenance phase ranges anywhere from around 2 to 18 years.

The most common chronic phase complications are more broadly covered in the treatment section because once a patient is fortunate enough to live through the acute phase of SCI, there is more of a continuum of care that makes up the chronic phase rather than just moving into what one would call the chronic phase. The major issues in the chronic phase include many of the issues already covered in the acute phase but are the cardiovascular system with both chronic and recurrent DVTs and PEs, the pulmonary system, the gastrointestinal system, the genitourinary system, skeletal conditions including too much bone-like heterotopic ossification or too little bone-like osteoporosis and osteopenia with pathologic fractures, the musculotendinous system with overuse injuries, progression of the SCI like in syringomyelia, progression of disability with any or all of the earlier conditions and/or just the aging process, and the integumentary system with a continued and repeated pressure injury. All of these will be expanded upon in the treatment section.

Functional Disabilities

Cervical (C1–C3) Complete. Persons with cervical SCI above the neurologic level of C5 have impairment in the movement of the head, neck, and muscles of respiration, creating a dependence on mechanical ventilation for respiration. Impairment in swallowing and inability to clear secretions is common. Impairment in verbal communication leads to disability in communication. Persons will require full assistance for transfers and turning in bed to prevent pressure injury and full assistance for all self-care and activities of daily living (ADLs) including bowel and bladder management. They will be non-ambulatory and require a power wheelchair for household and community ambulation. They require 24-hour attendant care to assist with these impairments and disabilities. Those who are ventilator dependent must have someone available to respond to alarms 24 hours per day.

Cervical (C4) Complete. Persons with a complete C4 neurological level of injury will have partial preservation of the upper trapezius, diaphragm, and cervical paraspinal muscles. They will require assistance with respiration and may or may not be able to breathe without the assistance of a ventilator. They require total assistance with bed mobility, wheelchair/bed transfers, pressure relief and positioning, and ADLs including bowel and bladder programs. For mobility, persons require a power wheelchair. They require 24-hour attendant care to assist with impairments and disabilities.

Cervical (C5) Complete. Persons with a complete C5 neurological level of injury will have partial preservation of upper extremity muscles including the deltoid, biceps, brachialis, brachioradialis, and serratus anterior. They will require total assistance with bowel and bladder programs, bed and wheelchair transfers, bathing, upper and lower body dressing, and homemaking tasks. They may require some assistance with respiratory secretion management. Total assistance is required to set up for eating, then it is possible for independent eating with appropriate equipment. They are expected to require up to 10 hours per day for personal care and 6 hours per day for home care.

Cervical (C6) Complete. Persons with a complete C6 level of injury are expected to have innervation of the previously mentioned muscles and partial innervation of the radial extensors and forearm supinators. Impairments are expected in wrist flexion, elbow extension, hand movement, and total paralysis of the trunk and lower extremities. Expected disabilities include partial to total assistance in bowel and bladder management, uneven bed/wheelchair transfers, and lower body dressing. Partial assistance is expected for bed mobility, eating, grooming, bathing, and homemaking tasks. They are expected to require up to 6 hours/day of personal care and 4 hours/day of home care.

Cervical (C7–C8) Complete. Persons with a complete C7–C8 level of injury are expected to have innervation of the previously mentioned muscles in addition to partial innervation of elbow extensors, wrist extensors, wrist flexors, and thumb and finger flexors/extensors. Impairments include paralysis of the trunk and lower extremities, handgrip, and hand dexterity. Expected disabilities include requiring partial assistance with bowel and bladder program management, bed mobility, bed/wheelchair transfers, bathing, community wheelchair mobility, transportation, and homemaking tasks. They are expected to require up to 6 hours/day of personal care and 2 hours/day of home care.

Thoracic (T1–T9) Complete. Persons with a complete T1–T9 level of injury are expected to have innervation of the upper extremities with partial innervation of the trunk. Impairments decrease endurance due to partial innervation of muscles of respiration and total paralysis of the lower extremities. Typically, they are unable to stand independently and may require assistance with housekeeping tasks that include heavy lifting such as laundry and moving objects around the home. They are expected to require up to 3 hours/day of home care.

Thoracolumbar (T10–L1) Complete. Persons with a complete T10–L1 level of injury are expected to have complete paralysis of the lower extremities. For independent transportation, they may require a car equipped with hand controls based on their lower extremity impairment. They will require assistance with tasks that involve heavy lifting. They are expected to require up to 2 hours/day of home care.

Lumbosacral (L2–S5) Complete. Persons with a complete L2–S5 level of injury are expected to have partial paralysis of the lower extremities. They may be partial household and community ambulators with assistance from crutches of knee-ankle-foot orthosis versus a wheelchair for long-distance community ambulation.

Psychosocial Disabilities

Anxiety and Depression

The large and permanent impact SCI has on the reduction of function may require larger psychosocial adaptation compared to chronic disease, with a smaller impact on physical functioning. The negative psychosocial impact stemming from the reduction of future expectations causes the incidence of depressive disorders to be up to five times as high in adults with SCI compared to the general population (Kemp, 2002). Other studies have suggested the high incidence of chronic pain in patients with SCI correlates with higher rates of anxiety and depressive disorders (Lim et al., 2017).

Family and Relationships

Sexual and marital relationships will also be affected after SCI. The disability's impact on family dynamics must be considered. The divorce rate after SCI is noted to be up to twice as high compared to the general population (Berkowitz et al., 1998). Mental health resources for spouses and family are to be considered during the readjustment period after an SCI. Access to support groups and patient-family education should be emphasized (Lynch & Cahalan, 2017).

Suicide

The rate of suicide is two to six times higher in those with SCI compared to the general population in the United States (Cao et al., 2014). Major identified risk factors for suicidal behavior in the SCI population are previous psychiatric diagnosis and severe chronic pain (DeVivo et al., 2002; Ahuja et al., 2017). Those with SCI should be assessed and provided mental health resources and intervention as needed.

Caregiver Burden

The rate of caregiver burden is high for those supporting individuals with SCI. Several studies have found that the majority of caregivers experience some degree of burden, with no caregivers endorsing little to no burden (Castellano-Tejedor, 2017). Symptoms of caregiver burden that have been described include burnout, high levels of stress, fatigue, and resentment. There are also time constraints from social and vocational opportunities for caregivers that may affect marital relationships and overall quality of life. The degree of caregiver burden can be alleviated by the assistance from home attendants to help with ADLs. It is also recommended caregivers be supplied with tools and coping strategies to manage these stressors.

Rehabilitation Potential (Expected Level of Improvement)

The overall level of the expected recovery of an SCI decreases as the severity of the neurological injury increases. For persons diagnosed with a complete level of injury, approximately 10%–15% will convert to an incomplete level of injury. For persons with an initial grade of an incomplete lesion, approximately one-third of AIS B will convert to AIS C, and up to two-thirds with an initial grade of AIS C will convert to AIS D or E. It should be noted that very few persons will improve to normal neurological levels. Prediction models have identified persons with greater levels of improvement in functional status to have less severe initial AIS grades and AIS motor scores of greater than 50 years old at the time of injury. Poor prognostic factors for improvement in functional recovery include older age and spinal cord edema or hemorrhage identified on magnetic resonance imaging. Approximately 80%–90% of complete level injuries, as measured in neurologic assessment in the first week of injury, will remain complete injuries. The following is a review of functional loss at varying spinal levels and the treatment that may be applied to restore some function loss:

1. C1–C3: Using phrenic nerve pacer and/or ventilator to assist with breathing.
2. C3–C4: Patients may be candidates for nerve transfer to improve upper extremity function.
3. C5–C6: May improve the ability to grab objects and improve the function of the triceps muscle. With assistance may independently eat, drink, and groom themself. Assistive devices may aid in self-direct transfers.
4. Persons with a C6 level of neurologic level of injury may be able to independently provide pressure relief and skin checks.
5. C7–C8: Can improve the ability to grasp objects and target fine finger movements.
6. T1: Potential to grab objects and perform natural hand movements.
7. T2–T9: May be candidates for nerve transfer to improve sensation to the lower extremity. May be a candidate for a spinal cord stimulator to improve lower extremity function. Expected for patients to be independent in basic ADLs, bowel and bladder function, and transfers. Expected to be independent with a wheelchair for mobility. Patients should be able to stand using a frame, tilt table, or standing wheelchair for exercise purposes.

8. T10–T12: Patients are expected to be independent in basic ADLs, bowel and bladder function, and transfers. Patients may rarely be household ambulators with orthoses. (It is this
author's opinion that household ambulation is difficult to achieve, and more likely ambulation is used as a therapeutic exercise with maximum assistance.) Persons can potentially
ambulate outdoors.

9. L1–L2: Patients are expected to be independent in basic ADLs, bowel and bladder function,
and transfers. May be a candidate for nerve transfer to facilitate hip extension to improve
community ambulation. Patients may sometimes be household ambulators with orthoses.

10. L3–L4: Patients are expected to be independent in basic ADLs, bowel and bladder function,
and transfers. May be a candidate for nerve transfer to facilitate knee extension to improve
community ambulation.

11. L5–S1: Patients are expected to be independent in basic ADLs, bowel and bladder function,
and transfers. May be a candidate for nerve or tendon transfer to facilitate ankle stability
and community ambulation.

Evaluation Standards

Acute Phase

Evaluation of an individual with SCI during the acute phase of injury includes initial medical
and neurologic stabilization as well as evaluation and maintenance of spinal stability. During the
acute phase of injury, hemodynamic stability must be monitored in the inpatient setting.

Post-Acute Phase: Inpatient Rehabilitation

Once the patient has been stabilized and reached a stable neurologic level, evaluation includes
defining the spinal cord level as noted earlier, assessing the patient for spasticity, bowel-
bladder function, and other SCI complications as described previously. Creating a treatment
plan for cardiovascular needs, neurologic complications such as autonomic dysreflexia, neurogenic bowel and bladder, and insensate skin are key components of the rehabilitation phase.
The rehabilitation program also includes evaluation of respiratory abilities and pulmonary
toileting, DVT prevention, psychosocial assessment, and functional goal assessment and
management.

Scales used to assess functional status include the functional independence measure (FIM)
score. The FIM is an 18-item measurement system that rates tasks on a 7-point ordinal scale
ranging from total assistance to complete independence. The items assessed include eating,
grooming, bathing, upper body dressing, lower body dressing, toileting, bladder management,
bowel management, toilet transfer, shower transfer, locomotion, stairs, cognitive comprehension, expression, social interaction, problem-solving, and memory. The Berg balance scale is a
14-item assessment used to determine the ability or inability to balance. This may be used during physiotherapy assessments when assessing functional ability.

Maintenance

Maintenance involves routine follow-up with a physiatrist to manage short- and long-term complications of SCI as discussed in the acute and potential complications section earlier as well as
the treatment section that follows.

Treatment and Medical Management

Acute Phase

The acute phase of treatment focuses on the basic resuscitation of a patient after injury by first responders. During the initial presentation, the medical team will assess and maintain the airway and ensure the patient is hemodynamically stable. Cervical spine injury often requires emergent intubation and should be performed carefully in the setting of suspected spinal trauma to avoid secondary SCI. Spinal shock occurs hours to days after spinal injury and presents as depression of voluntary movement and spinal reflexes below the level of injury. Neurogenic shock may also occur secondary to disruption of the sympathetic nervous system below the level of injury, usually T6 or below, and results in hypotension and bradycardia. If hemodynamically unstable, these injuries are treated with volume resuscitation and inotropic medications if needed to maintain a mean arterial pressure greater than 85 mmHg.

Spinal stability secondary to fracture and/or ligamentous injury will be assessed, and if there is spinal instability, this will be assessed and treated by a neurosurgery team. There are improved neurologic outcomes in patients who undergo surgical decompression within 24 hours (Fehlings et al., 2012). In the case of SCI secondary to trauma, concomitant brain injury, organ damage, and skeletal damage/fracture must be surveyed and treated.

Rehabilitation Phase

In the rehabilitation phase treatment is focused on optimizing recovery and providing specialty services including spasticity management, upper extremity restoration, wheelchair evaluation, gait training, diaphragmatic pacing, assistive technology, sexuality and fertility management, neurogenic bladder and bowel management, community re-entry and recreation therapy, family support, and patient and family education.

Cardiovascular System

Orthostatic hypotension is defined by a decrease in systolic blood pressure of 20 mmHg and a decrease in diastolic blood pressure of 10 mmHg when changing position from supine to upright. Signs and symptoms of orthostatic hypotension include lightheadedness, dizziness, feeling faint, blurred vision, fatigue, and syncope. Treatments include non-pharmacological and pharmacologic interventions, with the goal of treatment being to decrease excessive venous pooling in the lower extremities that leads to decreased stroke volume and cardiac output. Ineffective treatment of orthostatic hypotension will limit a person's ability to participate in a therapy program and time spent interacting with the community. Modality treatments for orthostatic hypotension include compression hose, abdominal binders, reclining chair, elevated leg rest, and progressive elevation on a tilt table with a physical therapist monitoring table function and patient tolerance. The medications prescribed for orthostatic hypotension include ephedrine, tyramine, Florinef, ergotamine, and Proamatine (midodrine).

Autonomic dysreflexia is defined as a sudden increase in systolic and diastolic blood pressure of 20–40 mmHg. Treatment includes having a personal attendant nearby to recognize symptoms, sit the person upright, loosen clothing, irrigate or catheterize the person, and assess for fecal impaction. If the cause/noxious stimulus is not identified and the blood pressure remains elevated, the person may need to be admitted to the hospital for management of blood pressure. Treatment for autonomic dysreflexia includes antihypertensives with rapid onset and short duration such as nifedipine and nitroglycerin ointment. If a person has taken sildenafil in the past 24 hours, an alternative antihypertensive such as prazosin or captopril may be used.

Pulmonary System

SCI leads to impairment in the muscles of the respiratory system, and respiratory complications are a major cause of morbidity and mortality in this population. Patients with high levels are at high risk for pneumonia. Treatment for pneumonia may be continued from the acute hospitalization or may be initiated in the acute rehabilitation setting. Treatment for pneumonia includes antibiotics, updraft agents, theophylline, mucolytic drugs, and beta inhalers. For long-term prevention, tetraplegics should receive an annual influenza vaccine and pneumococcal vaccine that should be initiated in the acute rehabilitation setting.

Respiratory muscle strength training in rehabilitation is effective in increasing respiratory muscle strength for patients with cervical SCI (Berlowitz & Tamplin, 2013). Further treatment for the prevention of pneumonia and atelectasis includes manual assisted coughing, insufflation-exsufflation treatment, intermittent positive pressure breathing (IPPB), chest physiotherapy, continuous positive airway pressure (CPAP), and bilevel positive airway pressure (BiPAP). If mucus plugging persists despite these interventions and becomes severe, a bronchoscopy may be indicated to clear the airway of secretions.

Medical Management

Long-acting and short-acting beta-agonists are used to reduce respiratory complications in tetraplegics and lower-level injuries prone to respiratory complications. These medications provide bronchodilation, reduce atelectasis, and improve forced expiratory volume in 1 second (FEV_1) (Spungen et al., 1993). Mucolytics such as nebulized sodium bicarbonate or acetylcysteine may mobilize secretions. Hydrating agents such as nebulized sodium chloride may also be used to mobilize secretions. Indications for mechanical ventilation include respiratory failure or intractable atelectasis.

Phrenic nerve pacer. Optimization and placement of a phrenic pacer may occur in the acute rehabilitation setting and is indicated for patients with diaphragmatic impairment. The benefits of a phrenic pacer are improved speech and smell, ease of transfer and mobility, reduced respiratory infections, reduced secretions, and possible decannulation (Sweis & Biller, 2017). The high-level spinal cord equipment includes a home ventilator, respiratory monitor, suctioning equipment, pulse oximeter, backup ventilator, home generator system, and Ambu bag.

Gastrointestinal System

The treatment for neurogenic bowel is dependent on if there is reflexive or areflexic bowel. Upper motor neuron (reflexive bowel) is defined as increased colonic wall tone and loss of voluntary control of the external anal sphincter, causing it to remain tight/closed. Stool evacuation occurs via reflex activity by stimulus into the rectum. Lower motor neuron (areflexic bowel) is defined as loss of colonic wall peristalsis causing decreased stool propulsion and decreased tone of the external anal sphincter.

Medical Management

Glycerin and bisacodyl are commonly used active ingredients in suppositories for bowel care. Potential surgical treatment includes placement of a stoma. The decision for placement of a colostomy/ileostomy is made on a patient-case basis and dependent on the individual's goals of care. Chronic constipation is a common chronic condition in SCI. Treatment includes counseling on an adequate diet with proper fiber and fluid intake as well as an appropriate daily activity. If not improved with these recommendations, a trial of laxative agents is necessary, including osmotic agents, lubricants, and enemas.

Equipment. Bathroom equipment includes bowel care/shower chairs, benches, raised commode seats, and standard toilet seats with padding. Those without adequate hand functioning may require gloving, digital bowel stimulator, or suppository inserter. Mechanical lifts and or/ transfer boards may be necessary for bathroom transfers. Patients with severe spasticity may require safety straps on the previously mentioned equipment as well to prevent falls.

Urogenital and Renal System

Neurogenic bladder is a disorder of bladder storage and emptying that may cause complications in the upper and lower urinary tract. The goals when designing a treatment program for neurogenic bladder are to preserve the upper urinary tract, reduce complications such as infection, and preserve lifestyle.

Intermittent Catheterization

For patients with intact hand function, intermittent catheterization should be considered. Intermittent catheterization should be avoided in persons with abnormal urethral anatomy, bladder capacity less than 200 mL, poor cognition, and unwillingness to catheterize. Failure to self-catheterize routinely throughout the day (four to six times daily) may lead to bladder overdistension and lead to urinary complications from high bladder pressure. Potential complications of intermittent catheterization include urinary tract infections, bladder overdistension, urinary incontinence, urethral trauma, urethral false passage, urethral stricture, autonomic dysreflexia, and bladder stones. If persons are planning to travel where toilet facilities are not available, a touchless catheter with a collection device is an alternative to an intermittent catheter.

Indwelling Catheterization

An indwelling catheter is a method of bladder management where a catheter is inserted into the bladder and connected to a storage device for an extended period of time. An indwelling catheter may be urethral or suprapubic. Indwelling urethral catheters are replaced every 2–4 weeks by the person or by a caregiver. The risk of catheter encrustation or blockage increases the longer a catheter is left in place. For persons with a history of bladder stone or catheter blockage, the indwelling urethral catheter should be exchanged more frequently, every 1–2 weeks. A 14–16 French catheter is generally recommended.

Indwelling suprapubic catheters are inserted by a specialized physician or health care provider. After successful insertion, the catheter is exchanged every 4 weeks by a trained caregiver. For persons with a history of catheter encrustation or blockage, the catheter should be exchanged every 1–2 weeks. Suprapubic tubes must be replaced immediately upon removal or the bladder tract/stoma will close. Renacidin is an irrigation solution for use within the lower urinary tract for the dissolution of bladder calculi and prevention of urethral encrustations.

Equipment

A catheter belt or device is required to secure an indwelling suprapubic or urethral catheter to the leg or abdomen. Equipment for indwelling catheters includes urinary collection devices or drainage bags. A leg bag is worn during the day and can be concealed under clothing. A night drainage bag is a larger leg bag that can collect all urine that drains from the bladder overnight. Catheter tips may irritate the bladder causing discomfort, urinary leakage, or triggering autonomic dysreflexia. In this case, anticholinergic medication such as oxybutynin may be prescribed to prevent involuntary detrusor contractions. Male patients with reduced hand function who wish to catheterize independently may benefit from an eagle board to achieve independent self-catheterization.

Detrusor Sphincter Dyssynergia

Alpha-adrenergic blockers are used to lower urethral resistance and improve voiding in persons with detrusor sphincter dyssynergia and low bladder pressure. Transurethral, transperineal, or bladder wall botulinum toxin may also be used to treat detrusor sphincter dyssynergia. Botulinum toxin injections lose effectiveness after 3–6 months due to nerve resprouting, and there is no limit to the number of injections that may be required to maintain effectiveness. Botulinum toxin injection is performed under cystoscope guidance by a specialized physician.

Surgical Management

A urethral stent is an option for persons with detrusor sphincter dyssynergia. It may be considered for those who do not have hand skills or a caregiver to provide intermittent catheterization, have a history of autonomic dysreflexia, or failed/have an intolerance to oral medications. For consideration of a urethral stent, the candidate must be able to put and keep in place a condom/external urinary catheter. Follow-up is recommended every 6 months after placement to monitor for obstruction (Seoane-Rodríguez et al., 2007).

Transurethral sphincterotomy (TURS) involves transurethral resection of the external urethral sphincter. After TURS the person will experience urinary incontinence managed with an external catheter connected to a leg bag requiring changing once per day. This reduces caregiver time and increases the independence of the person.

Electrical stimulation of the sacral parasympathetic nerves involves surgically implanting electrodes on the sacral nerve roots that attach to a stimulator implanted in the abdomen or chest. This procedure is combined with a rhizotomy to reduce reflex incontinence and increase bladder capacity. This method of neurogenic bladder treatment may reduce urologic complications and the long-term costs of bladder management.

Bladder augmentation is a surgical procedure that increases bladder capacity by augmenting the bladder with intestinal segments. As a result, bladder volume pressure is decreased and urinary continence is restored. This surgical option may be considered for women who are unable to use an external collecting catheter required for the surgical procedures described earlier.

Integumentary System

Treatment for pressure injury includes adequate seating and positioning. A pressure-redistribution bed is indicated in persons at risk or who have pressure injury. A high air-loss (air fluidized) support bed is indicated for those who have pressure injury on multiple turning surfaces or a recent skin graft. For patients unable to independently provide pressure relief while in a wheelchair, a power weight-shifting wheelchair is indicated. For persons with a pressure injury, sitting time should be limited and a gel or air surface should be used at all times when sitting. Standing wheelchairs can assist those with pelvic pressure injuries remobilize. For protection during ADLs, a padded toilet seat and bathing equipment should be ordered as well as padding and skin protection devices for recreational equipment and all wheelchairs. Deep stage III and stage IV pressure injury may require surgical referral for reconstruction.

Musculoskeletal System

Treatment for spasticity includes a full range of motion to all involved joints at least twice a day with prolonged terminal stretch by a personal attendant or therapist. Treatments for spasticity not improved with stretching include baclofen, Dantrium, and Valium. For spasticity refractory to oral medications, botulinum toxin injection and intrathecal baclofen pump can be considered.

Heterotopic ossification treatment includes early recognition using an x-ray or dual energy x-ray absorptiometry (DEXA) scan of the hip. Bisphosphonates are the first-line therapy treatment. Radiation therapy and surgical management may be considered for severe restriction of range of motion that interferes with ADLs.

Post-Rehabilitation Follow-Up

Cardiometabolic: The rate of cardiovascular disease is elevated in persons with SCI. This is likely related to the sedentary lifestyle many with SCI have due to decreased function, elevating the risk factors for the cardiometabolic disorder. When other risk factors are controlled, SCI patients are twice as likely to develop coronary artery disease (CAD) (Duckworth et al., 1983) have pointed to the leading cause of death for persons with incomplete SCI as ischemic heart disease. Patients should be screened for obesity, hypertension, prediabetes, and diabetes annually.

Recommendations for dyslipidemia include routine surveillance at a minimum of every 3 years in asymptomatic adults with SCI. For persons with risk factors present or dyslipidemia, annual screening is recommended. Treatment of dyslipidemia should include at a minimum a moderate-intensity statin.

Recommendations for prediabetes and diabetes screening includes testing at a minimum every 3 years if tests are normal. Testing follows the American Diabetes Association guidelines for monitoring A1C or fasting plasma glucose. Metformin is the primary pharmacotherapy treatment unless it is contraindicated or not tolerated by the patient. Persons may require referral to an endocrinology specialist.

Physician surveillance should include lifestyle interventions such as nutrition and physical activity assessment and recommendations. It is recommended that persons with SCI participate in a minimum of 150 minutes of physical exercise per week. To meet this recommendation, they may be provided with motorized training equipment based on their functional ability. Exercise is beneficial to restore high-density lipoprotein (HDL) and low-density lipoprotein (LDL) ratios.

Potential Complications

Sexual Dysfunction

Male erectile and ejaculatory functions are complex physiologic activities that require interaction between vascular, nervous, and endocrine systems. Whereas erections are controlled by the parasympathetic nervous system, ejaculations are controlled by the sympathetic nervous system. Men with SCI may obtain reflexogenic or psychogenic erections. The former can occur independently of conscious awareness and supraspinal input and is secondary to manual stimulation of the genital region. The latter is secondary to cortical modulation of the sacral reflex arc—the brain interprets erotic stimuli. In general, erections are more likely with incomplete lesions (both upper motor neuron [UMN] and lower motor neuron [LMN]) than complete lesions. Many times, men with SCI can only maintain an erection while the penis is stimulated, and the quality of the erection is insufficient for sexual satisfaction. As such, the erection must be augmented or induced. Methods to induce erections include oral therapy (e.g., sildenafil, tadalafil), intracavernosal injection therapy (e.g., papaverine, alprostadil, phentolamine), penile vacuum device, transurethral devices (e.g., alprostadil), and/or penile implants. The ability to ejaculate is less than the ability to obtain an erection.

The rate of ejaculation varies depending on the location and nature of the neurologic injury:

- Complete UMN lesions: ejaculation rate is estimated at 2%
- Incomplete UMN lesions: ejaculation rate is estimated at 32%
- Complete LMN lesions: ejaculation rate is estimated at 18%
- Incomplete LMN lesions: ejaculation rate is estimated at 70%

Methods to induce ejaculation include:

- Intrathecal neostigmine
- Subcutaneous physostigmine
- Direct aspiration of sperm from vas deferens
- Vibratory stimulation—can be used at home
- Electroejaculation: most popular in the United States

Heterotopic Ossification

Heterotopic ossification (HO) is the formation of bone in the soft tissue surrounding peripheral joints. HO can range from mild disease, defined as an incidental finding on radiographs, to severe disease, causing a significant reduction in the range of motion at the joint. Severe disease is present in up to 20%–30% of patients with SCI and can impair the ability to perform ADLs such as dressing, bathing, and transfers. Loss of range of motion may also cause pressure sores and pain secondary to an inadequate sitting position. HO is most often diagnosed between 1 and 6 months of injury. The gold standard for diagnosis is a three-phase 99m technetium bone scan, which can detect HO up to 2 weeks after SCI. Bisphosphonates and non-steroidal anti-inflammatory drugs (NSAIDs) have been shown to slow the progression of HO when used in the early phase of bone formation. Surgical resection of HO is a treatment option for severe disease interfering with the ability to achieve adequate positioning. Complications of surgery include fracture, infection, and hemorrhage with a high recurrence rate.

Osteoporosis/Osteoporotic Fracture

Osteoporosis is defined as a systemic disorder of the skeleton characterized by reduced bone mass and deterioration of the skeletal microarchitecture. Normal bone architecture is dependent on daily weight-bearing exercises to maintain the bone remodeling process. The loss of mobility in SCI predisposes to diffuse osteopenia and/or osteoporosis, and decreased bone formation may be seen in the first 2 weeks after injury. The DEXA scan is the gold standard for evaluating bone mineral density and the diagnosis of osteoporosis. Laboratory testing should include 25 hydroxyvitamin D, thyroid-stimulating hormone, parathyroid hormone, free testosterone (males), calcium, alkaline phosphatase, phosphorus, albumin, and creatinine. Treatments include weight-bearing exercises to induce mechanical loading on the bone. This can be achieved with body weight–supported treadmill training and tilt table standing in conjunction with a physical therapist. Medications for the prevention of osteoporosis and osteoporotic fracture include supplementation with calcium and vitamin D. Denosumab, a monoclonal antibody, has recently been found to increase bone mineral density in the SCI population (Varacallo et al., 2021).

Overuse Injuries

Chronic microtraumatic injuries interfere with the ability of the tissue to repair itself and may lead to the deposition of scar tissue in place of bone, muscle, or ligament. Upper extremity overuse injuries in the SCI population are common due to the reliance of the upper extremities for ambulation via wheelchair as well as ADLs. Shoulder injuries and pain are the most common and include impingement syndrome, rotator cuff tendonitis, bicipital tendonitis, and labral injuries. Diagnosis includes clinical evaluation by a physician as well as ultrasound, magnetic resonance imaging (MRI), and arthrography. Treatment may include a physiotherapy exercise program tailored to the injury, corticosteroid injection to the affected area, or surgical reconstruction if severe and failed conservative management.

Injuries at the elbow and the wrist may include lateral epicondylitis, ulnar neuropathy at the elbow, De Quervain's tenosynovitis, and carpal tunnel syndrome. Diagnosis includes radiographic imaging, ultrasound imaging, and/or MRI. Treatment may include a physiotherapy exercise program tailored to the injury, corticosteroid injection to the affected area, or surgical reconstruction if severe and failed conservative management.

Syringomyelia

Syringomyelia, also known as a syrinx, is defined as the development of a fluid-filled cyst within the gray matter of the spinal cord. The development of this syrinx within the spinal canal may cause progressive weakness, pain, and/or spasticity. This complication of SCI may occur in both paraplegic and tetraplegic individuals. The results of this complication may lead to new functional decline and physical impairments as a result of sensory impairment, motor function loss, or sphincter dysregulation. MRI is the imaging modality of choice to identify syringomyelia and is indicated in cases of SCI with a change in functional status. Evaluation by a neurosurgeon and surgical decompression are indicated in cases with associated motor weakness.

Expected Length of Disability

SCI is a result of insult to the spinal cord or cauda equina causing permanent changes to strength, sensation, autonomic function, and bowel/bladder function. The severity of the initial injury can be used to prognosticate the degree of functional recovery for those with traumatic SCI. Clinical outcomes may be prognosticated based on the neurologic level of injury as defined by the ASIA criteria. Preservation of pinprick sensation at the S4–S5 sacral dermatome within 1 week post-injury has been shown to prognosticate the ability to ambulate, with 75% of individuals with sacral sparing ambulating after recovery. Up to 30%–45% of individuals with an initial score of ASIA B ambulate short distances with assistance. Very few individuals with an initial score of ASIA A ambulate. Other factors associated with poor functional recovery include the presence of spinal cord hemorrhage, a long segment of spinal cord edema, and high cervical lesions.

Specific Categories of Need

Medical Physicians and Subspecialists

Following discharge from a hospital or inpatient rehabilitation facility, people living with SCI require long-term follow-up with primary providers and occasionally may require office visits with subspecialty providers. To monitor immediate post-discharge needs, the patient should schedule an appointment with his or her SCI physician within 2–4 weeks of discharge. For the first year, subsequent appointments may be every 1–3 months to address needs pertaining to transition to home, work, and return to the community. After the first year, this may be extended to every 6–12 months. The SCI patient should see an SCI physician at least once a year. Patients with SCI should also have a routine follow-up with their primary care physician for monitoring of general health and preventative care. Referrals to additional subspecialist providers may be requested by either the primary care physician or the SCI physician. These subspecialists include neurology, neurosurgery, orthopedic/spine surgery, urology, gastroenterology, dermatology/plastic surgery/wound care, psychiatry, and pain management. Patients with neurogenic bladder should follow up with a urologist annually.

Physical, Occupational, and Speech Therapy

In the immediate post-discharge period, home care with home physical therapy and occupational therapy benefits the patient's transition to home and return to the community. Additional therapy sessions and modifications may be required to assist with the transition back to work. Speech-language pathology (speech therapy) is necessary for patients with difficulty eating by mouth.

Respiratory Therapy

People with SCI who are ventilator-dependent, more common in high-level cervical spine injuries, must be set up with a respiratory care company that ideally will provide an experienced respiratory therapist to assist with ventilatory needs and to train the patient and family on the use of a home or portable ventilator.

Neuropsychology

Neuropsychologists play an integral role in addressing adjustment disorders and coping. The impact of an SCI on mental health should not be overlooked. Neuropsychologists also assist with underdiagnosed residual cognitive deficits (memory, visuospatial skills, attention/executive functioning, processing speed) in the SCI population (Dowler et al., 1995).

Social Worker

Following discharge from a hospital or inpatient rehabilitation facility, people living with SCI may have continued needs such as durable medical equipment (e.g., motorized wheelchair, transfer board, tub bench, raised toilet seat, hospital bed), home modifications (shower rails, chair lift), and transportation services (access-a-ride, modifications to personal vehicle). The social worker works with the rest of the rehabilitation team to help the patient obtain all of the this, especially if there are financial difficulties.

Nutrition

Nutritional counseling is beneficial for overall general health. It is especially important in the healing of patients with pressure injuries (bed sores).

Skilled Nursing Care/Home Health Aide

Select patients may require skilled nursing services to help with medication management and wound care. Those who require less intensive nursing needs may benefit from the services of a home health aide.

Research and Innovation

There is continued innovation and research in SCI. The use of exoskeletons for ambulation training has been shown to benefit bowel and bladder function. For patients with high cervical spine injuries and limited upper and lower extremity mobility, environmental control with voice/eye commands is beneficial.

References

Ahuja, C. S., Nori, S., Tetreault, L., Wilson, J., Kwon, B., Harrop, J., Choi, D., & Fehlings, M. G. (2017). Traumatic spinal cord injury-repair and regeneration. *Neurosurgery, 80*(3S), S9–S22. https://doi-org. proxy.library.vcu.edu/10.1093/neuros/nyw080

Berlowitz, D. J., & Tamplin, J. (2013). Respiratory muscle training for cervical spinal cord injury. *The Cochrane Database of Systematic Reviews, 7,* CD008507. https://doi-org.proxy.library.vcu. edu/10.1002/14651858.CD008507.pub2

Berkowitz, M., O'Leary, P., Kruse, D., & Harvey, C. (1998). *Spinal cord injury: An analysis of medical and social costs.* Demos Medical Publishing, Inc.

Bonner, S., & Smith, C. (2013). Initial management of acute spinal cord injury. *Continuing Education in Anaesthesia, Critical Care & Pain, 13*(6), 224–231.

Cao, Y., Massaro, J. F., Krause, J. S., Chen, Y., & Devivo, M. J. (2014). Suicide mortality after spinal cord injury in the United States: Injury cohorts analysis. *Archives of Physical Medicine and Rehabilitation, 95*(2), 230–235. https://doi.org/10.1016/j.apmr.2013.10.007. Epub October 23, 2013. PMID: 24161272.

Cardozo, C. P. (2007). Respiratory complications of spinal cord injury. *The Journal of Spinal Cord Medicine, 30*(4), 307.

Castellano-Tejedor, C., & Lusilla-Palacios, P. (2017). A study of burden of care and its correlates among family members supporting relatives and loved ones with traumatic spinal cord injuries. *Clinical Rehabilitation, 31*(7), 948–956. https://doi-org.proxy.library.vcu.edu/10.1177/0269215517709330

Chan, T. L. H., Cowan, R., Hindiyeh, N., Hashmi, S., Lanzman, B., & Carroll, I. (2020). Spinal cerebrospinal fluid leak in the context of pars interarticularis fracture. *BMC Neurology, 20*(1), 1–7.

Claydon, V. E., Steeves, J. D., & Krassioukov, A. (2006). Orthostatic hypotension following spinal cord injury: Understanding clinical pathophysiology. *Spinal Cord, 44*(6), 341–351.

DeVivo, M., Chen, Y., Mennemeyer, S., & Deutsch, A. (2011). Costs of care following spinal cord injury. *Topics in Spinal Cord Injury Rehabilitation, 16*(4), 1–9. https://doi.org/10.1310/sci1604-1

DeVivo, M. J., Go, B. K., & Jackson, A. B. (2002). Overview of the national spinal cord injury statistical center database. *The Journal of Spinal Cord Medicine, 25*(4), 335–338.

Dowler, R. N., O'Brien, S. A., Haaland, K. Y., Harrington, D. L., Feel, F., & Fiedler, K. (1995). Neuropsychological functioning following a spinal cord injury. *Applied Neuropsychology, 2*(3–4), 124–129.

Duckworth, W. C., Jallepalli, P., & Solomon, S. S. (1983). Glucose intolerance in spinal cord injury. *Archives of Physical Medicine and Rehabilitation, 64*(3), 107–110.

Fehlings, M. G., Vaccaro, A., Wilson, J. R., Singh, A., W Cadotte, D., Harrop, J. S., Aarabi, B., Shaffrey, C., Dvorak, M., Fisher, C., Arnold, P., Massicotte, E. M., Lewis, S., & Rampersaud, R. (2012). Early versus delayed decompression for traumatic cervical spinal cord injury: Results of the surgical timing in acute spinal cord injury study (STASCIS). *PLOS One, 7*(2), e32037. https://doi-org.proxy.library.vcu. edu/10.1371/journal.pone.0032037

Geerts, W., Cook, D., Selby, R., & Etchells, E. (2002). Venous thromboembolism and its prevention in critical care. *Journal of Critical Care*, *17*(2), 95–104.

Gould, M. K., Garcia, D. A., Wren, S. M., Karanicolas, P. J., Arcelus, J. I., Heit, J. A., & Samama, C. M. (2012). Prevention of VTE in nonorthopedic surgical patients: Antithrombotic therapy and prevention of thrombosis: American College of Chest Physicians Evidence-Based Clinical Practice Guidelines. *Chest*, *141*(2), e227S–e277S.

Hector, S. M., Biering-Sørensen, T., Krassioukov, A., & Biering-Sørensen, F. (2013). Cardiac arrhythmias associated with spinal cord injury. *Journal of Spinal Cord Medicine*, *36*(6), 591–599.

Jegede, A. B., Rosado-Rivera, D., Bauman, W. A., Cardozo, C. P., Sano, M., Moyer, J. M., . . . & Wecht, J. M. (2010). Cognitive performance in hypotensive persons with spinal cord injury. *Clinical Autonomic Research*, *20*, 3–9.

Kemp, L. A. (2002). Care and services for spinal injured people with, and without, neurological deficit. *Disability and Rehabilitation*, *24*(15), 810–816.

Kim, J. M., Losina, E., Bono, C. M., Schoenfeld, A. J., Collins, J. E., Katz, J. N., & Harris, M. B. (2012). Clinical outcome of metastatic spinal cord compression treated with surgical excision±radiation versus radiation therapy alone: A systematic review of literature. *Spine*, *37*(1), 78–84.

Lim, S. W., Shiue, Y. L., Ho, C. H., Yu, S. C., Kao, P. H., Wang, J. J., & Kuo, J. R. (2017). Anxiety and depression in patients with traumatic spinal cord injury: A nationwide population-based cohort study. *PLOS One*, *12*(1), e0169623. https://doi.org/10.1371/journal.pone.0169623. PMID: 28081205; PMCID: PMC5231351.

Lynch, J., & Cahalan, R. (2017, November). The impact of spinal cord injury on the quality of life of primary family caregivers: A literature review. *Spinal Cord*, *55*(11), 964–978. https://doi.org/10.1038/sc.2017.56. Epub June 27, 2017. PMID: 28653672.

Mackiewicz-Milewska, M., Jung, S., Kroszczyński, A. C., Mackiewicz-Nartowicz, H., Serafin, Z., Cisowska-Adamiak, M., Pyskir, J., Szymkuć-Bukowska, I., Hagner, W., & Rość, D. (2016). Deep venous thrombosis in patients with chronic spinal cord injury. *The Journal of Spinal Cord Medicine*, *39*(4), 400–404. https://doi-org.proxy.library.vcu.edu/10.1179/2045772315Y.0000000032

Merritt, C. H., Taylor, M. A., Yelton, C. J., & Ray, S. K. (2019). Economic impact of traumatic spinal cord injuries in the United States. *Neuroimmunology and Neuroinflammation*, *6*, 9.

Murray, L. M., & Knikou, M. (2019). Transspinal stimulation increases motoneuron output of multiple segments in human spinal cord injury. *PLoS One*, *14*(3), e0213696.

Nanclares, B. V. C., Padilla-Zambrano, H. S., El-Menyar, A., Moscote-Salazar, L. R., Galwankar, S., Pal, R., . . . & Romario, M. F. (2019). WACEM consensus paper on deep venous thrombosis after traumatic spinal cord injury. *Journal of Emergencies, Trauma, and Shock*, *12*(2), 150.

Schilero, G. J., Bauman, W. A., & Radulovic, M. (2018). Traumatic spinal cord injury. *Clinics in Chest Medicine*, *39*(2), 411–425. https://doi.org/10.1016/j.ccm.2018.02.002

Seoane-Rodríguez, S., Sánchez, R., Losada, J., Montoto-Marqués, A., Salvador-de la Barrera, S., Ferreiro-Velasco, M. E., Alvarez-Castelo, L., Balsa-Mosquera, B., & Rodríguez-Sotillo, A. (2007). Long-term follow-up study of intraurethral stents in spinal cord injured patients with detrusor-sphincter dyssynergia. *Spinal Cord*, *45*(9), 621–626. https://doi.org/10.1038/sj.sc.3102011. Epub January 9, 2007. PMID: 17211463.

Spungen, A. M., Dicpinigaitis, P. V., Almenoff, P. L., & Bauman, W. A. (1993). Pulmonary obstruction in individuals with cervical spinal cord lesions unmasked by bronchodilator administration. *Paraplegia*, *31*(6), 404–407. https://doi.org/10.1038/sc.1993.67

Sweis, R., & Biller, J. (2017). Systemic complications of spinal cord injury. *Current Neurology and Neuroscience Reports*, *17*, 1–8.

Vaikuntam, B. P., Middleton, J. W., McElduff, P., Connelly, L., Pearse, J., Stanford, R., Walsh, J., & Sharwood, L. N. (2019). Identifying predictors of higher acute care costs for patients with traumatic spinal cord injury and modeling acute care pathway redesign: A record linkage study. *Spine*, *44*(16), e974–e983. https://doi-org.proxy.library.vcu.edu/10.1097/BRS.0000000000003021

Varacallo, M., Davis, D. D., & Pizzutillo, P. (2021). Osteoporosis in spinal cord injuries. In *StatPearls*. StatPearls Publishing. Updated December 2, 2020. www.ncbi.nlm.nih.gov/books/NBK526109/

Whiteneck, G. G., & Jawad, M. H. (1993). *Aging with spinal cord injury*. Demos Medical Publishing.

Winkler, T., & Weed, R. O. (2004). Life care planning for spinal cord injury. In R. Weed (Ed.), *Life care planning and case management handbook* (pp. 517–574). CRC Press.

13 Spinal Disorders

Bharat C. Patel, Matthew Janzen, Ashley Plonk, and Krishn Patel

The annual prevalence of neck pain among adults ranges from 12.1% to 71.5%, and among children, it ranges from 34.5% to 71.5%, with most estimates of annual prevalence between 30% and 50%. Neck pain limiting activities is less common, with 12-month prevalence ranging from 2% to 11%. Côté et al. (1998) reported that the annual prevalence of neck pain in workers varied from 27.1% in Norway to 47.8% in Quebec, Canada. Moreover, each year, between 11% and 14.1% of workers were limited in their activities because of neck pain. Bovim et al. (1994) showed an overall prevalence of neck pain in the past year of 34.4%, with a total of 13.8% reporting neck pain that lasted for more than six months. Côté et al. illustrated various grades of chronic neck pain, with 5% of patients suffering from grades III and IV neck pain, which was associated with high pain intensity and disability (Manchikanti et al., 2011a, 2009a; Hartvigsen et al., 2006; Côté et al.).

The proportion of patients suffering from chronic upper or mid back pain secondary to thoracic disorders is relatively small compared to those suffering from low back and neck pain. In interventional pain management settings, thoracic pain has been reported in 3% to 23% of patients. Leboeuf-Yde et al. (2009) estimated the prevalence of thoracic pain in 13% of the general population in contrast to 43% with low back pain and 44% with neck pain during the past year. Despite the lower prevalence, the degree of disability resulting from thoracic pain disorders was similar to that of the other regions. This supports the view that although mechanical thoracic spinal pain is less common, it can be as disabling as lumbar or cervical pain (Manchikanti et al., 2011b; Singer & Edmondston, 2000; Manchikanti et al., 2009a, 2009b, 2004; Edmondston et al., 1997).

While the annual prevalence of chronic low back pain ranges from 15% to 45%, the point prevalence is 30%, and the age-related prevalence of the presence of low back pain is approximately 15% in adults and 27% in the elderly. Remarkably, studies have shown an increasing prevalence of chronic pain, specifically low back pain (Singer & Edmondston, 2000; Leboeuf-Yde et al.; Manchikanti et al., 2009a, 2009b, 2011c; Govind, 2004; Lawrence et al., 1998; Freburger et al., 2009).

Disorder (Disease) Definition

Strain

A strain is a common injury of muscle or tendon tissue. The fibers of the muscle or tendon in a strain are stretched or torn, resulting in acute pain. Strains usually occur with strenuous activity but can also result from trauma. Strains are more frequent in muscles that cross two joints, contain higher ratios of fast-twitch fibers, and function primarily in an eccentric manner (Noonan & Garrett, 1999). There are numerous classification systems for grading strains, which

DOI: 10.4324/b23293-13

usually involve a three-tier system based on multiple factors such as pain, swelling, ecchymosis, disability, range of motion, strength, palpable defect, and mechanism of injury. There is also a classification system that uses ultrasound and magnetic resonance imaging (MRI) based on the appearance of the tissue and the proportion of the fibers involved (Grassi et al., 2016). The diagnosis is often made based on the patient's history and physical examination. Imaging with MRI or ultrasound can aid in diagnosing strains when the clinical evaluation is unclear. However, MRI scans may be negative due to the fact that MRI alone cannot precisely measure the extent of the muscle structural damage. When positive, MRI may at times reveal evidence of edema. Ultrasound findings, however, are often negative as well and at times, transient hyperecoic or hypoecoic changes may occur after 3-5 days (Maffulli et al., 2013).

Sprain

A sprain is an injury to a ligament, the tissue connecting bones and supporting the function of joints. The fibers of a ligament are abnormally stretched or torn in a sprain. Sprains can result in pain, swelling, ecchymosis, joint instability, impaired range of motion, and disability (Behrsin & Briggs, 1988).

Fracture

A fracture is a partial or complete break in the continuity of a bone. Spinal fractures can occur in healthy bones due to high impact forces, while minor forces can cause fractures in bones weakened by pathological processes such as osteoporosis, infection, or tumor (Kendler et al., 2016). There are a variety of spinal fractures, including compression, burst, flexion-distraction, transverse process, and fracture-dislocation. Many classification systems exist for spinal fractures based on the location within the spine, location within the bone, mechanism of injury, and stability. The Denis classification system is one method of categorizing fractures based on dividing the spinal vertebrae along the anterior-posterior axis into three columns (anterior, middle, posterior). The middle column consists of the posterior third of the vertebral body, annulus, and posterior longitudinal ligament (Denis, 1983). Fractures involving the middle column have increased concern for instability (Bedbrook, 1971).

Herniated Disc

Intervertebral discs are composed of a fibrocartilage outer ring, called the annulus fibrosis, then a gelatinous core called the nucleus pulposus. The discs are located between the vertebral bodies, which form a joint while also acting as a cushion to absorb forces and allow movement in the spine between adjacent vertebrae. A disc herniation occurs when annulus fibrosis deforms, allowing a portion of the nucleus pulposus to move beyond its normal boundaries within the intervertebral space. A herniation is often associated with degeneration of the disc; however, overloading forces can also result in herniation in the absence of degenerative changes (Lotz & Chin, 2000). Herniations can be divided into protrusions, in which the herniated portion is narrower than the base, and extrusions, in which the herniated portion is wider than the base. Herniation can occur horizontally in the anatomical transverse plane or vertically in the sagittal plane. Vertical herniations into the adjacent vertebral body endplate are known as Schmorl's nodes (Kyere et al., 2012). The impact of a herniation varies depending on the size and location of the herniation in relation to the other surrounding tissue structures. Herniation can cause axial and/or radicular pain due to associated inflammation and nerve root compression (Schwarzer et al., 1995; Yang et al., 2015).

Degenerative Disc Disease

Degenerative disc disease is a commonly used term with a range of definitions. Generally, the term refers to pain related to the degeneration of one or more intervertebral discs. The term sometimes also includes osteoarthritis of the spine or spondylosis (Battié et al., 2019). The degenerative process may begin as early as adolescence, significantly sooner than the degeneration of most other musculoskeletal structures (Colombini et al., 2008). Disc degeneration has been shown to be associated with disc desiccation, increased acidity, and numerous genetic factors (Colombier et al., 2014; Cuesta et al., 2014). The composition of the disc changes, leading it to lose elasticity and the ability to withstand applied forces, causing the discs to bulge and leading to the loss of height (Grignon et al., 2000). The degenerative changes of the disc are linked to damage to surrounding muscles, ligaments, joints, and other tissues. As discs lose height, the adjacent vertebrae become closer and more force is applied to the facet joints resulting in osteoarthritic changes. Spinal ligaments also hypertrophy and buckle due to disc degeneration, which can further contribute to stenosis and potential compression of neural structures (Berry et al., 2019).

Radiculopathy

Radiculopathy is a condition caused by injury to a nerve root resulting in symptoms located in the distribution of those nerve fibers. Symptoms of radiculopathy can include numbness, tingling, paresthesia, abnormal reflexes, pain, and weakness. Pain from radiculopathy is often described as electric, sharp, shooting, or burning. Sensory changes in radiculopathy generally follow a dermatomal pattern. Weakness or muscle changes in the radiculopathy may follow a myotomal pattern. Radiculopathy is usually caused by compression of a nerve root from a bulging or herniated disc, bone spurs, facet or ligament hypertrophy or buckling, spondylolisthesis, neoplasm, or infectious process (Iyer & Kim, 2016; Matz et al., 2016).

Spondylolisthesis

Spondylolisthesis is a spinal condition occurring when one vertebra shifts out of alignment with the adjacent vertebra. Anterolisthesis is a spondylolisthesis that occurs when a vertebra moves anteriorly relative to the vertebra beneath it. Retrolisthesis occurs when a vertebra moves posterior relative to the vertebra beneath it. Etiologies of spondylolisthesis are commonly categorized as degenerative, dysplastic, isthmic, pathologic, or traumatic. Degenerative spondylolisthesis involves the deterioration of spinal structures responsible for stabilizing the vertebral column (Kreiner et al., 2016). Dysplastic spondylolisthesis results from congenital abnormalities of facet joints and their alignment. Isthmic spondylolisthesis is due to defects in the portion of the bone between the superior and inferior facets, called the pars interarticularis (Löwe et al., 1996). Pathologic spondylolisthesis can occur from systemic or localized conditions such as a bone or connective tissue disorder, neoplasm, infection, or iatrogenic process. Traumatic spondylolisthesis results from a fracture of the facets or pars interarticularis. Fracture of the pars interarticularis is also referred to as spondylolysis. Spondylolisthesis is commonly graded based on the proportion of the vertebral body out of anterior-posterior alignment with the adjacent vertebra. One of the most common grading systems for spondylolisthesis is Meyerding's classification, which consists of five grades with grade 1 being 1% to 25% slippage, grade 2 being up to 50% slippage, grade 3 being up to 75% slippage, grade 4 being up to 100% slippage, and grade 5 being greater than 100% slippage (Löwe et al.).

Stenosis

Stenosis is the narrowing of the spinal canal or one or more bony openings or foramina in the spine. The narrowing can cause pressure on nerves resulting in pain, numbness, weakness, and other neurological impairments. Blood vessels can also be compressed by stenosis leading to spinal cord injuries from infarction (Genevay & Atlas, 2010). Stenosis may occur in the central canal, lateral recess, or neural foramen. The central canal is the midline opening posterior to the vertebral body and anterior to the lamina, which contains the spinal cord in the cervical and thoracic areas and the cauda equina in the lumbar area. The lateral recess is located anterior to the superior articular facet, medial to the pedicle, and posterior to the vertebral body. The neural foramina are the lateral openings posterior to the vertebral bodies and inferior to the pedicle. Spinal nerve roots pass through the lateral recess and neural foramina.

Acute and Potential Complications

Range of Motion

Most spinal disorders may lead to decreased range of motion of the affected spinal segments. Reduced range of motion of the spine is usually secondary to muscle spasms, muscular tenderness, or increased pain with spinal movements due to pain from facet joints, discs, and or spinal ligaments.

Neurological Deficits

Various spinal disorders may lead to numbness and tingling in the extremities, loss of sensations in the extremities, and/or weakness of the muscles and muscle spasticity. They may lead to frequent falls, neurogenic bowel, or neurogenic bladder disorders. The severity of the neurological deficits depends on the severity of the specific spinal disorder.

Cervical Spondylotic Myelopathy

A severe cervical spondylotic disorder can lead to cervical spondylotic myelopathy. If not treated, it can also lead to quadriplegia and severe disability. Patients may become totally dependent and non-ambulatory with possible neurogenic bladder and bowel disorders. It may cause progressive muscular weakness in the upper extremities leading to loss of capability to perform fine motor movements. It may also lead to progressive weakness of the lower extremity muscles, loss of various sensations including joint proprioception, gait abnormalities, and frequent falls. Some patients will require cervical spine surgery as part of the treatment. The potential surgical complications are pseudarthrosis, restenosis, spinal instability, postoperative radiculopathy, postoperative kyphotic deformity, dysphagia, and axial neck pain. Adjacent level degeneration manifesting in the development of new symptoms occurs in up to 2.9% of anterior cervical discectomy-fusion (ACDF) patients per year after surgery and in up to 25% of patients ten years following surgery. The reoperation rate following ACDF ranges from 7% to 9% (Fast & Dudkiewicz, 2019; Nouri et al., 2015; Misawa et al., 2005; Fehlings et al., 2012; Young et al., 2019).

Cervical Spondylosis/Facet Joint Arthropathy

Cervical spondylosis can lead to chronic axial cervical pain and potential neurological deficits that may compromise quality of life and interfere with activities of daily living. The complications can occur from the treatments for facet joint pain. Neuritis is the most common complication after the radiofrequency ablation procedure. It occurs in less than 5% of procedures. Medial branches also innervate the multifidi muscles, which are dynamic stabilizers of the spine. Still, no short- or long-term sequelae have been reported in addition to the absence of segmental atrophy of the multifidi at long-term follow-up. Inadvertent damage to the ventral motor nerve root, superficial skin burns, or paresthesias are usually rare and are most likely secondary to incorrect needle placement or malfunction of the radiofrequency equipment (Kirpalani & Mitra, 2008; Braddom et al., 2011; Kornick et al., 2004; Dreyfuss et al., 2009).

Cervical Radiculopathy

Cervical radiculopathy may lead to chronic pain syndrome, temporary or persistent neurological deficits, and disability. Large cervical disc herniation may cause cervical myelopathy and spinal cord injury. Medications used to treat cervical radiculopathy can result in side effects such as peptic ulcers, gastroesophageal reflex disorder (GERD), nephritis, renal failure, central nervous system (CNS) suppression, endocrine side effects including hyperglycemia, hypothalamus-pituitary-adrenal axis suppression, and amenorrhea. Narcotics can result in nausea, constipation, respiratory suppression, mental status changes, suppressed endogenous opioids, dependency, tolerance, and abuse. Manipulation can result in vertebral artery dissection, carotid dissection, stroke, and recurrence of herniation and injury to the ventral nerve root as well as facet joint injury. Physical therapy may result in exacerbation of symptoms. Interventional pain management injections may result in adverse effects like vasovagal reaction, transiently increased pain, facial flushing, hyperglycemia, and vaginal spotting, all of which are self-limiting. Nerve injury, vascular insult, epidural hematoma, and spinal cord injury are rare but possible complications of spinal injections (Mostoufi, 2019; Caridi et al., 2011; Murphey et al., 1973; Abdi et al., 2007; Parenti et al., 1999; Pountos et al., 2016).

Cervical Spinal Stenosis

Untreated cervical spinal stenosis may lead to moderate to severe disability, mainly due to potentially irreversible neurological deficits such as loss of sensation, worsening of muscle weakness, bladder and bowel dysfunction, and quadriplegia. Untreated and worsening cervical spinal stenosis may lead to cervical myelopathy. Aggressive or improper physical or occupational therapy treatments can further injure the already injured spinal cord and the exiting nerve roots. Aggressive cervical traction may lead to signs and symptoms of cervical myelopathy and radiculopathy. Prolonged use of a cervical collar can cause atrophy of cervical musculature. Vertebral artery dissection and severe neurologic sequelae may result from forceful cervical manual techniques. Interlaminar epidural steroid injections may cause complications such as dural puncture and subsequent development of a post-dural puncture headache, spinal cord injury, stroke, and brainstem infarct. Spinal infection, hematoma, nerve injury, and spinal cord injury are rare but serious complications of interventional pain procedures and cervical spine surgery (Melenger & Okafor, 2019; Kavanagh et al., 2012; Edwards et al., 1999).

Vertebral Compression Fractures

Vertebral compression fractures may lead to neurologic complications, including nerve or spinal cord damage, continuous pain, instability, worsening kyphosis of the spine, difficulties with deep breathing, and increased risks of pulmonary complications such as pneumonia. Vertebroplasty or kyphoplasty is usually the treatment of choice. Complications of vertebroplasty or kyphoplasty procedures can include infection, bleeding, fracture in the treated or adjacent vertebrae, and systemic issues such as cement embolism. Cement leaks can occur in the surrounding tissues; damage to the spinal cord, spinal nerve, or vascular compression can occur (Hanson, 2019; Kim & Vaccaro, 2006; McCarthy & Davis, 2016).

Thoracic Spinal Disorders

Thoracic spinal disorders may lead to chronic pain, chronic thoracic radiculopathy, muscular weakness, and progressive thoracic spinal cord compression that may lead to paraplegia, neurogenic bowel and bladder, and muscular spasticity (Rosenberg & Pimentel, 2019; Brown et al., 1992; Leininger et al., 2011; O'Connor et al., 2002).

Lumbar Spondylotic Disease

Lumbar spondylotic diseases include lumbar degenerative disc disease and facet arthropathy, which can be progressive and may lead to chronic axial low back pain, subarticular spinal stenosis, or foraminal stenosis. In addition, central spinal stenosis and radiculopathy may be associated with neurological deficits. Intervention-based procedures carry risks of complications such as minor bleeding or bruising, procedure-related discomfort, and vasovagal reactions. Intra-articular steroid injections also carry with them related side effects from corticosteroids. Radiofrequency ablation has potential complications such as neuritis and unintended nerve damage (Schneider & Maybin, 2019; Mooney & Robertson, 1976; Schwarzer et al., 1994).

Lumbar Disc Herniation

Lumbar disc herniation can cause compression of nerve roots, leading to acute or chronic radiculopathy, numbness and tingling, loss of sensations, and muscle weakness. It may also cause paralysis such as cauda equina syndrome and conus medullaris syndrome. It may cause lower limb weakness and involvement of bowel and bladder function. It may also lead to chronic low back pain. Epidural steroid injections can result in epidural abscess and epidural hematoma. The injection can produce localized pain, and it has also been shown to result in spinal headaches from piercing the dura and a resultant spinal fluid leak. Surgical complications include infection, nerve root injury, paralysis, localized back pain, and the usual postoperative complications (e.g., thrombophlebitis, bladder infection). More serious surgical complications include nerve root or cauda equina injury, arachnoiditis, and post-laminectomy pain syndromes. These complications may lead to repeated surgery, which may become more extensive (Ellenberg & Ellenberg, 2019; Quraishi, 2012; Riew et al., 2006; Legrand et al., 2007).

Lumbar Spondylosis and Spondylolisthesis

Lumbar spondylosis may progress to lumbar spondylolisthesis. Spondylolisthesis can progress and result in spinal nerve compression, spinal stenosis, leg muscle weakness, loss of sensation in the legs, and chronic pain due to the progression of facet arthropathy and degenerative disc disease (Rainville & Mahmood, 2019; Rainville & Mazzaferro, 2001; Rainville et al., 2009; Scheepers et al., 2015; Lee et al., 2015).

Lumbar Spinal Stenosis

Patients with progressive worsening lumbar spinal stenosis may experience worsening axial back pain and/or lower extremity pain as well as loss of lower extremity sensation and muscle weakness, which can lead to frequent falls. It can also lead to decreased walking tolerance, known as neurogenic claudication. It may also cause neurogenic bladder, cauda equina syndrome, and conus medullaris syndrome. Quantified data on complications associated with nonsurgical interventional procedures, including epidural steroid injections, are limited. A retrospective study of 207 patients receiving transformational epidural steroid injections reported the following adverse events: transient non-positional headaches that resolved within 24 hours (3.1%), increased back pain (2.4%), facial flushing (1.2%), increased leg pain (0.6%), vasovagal reaction (0.3%), increased blood glucose concentration in insulin-dependent diabetes (0.3%), and intraoperative hypertension (0.3%). Other potential complications are infection at the injection site, dural puncture potentially with associated spinal headache, chemical or infectious meningitis, epidural hematoma, intravascular penetration, anaphylaxis, and nerve root or spinal cord injury leading to paresis or paralysis. Complications of decompressive surgery include infection (0.5% to 3%), epidural hematoma, vascular injury (0.02%), thromboembolism including pulmonary embolism (0.5%), dural tears (<1% to 15%), nerve root injury, postsurgical spinal instability, nonunion or hardware failure, adjacent segment degeneration, recurrence of symptoms (10% to 15%), and death (0.35% to 2%) (Isaac & Sarno, 2019; Atlas et al., 2000; Deyo et al., 1993; Botwin et al., 2000; Huntoon & Martin, 2004).

Sacroiliac Joint Pain

Like other causes of chronic pain, sacroiliac joint pain can produce pain-related insomnia, depression, anxiety, globalization of pain, kinesiophobia, and disability. Degenerative causes of sacroiliac pain are more prevalent in women, whereas inflammatory causes predominate in men. Manipulation therapy or therapeutic exercise can increase pain in some patients. An intra-articular steroid injection can be associated with a temporary increase in pain and local bleeding. Potential systemic steroid effects include an increase in serum blood glucose concentration, hypertension, psychosis, and fluid retention. A local steroid injection can cause fatty atrophy, infection, and skin depigmentation (Isaac & Brassil, 2019; Dreyfuss et al., 2004; Patel et al., 2012).

Functional Disabilities

Sacral S2, S3, and S4

Spinal disorders occurring at sacral levels S2, S3, and S4 are uncommon. If severe enough, spinal disorders occurring at the sacral level may cause bowel and bladder dysfunction. They may cause pudendal nerve neuropathy and loss of sensation in the perineal area. The patient will remain independent with mobility (Deutsch & Sawyer, 1996; Stolov & Clowers, 1981; Blackwell et al., 2001).

Lumbosacral L5 and S1

Spinal disorders at lumbosacral levels L5 and S1 may cause bowel and bladder dysfunction. They may also cause impairment of ambulation secondary to pain, muscle weakness, and impairment of sensation. With treatments, bladder and bowel function can become independent. Total independence in ambulation can be restored with the assistance of a cane, crutches, or short leg braces. If the patient develops a partial or complete foot drop, an ankle-foot orthosis is required to help ambulation and prevent falls. Prolonged standing and walking may be impaired. A wheelchair may not be necessary (Deutsch & Sawyer, 1996; Stolov & Clowers, 1981; Blackwell et al., 2001).

Lumbar L1, L2, L3, and L4

Spinal disorders occurring at lumbar levels L1, L2, L3, and L4 may impair bowel and bladder function. It may also lead to impairment of ambulatory functions secondary to pain, muscle weakness, and loss of sensation. With treatments, bladder and bowel functions can become independent. Ambulation can become independent for short distances, and a wheelchair may be necessary (Deutsch & Sawyer, 1996; Stolov & Clowers, 1981; Blackwell et al., 2001).

Thoracic

Spinal disorders at thoracic levels are less common and usually do not cause significant disabilities. Spinal cord injury may occur at an affected level if the disorder is severe enough. Thoracic disorders can lead to chronic thoracic pain and radiculopathy resulting in decreased ambulation tolerance and decreased sitting and standing tolerance. Spinal cord injury secondary to thoracic spinal disorders will cause impairment of personal hygiene, ambulation, transfers, dressing, and driving. Thoracic spinal disorders may also cause bladder and bowel dysfunction (Deutsch & Sawyer, 1996; Stolov & Clowers, 1981; Blackwell et al., 2001).

Cervical C7, C8, and T1 Levels

Spinal disorders at these spinal levels may cause personal hygiene, dressing, driving, and cooking impairment. This is due to the weakness of the forearm and hand muscles and loss of sensation in the forearm and hands. If the patient develops a wrist drop, wrist orthoses may be necessary (Deutsch & Sawyer, 1996; Stolov & Clowers, 1981; Blackwell et al., 2001).

Cervical C3, C4, C5, and C6 Levels

Spinal disorders at these levels may cause personal hygiene, dressing, driving, and cooking impairment. This is caused due to weakness of upper extremity muscles and loss of sensation in the upper extremities. Spinal cord injury at these levels will cause impairment of all other functions. Although a small number of patients may achieve modified independence in most functions, independent living is not practical. These patients require partial to total physical assistance for personal hygiene. Transfer activity requires partial to total assistance, and dressing requires partial to total physical assistance. Complete independence in eating, sitting, and driving can be achieved for spinal cord injury at or below the C6 level. Spinal cord injury above the C6 level will result in impairment of nearly all functions. Motorized wheelchair ambulation is required. Personal hygiene, transfers, dressing, writing, and driving will require assistance. Spinal cord injury above the C5 level will likely require training in the special use of upper respiratory equipment (Deutsch & Sawyer, 1996; Stolov & Clowers, 1981; Blackwell et al., 2001).

Psychosocial Disabilities

Research has established that patients' attitudes, beliefs, expectations, and coping resources can increase or diminish pain intensity and pain-related disability. Depression is the strongest predictor of health state across diseases and cultures. Health anxiety is also an important risk factor for chronic pain and disability. An additional correlation in disability pain is anger, which may affect pain through biological mechanisms with increased arousal and may interfere with pain acceptance and treatment adherence. Anger can take the form of frustrations related to the persistence of symptoms, lack of an established etiology or other aspects of uncertainty, treatment failures, workers' compensation or other disability claims, and problems with finances and family relationships. Behaviors may also be maintained and reinforced by the rewards of avoiding the pain sensation, obtaining opioid medication, and avoidance of undesirable activities such as work. Pain avoidance behaviors can exacerbate pain intensity and pain-related disability. Avoidance activity is anticipatory anxiety about pain, which may act as a conditioned stimulus for pain maintained after healing. Avoiding painful activities perpetuates and reinforces the belief that pain is an indicator of tissue damage and therefore retards healing.

Catastrophizing refers to a catastrophically injured person assuming that the worst will happen or is still to come from trauma. Often, it involves the individual believing that they are in a worse situation than they are or exaggerating the difficulties they face. For example, someone with a spinal cord injury may believe that they may never return to work or that their familial role will change dramatically. The tendency to catastrophize during painful stimulation contributes to more intense pain experience and increased emotional distress. Catastrophizing has been broadly conceived as an exaggerated negative "mental set" brought to bear during painful experiences. Even though findings have been consistent in showing a relation between catastrophizing and pain, research in this area continues to be performed. There are multiple ways to cope with pain, and there are different ways to regulate emotions associated with chronic diseases (Murphey et al., 1973). Because most patients with chronic diseases are unable to "solve" their persisting pain conditions by themselves (in terms of recovery or repair and finding distance to negative emotions associated with pain), they have to find strategies to adapt to a long-lasting course of the disease (Murphey et al.).

Consequently, a patient's coping with chronic pain is an ongoing process that includes appraisals of stress; cognitive, behavioral, and emotional responses; and subsequent reappraisals of stress. Thus, patients have to find ways to maintain physical, emotional, and spiritual health despite often long-lasting courses. Factors have been identified that protect against the debilitating impact of painful injury or disease in the development of disability. Key protective factors include:

1. A strong sense of self-efficacy or confidence in one's ability to follow a course of action to accomplish desired outcomes (e.g., control of pain). Effective use of cognitive, affective, and behavioral coping skills, such as muscle relaxation, distraction, commitment to activity, and an ability to redefine situations in less catastrophic ways.
2. A readiness or willingness to engage in active roles that are contradictory to lapsing into more adaptive patterns of thinking, feeling, and behaving. A capacity for accepting certain limitations or handicaps, thereby avoiding one's life being consumed by unsuccessful efforts to eliminate pain.
3. The social environment is often a significant source of stress reactivity, with vocational, familial, and other sources of social stress able to exacerbate pain. A dramatic increase has been shown in medical visits, analgesic use, and hospital admissions to coincide with significant life events, including conflicts with employers, insurers, lawyers, and financial distress. Being compelled to abandon usual roles, such as a worker, family member, or friend, also leads to deteriorating social relationships. Stress and strain in interactions with others, lapsing into the sick person or invalid role, and social isolation are common problems for people with chronic pain.
4. Psychosocial disability is one of the most misunderstood areas regarding patients suffering disabilities. Psychosocial disability refers to difficulties that an individual faces in being able to perform activities of daily living (ADLs) because of the impairments that they cause. These psychosocial disabilities can exclude patients from being able to participate in employment opportunities, personal relationships, and recreational activities. Psychosocial disabilities may also restrict a patient's ability to concentrate, interact with others, manage stress, and cope with stress in their lives.

Studies have shown that patients with chronic spinal pain are associated with a higher likelihood of psychological disorders such as anxiety, depression, kinesiophobia, and catastrophizing.

A connection to the increase in psychosocial states of mind has been correlated to a biochemical sequence of events that eventually lead to greater spinal pain and greater disability. When a patient exhibits these psychosocial disabilities, they have also been shown to have a deterioration in daily activities and exercise. Anxiety is associated with higher levels of spinal pain and an increase in other musculoskeletal pain conditions. Depression also seems to correlate with spinal pain and disabilities; studies have shown a strong predictor between daily spinal pain and depression in patients. Even though anxiety and depression have been found to correlate with spinal pain, none of these factors can predict pain intensity. Numerous studies have documented a strong association between chronic pain and psychopathology. Chronic pain is most often associated with depressive disorders, anxiety disorders, somatoform disorder, substance use disorders, and personality disorders (Dimitriadis et al., 2015; Harvey et al., 2016; Manchikanti & Fellows, 2011; Craig & Versloot, 2010; Vranceanu et al., 2009; DeGood & Tait, 2001; Jensen et al., 1991; Sullivan et al., 2001; Büssing et al., 2010; Morley et al., 1999; McCracken & Eccleston, 2005; Dubin et al., 2010; Brown & Nicassio, 1987; Ramirez-Maestre et al., 2008; Moore & Brødsgaard, 1999; Roth et al., 2008; Means-Christensen et al., 2008; Dersh et al., 2002).

Rehabilitation Potential

The rehabilitation potential of spinal conditions varies depending on injury type, location, severity, comorbidities, and multiple psychosocial factors (Casiano et al., 2020). Low back pain and associated disability improve in the majority of cases in the first month (Pengel et al., 2003). Factors associated with increased risk of chronic low back pain include somatization, depressive mood, and psychological distress (Pincus et al., 2002). Neck pain is less likely to resolve quickly, with over 50% of patients continuing to report symptoms after one year. Multiple factors are associated with a worse prognosis for neck pain, with the strongest associations being a history of other musculoskeletal disorders, older age, baseline disability, and baseline pain (Carroll et al., 2008; Walton et al., 2013; McLean et al., 2007). Exercising as a lifestyle habit before the onset of neck pain was associated with an improved prognosis (Walton et al.). Injuries with muscle strains generally have excellent recovery with conservative rehabilitation, with only large tears requiring surgery (Maffulli et al., 2014).

Evaluation Standards

Acute Phase

The evaluation of spinal conditions is often initially conducted in the emergency department/ urgent care or primary care setting. The evaluation of spine conditions should include obtaining a detailed history and physical examination. The history and physical exam will assess for red flags and guide the next steps in the patient's care. Pertinent aspects of the history include prior or current spinal conditions, osteoporosis/osteopenia, immunosuppression, cancer, intravenous drug use, unintentional weight loss, fevers, chills, night sweats, worse pain at night, and recent infections. Concern for infection or tumor should be evaluated promptly without delay, as this may significantly increase the potential morbidity and mortality of such conditions. Laboratory testing is critical in the assessment of potential infectious etiologies. Testing may include a complete blood count (CBC), erythrocyte sedimentation rate (ESR), C-reactive protein (CRP), and sets of blood cultures. The history and physical must also assess for impairments with bowel or bladder function, sensation, coordination, and strength. These can be signs of worsening neurological injury, requiring urgent additional workup, including advanced imaging (MRI or computed tomography [CT] scan if MRI is contraindicated) and potential neurosurgical consultation. In patients with an increased risk of fracture, including age greater than 50, history of osteopenia/osteoporosis, previous spinal fracture, chronic steroid use, or recent trauma, x-rays should be considered as part of the initial workup. Flexion and extension x-ray views should be obtained if there is a concern for potential spinal instability (Casiano et al., 2020; Patel et al., 2016).

Post-Acute Phase

Primary care providers' experience and comfort with managing spinal conditions can vary greatly. While most primary care providers are well trained in the initial management of many spinal conditions, more complex patients may benefit from earlier referral to spine specialists, including physiatrists, orthopedists, or neurosurgeons. Spinal conditions that worsen or fail to improve with conservative treatment for over six weeks may require further workup with advanced imaging if it has not already been obtained (Patel et al., 2016). Nerve conduction studies (NCSs) and electromyography (EMG) are tests to assess the health of nerves and muscles. These tests can aid in localizing and determining the etiology of neurological symptoms such as impaired strength or sensation. The NCS or the EMG study should not be performed until at least 2 to 3 weeks after the onset of symptoms, as some findings may not be detectable for a couple of weeks (Patel et al.; Chichkova et al., 2010).

Maintenance

Spinal conditions should be monitored closely for worsening or recurrence of symptoms, including pain, impaired sensation or strength, and changes in bowel or bladder function. New or worsening symptoms should be evaluated by the provider caring for the patient's spinal condition or in the emergency department for severe or red flag symptoms. The frequency of repeat testing and imaging varies greatly depending on multiple factors, including the type of condition, severity of symptoms, and treatments. Before undergoing interventional procedures, recent imaging must be evaluated for procedure planning. Application of the NCS/EMG studies may help evaluate the etiology of new or worsening symptoms, especially when previous studies are available for comparison to highlight changes (Chichkova et al., 2010).

Treatment

Acute Phase

Treatments for spinal disorders vary greatly depending on the type of injury and severity. All treatment options have associated risks and benefits that should be thoroughly discussed with patients so that a treatment plan can be constructed based on the patient's health, goals, and preferences. Conditions involving significant compression on the spinal cord or nerves may require emergent surgical decompression. Similarly, conditions associated with substantial instability of the spine may require urgent surgical fusion. Spinal conditions that do not impose a risk for neurological damage can initially be treated with conservative methods with the lowest risks, including activity modification, heat, and ice. Patients may consider adding non-narcotic topical medications such as lidocaine, menthol, and diclofenac. Oral medications may be considered based on a patient's health, including acetaminophen, nonsteroidal anti-inflammatories (NSAIDs), and muscle relaxants. Narcotic pain medication, including opioids, may be considered for severe pain refractory to other treatments when both the patient and prescribing physician feel the potential benefits outweigh the potential risks (Casiano et al., 2020; John M. Eisenberg Center for Clinical Decisions and Communications Science, 2016).

Rehabilitation Phase

Spinal injuries that do not resolve quickly with initial conservative care may require progression to more involved rehabilitation treatments. Physical therapy helps treat numerous spinal conditions. Patients must have a prescription from their treating physician to participate in physical therapy. The therapy prescription should include the diagnosis, safety precautions, treatment type, frequency, and duration. Education and protection of injured tissue is the most important component of any spinal care program that includes proper body mechanics for movement and ADLs. Physical modalities help control pain and inflammation along with relative rest. Physical modalities used during acute phase treatment are superficial cold or cryotherapy, superficial heat, deep heat/shortwave diathermy, therapeutic electrical stimulation such as a transcutaneous electrical nerve stimulation (TENS) unit, laser therapy, phonophoresis, iontophoresis, manual therapy, mechanical therapy like traction, use of corsets, and therapeutic exercises. Therapy is usually performed at outpatient facilities but often includes providing patients with a home exercise program (HEP) they can perform on their own (Jorgensen et al., 2018; O'Connell et al., 2016; Shipton, 2018; Sterling et al., 2019).

Subacute Phase

The subacute phase of rehabilitation aims to achieve a full, pain-free range of motion for injured and adjacent motion segments of the spine. Massage, stretching, traction, and other myofascial release techniques can be beneficial to improving range of motion and restoring optimal joint mobility. Therapeutic exercises are prescribed to increase the dynamic stabilization of the spine to control pain, optimize repair and regeneration of the injured soft tissues, and eliminate repetitive injury. Aquatic rehabilitation may be used along with other therapeutic exercises.

Post-Rehabilitation Follow-Up

Patients should follow up with their treating providers at regular intervals during and after completing a rehabilitation program so that their progress can be monitored and issues can be addressed. Patients may not tolerate rehabilitation programs due to pain or health and safety concerns. Attempts should be made to modify the program to facilitate a patient's ability to participate safely; however, other treatments should be investigated if all reasonable modifications fail. If a patient cannot participate in a rehabilitation program or fails to sufficiently improve with a rehabilitation program, more invasive treatments such as injections or surgeries may be considered. Injection treatments can include a range of substances such as saline, dextrose, local anesthetics, botulinum toxin, phenol, cortisone, platelet-rich plasma (PRP), and stem cells. The target of injection treatments can include muscles, tendons, ligaments, nerves, intervertebral discs, and joints. Surgical treatments of the spine include discectomy, synthetic disc replacement, laminectomy, open reduction and internal fixation, and fusion (Chou et al., 2009).

Expected Length of Disability

The length of disability for spinal conditions can fully range from permanent to no disability. Numerous factors impact the duration of disability, which depends on the type of injury, location, severity, comorbidities, associated injuries, contraindications to treatments, psychosocial factors, and job/employment characteristics (Casiano et al., 2020; Steenstra et al., 2005). Approximately two-thirds of patients with low back pain return to work within a month, 85% return within six months, and 93% return beyond six months (Wynne-Jones et al., 2014). Longer absence from work is associated with an increased risk of permanent disability (Waddell & Burton, 2006; Hashemi et al., 1998).

Specific Categories of Need

Life care plans utilize "Category of Need" charts to identify the need of the injured person detailing the equipment, medical and rehabilitation services, medications, home modifications, attendant care, home health care services, and vocational services, to name a few needs, over their remaining life span (Maniha & Watson, 2019). The following are some of the categories of need that may be applied to various spinal disorders:

1. Impaired gait and balance are frequent consequences of pain and neurological deficits associated with spinal conditions. Depending on the degree of impairment, the patients may require a cane for a small amount of added stability, a walker for greater support, or a wheelchair as a source of mobility if ambulation is further limited. The patient may require spinal orthoses such as a flexible or rigid lumbar corset, lumbar belt, sacroiliac joint belt, or corset.
2. The wrist drop may occur secondary to cervical spine disorder, and the patient may require the use of a wrist orthosis. The foot drop is a condition in which the ankle cannot properly dorsiflex, which can be due to several causes, including injury to the lower lumbar nerve roots. An ankle-foot-orthosis (AFO) is a category of brace that can help to support the ankle joint and improve the function of patients with foot drop (Carolus et al., 2019).
3. Fractures and instability in the spine often require treatment in the form of additional stabilization. Stabilization can be supplemented with external bracing initially while the patient is healing or until more definitive treatment can be provided. Standard braces for the neck include Aspen cervical collars, Miami J collars, and Philadelphia collars. The cervical spine sometimes requires more stability than a collar can provide, in which case a halo brace may be applied (Karimi et al., 2016; Richter et al., 2001). A thoracic lumbar sacral orthosis (TLSO) often provides bracing for the middle and lower back. Permanent sources of stability can come from surgical procedures such as spinal fusion or kyphoplasty (Leone et al., 2007; Muggleton et al., 2000; Patel et al., 2020).

Conclusion

Spinal disorders are common and cause significant disability and other consequences. Intervertebral discs, facet joints, occipital and axial joints, ligaments, fascia, muscles, and nerve root dura are capable of transmitting pain in the spine with resulting symptoms of neck and back pain, upper and lower extremity pain, and cervicogenic headache leading to physical as well as psychosocial disabilities. A severe spinal disorder may cause a spinal cord injury such as central or anterior cord syndrome, cauda equina syndrome, or conus medullaris syndrome. The patients may develop quadriplegia to paraplegia with a severe progressive spinal disorder leading to severe disabilities. The psychosocial aspects of disabling chronic pain include cognitive (e.g., beliefs, expectations, and coping style), affective (e.g., depression, anxiety, heightened concern about illness, and anger), behavioral (e.g., avoidance), and social (e.g., secondary gain and cultural aspects) factors.

Appendix 13A

Glossary for All Health Care Practitioners

1. **Catastrophizing:** When someone assumes that the worst will happen. Often, it involves the individual believing that he or she is in a worse situation than they really are or exaggerating the difficulties he or she faces. For example, someone with a spinal cord injury may believe that he or she may never return to work or that their familial role with change. www.healthline.com/health/anxiety/catastrophizing#:~:text=Catastrophizing%20is%20 when%20someone%20assumes,they'll%20fail%20an%20exam.

2. **Cauda equina:** The collection of nerves at the end of the spinal cord is known as the cauda equina, due to its resemblance to a horse's tail. The spinal cord ends at the upper portion of the lumbar (lower back) spine. The individual nerve roots at the end of the spinal cord that provide motor and sensory function to the legs and the bladder continue along in the spinal canal. The cauda equina is the continuation of these nerve roots in the lumbar and sacral region. These nerves send and receive messages to and from the lower limbs and pelvic organs. www.aans.org/en/Patients/Neurosurgical-Conditions-and-Treatments/Cauda-Equina-Syndrome#:~:text=The%20cauda%20equina%20is%20the,roots%20of%20 the%20cauda%20equina.

3. **Denis classification system:** This is a spinal injury classification system based on radiological findings and proposed tissues affected. U.S. orthopedic surgeon Francis Denis devised the concept from a retrospective review of 412 thoracolumbar spine injuries and observations on spinal instability (see references). Denis divides the spinal motion segment into three columns. In the author's own words: "The posterior column consists of what Holdsworth described as the posterior ligamentous complex. The middle column includes the posterior longitudinal ligament, posterior annulus fibrosus, and posterior wall of the vertebral body. The anterior column consists of the anterior vertebral body, anterior annulus fibrosus, and anterior longitudinal ligament." www.scientificspine.com/spine-scores/denis-classification.html

4. **Disc desiccation:** Disc desiccation is one of the most common features of degenerative disc disease. It refers to the dehydration of the discs. The vertebral discs are full of fluid, which keeps them both flexible and sturdy. As people age, the discs begin to dehydrate or slowly lose their fluid. The disc's fluid is replaced by fibrocartilage, the tough, fibrous tissue that makes up the outer portion of the disc. www.healthline.com/health/disc-desiccation

5. **Dysplastic:** A specific type of nevus (mole) that looks different from a common mole. Dysplastic nevi are mostly flat and often larger than common moles and have irregular borders. A dysplastic nevus can contain different colors, which can range from pink to dark brown. Parts of the mole may be raised above the skin surface. A dysplastic nevus may develop into melanoma (a type of skin cancer), and the more dysplastic nevi a person has, the higher the

risk of melanoma. A dysplastic nevus is sometimes called an atypical mole. www.cancer.gov/publications/dictionaries/cancer-terms/def/dysplastic-nevus

6. **Ecchymosis:** Ecchymoses are purpuric flat patches on the skin, commonly known as bruises. Ecchymoses typically are ≥1 cm in size and are caused by a greater volume of extravasated blood than in petechiae. Thus, ecchymoses tend to take longer to resolve (one to three weeks). Petechiae in a patient with an underlying coagulopathy can quickly evolve into ecchymoses, sometimes within minutes. Ecchymoses resulting from infection are uncommon in children. When ecchymoses occur, they are most frequently due to *Neisseria meningitidis* bloodstream infection with coagulopathy. Other reported causes include other gram-negative bacteria, gram-positive bacteria (*Staphylococcus aureus, Streptococcus pyogenes,* and *Streptococcus pneumoniae*), viruses (dengue and other hemorrhagic fevers), and *Rickettsia rickettsii* (Rocky mountain spotted fever). www.sciencedirect.com/topics/medicine-and-dentistry/ecchymosis

7. **Iatrogenic process:** When medical or surgical treatment causes a new illness or injury, the result is considered to be iatrogenic. People going for medical care, for example, may have a fear that something could go wrong as a result of the treatment. An iatrogenic event can either complicate one's existing medical condition or cause health issues unrelated to the illness for which the individual sought treatment in the first place. These types of situations are rarely intentional, though medical providers are human and mistakes can be made. www.verywellhealth.com/what-is-iatrogenic-2615180

8. **Isthmic:** The isthmus from the medical perspective and terminology is a narrow organ, passage, or piece of tissue connecting two larger parts. An orthopedic example is found in isthmic spondylolisthesis. This spinal condition is where one vertebra slips forward over the vertebra below. It is caused by a defect or fracture of the pars interarticularis, a bone that connects the upper and lower facet joints. A patient may have inherited the defect or obtained a fracture by the accumulative effects of spinal stress. www.cancer.gov/publications/dictionaries/cancer-terms/def/isthmus and https://uvahealth.com/services/spine/isthmic-spondylolisthesis

9. **Neural foramen:** A neural foramen is an opening on either side of the spinal column at each intervertebral level through which the spinal nerve roots traverse while surrounded by arteries, veins, and epidural fat. The neural foramina are formed at the lateral aspects of the vertebral canal. Neural foraminal stenosis refers to the narrowing of the small openings between each vertebra in the spine, called foramen, which nerve roots pass through. A type of spinal stenosis, neural foraminal stenosis does not always cause symptoms, but if a nerve gets compressed in the gap, this will be painful. www.medicalnewstoday.com/articles/319792#:~:text=Neural%20foraminal%20stenosis%20refers%20to,gap%2C%20this%20will%20be%20painful.

10. **Osteoporosis:** Osteoporosis, "porous bones," is a disease that causes bones to become brittle and susceptible to fractures. These fractures typically occur in the hip, spine, and wrist. A fracture or broken bone can have a huge effect on one's life, causing disability, pain, or loss of independence. Fractures can make it very difficult to do daily activities without help. Unfortunately, the International Osteoporosis Foundation currently estimates that one in three women and one in five men over age 50 will suffer an osteoporotic fracture. www.algaecal.com/osteoporosis-treatment/?ph=sem-content&campaignid=11024886153&adgroupid=110631259080&adid=529809327266&gclid=Cj0KCQjwzLCVBhD3ARIsAPKYTcQYr2ZwiU0ABD2z2FKLapVzQz3LauMbiOpHg8yyVeqavqijA73Dp8IaAswoEALw_wcB

11. **Osteopenia:** Osteopenia is a loss of bone mineral density (BMD) that weakens bones. It's more common in people older than 50, especially women. Osteopenia has no signs

or symptoms, but a painless screening test can measure bone strength. Certain lifestyle changes can help preserve bone density and prevent osteoporosis. Osteopenia usually doesn't cause any signs or symptoms until it progresses to osteoporosis. Rarely, some people with osteopenia may experience bone pain or weakness. The condition is usually detected when a person has a BMD screening. https://my.clevelandclinic.org/health/diseases/21855-osteopenia#:~:text=Osteopenia%20is%20a%20loss%20of,bone%20density%20and%20prevent%20osteoporosis.

12. **Paresthesia:** Paresthesia refers to a burning or prickling sensation that is usually felt in the hands, arms, legs, or feet, but can also occur in other parts of the body. The sensation, which happens without warning, is usually painless and described as tingling or numbness, skin crawling, or itching.

   Most people have experienced temporary paresthesia—a feeling of "pins and needles"—at some time in their lives when they have sat with their legs crossed for too long or fallen asleep with an arm crooked under their head. It happens when sustained pressure is placed on a nerve. The feeling quickly goes away once the pressure is relieved.

   Chronic paresthesia is often a symptom of an underlying neurological disease or traumatic nerve damage. Paresthesia can be caused by disorders affecting the central nervous system, such as stroke and transient ischemic attacks (mini-strokes), multiple sclerosis, transverse myelitis, and encephalitis. A tumor or vascular lesion pressed up against the brain or spinal cord can also cause paresthesia. Nerve entrapment syndromes, such as carpal tunnel syndrome, can damage peripheral nerves and cause paresthesia accompanied by pain. Diagnostic evaluation is based on determining the underlying condition causing the paresthetic sensations. An individual's medical history, physical examination, and laboratory tests are essential for the diagnosis. Physicians may order additional tests depending on the suspected cause of the paresthesia. www.ninds.nih.gov/health-information/disorders/paresthesia

References

Abdi, S., Datta, S., Trescot, A. M., Schultz, D. M., Adlaka, R., Atluri, S. L., Smith, H. S., & Manchikanti, L. (2007). Epidural steroids in the management of chronic spinal pain: A systematic review. *Pain Physician, 10*(1), 185–212.

Atlas, S. J., Keller, R. B., Robson, D., Deyo, R. A., & Singer, D. E. (2000). Surgical and nonsurgical management of lumbar spinal stenosis: Four-year outcomes from the Maine lumbar spine study. *Spine, 25*(5), 556–562. https://doi.org/10.1097/00007632-200003010-00005

Battié, M. C., Joshi, A. B., Gibbons, L. E., & ISSLS. (2019). Degenerative spinal phenotypes group degenerative disc disease: What is in a name? *Spine, 44*(21), 1523–1529. https://doi.org/10.1097/BRS.0000000000003103

Bedbrook, G. M. (1971). Stability of spinal fractures and fracture dislocations. *Paraplegia, 9*(1), 23–32. https://doi.org/10.1038/sc.1971.3

Behrsin, J. F., & Briggs, C. A. (1988). Ligaments of the lumbar spine: A review. *Surgical and Radiologic Anatomy: SRA, 10*(3), 211–219. https://doi.org/10.1007/BF02115239

Berry, J. A., Elia, C., Saini, H. S., & Miulli, D. E. (2019). A review of lumbar radiculopathy, diagnosis, and treatment. *Cureus, 11*(10), e5934. https://doi.org/10.7759/cureus.5934

Blackwell, T., Krause, J., Winkler, T., & Stiens, S. (2001). *Spinal cord injury desk reference* (pp. 157–160). Demos Medical Publishing.

Botwin, K. P., Gruber, R. D., Bouchlas, C. G., Torres-Ramos, F. M., Freeman, T. L., & Slaten, W. K. (2000). Complications of fluoroscopically guided transforaminal lumbar epidural injections. *Archives of Physical Medicine and Rehabilitation, 81*(8), 1045–1050. https://doi.org/10.1053/apmr.2000.7166

Bovim, G., Schrader, H., & Sand, T. (1994). Neck pain in the general population. *Spine, 19*(12), 1307–1309. https://doi-org.proxy.library.vcu.edu/10.1097/00007632-199406000-00001

Braddom, R. L., Chan, L., & Harrast, M. A. (2011). *Physical medicine and rehabilitation* (4th ed., pp. xxiv, 1506). Saunders, Elsevier.

Brown, C. W., Deffer, P. A., Jr, Akmakjian, J., Donaldson, D. H., & Brugman, J. L. (1992). The natural history of thoracic disc herniation. *Spine*, *17*(Suppl 6), S97–S102. https://doi-org.proxy.library.vcu.edu/10.1097/00007632-199206001-00006

Brown, G. K., & Nicassio, P. M. (1987). Development of a questionnaire for the assessment of active and passive coping strategies in chronic pain patients. *Pain*, *31*, 53–64.

Büssing, A., Ostermann, T., Neugebauer, E. A., & Heusser, P. (2010). Adaptive coping strategies in patients with chronic pain conditions and their interpretation of disease. *BMC Public Health*, *10*, 507. https://doi.org/10.1186/1471-2458-10-507

Caridi, J., Pumberger, M., & Hughes, A. (2011). Cervical radiculopathy: A review. *HSS Journal*, *7*(3), 265–272.

Carolus, A. E., Becker, M., Cuny, J., Smektala, R., Schmieder, K., & Brenke, C. (2019). The interdisciplinary management of foot drop. *Deutsches Arzteblatt International*, *116*(20), 347–354. https://doi.org/10.3238/arztebl.2019.0347

Carroll, L. J., Holm, L. W., Hogg-Johnson, S., Côté, P., Cassidy, J. D., Haldeman, S., Nordin, M., Hurwitz, E. L., Carragee, E. J., van der Velde, G., Peloso, P. M., Guzman, J., & Bone and Joint Decade 2000–2010 Task Force on Neck Pain and Its Associated Disorders (2008). Course and prognostic factors for neck pain in whiplash-associated disorders (WAD): Results of the bone and joint decade 2000–2010 task force on neck pain and its associated disorders. *Spine*, *33*(4 Suppl), S83–S92. https://doi.org/10.1097/BRS.0b013e3181643eb8

Casiano, V. E., Dydyk, A. M., & Varacallo, M. (2020). Back pain. In *StatPearls*. StatPearls Publishing. Updated October 24, 2020. www.ncbi.nlm.nih.gov/books/NBK538173/

Chichkova, R. I., & Katzin, L. (2010). EMG and nerve conduction studies in clinical practice. *Practical Neurology, Bryn Mawr Communications*. https://practicalneurology.com/articles/2010-jan-feb/emg-and-nerve-conduction-studies-in-clinical-practice

Chou, R., Loeser, J. D., Owens, D. K., Rosenquist, R. W., Atlas, S. J., Baisden, J., Carragee, E. J., Grabois, M., Murphy, D. R., Resnick, D. K., Stanos, S. P., Shaffer, W. O., Wall, E. M., & American Pain Society Low Back Pain Guideline Panel (2009). Interventional therapies, surgery, and interdisciplinary rehabilitation for low back pain: An evidence-based clinical practice guideline from the American pain society. *Spine*, *34*(10), 1066–1077. https://doi.org/10.1097/BRS.0b013e3181a1390d

Colombier, P., Clouet, J., Hamel, O., Lescaudron, L., & Guicheux, J. (2014). The lumbar intervertebral disc: From embryonic development to degeneration. *Joint Bone Spine*, *81*(2), 125–129. https://doi.org/10.1016/j.jbspin.2013.07.012

Colombini, A., Lombardi, G., Corsi, M. M., & Banfi, G. (2008). Pathophysiology of the human intervertebral disc. *The International Journal of Biochemistry & Cell Biology*, *40*(5), 837–842. https://doi.org/10.1016/j.biocel.2007.12.011

Côté, P., Cassidy, J. D., & Carroll, L. (1998). The Saskatchewan health and back pain survey: The prevalence of neck pain and related disability in Saskatchewan adults. *Spine*, *23*, 1689–1698.

Craig, K. D., & Versloot, J. (2010). Psychosocial perspectives on chronic pain. In M. E. Lynch, K. D. Craig, & P. W. H. Peng (Eds.), *Clinical pain management* (pp. 24–31). Wiley-Blackwell. https://doi.org/10.1002/9781444329711.ch4

Cuesta, A., Del Valle, M. E., García-Suárez, O., Viña, E., Cabo, R., Vázquez, G., Cobo, J. L., Murcia, A., Alvarez-Vega, M., García-Cosamalón, J., & Vega, J. A. (2014). Acid-sensing ion channels in healthy and degenerated human intervertebral disc. *Connective Tissue Research*, *55*(3), 197–204. https://doi.org/10.3109/03008207.2014.884083

DeGood, D. E., & Tait, R. C. (2001). Assessment of pain belief and pain coping. In D. C. Turk & R. Melzack (Eds.), *Handbook of pain assessment* (2nd ed., pp. 320–345). Guilford Press.

Denis, F. (1983). The three-column spine and its significance in the classification of acute thoracolumbar spinal injuries. *Spine*, *8*(8), 817–831. https://doi.org/10.1097/00007632-198311000-00003

Dersh, J., Polatin, P. B., & Gatchel, R. J. (2002). Chronic pain and psychopathology: Research findings and theoretical considerations. *Psychosomatic Medicine*, *64*, 773–786.

Deutsch, P., & Sawyer, H. (1996). *A guide to rehabilitation*. AHAB Press.

Deyo, R. A., Ciol, M. A., Cherkin, D. C., Loeser, J. D., & Bigos, S. J. (1993). Lumbar spinal fusion: A cohort study of complications, reoperations, and resource use in the medicare population. *Spine*, *18*(11), 1463–1470.

Dimitriadis, Z., Kapreli, E., Strimpakos, N., & Oldham, J. (2015). Do psychological states associate with pain and disability in chronic neck pain patients? *Journal of Back and Musculoskeletal Rehabilitation*, *28*(4), 797–802. https://doi.org/10.3233/BMR-150587

Dreyfuss, P., Dreyer, S. J., Cole, A., & Mayo, K. (2004). Sacroiliac joint pain. *Journal of the American Academy of Orthopaedic Surgery, 12*, 255–265. PMID: 15473677.

Dreyfuss, P., Stout, A., Aprill, C., Pollei, S., Johnson, B., & Bogduk, N. (2009). The significance of multifidus atrophy after successful radiofrequency neurotomy for low back pain. *PM & R: The Journal of Injury, Function, and Rehabilitation, 1*(8), 719–722. https://doi-org.proxy.library.vcu.edu/10.1016/j.pmrj.2009.05.014

Dubin, R., & King-VanVlack, C. (2010). The trajectory of chronic pain: Can a community-based exercise/education program soften the ride? *Pain Research & Management, 15*(6), 361–368. https://doi.org/10.1155/2010/617129

Edmondston, S. J., & Singer, K. P. (1997). Thoracic spine: Anatomical and biomechanical considerations for manual therapy. *Manual Therapy, 2*(3), 132–143. https://doi.org/10.1054/math.1997.0293

Edwards, R. J., Cudlip, S. A., & Moore, A. J. (1999). Surgical treatment of cervical spondylotic myelopathy in extreme old age. *Neurosurgery, 45*(696), 30.

Ellenberg, M., & Ellenberg, M. (2019). *Essentials of physical medicine and rehabilitation* (pp. 257–263). Elsevier.

Fast, A., & Dudkiewicz, I. (2019). *Essentials of physical medicine and rehabilitation* (pp. 3–7). Elsevier.

Fehlings, M. G., Smith, J. S., Kopjar, B., Arnold, P. M., Yoon, S. T., Vaccaro, A. R., Brodke, D. S., Janssen, M. E., Chapman, J. R., Sasso, R. C., Woodard, E. J., Banco, R. J., Massicotte, E. M., Dekutoski, M. B., Gokaslan, Z. L., Bono, C. M., & Shaffrey, C. I. (2012). Perioperative and delayed complications associated with the surgical treatment of cervical spondylotic myelopathy based on 302 patients from the AOSpine North America cervical spondylotic myelopathy study. *Journal of Neurosurgery, Spine, 16*(5), 425–432. https://doi-org.proxy.library.vcu.edu/10.3171/2012.1.SPINE11467

Freburger, J. K., Holmes, G. M., Agans, R. P., Jackman, A. M., Darter, J. D., Wallace, A. S., Castel, L. D., Kalsbeek, W. D., & Carey, T. S. (2009). The rising prevalence of chronic low back pain. *Archives of Internal Medicine, 169*(3), 251–258. https://doi.org/10.1001/archinternmed.2008.543

Genevay, S., & Atlas, S. J. (2010). Lumbar spinal stenosis: Best practice & research. *Clinical Rheumatology, 24*(2), 253–265. https://doi.org/10.1016/j.berh.2009.11.001

Govind, J. (2004). Lumbar radicular pain. *Australian Family Physician, 33*, 409–412.

Grassi, A., Quaglia, A., Canata, G. L., & Zaffagnini, S. (2016). An update on the grading of muscle injuries: A narrative review from clinical to comprehensive systems. *Joints, 4*(1), 39–46. https://doi.org/10.11138/jts/2016.4.1.039

Grignon, B., Grignon, Y., Mainard, D., Braun, M., Netter, P., & Roland, J. (2000). The structure of the cartilaginous end-plates in elder people. *Surgical and Radiologic Anatomy: SRA, 22*(1), 13–19. https://doi.org/10.1007/s00276-000-0013-7

Hanson, T. (2019). *Essentials of physical medicine and rehabilitation* (pp. 228–233). Elsevier.

Hartvigsen, J., Frederiksen, H., & Christensen, K. (2006). Back and neck pain in seniors-prevalence and impact. *European Spine Journal, 15*, 802–806.

Hashemi, L., Webster, B. S., & Clancy, E. A. (1998). Trends in disability duration and cost of workers' compensation low back pain claims (1988–1996). *Journal of Occupational and Environmental Medicine, 40*(12), 1110–1119. https://doi.org/10.1097/00043764-199812000-00011

Harvey, C., Brophy, L., Parsons, S., Moeller-Saxone, K., Grigg, M., & Siskind, D. (2016). People living with psychosocial disability: Rehabilitation and recovery-informed service provision within the second Australian national survey of psychosis. *The Australian and New Zealand Journal of Psychiatry, 50*(6), 534–547. https://doi.org/10.1177/0004867415610437

Huntoon, M. A., & Martin, D. P. (2004). Paralysis after transforaminal epidural injection and previous spinal surgery. *Regional Anesthesia Pain Medicine, 29*, 494–495. PMID: 15372396.

Isaac, Z., & Brassil, M. (2019). *Essentials of physical medicine and rehabilitation* (pp. 284–290). Elsevier.

Isaac, Z., & Sarno, D. (2019). *Essentials of physical medicine and rehabilitation* (pp. 277–283). Elsevier.

Iyer, S., & Kim, H. J. (2016). Cervical radiculopathy. *Current Reviews in Musculoskeletal Medicine, 9*(3), 272–280. https://doi.org/10.1007/s12178-016-9349-4

Jensen, M. P., Turner, J. A., Romano, J. M., & Karoly, P. (1991). Coping with chronic pain: A critical review of the literature. *Pain, 47*(3), 249–283. https://doi.org/10.1016/0304-3959(91)90216-K

John M. Eisenberg Center for Clinical Decisions and Communications Science. (2016, November 15). Noninvasive treatments for low back pain: Current state of the evidence. In *Comparative effectiveness review summary guides for clinicians*. Agency for Healthcare Research and Quality (US). Updated 2007. www.ncbi.nlm.nih.gov/books/NBK396522

Jorgensen, J. E., Afzali, T., & Riis, A. (2018). Effect of differentiating exercise guidance based on a patient's level of low back pain in primary care: A mixed-methods systematic review protocol. *British Medical Journal, 8*(1), e019742. https://doi.org/10.1136/bmjopen-2017-019742

Karimi, M. T., Kamali, M., & Fatoye, F. (2016). Evaluation of the efficiency of cervical orthoses on cervical fracture: A review of literature. *Journal of Craniovertebral Junction & Spine, 7*(1), 13–19. https://doi.org/10.4103/0974-8237.176611

Kavanagh, R. G., Butler, J. S., O'Byrne, J. M., & Poynton, A. R. (2012). Operative techniques for cervical radiculopathy and myelopathy. *Advances in Orthopedics*, 794087. https://doi.org/10.1155/2012/794087

Kendler, D. L., Bauer, D. C., Davison, K. S., Dian, L., Hanley, D. A., Harris, S. T., McClung, M. R., Miller, P. D., Schousboe, J. T., Yuen, C. K., & Lewiecki, E. M. (2016). Vertebral fractures: Clinical importance and management. *The American Journal of Medicine, 129*(2). https://doi.org/10.1016/j.amjmed.2015.09.020

Kim, D. H., & Vaccaro, A. R. (2006). Osteoporotic compression fractures of the spine; current options and considerations for treatment. *The Spine Journal: Official Journal of the North American Spine Society, 6*(5), 479–487. https://doi.org/10.1016/j.spinee.2006.04.013

Kirpalani, D., & Mitra, R. (2008). Cervical facet joint dysfunction: A review. *Archives of Physical Medicine and Rehabilitation, 89*(4), 770–774. https://doi-org.proxy.library.vcu.edu/10.1016/j.apmr.2007.11.028

Kornick, C., Kramarich, S. S., Lamer, T. J., & Todd Sitzman, B. (2004). Complications of lumbar facet radiofrequency denervation. *Spine, 29*(12), 1352–1354. https://doi.org/10.1097/01.brs.0000128263.67291.a0

Kreiner, D. S., Baisden, J., Mazanec, D. J., Patel, R. D., Bess, R. S., Burton, D., Chutkan, N. B., Cohen, B. A., Crawford, C. H., III, Ghiselli, G., Hanna, A. S., Hwang, S. W., Kilincer, C., Myers, M. E., Park, P., Rosolowski, K. A., Sharma, A. K., Taleghani, C. K., Trammell, T. R., Vo, A. N., ... Williams, K. D. (2016). Guideline summary review: An evidence-based clinical guideline for the diagnosis and treatment of adult isthmic spondylolisthesis. *The Spine Journal: Official Journal of the North American Spine Society, 16*(12), 1478–1485. https://doi.org/10.1016/j.spinee.2016.08.034

Kyere, K. A., Than, K. D., Wang, A. C., Rahman, S. U., Valdivia-Valdivia, J. M., La Marca, F., & Park, P. (2012). Schmorl's nodes. *European Spine Journal: Official Publication of the European Spine Society, the European Spinal Deformity Society, and the European Section of the Cervical Spine Research Society, 21*(11), 2115–2121. https://doi.org/10.1007/s00586-012-2325-9

Lawrence, R. C., Helmick, C. G., Arnett, F. C., Deyo, R. A., Felson, D. T., Giannini, E. H., Heyse, S. P., Hirsch, R., Hochberg, M. C., Hunder, G. G., Liang, M. H., Pillemer, S. R., Steen, V. D., & Wolfe, F. (1998). Estimates of the prevalence of arthritis and selected musculoskeletal disorders in the United States. *Arthritis Rheum, 41*(5), 778–799. https://doi.org/10.1002/1529-0131(199805)41:5<778::AID-ART4>3.0.CO;2-V. PMID: 9588729.

Leboeuf-Yde, C., Nielsen, J., Kyvik, K. O., Fejer, R., & Hartvigsen, J. (2009). Pain in the lumbar, thoracic, or cervical regions: Do age and gender matter? A population-based study of 34,902 Danish twins 20–71 years of age. *BioMed Central (BMC) Musculoskeletal Disorders, 10*, 39. https://doi.org/10.1186/1471-2474-10-39

Lee, G. W., Lee, S. M., Ahn, M. W., Kim, H. J., & Yeom, J. S. (2015). Comparison of surgical treatment with direct repair versus conservative treatment in young patients with spondylolysis: A prospective, comparative, clinical trial. *Spine Journal, 15*, 1545–1553. PMID: 25687414.

Legrand, E., Bouvard, B., Audran, M., Fournier, D., Valat, J. P., & Spine Section of the French Society for Rheumatology. (2007). Sciatica from disk herniation: Medical treatment or surgery? *Joint Bone Spine, 74*(6), 530–535. https://doi.org/10.1016/j.jbspin.2007.07.004

Leininger, B., Bronfort, G., Evans, R., & Reiter, T. (2011). Spinal manipulation or mobilization for radiculopathy: A systematic review. *Physical Medicine and Rehabilitation Clinics of North America, 22*(1), 105–125. https://doi.org/10.1016/j.pmr.2010.11.002

Leone, A., Guglielmi, G., Cassar-Pullicino, V. N., & Bonomo, L. (2007). Lumbar intervertebral instability: A review. *Radiology, 245*(1), 62–77. https://doi.org/10.1148/radiol.2451051359

Lotz, J. C., & Chin, J. R. (2000). Intervertebral disc cell death is dependent on the magnitude and duration of spinal loading. *Spine, 25*(12), 1477–1483. https://doi.org/10.1097/00007632-200006150-00005

Löwe, A., Hopf, C., & Eysel, P. (1996). Die Bedeutung der exakt lateralen Röntgendokumentation bei der Meyerding Graduierung von spondylolisthesen [Significance of exact lateral roentgen documentation in Meyerding's grading of spondylolistheses]. *Zeitschrift für Orthopädie und ihre Grenzgebiete, 134*(3), 210–213. https://doi.org/10.1055/s-2008-1039750

Maffulli, N., Del Buono, A., Oliva, F., Giai Via, A., Frizziero, A., Barazzuol, M., Brancaccio, P., Freschi, M., Galletti, S., Lisitano, G., Melegati, G., Nanni, G., Pasta, G., Ramponi, C., Rizzo, D., Testa, V., &

Valent, A. (2014). Muscle injuries: A brief guide to classification and management. *Translational Medicine @ UniSa*, *12*, 14–18.

Manchikanti, L., Boswell, M. V., Singh, V., Benyamin, R. M., Fellows, B., Abdi, S., Buenaventura, R. M., Conn, A., Datta, S., Derby, R., Falco, F. J., Erhart, S., Diwan, S., Hayek, S. M., Helm, S., Parr, A. T., Schultz, D. M., Smith, H. S., Wolfer, L. R., Hirsch, J. A., . . . ASIPP-IPM (2009b). Comprehensive evidence-based guidelines for interventional techniques in the management of chronic spinal pain. *Pain Physician*, *12*(4), 699–802.

Manchikanti, L., Boswell, M. V., Singh, V., Pampati, V., Damron, K. S., & Beyer, C. D. (2004). Prevalence of facet joint pain in chronic spinal pain of cervical, thoracic, and lumbar regions. *BMC Musculoskeletal Disorders*, *5*, 15. https://doi-org.proxy.library.vcu.edu/10.1186/1471-2474-5-15

Manchikanti, L., Falco, F., & Benyamin, R. (2011a). Pain medicine and interventional pain management: A comprehensive review. In *Clinical aspects* (pp. 36–37). ASIPP Publishing.

Manchikanti, L., & Fellows, B. (2011). Pain medicine and interventional pain management: A comprehensive review. In *Foundations* (pp. 55–66). ASIPP Publishing.

Manchikanti, L., Hirsch, J., Datta, S., & Falco, F. (2011c). Pain medicine and interventional pain management: A comprehensive review. In *Clinical aspects* (pp. 88–89). ASIPP Publishing.

Manchikanti, L., Singh, V., & Datta, S. (2011b). Pain medicine and interventional pain management: A comprehensive review. In *Clinical aspects* (pp. 61–62). ASIPP Publishing.

Manchikanti, L., Singh, V., Datta, S., Cohen, S. P., Hirsch, J. A., & American Society of Interventional Pain Physicians. (2009a). Comprehensive review of epidemiology, scope, and impact of spinal pain. *Pain Physician*, *12*(4), e35–e70.

Maniha, A., & Watson, L. (2019). Life care planning resources. In R. Weed & D. Berens (Eds.), *Life care planning and case manager handbook* (4th ed., pp. 729–757). Routledge.

Matz, P. G., Meagher, R. J., Lamer, T., Tontz, W. L., Jr, Annaswamy, T. M., Cassidy, R. C., Cho, C. H., Dougherty, P., Easa, J. E., Enix, D. E., Gunnoe, B. A., Jallo, J., Julien, T. D., Maserati, M. B., Nucci, R. C., O'Toole, J. E., Rosolowski, K., Sembrano, J. N., Villavicencio, A. T., & Witt, J. P. (2016). Guideline summary review: An evidence-based clinical guideline for the diagnosis and treatment of degenerative lumbar spondylolisthesis. *The Spine Journal: Official Journal of the North American Spine Society*, *16*(3), 439–448. https://doi.org/10.1016/j.spinee.2015.11.055

McCarthy, J., & Davis, A. (2016). Diagnosis and management of vertebral compression fractures. *American Family Physician*, *94*(1), 44–50.

McCracken, L. M., & Eccleston, C. (2005). A prospective study of acceptance of pain and patient functioning with chronic pain. *Pain*, *118*(1–2), 164–169. https://doi-org.proxy.library.vcu.edu/10.1016/j.pain.2005.08.015

McLean, S. M., May, S., Moffett, J. K., Sharp, D. M., & Gardiner, E. (2007). Prognostic factors for progressive non-specific neck pain: A systematic review. *Physical Therapy Reviews*, *12*(3), 207–220.

Means-Christensen, A. J., Roy-Byrne, P. P., Sherbourne, C. D., Craske, M. G., & Stein, M. B. (2008). Relationships among pain, anxiety, and depression in primary care. *Depression and Anxiety*, *25*(7), 593–600. https://doi-org.proxy.library.vcu.edu/10.1002/da.20342

Melenger, A., & Okafor, C. E. (2019). *Essentials of physical medicine and rehabilitation* (pp. 33–38). Elsevier.

Misawa, T., Kamimura, M., Kinoshita, T., Itoh, H., Yuzawa, Y., & Kitahara, J. (2005). Neurogenic bladder in patients with cervical compressive myelopathy. *Journal of Spinal Disorders & Techniques*, *18*(4), 315–320. https://doi-org.proxy.library.vcu.edu/10.1097/01.bsd.0000166638.31398.14

Mooney, V., & Robertson, J. (1976). The facet syndrome. *Clinical Orthopaedics and Related Research*, *115*, 149–156.

Moore, R., & Brødsgaard, I. (1999). Cross-cultural investigations of pain. In I. K. Crombie, P. R. Croft, S. J. Linton, L. LeResche, & M. Von Korff (Eds.), *Epidemiology of pain* (pp. 53–80). IASP Press.

Morley, S., Eccleston, C., & Williams, A. (1999). Systematic review and meta-analysis of randomized controlled trials of cognitive behaviour therapy and behaviour therapy for chronic pain in adults, excluding headache. *Pain*, *80*, 1–13.

Mostoufi, S. A. (2019). *Essentials of physical medicine and rehabilitation* (pp. 22–28). Elsevier.

Muggleton, J. M., Kondracki, M., & Allen, R. (2000). Spinal fusion for lumbar instability: Does it have a scientific basis? *Journal of Spinal Disorders*, *13*(3), 200–204. https://doi.org/10.1097/00002517-200006000-00002

Murphey, F., Simmons, J. C. H., & Brunson, B. (1973). Ruptured cervical discs 1939–1972. *Clinical Neurosurgery*, *20*, 9–17. PMID: 4762825.

Noonan, T. J., & Garrett, W. E., Jr (1999). Muscle strain injury: Diagnosis and treatment. *The Journal of the American Academy of Orthopaedic Surgeons*, *7*(4), 262–269. https://doi.org/10.5435/00124635-199907000-00006

Nouri, A., Tetreault, L., Singh, A., Karadimas, S. K., & Fehlings, M. G. (2015). Degenerative cervical myelopathy: Epidemiology, genetics, and pathogenesis. *Spine*, *40*(12), e675–e693. https://doi-org.proxy.library.vcu.edu/10.1097/BRS.0000000000000913

O'Connell, N. E., Cook, C. E., Wand, B. M., & Ward, S. P. (2016). Clinical guidelines for low back pain: A critical review of consensus and inconsistencies across three major guidelines: Best practice & research. *Clinical Rheumatology*, *30*(6), 968–980. https://doi.org/10.1016/j.berh.2017.05.001

O'Connor, R. C., Andary, M. T., Russo, R. B., & DeLano, M. (2002). Thoracic radiculopathy. *Physical Medicine and Rehabilitation Clinics of North America*, *13*(3), 623, viii. https://doi.org/10.1016/s1047-9651(02)00018-9

Parenti, G., Orlandi, G., & Bianchi, M. (1999). Vertebral and carotid artery dissection following chiropractic cervical manipulation. *Neurosurgeon Reviews*, *22*(2–3), 127–129. PMID: 10547013.

Patel, A., Petrone, B., & Carter, K. R. (2020). Percutaneous vertebroplasty and kyphoplasty. In *StatPearls*. StatPearls Publishing. Updated January 2020. Retrieved September 22, 2020, from www.ncbi.nlm.nih.gov/books/NBK525963/

Patel, N. D., Broderick, D. F., Burns, J., Deshmukh, T. K., Fries, I. B., Harvey, H. B., Holly, L., Hunt, C. H., Jagadeesan, B. D., Kennedy, T. A., O'Toole, J. E., Perlmutter, J. S., Policeni, B., Rosenow, J. M., Schroeder, J. W., Whitehead, M. T., Cornelius, R. S., & Corey, A. S. (2016). ACR appropriateness criteria low back pain. *Journal of the American College of Radiology: JACR*, *13*(9), 1069–1078. https://doi.org/10.1016/j.jacr.2016.06.008

Patel, N. D., Gross, A., Brown, L., & Gekht, L. (2012). A randomized, placebo-controlled study to assess the efficacy of lateral branch neurotomy for chronic sacroiliac joint pain. *Pain Medicine*, *13*, 383–398. PMID: 22299761.

Pengel, L. H., Herbert, R. D., Maher, C. G., & Refshauge, K. M. (2003). Acute low back pain: A systematic review of its prognosis. *British Medical Journals (Clinical Research Ed.)*, *327*(7410), 323. https://doi.org/10.1136/bmj.327.7410.323

Pincus, T., Burton, A. K., Vogel, S., & Field, A. P. (2002). A systematic review of psychological factors as predictors of chronicity/disability in prospective cohorts of low back pain. *Spine*, *27*(5), e109–e120. https://doi.org/10.1097/00007632-200203010-00017

Pountos, I., Panteli, M., Walters, G., Bush, D., & Giannoudis, P. V. (2016). Safety of epidural corticosteroid injections. *Drugs in R&D*, *16*(1), 19–34. https://doi.org/10.1007/s40268-015-0119-3

Quraishi, N. A. (2012). Transforaminal injection of corticosteroids for lumbar radiculopathy: Systematic review and meta-analysis. *European Spine Journal: Official Publication of the European Spine Society, the European Spinal Deformity Society, and the European Section of the Cervical Spine Research Society*, *21*(2), 214–219. https://doi.org/10.1007/s00586-011-2008-y

Rainville, J., & Mahmood, U. (2019). *Essentials of physical medicine and rehabilitation* (pp. 269–276). Elsevier.

Rainville, J., & Mazzaferro, R. (2001). Evaluation of outcomes of aggressive spine rehabilitation in patients with back pain and sciatica from previously diagnosed spondylolysis and spondylolisthesis. *Archives of Physical Medicine and Rehabilitation*, *82*, 1309–2001.

Rainville, J., Nguyen, V., & Suri, P. (2009). Effective conservative treatment for chronic low back pain. *Seminars in Spine Surgery*, *21*, 257–263. PMID: 20161564.

Ramirez-Maestre, C., Esteve, R., & Lopez, A. E. (2008). Cognitive appraisal and coping in chronic pain patients. *European Journal of Pain*, *12*, 749–756.

Richter, D., Latta, L. L., Milne, E. L., Varkarakis, G. M., Biedermann, L., Ekkernkamp, A., & Ostermann, P. A. (2001). The stabilizing effects of different orthoses in the intact and unstable upper cervical spine: A cadaver study. *The Journal of Trauma*, *50*(5), 848–854. https://doi.org/10.1097/00005373-200105000-00012

Riew, K. D., Park, J. B., Cho, Y. S., Gilula, L., Patel, A., Lenke, L. G., & Bridwell, K. H. (2006). Nerve root blocks in the treatment of lumbar radicular pain: A minimum five-year follow-up. *The Journal of Bone and Joint Surgery: American Volume*, *88*(8), 1722–1725. https://doi.org/10.2106/JBJS.E.00278

Rosenberg, D., & Pimentel, D. (2019). *Essentials of physical medicine and rehabilitation* (pp. 234–237). Elsevier.

Roth, R. S., Geisser, M. E., & Bates, R. (2008). The relation of post-traumatic stress symptoms to depression and pain in patients with accident-related chronic pain. *Journal of Pain*, *9*, 588–596.

Scheepers, M. S., Streak Gomersall, J., & Munn, Z. (2015). The effectiveness of surgical versus conservative treatment for symptomatic unilateral spondylolysis of the lumbar spine in athletes: A systematic review. *JBI Database of Systematic Reviews and Implementation Reports*, *13*(3), 137–173. https://doi.org/10.11124/jbisrir-2015-1926

Schneider, B., & Maybin, S. A. (2019). *Essentials of physical medicine and rehabilitation* (pp. 252–256). Elsevier.

Schwarzer, A. C., Aprill, C. N., Derby, R., Fortin, J., Kine, G., & Bogduk, N. (1994). Clinical features of patients with pain stemming from the lumbar zygapophysial joints. Is the lumbar facet syndrome a clinical entity? *Spine*, *19*(10), 1132–1137. https://doi.org/10.1097/00007632-199405001-00006

Schwarzer, A. C., Aprill, C. N., Derby, R., Fortin, J., Kine, G., & Bogduk, N. (1995). The prevalence and clinical features of internal disc disruption in patients with chronic low back pain. *Spine*, *20*(17), 1878–1883. https://doi.org/10.1097/00007632-199509000-00007

Shipton, E. A. (2018). Physical therapy approaches in the treatment of low back pain. *Pain and Therapy*, *7*(2), 127–137. https://doi.org/10.1007/s40122-018-0105-x

Singer, K. P., & Edmondston, S. J. (2000). Introduction: The enigma of the thoracic spine. In K. P. Singer & S. J. Edmondston (Eds.), *Clinical anatomy and management of thoracic spine* (Vol. 2, pp. 3–13). Butterworth Heinemann.

Steenstra, I. A., Verbeek, J. H., Heymans, M. W., & Bongers, P. M. (2005). Prognostic factors for duration of sick leave in patients sick listed with acute low back pain: A systematic review of the literature. *Occupational and Environmental Medicine*, *62*(12), 851–860. https://doi.org/10.1136/oem.2004.015842

Sterling, M., de Zoete, R., Coppieters, I., & Farrell, S. F. (2019). Best evidence rehabilitation for chronic pain part 4: Neck pain. *Journal of Clinical Medicine*, *8*(8), 1219. https://doi.org/10.3390/jcm8081219

Stolov, W., & Clowers, M. (1981). *Handbook of severe disability*. Rehabilitation Services Administration, U.S. Department of Education, Contract No. 105-76-4115.

Sullivan, M. J., Thorn, B., Haythornthwaite, J. A., Keefe, F., Martin, M., Bradley, L. A., & Lefebvre, J. C. (2001). Theoretical perspectives on the relation between catastrophizing and pain. *The Clinical Journal of Pain*, *17*(1), 52–64. https://doi-org.proxy.library.vcu.edu/10.1097/00002508-200103000-00008

Vranceanu, A. M., Barsky, A., & Ring, D. (2009). Psychosocial aspects of disabling musculoskeletal pain. *Journal of Bone and Joint Surgery: American Volume*, *91*, 2014–2018.

Waddell, G., & Burton, A. K. (2006). *Is work good for your health and well-being?* TSO (The Stationery Store).

Walton, D. M., Carroll, L. J., Kasch, H., Sterling, M., Verhagen, A. P., Macdermid, J. C., Gross, A., Santaguida, P. L., Carlesso, L., & ICON. (2013). An overview of systematic reviews on prognostic factors in neck pain: Results from the international collaboration on neck pain (ICON) project. *The Open Orthopaedics Journal*, *7*, 494–505. https://doi-org.proxy.library.vcu.edu/10.2174/1874325001307010494

Wynne-Jones, G., Cowen, J., Jordan, J. L., Uthman, O., Main, C. J., Glozier, N., & van der Windt, D. (2014). Absence from work and return to work in people with back pain: A systematic review and meta-analysis. *Occupational and Environmental Medicine*, *71*(6), 448–456. https://doi.org/10.1136/oemed-2013-101571

Yang, H., Liu, H., Li, Z., Zhang, K., Wang, J., Wang, H., & Zheng, Z. (2015). Low back pain associated with lumbar disc herniation: Role of moderately degenerative disc and annulus fibrous tears. *International Journal of Clinical and Experimental Medicine*, *8*(2), 1634–1644.

Young, J. A., Welch, S., & Frontera, W. (2019). *Essentials of physical medicine and rehabilitation* (pp. 8–11). Elsevier.

14 Peripheral Neuropathies

Gary E. Kraus

Peripheral neuropathy is a common neurological problem and encompasses a variety of functional, anatomical, and pathological disturbances (Thompson & Thomas, 2005). Patients suffering from chronic pain of neuropathic origin experience worsened health and greater disability than those not suffering from this type of pain. Disorders of the peripheral nervous system, including sensory disturbance, are commonly seen in adults. According to Watson and Dyck (2015) in citing the works of Martyn and Hughes (1997) and the Italian General Practitioner Study Group (1995), peripheral neuropathy has a prevalence of 2.4% in the general population and increases with age to an estimated 8% in those over 55 years of age. Nerve fibers affected by peripheral neuropathy may serve motor, sensory, or autonomic functions; the fibers may be large or small; the distribution of neuropathic involvement may be proximal, distal, or multifocal; and the onset of symptoms may be acute (less than 3 weeks), subacute (3 weeks to 3 months), or chronic (over 3 months) (Younger, 2004). Peripheral neuropathy may occur as a result of several common and many rare diseases, but the most common cause is diabetes (England & Asbury, 2004). As cited by Martyn and Hughes (1997), Palumbo found that within 5 years of diagnosis, 4% of diabetic patients had developed peripheral neuropathy, and the prevalence had risen to 15% by 20 years after diagnosis. It is more frequently seen in patients with diabetes mellitus, human immunodeficiency virus infection, dysproteinemic disorders, and those receiving chemotherapy. Peripheral nerves may be affected by nerve disorders occurring individually or as a group; in similar or distant regions of the body; as a result of various adverse conditions including trauma, entrapment, inflammation, compression on nerves, traction or stretching of nerves, ischemia to nerves, tumors (local or systemic), infection, metabolic abnormalities, systemic disease, medications, autoimmune disorders, iatrogenic causes, and inherited conditions; and many other reasons (National Institute of Neurological Disorders and Stroke, n.d.; Pindrik & Belzberg, 2014; Scott et al., 2013). The most common pattern of clinical symptoms is those of length-dependent peripheral neuropathy, in which symptoms begin symmetrically and in the longest nerves at their terminal portions, such as the distal foot, and progress to ascend from there. Most peripheral neuropathies are predominantly sensory and length-dependent (Watson & Dyck, 2015). The most common neuropathy is sensorimotor distal symmetric polyneuropathy, associated with a stocking sensory loss with variable distal weakness. There may be impairment of balance, gait, dexterity of the hands and feet, and reflexes. It may be classified clinically, electrodiagnostically, and histopathologically (Younger, 2004). Diseases of the peripheral nervous system may involve muscles (myopathies), nerves (neuropathies, with axons and myelin being affected), and neuromuscular junctions (Choi & Di Maria, 2021).

The subject of peripheral neuropathy; its anatomy; and physiology, classification, evaluation, treatment, and prognosis is an extremely broad topic, and the intent of this chapter is to present a summary review, not an exhaustive analysis of the subject.

DOI: 10.4324/b23293-14

Anatomy of Peripheral Nerves and End Organs

Gross Anatomy of Peripheral Nerves

The peripheral nervous system encompasses the spinal nerves including their roots and rami, peripheral nerves, and peripheral portions of the autonomic nervous system, including the cranial nerves III through XII (with the exception of the first and second cranial nerves, which are extensions of the central nervous system and are myelinated by oligodendrocytes, as Rueda-Lopes (2021) cited Marques (2021), which are myelinated by Schwann cells. Leaving the spinal cord at various levels (segments) are filaments that become the dorsal and ventral roots, which enter a dural sac separated by a septum. The dorsal root contains a spinal ganglion, peripheral to which the dorsal and ventral roots join to become a spinal nerve, which then gives off a dorsal ramus that supplies the back, and a ventral ramus (known as primary ramus) that supplies the limbs and ventrolateral portions of the body wall. Those ventral rami in the cervical region join to form the brachial plexus, and those in the lumbosacral region join to form the lumbosacral plexus. The ventral rami of a spinal nerve joins those of other spinal nerves in the plexus, and its component funiculi will enter several peripheral nerves which emerge from the plexus, resulting in each ventral ramus contributing to several peripheral nerves, and each peripheral nerve being supplied by fibers from several ventral rami. Peripheral nerves typically have five categories of branches: 1) muscular (motor, sensory, and autonomic fibers to muscles, connective tissue, tendons, joints); 2) cutaneous or mucosal (sensory and autonomic fibers supplying subjacent joints, ligaments, and tendons); 3) articular (where a nerve crosses a joint); 4) vascular (sensory and autonomic fibers to adjacent blood vessels); and 5) terminal (any of the previously mentioned items).

The portion of skin that has sensation supplied by sensory fibers of a single dorsal root through its dorsal and ventral rami is known as a dermatome. There is overlap in the sensory nerve supply of each dermatome, so that a section of a single root will not produce complete anesthesia in that dermatome, but rather a hypoalgesia. While the cutaneous distribution of peripheral and spinal nerves is identical over the trunk of the body, that is not true with respect to the limbs, where there is less overlap between peripheral nerves than the overlap seen with spinal nerves. For this reason, division of a peripheral nerve will result in more significant weakness or paralysis of the muscles innervated by that nerve, autonomic dysfunction will occur, and sensation will be lost more so in the central portion of the distribution of the nerve than at its periphery of distribution (Gardner & Bunge, 2005).

The autonomic nervous system, also known as the visceral or vegetative nervous system, supplies motor nerve fibers to cardiac muscle, smooth muscle, and glands. The preganglionic axons leave the brainstem and spinal cord over certain cranial nerves and ventral roots to travel to peripheral autonomic ganglia, where they synapse onto postganglionic cells, which then distribute fibers to cardiac muscle, smooth muscle, and certain gland cells. The autonomic nervous system, based on anatomic classification, is grouped into sympathetic, parasympathetic, and enteric systems or divisions, with viscera generally being supplied by both sympathetic and parasympathetic divisions, and the enteric system is limited to the wall of the bowel. Most sympathetic preganglionic fibers leave the spinal nerves or ventral rami and course through the rami communicantes to reach the sympathetic trunks, which are located on each side of the vertebral column, where they mostly synapse in the ganglia of the trunk and in accessory ganglia or continue through to reach the prevertebral plexus ganglia. Postganglionic fibers originating in the ganglia of the trunk may then go directly to adjacent viscera and blood vessels, while others will go through the rami communicantes to return to the spinal nerves and dorsal and ventral rami.

Ultimately, fibers of the ventral and dorsal rami will supply sweat glands, smooth muscle of hair follicles, and smooth muscle motor fibers of blood vessels of the limbs and walls of the trunk. The parasympathetic nervous system, which contains preganglionic fibers that arise from the brainstem (through cranial nerves III, VII, IX, X, and XI) and from the sacral cord (through the second and third or third and fourth ventral roots), contains ganglion cells that are typically in or near the organ to be innervated, resulting in short postganglionic fibers. The parasympathetic ganglia of the cranial nerves are known as the cephalic or cranial parasympathetic ganglia (ciliary, pterygopalatine, otic, and submandibular) and send postganglionic fibers to innervate the eye, lacrimal and salivary glands, and oral and nasal cavities (mucous and serous glands). The vagus nerve (cranial nerve XI) has preganglionic fibers that travel to ganglion cells in or near the walls of the neck, thorax, and abdomen. The sacral plexus preganglionic parasympathetic fibers, which leave the plexus as pelvic splanchnic nerves, enter the inferior hypogastric plexus to reach ganglion cells in the walls of pelvic organs. The enteric nervous system, which travels the length of the gastrointestinal system from the esophagus to the rectum, consists of two plexuses of ganglion cells with interconnecting fibers. Meissner's plexus is more internally located in the gut wall submucosa, and Auerbach's plexus (myenteric plexus) is more externally located between the external longitudinal and internal circular smooth muscle layers of the gut wall (Gardner & Bunge, 2005).

Microscopic Anatomy of Peripheral Nerves

There is a hierarchy to the anatomy of nerves, with the individual axon either surrounded by myelin (in myelinated nerves) or not having encircling myelin (unmyelinated) and then being surrounded by endoneurium. These endoneurium-surrounded structures run in parallel with each other to form groups called fascicles, which are surrounded by perineurium. Perineurium-covered structures are then grouped together and covered in turn by an epineurium, which covers the peripheral nerve. The epineurium is composed of supportive cells and a collagenous connective tissue matrix. Individual nerve fibers consist of an axon with its associated Schwann cells, and the fibers are grouped together in bundles or fascicles, which themselves are delineated from each other by the perineural sheath (perineurium) (Mihailoff & Haines, 2018; Pindrik & Belzberg, 2014).

Axons and Schwann cells make up roughly 50% of the space within the perineurium, with endoneurial fluid and collagen taking up another 20%–30%, and the remainder containing fibroblasts, macrophages, mast cells, and small blood vessels. The endoneurium surrounds the axon/Schwann cell, and these are grouped together along with interstitial cellular elements and connective tissue within a nerve fascicle (Younger, 2004). Spinal roots do not have an epineurium. Berthold et al. (2005) and Clarke and Bearn (1972) cited Fontana (1781, Vol. 2, pp. 194–203) describing "spiral bands of Fontana" which allow stretching of nerves by up to 20% without damaging the nerve fibers.

Peripheral nerves contain myelinated and unmyelinated axons. A peripheral myelinated nerve fiber has a single continuous axon, which is wrapped in a serial manner with a set of Schwann cells, with the point of contact between adjacent Schwann cells that is known as the node of Ranvier being a short approximately 1-micron-long segment of myelin-free fiber. The compaction of the spiral wrapping of Schwann cell layers around an axon forms myelin. Once Schwann cells have developed and established a one-to-one relationship with an axon, they no longer undergo mitotic division unless a pathologic process occurs (Berthold et al., 2005). Schwann cells play a critical role in the development, maintenance, and regeneration of peripheral nerves and work in conjunction with nerve growth factors to help with peripheral nerve regeneration.

Schwann cells secrete nerve growth factors and neurotrophins and help guide sprouting axons of damaged nerves to their final destination (Pindrik & Belzberg, 2014). The significant length of peripheral axons may contribute to their vulnerability. Injury to an axon or the cell body can result in Wallerian degeneration, in which case there is degeneration of the axon and myelin distal to the injury, as well as to the cell body (Birch, 2011). Wallerian degeneration has been found to start at 4 days after an injury, to be complete in about 50% of injured axons at 7 days after an injury, and to be complete in most nerves at 8 days (Eder et al., 2017). In 1850, Augustus Waller (1851) observed, after sectioning the hypoglossal nerve in frogs,

> during the four first days, after section of the hypoglossal nerve, no change is observed in its structure. On the fifth day the tubes appear more varicose than usual . . . about the tenth day . . . the white matter of SCHWANN cannot be detected . . . after twelve or fifteen days many of the tubules have ceased to be visible.
>
> (p. 376)

In addition, changes in the endoneurial connective tissue and the vascular supply of nerves may result in peripheral neuropathy (Katona & Weis, 2017).

Classification of Nerve Injury

Peripheral nerves can be injured at the time of trauma or in a delayed manner secondarily as a result of edema, ischemia, infection, or scar formation. Mechanisms of nerve injury include stretch injury to a nerve, avulsion of a nerve from the spinal cord, nerve transections, crush injury to a nerve, and damage from compartment syndrome of vascular compromise which leads to nerve ischemia. When axons and structural components are damaged, Wallerian degeneration occurs. Seddon (1942, 1943) described three morphological changes to nerves that occur with injury, each with a characteristic clinical behavior. Neurapraxia refers to an injury with a "short-lived paralysis," in which motor and sensory loss occurs, despite axonal continuity, but there is an excellent prognosis for recovery. Axonotmesis refers to damage to the axons but the sheath and supporting structures are not completely divided, resulting in a good prognosis for recovery, although slower than with neurapraxia. Neurotmesis refers to a nerve (axons and supporting structures) that is completely severed. (Seddon, 1942, 1943). Sunderland (1951) and DiPonio et al. (2005) updated the classification with respect to second-, third- and fourth-degree injuries corresponding to various severities of axonotmesis.

Classification of Peripheral Neuropathy

Different patterns of peripheral nerve involvement may exist. Mononeuropathy multiplex describes the involvement of two or more nerves by a neuropathic disorder. Involvement of myelinated mixed motor and sensory nerves is referred to as large fiber neuropathy. Axonopathy describes a disorder in which axons are mainly affected, whereas a demyelinating neuropathy refers to primary involvement of the myelin sheath covering an axon. Involvement of the unmyelinated axons, which subserve pain, temperature reception, vasomotor, sudomotor, autonomic function, and hair follicles, is referred to as small fiber neuropathy. Sensory loss attributed to involvement of the dorsal root ganglia is referred to as ganglionopathy, whereas anterior horn cell disease is described as neuronopathy (Younger, 2004). Cranial nerves may be involved in isolation or in combination with a generalized polyneuropathy (Thompson & Thomas, 2005).

Neuropathy may be characterized as involving:

- A single nerve (mononeuropathy); typical causes include trauma, focal compression, and entrapment.
- A segmental nerve (radiculopathy).
- A group of nerves in close anatomic proximity (monomelic/regional/multisegmental) resulting in polyradiculopathy, plexopathy, polyradiculoneuropathy, or radiculoplexopathy.

The radiculopathy component of these terms is used if there is significant involvement of spinal nerve roots in addition to peripheral nerve trunks (polyradiculoneuropathy).

This may be related to vasculitis, sarcoidosis, lymphoma, and other systemic diseases where several noncontiguous individual nerves are affected by the same neuropathic disorder, either simultaneously or serially (mononeuropathy multiplex, multifocal neuropathy). diffuse and symmetric involvement of nerves (polyneuropathy); most common cause is diabetes mellitus (Herskovitz et al., 2010; England & Asbury, 2004).

Evaluation of Patients With Peripheral Neuropathy

Peripheral neuropathies are evaluated by taking a patient history, performing a physical examination, and subsequently possibly obtaining electrodiagnostic testing, imaging, and other studies. From the history, onset and duration of symptoms are important factors, as well as functional limitations. Symptoms may include motor (weakness, cramps, etc.), sensory (numbness, pain, dysesthesia, etc.), and autonomic (constipation, anhidrosis, orthostasis, etc.) complaints, as well as gait imbalance and falls. The history should include questions about family history, social history (occupation, toxic exposure, illicit drug use, etc.), neurotoxic medications, and a review of systems (systemic disorders, malignancy, etc.). The physical examination should focus on motor (weakness, atrophy, tremor) and sensory (pain, temperature, vibration and position loss) findings, reflex changes, autonomic signs (orthostasis, tachycardia), gait difficulty, and lesions on the body (skin, gums, nails, hair) (Herskovitz et al., 2010).

In the evaluation of peripheral neuropathy, it is important while taking a history to note the symptoms and their temporal progression. Patients suffering from peripheral neuropathy may present with sensory symptoms (including numbness and tingling, clumsiness, pain [burning sensations, prickly paresthesias, lightning or lancinating pain, electric shock, shooting, stabbing, painful tingling, pressing, itching, pricking]), motor symptoms (weakness), autonomic symptoms (impotence, sweat abnormalities, orthostatic hypotension), or neuropathic pain (burning, stabbing, electrical in nature) (Watson & Dyck, 2015; Younger, 2004; de Souza et al., 2016). Patients typically present with signs and symptoms of sensory changes before motor or autonomic changes occur (Doughty & Seyedsadjadi, 2018). The medical history evaluation should look for possible causes in the past such as a recent viral illness, immunization, change in or new medications, toxic environmental exposure, and underlying illness (Younger, 2004). In the search for the cause of a peripheral neuropathy, the list of potentially relevant diseases is extremely large, as almost every organ system might be involved (Grant & Benstead, 2005).

Pertinent areas of patient evaluation in the search for a cause of peripheral neuropathy include but are not limited to:

- *Constitutional symptoms*: weight loss, malaise, fever, infection, amyloidosis, malignancy, diabetes, hypothyroidism, etc.
- *Gastrointestinal symptoms*: early satiety, cramps, diarrhea, constipation: rule out heavy metal toxicity, acute intermittent porphyria, diabetic autonomic neuropathy (gastroparesis),

paraneoplastic disorders; individuals with inflammatory bowel disease may develop a neuropathy
- *Oral cavity*: lead lines along the border of the gums, etc.
- *Skin diseases* (decreased sensation leading to unrecognized trauma and systemic illness such as diabetes causing slow healing)
- Inspection of nails and hair to evaluate for toxic poisoning
- *Ocular manifestations*: diabetes and other diseases
- *Hearing loss*: nutritional deficiency and hereditary causes of neuropathy
- *Renal dysfunction*: Fabry's disease, diabetes, etc.
- *Musculoskeletal deformities of the feet*: pes cavus (indicates muscle weakness and imbalance beginning early in life, prior to completion of bony development)
- *Neuropsychological changes* such as delirium may suggest heavy metal toxicity, etc.

Clinical features that help in the assessment of neuropathy include:

- The anatomic pattern of which portions of the body are affected (such as distal, proximal, or multifocal)
- Timing of onset (acute, subacute or chronic)
- Sensory vs motor involvement, or both
- Reflex changes
- Gait changes
- Timing of recovery (Herskovitz et al., 2010)

The physical examination of the patient suffering from peripheral neuropathy should evaluate for a possible underlying systemic disorder. A general examination focusing on evaluation of the eyes, skin, lymph nodes, liver, spleen, bladder, testes, cardiopulmonary function, joint function, and gynecologic and rectal examination will help to screen for systemic pathology and possible malignancy. Examination of the peripheral nervous system should evaluate for sensory and motor function. Sensory evaluation should include assessment of light touch, detection of passive joint movement, vibratory sensation, discrimination of pinprick and cold temperature sensation, stance, gait, and coordination. Examination of peripheral motor function evaluates for deformity of the foot, hand, and spine, as well as muscle wasting and fasciculations and strength testing.

The autonomic nervous system may be evaluated through examination for orthostatic change in blood pressure, pupillary response to light and accommodation, patterns of sweating and hair loss, and other findings (Younger, 2004). Horner's syndrome may develop from lesions involving the first thoracic root or the cervical sympathetic chain. Anhidrosis may be present in the cutaneous territory of a peripheral nerve when a mononeuropathy is involved. Difficulties with genitourinary function may be seen in patients with diabetic and amyloid neuropathy. (Thompson & Thomas, 2005).

Skeletal deformities may be present if chronic neuropathies develop before cessation of growth, resulting in possible foot, hand, and spinal deformities. A claw hand and clawing of the toes may be seen on examination, and kyphoscoliosis may be present. When pes cavus or a spinal deformity is present, it indicates that the neuropathy had an onset in childhood. Trophic ulcers and neuropathic joint degeneration may occur, as the loss of pain sensation may expose tissues to risk of repeated trauma. In patients with diabetes, ischemia and risk of diabetic tissues suffering infection may be significant. Thickened, palpable, or visible enlargement of nerve trunks may be encountered in a variety of peripheral neuropathies (Thompson & Thomas, 2005).

Electrodiagnostic testing (electromyography/nerve conduction study [EMG/NCS]) helps to differentiate between predominant axonopathy, myelinopathy (demyelinating), mixed axonal-demyelinating, or neuronopathy (ganglionopathy). While EMG/NCS assesses the function and integrity of large, myelinated A beta nerve fibers, it does not assess small nerve fibers such as C fibers and small unmyelinated A delta fibers (Herskovitz et al., 2010; Watson & Dyck, 2015).

Small fiber peripheral neuropathies may affect the autonomic nervous system. Epidermal skin biopsy may be performed to evaluate nerve fiber density. Quantitative autonomic tests include studies to evaluate cardiovagal function (response of heart rate to deep breathing, Valsalva maneuver, and upright stance), tilt table assessment of blood pressure control and pulse regulation, sudomotor evaluation with thermally and chemically induced sweating (quantitative sudomotor axon reflex test [QSART]), and assessment of sphincter and erectile dysfunction. (Herskovitz et al., 2010; Watson & Dyck, 2015; Younger, 2004). In patients with cranial nerve involvement, visual, brainstem auditory, and somatosensory evoked responses may be helpful to evaluate (Younger, 2004).

With the exception of assessment of small fiber neuropathy, nerve biopsy is typically not needed. Biopsies that may be considered include those of nerves (sural nerve and others), skin, and muscle motor nerves (Katona & Weis, 2017). Cerebrospinal fluid (CSF) analysis may help with the diagnosis of immune demyelinating neuropathy. Magnetic resonance imaging (MRI) may at times be used to identify nerve enlargement or enhancement. Despite extensive evaluation, Herskovitz et al. (2010) has cited Wolfe, Smith, Notermans, and Mcleod in stating that one third to one half of neuropathies will remain idiopathic or cryptogenic with respect to diagnosed etiology and that mostly the involvement is axonal, affecting sensory or sensorimotor or small fiber types. These are known as chronic idiopathic axonal polyneuropathy (CIAP) or small fiber neuropathy (SFN).

Other testing for the evaluation and diagnosis of peripheral neuropathy in order to evaluate for systemic diseases that may cause peripheral neuropathy include:

- Blood comprehensive metabolic panel (CMP)
- Complete blood count (CBC)
- Erythrocyte sedimentation rate (ESR)
- Glucose testing and its relation to diabetes
- Vitamin B_{12} levels
- Selective autoantibody tests
- Other tests (Herskovitz et al., 2010; Younger, 2004)

Focal Neuropathy (Mononeuropathy)

Entrapments

Carpal Tunnel Syndrome

Carpal tunnel syndrome (CTS) is a mononeuropathy caused by compression of the median nerve in the carpal tunnel at the wrist (England & Asbury, 2004). CTS is the most commonly encountered entrapment in clinical practice and results from compression of the median nerve at the wrist under the transverse carpal ligament. Episodic ischemia causes nocturnal paresthesia (Birch, 2011). Patients often report numbness, tingling, and pain in the hand, which may radiate into the forearm. Symptoms are often worse at night and with repetitive use. Weakness of thumb abduction and atrophy of the thenar eminence may be present with advanced cases. Physical examination findings may include decreased sensation affecting the first three digits of the hand, as well as the ulnar aspect of the fourth digit, as well as a positive Phalen's and Tinel's sign. Diagnostic testing with EMG/NCV (nerve conduction velocity) studies is essential, and evaluation of median neuropathy is one of the most common reasons for obtaining electrodiagnostic studies. The typical findings on NCS will reveal slow median nerve speed (motor and sensory) across the carpal tunnel space but normal at other portions of the nerve. Early on in the disease, it may be only the sensory nerve study that is abnormal, but the motor nerve study may be affected as the disease progresses. It is best to wait 4–6 weeks after the onset of symptoms before obtaining an EMG/NCS, as it takes time for Wallerian degeneration to occur and for the EMG component to show abnormalities (Choi & Di Maria, 2021). MRI imaging may be helpful, especially when the clinical picture is unclear (Scott et al., 2013; Callaghan et al., 2015).

Ulnar Neuropathy at the Elbow

Ulnar neuropathy is a mononeuropathy due to compression of the nerve at or near the elbow (England & Asbury, 2004). Ulnar neuropathy resulting from entrapment of the ulnar nerve at the elbow is the second most common entrapment syndrome of the upper extremity. It may result from external compression due to resting the elbow on a flat surface, as well as from a fracture of the elbow, recurrent subluxation of the ulnar nerve, or synovial cysts. Clinical features may include elbow pain and numbness, as well as symptoms of numbness and tingling involving the fifth and ulnar aspect of the fourth digits, and in severe cases, weakness may ensue. Physical examination findings may include applying pressure over the cubital tunnel to evaluate for symptoms. EMG/NCS testing should be performed, and radiographic x-rays may be performed to rule out bony deformities. While the motor nerve study will show focal slowing of the ulnar nerve across the elbow, the sensory nerve study may be normal, or it may show a reduced or absent sensory nerve action potential (SNAP) aptitude. (Scott et al., 2013; Callaghan et al., 2015; Choi & Di Maria, 2021).

Common Peroneal Neuropathy at the Fibular Head

The common peroneal nerve, which arises from the sciatic nerve in the distal thigh, is most vulnerable for compression where it winds around the fibular head and most commonly presents as foot drop. EMG/NCS studies may localize demyelination of the nerve segment traveling through the fibular tunnel. Plain radiographic x-rays may be performed to evaluate for fracture or dislocation, and MRI scanning may evaluate soft tissues (Scott et al., 2013).

Distal Tibial Neuropathy (Tarsal Tunnel Syndrome)

The tibial nerve, which arises from the sciatic nerve, descends to the medial malleolus and travels under the flexor retinaculum at the medial side of the ankle. Perimalleolar pain is the most common presenting symptom in patients with tarsal tunnel syndrome. EMG/NCS studies may be helpful, and plain radiographic x-rays may evaluate for fracture or dislocation. MRI may be used to examine the soft tissue structures (Scott et al., 2013).

Other Mononeuropathies

Facial Neuropathy

Facial neuropathy may present with acute weakness of the upper and lower portions of one side of the face and may be accompanied by decreased tearing, hyperacusis, and diminished taste from the anterior two thirds of the tongue (Callaghan et al., 2015).

Meralgia Paresthetica

Meralgia paresthetica is mononeuropathy that is sensory in nature, as it results from compression of the lateral femoral cutaneous nerve as it passes from the lumbosacral plexus toward the inguinal ligament to the anterior thigh, possibly resulting in pain and dysesthesia in the anterolateral thigh (Coffey & Gupta, 2022).

Polyneuropathy

Polyneuropathies are the most common type of disorder of the peripheral nervous system in adults. The diagnosis should identify treatable etiologies, as rapid intervention may be required for Guillain-Barré syndrome and vasculitis, and treatment regimens should be implemented for treatable etiologies such as inflammatory, endocrinological, toxic, nutrition-related, and tumor-related causes. The rate of onset is important to note, as it can be acute and rapid with Guillain-Barré syndrome, subacute with vasculitis, and chronic with diabetes. The cause of peripheral neuropathy remains elusive in up to 30% of cases (Sommer et al., 2018).

Distal symmetric polyneuropathy is the most common subtype of peripheral neuropathy, with diabetes being the most common cause, followed by alcohol intake and inherited disorders such as Charcot-Marie-Tooth disease (a motor and sensory neuropathy) (Dyck et al., 1981). Other causes include chronic kidney and liver disease, nutritional deficiencies (vitamin B_{12}, vitamin E, thiamine, copper, etc.), effects from medications (chemotherapeutic medications such as vincristine, cisplatin, Taxol, phenytoin, etc.), autoimmune disorders (rheumatoid arthritis, lupus, sarcoidosis, etc.), infectious causes (infectious, hepatitis), neoplastic etiologies (monoclonal gammopathy of unclear clinical significance [MGUS], multiple myeloma, etc.), and idiopathic reasons. Callaghan et al. (2015) cited Boulton, Dyck, Franklin, Maser, and Partanen in reporting a prevalence of distal symmetric polyneuropathy ranging from 10% to 34% in patients with type 1 diabetes and 8% to 25% in those with type 2 diabetes. Callaghan et al. (2015) further cited studies of Callaghan, Johannsen, and Lubec, noting that diabetes as an etiology accounts for 32–53% of cases of distal symmetric polyneuropathy. In some patients, only small nerve fibers will be affected, and electrodiagnostic testing may be normal. The most important component of the evaluation that patients typically report is numbness, tingling, and pain starting in their toes with a slow progression proximally, and this pattern is referred to as a stocking-glove distribution. Symptoms may occur in the fingertips usually after they have reached the level of the knees in the lower extremities. Weakness in the lower extremities usually occurs late in the progression of the disease and often starts with weakness of extension of the toe, followed by weakness of ankle dorsiflexion (Callaghan et al., 2015). When small fiber neuropathy is suspected, electrodiagnostic studies will not provide help with diagnosis, and quantitative skin testing or skin biopsy may help with the diagnosis (Sommer et al., 2018). Peripheral neuropathies may be immune-mediated. Patients should be suspected to have Guillain-Barré syndrome when they suffer an ascending paralysis following a gastrointestinal or respiratory infection, and rapid hospitalization and possible intensive care unit treatment may be needed. Close monitoring, with supportive care and use of intravenous immunoglobulins (IVIg) and plasmapheresis, may be needed. Chronic inflammatory demyelinating polyradiculoneuropathy (CIDP) often has a clinical presentation of symmetrical, mainly motor, polyradiculoneuropathy causing proximal and distal muscle weakness, areflexia, paresthesia, and sensory deficits and often has a chronic progressive course, although symptoms and the course of progression can vary (Sommer et al., 2018).

Multifocal Neuropathy, Multiple Mononeuropathy, and Mononeuropathy Multiplex

Mononeuropathy multiplex may cause an asymmetric, stepwise progression of sensory motor deficits and may involve more than one peripheral or cranial nerve. It is often associated with systemic or non-systemic vasculitis (polyarteritis nodosa, systemic lupus erythematosus, rheumatoid arthritis, Wegener's granulomatosis, Churg-Strauss syndrome). Approximately 75% of patients with vasculitic neuropathy will suffer involvement of the common peroneal nerve, often resulting in a painful foot drop (Matsuda et al., 2012).

Radiculopathy

Radiculopathy, with numbness, tingling, and pain occurring in a dermatomal distribution, with weakness similarly occurring in a myotomal pattern, can occur from peripheral neuropathy and can affect the lumbar nerve roots as well as those in the cervical spine (Callaghan et al., 2015). Radiculopathy may result from a nerve root being compressed on its course from within the spinal canal to its exiting the spinal canal, and sources of compression may include herniated discs, arthritic spurs, spondylolistheses, and any other causes of nerve compression. The most common disorder of spinal nerves in a clinical practice results from acute disc herniations, which may be superimposed upon intervertebral foraminal narrowing. Spondylosis can produce narrowing of the central canal and neural foramen. Spondylolistheses can also create compression on nerve roots. Radiculopathy can also arise as a result of radiation and may develop months or years after radiotherapy to the spine or other regions of the body. Another cause may be arachnoiditis, which may result from previous spine surgery (failed back syndrome) and other etiologies (Chalk, 2005).

Plexopathies

Lesions of the brachial and lumbosacral plexuses can occur. These plexuses are complex structures that derive their nerves from the spine (cervical, lumbar, sacral nerve roots). The brachial plexus, a complex anatomical structure, consists of various groupings of nerves into trunks (upper, middle, and lower), divisions (anterior and posterior), and cords (lateral, medial, and posterior) and originates from the cervical and thoracic roots (C5–T1). Causes such as trauma (the most common cause), infection, inflammation, neoplasm, compression (thoracic outlet compression), and iatrogenic and radiation-induced factors must be excluded before it may be considered idiopathic (Scott et al., 2013). Patients suspected of suffering from brachial plexus injuries should have cervical spine and chest radiographs to rule out fractures of the neck, clavicle, or ribs, all of which may be associated with a brachial plexus injury. A myelogram and post-myelogram computerized tomography (CT) scan of the cervical spine will be helpful to evaluate for brachial plexus avulsion injuries (primary roots may be torn/avulsed from the spinal cord as a result of traction), and MRI may be used as well. Findings may reveal a pseudomeningocele on CT myelography or MRI imaging (Spinner & Kline, 2000; Pindrik & Belzberg, 2014).

Causes of Peripheral Neuropathy

This section will differentiate 1) disease processes that may cause peripheral neuropathy and 2) causes of peripheral neuropathy based on anatomic distribution of affected nerves.

Causes of Peripheral Neuropathy Based on Disease Process

Most cases of peripheral neuropathy are either acquired or genetic in nature. Those that are acquired are either symptomatic from another disorder or condition or idiopathic. Following are several causes of peripheral neuropathy. The list is not exhaustive but reflects some of the more common causes.

Trauma

Nerves can be damaged as a result of direct trauma (open or closed), ischemia (compartment syndrome or external compressive events), traction or stretching, pressure, distortion, entrapment within fractures or joints, cold, heat, severance, electric shock, injection of noxious substances, and vibration injuries (Birch, 2011). Physical injury/trauma is the most common cause of acquired single-nerve injury and may result from automobile injuries, falls, sports, and medical procedures (National Institute of Neurological Disorders and Stroke, n.d.). Injuries to the nerves can result in crushing of nerves, compressing of nerves, and avulsing of nerves from the spinal cord. Herniated discs in the spine, resulting from significant or mild trauma or from repetitive motions, may compress upon nerves. Arthritic spurs may compress nerves, as may herniated discs (causing radiculopathy). Limb amputations may result in phantom limb pain. Compression of nerves at the wrist (median nerve compression in CTS) and elbow (ulnar nerve compression) may occur. As cited by Birch, Lundborg found that impairment to vascular flow to a nerve could be caused by an 8% elongation of a segment of a nerve, and all blood flow may be arrested by an elongation of 10–15% (Birch, 2011).

Injection injuries occur when the point of a needle lacerates the perineurium, and if the nerve is injected with commonly used substances such as steroids, anesthetic agents for local or intravenous use, anxiolytic medications such as diazepam, or antibiotics, the consequences may be severe. Commonly involved sites include the sciatic nerve in the buttock, the brachial plexus (neck and axilla), the radial nerve in the arm, and the median nerve at the elbow. The onset of pain is usually severe, local, and radiated, and progression may occur over hours. Typically, the symptoms that develop acutely at the time of the injury (although they may develop burning or paresthesias in a delayed manner) may include severe, painful electric shocks radiating distally in the limb in the distribution of the nerve (Birch, 2011; Spinner & Kline, 2000; Kline et al., 1998; Esquenazi et al., 2016). Other traumatic causes of peripheral nerve injury include the following:

- Complex regional pain syndrome (CRPS) is another source of pain. CRPS has historically been known as reflex sympathetic dystrophy (RSD), causalgia, and Sudeck's atrophy, among other names. It is a neuropathic pain disorder related to involvement of the autonomic nervous system (Harden & Bruehl, 2010).
- Vascular injuries may result in mass lesions (hematoma), arteriovenous fistula, pseudoaneurysm, etc., which compress upon nerves.
- Previous surgeries that may include failed back surgery (i.e., post-laminectomy and other spinal surgical procedures) and arachnoiditis.
- Injuries to the brachial plexus may occur as a result of trauma in adults and may result from an obstetric injury during birth.
- Central nervous system injury and other diseases producing distal pain (not a peripheral neuropathy but causing peripheral pain) that may include brain injury (especially thalamic injury), spinal cord injury, multiple sclerosis, and central nervous system tumors.

Metabolic and Toxic Neuropathies and Systemic Disorders

- Diabetes
- Thyroid gland dysfunction
- Uremia and liver failure–associated neuropathy
- Toxic neuropathies (alcohol use related, drug use, heavy metal related, nutritional related, chemotherapy induced, etc.)
- Vitamin deficiencies (vitamin B_{12}, etc.)
- Amyloidosis (amyloid deposits within nerves)
- Sarcoidosis (granuloma accumulation within nerves) (Roth et al., 2021; Callaghan et al., 2018)

Vascular Disorders

- Systemic vasculitis: polyarteritis nodosa, microscopic polyangiitis, Churg-Strauss syndrome, Wegener's granulomatosis
- Vasculitis associated with connective tissue diseases: rheumatoid arthritis, systemic lupus erythematosus, Sjögren's syndrome, scleroderma (Collins, 2005)
- Decreased blood and oxygen supply to peripheral nerves, possibly causing ischemic injury, may lead to nerve damage and may be contributed to by diabetes and smoking

Systemic Autoimmune Diseases

- Sjögren's syndrome
- Lupus
- Rheumatoid arthritis
- Antiphospholipid syndrome

Immune-Mediated Neuropathies and Related Disorders

- Guillain-Barré syndrome
- CIDP
- Vasculitic neuropathy
- Sarcoid neuropathy
- Infectious neuropathies
- Dysproteinemic neuropathies
- Paraneoplastic neuropathies (triggered by the immune system in response to cancer)

Certain Cancers and Benign Tumors

- Schwannoma
- Neurofibroma
- Ganglioneuroma
- Malignant peripheral nerve tumors (Giannini, 2005)
- Malignant apical lung neoplasm (typically non–small cell carcinoma, usually squamous cell or adenocarcinoma) may affect brachial plexus causing Pancoast's syndrome (Wilbouorn, 2005)
- Nerve involvement may occur as a result of either direct infiltration or pressure upon nerves

Chemotherapy Drugs

- 30–40% of those treated with these mediations may develop polyneuropathy

Radiation Therapy

- May cause nerve damage starting months or years after treatment. Significant peripheral neuropathy will likely occur with radiation doses exceeding 20 Gy (Vujaskovic, 1997).

Burn Injuries

- Thermal
- Electrical
- Chemical

Infections

- Viruses (varicella-zoster, West Nile virus, Epstein-Barr virus, cytomegalovirus, and herpes simplex target the sensory fibers)
- Lyme disease may cause a range of neuropathic symptoms
- Human immunodeficiency virus (HIV) can cause extensive damage to the central and peripheral nervous system
- Chagas disease
- Complex Regional Pain Syndrome (CRPS)

Hereditary

- Charcot-Marie-Tooth disease
- Acute intermittent porphyria
- Tyrosinemia
- Mitochondrial depletion syndromes
- Fabry disease
- Hereditary sensory and autonomic neuropathy
- Hereditary motor neuropathies and others (Katona & Weis, 2017; National Institute of Neurological Disorders and Stroke, n.d.; de Souza et al., 2016; Roth et al., 2021)

Causes of Peripheral Neuropathy Based on Anatomic Distribution of Affected Nerves

Systemic Polyneuropathy Causes

- Diabetes
- Toxin related
- Alcohol induced
- Drug induced (i.e., chemotherapy)
- Heavy metal poisoning
- Inflammatory
- Guillain-Barré syndrome
- Vasculitis
- CIDP
- Nutrition related
- Thiamine deficiency

- Cobalamin deficiency
- Vitamin E deficiency
- Cancer related
- Paraneoplastic syndromes
- Plexopathies from tumor infiltration
- Peripheral nerve compromise from tumor infiltration
- Infectious causes
- Leprosy
- HIV related
- Lyme disease
- Organ failure related
- Renal failure
- Hepatic failure
- Pulmonary failure
- Organ transplant related

Mononeuropathy Causes

- Entrapment neuropathies (i.e., CTS, ulnar neuropathy at the elbow)
- Trauma to a specific nerve

Multiple Mononeuropathies

- Leprosy
- Diabetic multiple mononeuropathies
- HIV-related neuropathies
- Sarcoidosis-related neuropathy (Waldman et al., 2017)

Cranial Nerves

- *Cranial nerves III, IV, and VI*: trauma, neoplasm, vascular disease and aneurysms (cranial nerve III compression resulting in a dilated pupil may be seen as a result of compression by a posterior communicating artery aneurysm), infections, and toxins (possibly in cavernous sinus) (Leavitt & Younge, 2005)
- *Cranial nerve V*: trauma, perineural spread of tumor, trigeminal schwannomas and other nerve tumors, toxins, idiopathic trigeminal neuropathy, trigeminal neuralgia (from vascular compression, tumors, etc.) (Hughes, 2005)
- *Cranial nerve VII*: idiopathic facial nerve paralysis (Bell's palsy), Ramsey Hunt syndrome, granulomatous disease, amyloidosis, trauma, diabetes mellitus, HIV, pregnancy, benign intracranial hypertension, tumor, inherited familial facial palsy, congenital/pediatric facial nerve paralysis, hemifacial spasm (Klein, 2005)
- *Cranial nerve VIII*: auditory neuropathy (autoimmune, infectious, toxic/metabolic, syndrome related), vestibular neuronitis, lesions compressing or infiltrating vestibulocochlear nerve, vestibular schwannoma, trauma, drugs, noise (Bamiou & Luxon, 2005)
- *Cranial nerves IX, X, XI, and XII*: intramedullary and extramedullary lesions, glossopharyngeal neuralgia (cranial nerve IX) (Thomas & Mathias, 2005)

Evaluation of Peripheral Neuropathy

Electromyography and Nerve Conduction Studies

EMG and NCS are used in the evaluation of patients suspected of having peripheral neuropathy in order to evaluate the characteristic electrophysiological findings in different types of peripheral nerve disorders. NCS and needle EMG are separate tests but are routinely used together in testing. The results should be evaluated with the clinical picture in mind, as an electrophysiological diagnosis does not necessarily determine the cause of the peripheral nerve abnormalities (such as determining whether polyneuropathy results from diabetes or from vitamin B_{12} deficiency). Electrodiagnostic studies utilizing both NCS and EMG provide for the evaluation of sensory and motor neurons, the neuromuscular junction, and individual muscles and aid in the diagnosis of neuromuscular disease (Choi & Di Maria, 2021). These studies do have limitations and should be used in conjunction with a careful history and physical examination (Spinner & Kline, 2000).

The EMG examination helps to assess whether weakness is related to neurogenic involvement or to myopathy. Crone cites Denny-Brown in finding that fibrillation potentials seen on EMG indicate ongoing denervation. A motor unit potential (MUP) is a compound potential generated by muscle fibers during voluntary activity or electrical stimulation, and evaluation of these potentials (duration, amplitude, and shape) is important in distinguishing neurogenic lesions from myopathy. It is not until 4–6 weeks after an acute neurogenic disorder, when reinnervation of muscle fibers by collateral sprouting from surviving motor axons takes place, that MUPs become abnormal (Crone & Krarup, 2013; Wohlfart, 1957).

NCSs only assess the function of large fiber myelinated alpha-motor and sensory fibers to evaluate axonal loss and help to distinguish whether the myelin versus the axon is affected. During a motor NCS, an electrical stimulus is applied to the skin overlying a nerve, and a compound muscle action potential (CMAP) is recorded over a muscle belly. The sum of motor unit action potentials is known as the CMAP. In sensory NCS, an electrical stimulus is applied to the surface of the skin and a response is recorded on the skin distally, overlying the nerve. The sum of action potentials from individual sensory fibers is known as the compound SNAP. Stimulus-response relationships are determined, where a stimulus is given and a response measured. Conduction time is measured by determining the latency between the start of the stimulus and the arrival of a response. Amplitude, distal latency, and conduction velocity help to determine whether the pathology is arising from the myelin sheath or the axon. Axonal neuropathy typically reveals a reduced CMAP amplitude but normal distal latency and conduction velocity, whereas a demyelinating neuropathy is characterized by increased distal latency and decreased conduction velocity (Choi & Di Maria, 2021).

Nerve compression or vascular lesions that cause disruption of axonal continuity may be associated with Wallerian degeneration of nerve fibers distal to the lesion. While it is often difficult using only NCS to localize a lesion causing disruption of axonal continuity, the addition of an EMG examination is often very helpful (Wohlfart, 1957). Choi and Di Maria cite Martyn, Kendall, Nardin, Barr, Tong, Boon, and the American Academy of Electrodiagnostic Medicine in finding that EMG may be very beneficial for distinguishing myopathies from neuropathies and is essential for evaluating radiculopathies. Fibrillations will be seen on EMG when radiculopathy exists for over 3 weeks, while they may not show any abnormalities if the test is performed less than 3 weeks after the onset of symptoms. Fibrillation and positive sharp waves appear 10–14 days after injury in proximal muscles and 3–4 weeks after injury in distal muscles (Campbell, 2008). EMG may show spontaneous fibrillations and positive sharp waves in cases of myopathy (Choi & Di Maria, 2021).

After traumatic injury to a nerve, although the NCS can reveal nerve damage, in the first few days after an injury, it may not be able to distinguish between neurapraxia, axonotmesis, and neurotmesis. Serial EMG/NCS studies performed every 1–3 months may be able to provide additional information. A combination of EMG/NCS helps to differentiate neurapraxia from a more severe grade of peripheral nerve injury, and it helps to define the location and severity of the lesion, exclude other lesions, and predict recovery (Spinner & Kline, 2000). When surgery is performed, intraoperative electrodiagnostic studies, implemented by stimulating surgically exposed nerves across a suspected lesion, may yield additional information about axonal continuity and whether axonal regrowth has started to occur. This can be performed before and after neurolysis and has been helpful in all but Sunderland's fifth-degree lesions (neurotmesis) (DiPonio et al., 2005). Use of intraoperative nerve action potentials allows for relatively early surgical evaluation of common lesions in continuity (Spinner & Kline, 2000).

With the combination of the mode of onset of symptoms of peripheral neuropathy and a detailed electrophysiological examination, it is generally possible to determine the etiology as being in one of several categories, depending upon the timing of onset (acute: less than 4 weeks; subacute: 4–8 weeks; slowly progressing: greater than 2 months); whether the neuropathy is mainly of a demyelination or axonal degeneration origin; and the anatomic distribution of nerve lesions. More specifically, the peripheral nerve disorders can be broken down into mononeuropathy, multiple mononeuropathy, polyneuropathy, and subsequently classified further depending upon whether the cause is axonal loss or demyelination and the timing of onset (Crone & Krarup, 2013; England & Asbury, 2004).

Evaluation of Autonomic Function

Small unmyelinated nerve fibers cannot be assessed by conventional neurophysiological studies because of their high threshold to electrical stimulation and the small amplitudes of their action potentials. C-sensory nerve fibers, which support temperature sensation, and postganglionic autonomic nerve fibers (sympathetic and parasympathetic) are unmyelinated. Testing for orthostatic hypotension may be helpful. Sudomotor function tests include the QSART, the sweat imprint, and the thermoregulatory sweat test, which evaluate the extent, distribution, and location of deficits in sympathetic cholinergic function (Vinik et al., 2003).

Imaging

Ultrasound. Ultrasonography uses sound waves that are sent from a transducer through a patient's skin to create images. Since many peripheral nerves are less than 1 mm in diameter, high image resolution (>12-Hz transducer) is needed for adequate nerve visualization. Nerves are viewed in both cross-sectional (axial) and longitudinal views. Cross-sectional area of nerves is a commonly used parameter in the evaluation of peripheral nerves, and intraneural blood flow can be measured using power Doppler. Ultrasound is often used in the evaluation of peripheral neuropathy and is often used as an adjunct to electrodiagnostic testing, especially when a lesion cannot be localized by that testing. It is useful in the evaluation of compression neuropathies (CTS, ulnar neuropathy at the elbow), traumatic nerve injuries, and brachial plexopathy (Gonzalez & Hobson-Webb, 2021). Ultrasound can also be used to evaluate muscles and evaluate for patterns of denervation (Simon et al., 2016).

Magnetic resonance imaging. MRI distinguishes between different tissues by distinguishing the physical properties of protons and water molecules. MRI can be used to visualize nerves as well as muscle (along with ultrasound) to provide additional information about denervation and patterns of muscles involved (Simon et al., 2016). Standard MRI reveals the outline of some nerves but has difficulty distinguishing between nerves and similar-appearing surrounding structures (Gonzalez & Hobson-Webb, 2021). Magnetic resonance neurography (MRN) describes a combination of qualitative and quantitative techniques used to image peripheral nerves and allows for improved visualization of nerve morphology (Gonzalez & Hobson-Webb). MRN is a tissue selective imaging modality that can be used to study peripheral nerves, and the information gained may be used to complement that obtained through a clinical examination and an EMG/NCS study. It has been found to be helpful when EMG/NCS studies and traditional MRI scanning is inconclusive to rule out tumors which may be affecting peripheral nerves or nerve plexuses, as well as for surgical decision making and planning for patients who have lesions or have suffered peripheral nerve trauma (Du et al., 2010).

Diffusion tensor tractography (DTT), which has been extensively applied to evaluating white matter tracts in the brain, may also be applied to peripheral nerves. While ultrasound and MRN may have difficulty differentiating between neurotmesis and axonotmesis, especially when the nerve remains in continuity, DTT has the potential to improve this diagnosis significantly. DTT has limitations with respect to spatial and contrast resolution and relatively low signal-to-noise ratio (Matsuda et al., 2012).

Traumatic Neuropathies

A major drawback in the use of electrodiagnostic studies to evaluate nerve trauma arises from the delay (typically several weeks after an injury) in which abnormalities in the nerve are detected, and even once changes do occur, differentiating partial from complete transections may be difficult. MRN shows an entire nerve in three dimensions and is useful in the setting of trauma, tumor, compressive lesions, and the evaluation of brachial plexus injuries (Gonzalez & Hobson-Webb, 2021; Holzgrefe et al., 2019).

Biopsy (Nerve and Skin)

Pathologic changes in a peripheral nerve biopsy specimen may provide insight into the cause of a peripheral nerve disorder. In order to avoid subjecting a patient to a serious neurological deficit, a segment of the sural, superficial peroneal sensory, or femoral intermedius nerve may be removed surgically. Adjacent muscle may be biopsied at the same procedure (Younger, 2004). As cited by England and Asbury (2004) regarding the works of Davies, Dyck, Bosboom, Deprez, Flachenecker, Gabriel, Said, Asbury, and Vallat, nerve biopsy is most useful in the evaluation of inflammatory disorders such as vasculitis, sarcoidosis, CIDP, infectious diseases such as leprosy, or infiltrative disorders such as amyloidosis or tumor. This procedure should only be used when the diagnosis is not clear after using other diagnostic tests.

Complications and Functional Disabilities Associated With Peripheral Neuropathy

Complications of peripheral neuropathy affect many body systems and can include all of the following:

- *Weakness*: muscle weakness may lead to inability to perform activities, muscle shortening, and contractures.
- *Sensory loss*: may involve diminished ability to perceive pain and touch, can compromise a patient's ability to protect an extremity from injury, more commonly affecting the feet than the upper extremities.

- *Autonomic dysfunction*: present in neuropathies affecting small fibers and plays a role in neurogenic pain and regional pain syndromes (CRPS), and patients may experience decreased sweating, orthostatic hypotension, gastroparesis, constipation, etc.
- *Neurogenic bowel and bladder*: complications include upper urinary tract infections, renal stones and damage, and skin breakdown.
- *Bladder and bowel incontinence.*
- *Sexual dysfunction.*
- *Consequences of immobility and deconditioning*: due to improper positioning and immobility, development of pressure neuropathies, pressure sores (decubitus ulcers), loss of strength, and decreased range of motion may occur.

Treatment of Peripheral Neuropathy

The goal in the evaluation of peripheral neuropathy is to identify the underlying etiology and implement treatments to address the cause if possible. While treatment generally helps to prevent further progression of the neuropathy, symptoms may generally not improve unless caught early in the disease process, when symptoms may improve or resolve. More commonly, the symptoms that have resulted from the pretreatment injury will linger, and treatment is aimed at managing symptoms (Watson & Dyck, 2015).

Medical causes of peripheral neuropathy, such as diabetes mellitus, hypothyroidism, renal insufficiency, vitamin B_{12} deficiency, and systemic vasculitis, should be directly treated. Neuropathies related to Guillain-Barré syndrome and CIDP may be treated with IVIg and plasmapheresis (Sommer et al., 2018). There is no specific treatment for many chronic neuropathies, including the hereditary neuropathies and chronic idiopathic axonal polyneuropathy (England & Asbury, 2004).

Neuropathic pain is common and may be difficult to treat. It may result from spontaneous activity and sensitization of damaged axons (Sommer et al., 2018). Neuropathic pain can be treated with antiepileptic drugs (gabapentin, carbamazepine, pregabalin), tricyclic antidepressants and serotonin and norepinephrine reuptake inhibitors (amitriptyline, nortriptyline, venlafaxine, duloxetine), and topical lidocaine (England & Asbury, 2004; Walk & Backonja, 2010). If additional treatment is needed, tramadol or opioids may be added (Herskovitz et al., 2010). Treatment generally starts with a low dose of medication and is modified in order to get the maximum response with the least adverse side effects (Khdour, 2020).

Foot care is important, as length-dependent peripheral neuropathy sensory symptoms often affect the feet, and ulceration or injury to the feet may occur without the patient being aware (Watson & Dyck, 2015). General treatments include weight reduction, good shoes, and ankle-foot orthoses as needed. Physical and occupational therapy may be of benefit to help with designing and implementing adaptive equipment for chronically disabled patients (England & Asbury, 2004).

Common Entrapment Neuropathies

Most patients who experience nerve entrapments have mild or intermittent symptoms. Conservative care is generally implemented initially, with surgery being indicated for patients with persistent pain or neurologic symptoms or in cases where electrodiagnostic studies show worsening despite rest, conservative treatment, and decreased use of the limb. Rapidly worsening deficits may also warrant early surgery. Conservative nonoperative care generally consists of a trial of nonsteroidal anti-inflammatory medications, avoidance of activities that may place the region of concern under stress or irritation of the affected nerve, splinting, and possibly local steroid injections. In addition, improvement or better control of contributory systemic disease such as diabetes may help to decrease symptoms. Surgical intervention for nerve entrapments typically involves a wide decompression of the affected nerve and possibly a transposition if needed. Spinner and Kline find that with the most common nerve compression syndromes, "excellent results can be expected for median nerve decompression at the wrist, good outcomes for ulnar nerve surgery at the elbow, and fairly good results for peroneal nerve decompression at the fibular neck" (Spinner & Kline, 2000, p. 690).

Carpal Tunnel Syndrome

CTS may be treated through nonsurgical as well as surgical management. Nonsurgical management may consist of rest, avoidance of precipitating factors, splinting, and the use of anti-inflammatory medications and local steroid injections. For cases that are refractory to nonsurgical management, surgery for decompression of the median nerve at the wrist may be considered.

Ulnar Neuropathy at the Elbow

The initial treatment of ulnar neuropathy is conservative, with avoidance of pressure on the elbow. Splints or cushions/elbow pads may be used. When neurological deficits are significant or progressive, surgery for decompression or submuscular transposition of the ulnar nerve may be considered (Scott et al., 2013).

Common Peroneal Neuropathy at the Fibular Head

Nonsurgical treatment may consist of nonsteroidal anti-inflammatory medications and activity modification or biomechanical correction. Surgery may be performed to release the nerve from compression due to overlying muscle and fascia or if compression at the fibular head is due to a ganglion cyst arising from the tibiofibular joint (Scott et al., 2013).

Distal Tibial Neuropathy (Tarsal Tunnel Syndrome)

Conservative management with avoidance of precipitating activities and the use of nonsteroidal anti-inflammatory medications may be helpful for pain control. Local corticosteroid injections may be used. When patients don't improve with conservative measures, surgical exploration to release the flexor retinaculum or to address a ganglion cyst or other structural abnormality may be considered (Scott et al., 2013).

Intravenous Immunoglobulin

For most peripheral neuropathies, including small fiber peripheral neuropathy, Guillain-Barré syndrome, CIDP, and other types, high-dose human IVIg is the treatment of choice. Plasmapheresis may also be utilized at times (Younger, 2004).

Spinal Cord Stimulation and Intrathecal Opioids for Pain Control

Despite treatments used to help patients suffering from neuropathic pain as a result of peripheral nerve injuries, relief from pain is sometimes inadequate, with the pain being unremitting and agonizing, causing physical and psychological disability in patients, interfering with personal and work life and activities of daily living. In a seminal work published in 1965, Melzak and Wall proposed and discussed a gate theory related to pain, in which they felt that a gate control system modulates sensory input from the skin before it evokes pain perception and response. They felt that the therapeutic implications are 1) "control of pain may be achieved by selectively influencing the large, rapidly conducting fibers . . . the gate may be closed by decreasing the small-fiber input and also by enhancing the large-fiber input" and 2) "a better understanding of the substantia gelatinosa may lead to new ways of controlling pain" (Melzack & Wall, 1965, p. 971). Shortly after this work was published, applications of neuromodulation were developed for use in people (Stuart & Winfree, 2009). It has been delivered with an implantable device through both spinal cord stimulation and peripheral nerve stimulation (Haque & Winfree, 2006; Shealy et al., 1967). In addition, if a trial period of intrathecal opioid therapy is successful, an intrathecal catheter delivering opioids from an implanted pump reservoir may provide pain improvement or relief with a low amount of systemic side effects (Koulousakis et al., 2007).

Spinal cord stimulation, which is the most commonly used implantable neurostimulation technique, has been used for more than 40 years for many types of pain syndromes and regional pain problems (failed back surgery syndrome, peripheral neuropathy, refractory chronic unstable angina pectoris, peripheral vascular disease, pain of spinal origin, CRPS), and outcomes and efficacy have varied over time as the technique has been modified (Lee & Pilitsis, 2006). Initially a trial stimulator is placed, and if there is a favorable response with pain improvement, a permanent implantation of electrodes (either paddle type or percutaneous electrodes) and an implantable pulse generator is performed (Stuart & Winfree, 2009).

Stimulation along a specific spinal nerve root or roots is known as spinal nerve root stimulation, and this technique provides for the selectivity of peripheral nerve stimulation by a variety of placements (intraspinal, transforaminal, extraforaminal) (Haque & Winfree, 2006).

If the electrode array can be placed along the desired peripheral nerve at least as easily as other forms of stimulation, then peripheral nerve stimulation is indicated when pain is confined to the distribution of a single or a limited number of peripheral nerves. For percutaneous nerve stimulation, electrodes are inserted in the epifascial plane above the muscle. For open peripheral nerve stimulation, a percutaneous or paddle lead is placed adjacent to the nerve, possibly placing a layer of fascia between the electrode and the nerve (Stuart & Winfree, 2009).

There are some pain syndromes that are not amenable to treatment by either spinal cord, peripheral nerve, or spinal nerve root stimulation, and therefore the technique of subcutaneous peripheral nerve stimulation has evolved. This technique may be used in conjunction with an implanted spinal cord stimulator or peripheral nerve stimulator. The technique for lead placement involves placement in the subcutaneous region where the pain is located under local anesthesia (Stuart & Winfree, 2009).

Treatment of Traumatic Mononeuropathies and Plexus Injuries

When a nerve is severed (neurotmesis), it is rare to have functional recovery without surgical intervention. After a nerve is surgically repaired through a direct end-to-end suture repair, regeneration may occur at the proximal end of the graft and the proximal end of the distal nerve stump. When the injury to the nerve is less severe than a complete disruption, but rather results in Sunderland's fourth- and third-degree lesions with sparing of the perineurium and epineurium (third-degree lesions) and epineurium (fourth degree lesions), the continuity improves the chances of successful regeneration, although scar or clots may block advancing neurites, resulting in formation of a neuroma in continuity. With a Sunderland second-degree lesion, since the endoneurial tubes are intact, the advancing neurites during regeneration follow these tubes to reinnervate the distal segments more easily. When neurapraxia occurs, axons and their support-ing structures are intact but there is segmental demyelination, resulting in a loss of motor and sensory function. While the prognosis for recovery is excellent, timing for recovery can take anywhere from minutes to hours or up to 3–6 months, depending upon the severity (DiPonio & McGillicuddy, 2005).

David Kline, at Louisiana State University Medical Center, has amassed a tremendous amount of experience in the surgical treatment of peripheral nerve injuries, and he and his team have written extensively on their experiences. Some of their outstanding work is referenced here. When there is an open wound associated with a traumatic nerve injury, immediate surgical exploration is required, and a sharply transected nerve may be repaired with an end-to-end anas-tomosis for the best chance of recovery. Early surgery (within 72 hours of injury) is indicated for clean open injuries in which a laceration (from glass, razor blade, etc.) may cause transection of a nerve, and an end-to-end suture repair is typically performed (Spinner & Kline, 2000). If the nerve transection resulted in jagged edges, they can be trimmed to expose a clean nerve prior to anastomosis. If, after retraction and trimming, the proximal and distal nerve endings are too far apart, a nerve graft (typically a sural nerve) may be interposed (DiPonio & McGillicuddy, 2005).

When a nerve has suffered a blunt transection (from auto metal, industrial machinery, pro-peller blade, chain saw, etc.), it is best to delay the repair by several weeks, at which time one can better determine the extent of proximal and distal neuromas. A nerve graft may be used if, after resecting the nerve ends back to healthy tissue, the distance is too great to allow a primary repair. An increasing neurologic deficit, typically associated with increasing pain, is another indication for early intervention. Compartment syndrome may result in ischemia to a peripheral nerve, and a fasciotomy may preserve and protect nerve function in addition to other soft tissues of the limb (Spinner & Kline, 2000).

When there is a closed injury, electrodiagnostic studies and somatosensory evoked poten-tials may help to assess the degree of nerve injury (neurapraxia, axonotmesis, neurotmesis) and whether there is continuity of the nerve. Serial studies may be of benefit. In cases of neurapraxic lesions, regenerating axons advance about 1 mm per day, and if there is little or no improve-ment in function, surgical exploration may be undertaken to evaluate for scar or neuroma in continuity or to determine whether a surgically improvable lesion is present. Surgery should not be undertaken if there is neurapraxia or axonotmesis, nerve root avulsion, or spinal cord injury or if over 2 years have passed since the time of injury (DiPonio & McGillicuddy, 2005). Patients with closed injuries should typically be followed for 2–5 months and should receive serial examinations and EMG/NCS studies to assess for clinical or electrophysiological signs of regeneration. If there are early signs of spontaneous recovery, nonoperative treatment may be continued. Patients suspected of having suffered a focal lesion in continuity (such as from a gunshot, contusion, or fracture) typically undergo a surgical exploration at 2–3 months after the injury, although those with suspected lengthier lesions may have surgery delayed until 3–5 months after injury. A long delay in repair may jeopardize end-organ integrity. As mentioned earlier, use of intraoperative nerve action potentials allows for relatively early evaluation of lesions in continuity. When surgical exploration of an injured nerve reveals scar tissue, an exter-nal neurolysis may be performed, which consists of removal of scar tissue in a circumferen-tial manner around the nerve, proceeding from healthy to scarred areas, releasing any areas of entrapment. Successful external neurolysis of a nerve has little risk of fascicular injury or vascular interruption. When external neurolysis is performed for a nerve that conducts a nerve action potential across the area of a lesion, there are occasionally immediate benefits of the procedure, with continued improvement over months or years. When a nerve is injured asym-metrically from a cross-sectional aspect, with a portion of the nerve showing significant injury but another being spared, an internal neurolysis may be performed, with the damaged portion separated from the healthy portion at a fascicular level. It is likely that the healthy portion will conduct a nerve action potential across it but the unhealthy portion will not. In this case, the unhealthy portion can be resected back to normal nerve tissue and repaired with a nerve graft. In general, during exploration of a traumatized nerve, when a gap exists from either a transection of the nerve or as a result of removing a nonconducting neuroma in continuity, an end-to-end epineural repair is attempted, provided that the gap is short and that there is sufficient slack on the nerve so that there will not be significant tension on the suture line and nerve. In order to help release tension, mobilization of the nerve or transposition of the nerve may be performed, which may provide several centimeters of additional length. When it is not possible to perform an end-to-end repair without undue tension on the suture line, a graft repair is performed, with the sural nerve, antebrachial cutaneous nerve, or occasionally superficial sensory radial nerve typically being harvested. Results are generally better when there is an end-to-end repair, as opposed to using an interpositioned nerve graft (Spinner & Kline, 2000).

Spinner and Kline have cited the works of Friedman, McGillicuddy, and Narakas in reporting that when it comes to the repair of brachial plexus injuries or combined preganglionic/postganglionic lesions (confirmed at surgery), reconstructions can be performed with nerve transfers (known as neurotization), which allow for the substitution of a nerve or plexus element that works for one that does not. Although preoperative clinical, electrodiagnostic, and imaging (myelographic or MRI studies) are helpful to assess for brachial plexus nerve root avulsion, open surgical exploration of the brachial plexus at a foraminal level is needed, with measurements of nerve action potentials to evaluate spinal nerves and trunks. Relative contraindications to surgery for peripheral nerve or brachial plexus injury include the presence of a plexus injury with significant neurologic deficit for more than 1 year and isolated C8 or T1 nerve root avulsions. Patients who are not candidates for neural reconstruction may still benefit from other reconstructive procedures, which may help regain function (Spinner & Kline, 2000).

Brachial plexus injuries that are obstetric palsies arising at birth are challenging to treat because of the difficulty predicting the natural history for an individual patient, as well as the likelihood of a spontaneous recovery. Those patients who show some recovery in the first few months will often have excellent results, but when recovery is not seen by 3–6 months after the injury, they are likely to suffer significant limitation in function. In those cases, surgery may be performed on the brachial plexus with the hope of improvement, although normal function is unlikely (Spinner & Kline, 2000).

When a lesion develops on a peripheral nerve in response to an offending cause, the lesion will worsen until the cause is removed. The rapidity of worsening will depend upon the cause. With a nerve is subject to severe compression by an encircling suture or compressive plate or to traction, compression, and ischemia from an expanding hematoma, correction of the offending agent should be performed within hours, with delay diminishing chances of full recovery (Birch, 2011).

In 2000, Spinner and Kline reported their experience at Louisiana State University Medical Center, with 3,000 nerve injuries and another 1,000 entrapments and tumors. In those patients who had a recordable nerve action potential, 90% recovered good function, including "those neural elements typically producing poor results when grafted, including lower roots, medial cord, and the ulnar nerve" (p. 690). They found that 70% of those who had direct suture repairs had good results, while those undergoing graft repairs had good results in 50% of cases, and those who had short grafts placed had better outcomes than those in whom the graft was over 3 inches in length. Children had better outcomes than adults, and those who underwent early surgery did better than those who had late surgery (Spinner & Kline, 2000).

In another study based upon outcomes of 1,019 brachial plexus lesions in patients who underwent surgery at the same institution over a 30-year period, the breakdown of causes were stretches/contusions (50% of cases), plexus tumors (16% of cases), thoracic outlet syndromes (16%), gunshot wounds (12%), and lacerations (7%). When surgery was indicated, depending upon the timing of surgery, type of injury or disease, and portions of the brachial plexus that were involved, functional outcomes following surgical repair were encouraging, although they found a decreased chance of functional recovery with delays in surgery for more than 6 months after the injury (Kim et al., 2003). The goal of nerve transfer in brachial plexus injuries is to promote elbow flexion, shoulder stability, and arm abduction (Pindrik & Belzberg, 2014).

Iatrogenic peripheral nerve injuries may be caused by medical interventions, and patients who have suffered an injury should be examined and appropriately treated as soon as possible. Among causes of iatrogenic nerve injury are operations on bone fractures, lymph node biopsy, carpal tunnel release, vascular surgery, orthopedic procedures, benign nerve sheath removal, hernia repair, radiation, wound exploration, resection of cysts, thoracic surgery, lipoma removal, injection injuries, and immobilization during anesthesia (Rasulić et al., 2017). Intraoperative positioning nerve injuries are rare, and while most patients will spontaneously improve, others may require more specialized treatment (Winfree & Kline, 2005).

Injection injuries to peripheral nerves may result in neuritic pain which at times responds to medications, but typically is unrelieved by sympathetic blocks. If severe neurologic deficit occurs and does not improve clinically or electrically within 3–5 months, surgery may be indicated. Surgery consists of an external neurolysis as well as nerve action potential recording. When there is a complete injury to a nerve, graft repairs are necessary to attempt to restore function.

In a series of 380 patients who suffered sciatic nerve injuries, injection injuries accounted for more than half of the cases that occurred at the buttock level. In most cases where only neurolysis was performed (due to a positive nerve action potential being recorded distal to the lesion), useful function was found in the peroneal division. In cases where there was no nerve action potential transmitted across the lesion, the affected segment of nerve was resected and repaired by end-to-end suture or grafts. In the peroneal division, only 36% of patients experienced a significant recovery after suture or graft repair, but a similar outcome was good to excellent when the repair was in the tibial division, even when lengthy grafts were required. When it came to exploring nerve lesions in the buttock, there is no ability within the early months other than intraoperative evaluation using nerve action potentials to determine which patients will be in the majority of those who do not require excision (require neurolysis only) versus those who do (Kline et al., 1998).

In a study of patients who had suffered iatrogenic radial nerve injuries due to injections, 23 out of 33 patients in the series underwent surgical intervention for treatment due to persistent pain or persistent neurological deficit. Either neurolysis, end-to-end repair, or graft repair was performed, depending upon intraoperative nerve action potentials. They found that patients who have suffered radial nerve injection injuries can achieve good functional outcomes when they undergo early and proper surgical management (Esquenazi et al., 2016).

Chronic Regional Pain Syndrome

CRPS is treated with nonsteroidal anti-inflammatory drugs, corticosteroids, COX-2 inhibitors, and free radical scavengers. Harden cites Stanton-Hicks, Burton, Bonica, and Evans in reporting the use of sympathetic nerve blocks, surgical sympathectomies, and spinal cord stimulators to treat CRPS (Harden & Bruehl, 2010).

Phantom pain may be treated with a variety of methods, including pharmacologic treatment, NMDA Receptor Antagonists, Anti-depressive agents, anticonvulsants, peripheral nerve blocks, Transcutaneous electrical nerve stimulation, spinal cord stimulation, and motor cortex stimulation (Culp & Abdi, 2022).

Brain Stimulation

Invasive procedures on the brain such as deep brain stimulation (DBS) and motor cortex stimulation (MCS), as well as percutaneous repetitive transcranial magnetic stimulation (rTMS) and transcranial direct current stimulation (tDCS), have had some effect on the treatment of chronic pain. Additional research is needed (Lefaucheur et al., 2008; Plow et al., 2012; Hamid et al., 2019; Attia et al., 2021).

Rehabilitation

Rehabilitation is generally indicated for the majority of patients suffering from peripheral neuropathy. Initially, assessment of a patient's capabilities and limitations is important. Factors to consider include pain and the physical limitations associated with it, weakness, personal issues (individual emotional stability and financial concerns), and limitations due to previous surgery (bracing, wound care, delicate anastomosis of nerves and tendons). Rehabilitation may include the following: modalities to help with pain and reduce inflammation (heat, ice, iontophoresis, transcutaneous stimulation, ultrasound); range-of-motion exercises (active and passive); resistance exercises (static and dynamic); splinting (to help to prevent further injury and contractures and stabilize joints and other at-risk structures); and cognitive and behavioral education (to properly use modalities and orthotics, decrease further injury, and establish realistic outcome expectations) (Scott et al., 2013). Exercises may be incorporated that will help patients to improve stability while standing and walking through training of balance, coordination, and proprioception. Goals may include increasing muscle strength and function, endurance, coordination and balance, speed and quickness, flexibility, and range of motion and prevention of deformities and contractures (Sommer et al., 2018; Dombovy, 2005). Among the elderly suffering from peripheral neuropathy of the lower limbs, responsiveness to rehabilitation was found to be greater for gait than for static balance, but exercise may have an effect on static balance (Caronni et al., 2019). Balance training has been found at times to be the most effective exercise intervention, with strength and endurance having less of an impact on patients suffering from peripheral neuropathy (Streckmann et al., 2014).

Physical therapy for open and closed peripheral nerve injuries helps to maintain strength and range of motion and to provide approaches to deal with altered mobility or activities of daily living. Prognosis for patients who have suffered a traumatic nerve injury and who have undergone surgical or conservative management is improved by a rehabilitative program designed to meet the patients' needs in maximizing their abilities, and it is also dependent on the patient's age, health, motivation, activity level, and social support. In young patients, reorganization of neural pathways and movement coordination can continue for 5 years (DiPonio et al., 2005).

Orthotic devices may be beneficial for the management of neuropathies. They serve the purposes of protection/immobilization (for stabilization of bony fragments and post-surgical repair of tendons, joints, and nerves), correction (to prevent or correct deformities and subluxations), and functional assistance (compensating for weak muscles or deformities). Dombovy felt that because of the need of a thorough understanding of biomechanics and anatomy, health care professionals who have a thorough understanding of these principles should be involved in the prescription, fabrication, and application of these orthoses (Dombovy, 2005).

The functional status of a patient suffering from peripheral neuropathy and its sequelae may be significantly impaired. A range of assistive and adaptive devices may be needed. Ambulation aids may help with patients suffering from weakness of the trunk or lower extremities, balance concerns, and weight-bearing difficulties. A physical therapy evaluation will help to make sure that the corrective device is ordered and properly used by the patient. In decreasing order, maximum stability is provided by a walker, axillary crutches, forearm crutches, two canes, a quad cane, and eventually a single-tipped cane. In neuropathies causing motor neuron disease, polyradiculoneuropathy, and neuropathies in which a patient has compromised cardiovascular capacity, a wheelchair may be needed. Dombovy felt that evaluation by a specialist may be needed if the physician is unfamiliar with the various wheelchair models and options, as there are more than 10,000 models of wheelchairs available (Dombovy, 2005). It is possible that alterations may have to be made in the patient's house. An evaluation by a physical and occupational therapist may be extremely beneficial. These can involve a change in eating utensils, pens, toothbrushes, and other similar items, which may need to have built-up handles. Long-handles shoehorns, reachers, and devices to assist donning socks may be required, as may be clothing and shoes with Velcro closures. Bathrooms may need to be modified with shower benches, grab bars, commodes, raised toilet seats, and handheld shower heads. Stair rails may be needed, and furniture may have to be rearranged. More involved modifications such as widening doorways and enlarging a bathroom to allow for wheelchair access and installing entrance ramps might have to be undertaken. Additional modifications of computer interfaces, telephone equipment, and other desk or workplace modifications might help a patient to return to productive and fulfilling work (Dombovy, 2005).

After undergoing surgery for peripheral nerve injury, serial clinical and electrophysiological examinations may be needed to document recovery. As physical therapy is important to implement before surgery, it is also important to continue after surgery, in a progressive manner, in order to promote strength and range of motion (Spinner & Kline, 2000).

Disability

Peripheral neuropathy is highly prevalent in the population and places patients at risk for suffering from pain, falls, ulcerations, and amputations (Callaghan et al., 2015). Patients aged 50–85 who suffer from diffuse polyneuropathy are found to have an increased risk of falling, which correlates with increased severity of peripheral neuropathy as well as with increased body mass index (BMI) (Richardson, 2002). Peripheral sensory neuropathy is an independent risk factor for lower extremity amputation in patients with diabetes (Alder et al., 1999).

In a study in which patients with upper extremity peripheral nerve disorders were evaluated, it was found that in order to decrease disability and improve quality of life, occupational therapists should help patients to maintain meaningful work and household roles and also assist with addressing pain and difficulties with intimate relationships and sleep. The patients evaluated were categorized into seven diagnostic groups: disorders of the 1) median nerve, 2) ulnar nerve, and 3) radial nerve, as well as 4) proximal nerve injury (axillary, long thoracic, suprascapular, or musculocutaneous), 5) dual-nerve compression (two or more different nerves), 6) thoracic outlet syndrome, and 7) brachial plexus injury (Stonner et al., 2017). Patients who experience chronic pain of predominantly neuropathic origin have worsened health and greater disability than individuals without pain or individuals who experience chronic pain that is not of a predominantly neuropathic origin (Smith et al., 2007).

Life Care Planning

The goal of life care planning as it pertains to an individual who is suffering from peripheral neuropathy may vary tremendously in nature and scope, given the multitude of organ systems that may be involved, the varying degrees of incapacity that may result, and the various treatment measures (conservative and surgical, orthotics, etc.) that may be needed to try to restore function and alleviate pain. A tremendous variety of health care providers may be needed. The details of what treatments will be needed will be determined by the anatomical nature of the organ systems involved, the degree of incapacity of an individual, the amount of pain they are experiencing, any restorative procedures that may be contemplated, and anticipated complications that may arise.

References

Adler, A. I., Boyko, E. J., Ahroni, J. H., & Smith, D. G. (1999). Lower-extremity amputation in diabetes: The independent effects of peripheral vascular disease, sensory neuropathy, and foot ulcers. *Diabetes Care, 22*(7), 1029–1035. https://doi.org/10.2337/diacare.22.7.1029

Attia, M., McCarthy, D., & Abdelghani, M. (2021). Repetitive transcranial magnetic stimulation for treating chronic neuropathic pain: A systematic review. *Current Pain and Headache Reports, 25*(7), 48. https://doi.org/10.1007/s11916-021-00960-5

Bamiou, D.-E., & Luxon, L. M. (2005). Diseases of the eighth cranial nerve. In P. J. Dyck & P. K. Thomas (Eds.), *Peripheral neuropathy* (pp. 1253–1272). Elsevier Inc.

Berthold, C. H., Fraher, J. P., King, R. H. M., & Rydmark, M. (2005). Microscopic anatomy of the peripheral nervous system. In P. J. Dyck & P. K. Thomas (Eds.), *Peripheral neuropathy* (pp. 35–91). Elsevier Inc.

Birch, R. (2011). *Surgical disorders of the peripheral nerves* (2nd ed.). Springer.

Callaghan, B. C., Gao, L., Li, Y., Zhou, X., Reynolds, E., Banerjee, M., Pop-Busui, R., Feldman, E. L., & Ji, L. (2018). Diabetes and obesity are the main metabolic drivers of peripheral neuropathy. *Annals of Clinical and Translational Neurology, 5*(4), 397–405. https://doi.org/10.1002/can3.531

Callaghan, B. C., Price, R. S., & Feldman, E. L. (2015). Distal symmetric polyneuropathy: A review. *JAMA, 314*(20), 2172–2181. https://doi.org/10.1001/jama.2015.13611

Campbell, W. W. (2008). Evaluation and management of peripheral nerve injury. *Clinical Neurophysiology: Official Journal of the International Federation of Clinical Neurophysiology, 119*(9), 1951–1965. https://doi.org/10.1016/j.clinph.2008.03.018

Caronni, A., Picardi, M., Pintavalle, G., Aristidou, E., Redaelli, V., Antoniotti, P., Sterpi, I., Tropea, P., & Corbo, M. (2019). Responsiveness to rehabilitation of balance and gait impairment in elderly with peripheral neuropathy. *Journal of Biomechanics, 94*, 31–38. https://doi.org/10.1016/j.jbiomech.2019.07.007

Chalk, C. (2005). Diseases of spinal roots. In P. J. Dyck & P. K. Thomas (Eds.), *Peripheral neuropathy* (pp. 1323–1337). Elsevier Inc.

Choi, J. M., & Di Maria, G. (2021). Electrodiagnostic testing for disorders of peripheral nerves. *Clinics in Geriatric Medicine, 37*(2), 209–221. https://doi.org/10.1016/j.cger.2021.01.010

Clarke, E., & Bearn, J. G. (1972). The spiral nerve bands of Fontana. *Brain: A Journal of Neurology, 95*(1), 1–20. https://doi.org/10.1093/brain/95.1.1

Coffey, R., & Gupta, V. (2022). Meralgia paresthetica. *In StatPearls*. StatPearls Publishing.

Collins, M. P. (2005). Neuropathies with systemic vasculitis. In P. J. Dyck & P. K. Thomas (Eds.), *Peripheral neuropathy* (pp. 2335–2404). Elsevier Inc.

Crone, C., & Krarup, C. (2013). Neurophysiological approach to disorders of peripheral nerve. *Handbook of Clinical Neurology, 115*, 81–114. https://doi.org/10.1016/B978-0-444-52902-2.00006-0

Culp, C., & Avdi, S. (2022). Current Understanding of Phantom Pain and its Treatment. *Pain Physician, 25*, 941–957.

de Souza, J. B., Carqueja, C. L., & Baptista, A. F. (2016). Physical rehabilitation to treat neuropathic pain. *Revista do Instituto de Medicina Tropical de Sao Paulo, 17*(Suppl 1), 85090.

DiPonio, L., Leonard, J. A., & McGillicuddy, J. E. (2005). Management of traumatic mononeuropathies. In M. B. Bromberg & A. G. Smith (Eds.), *Handbook of peripheral neuropathy* (pp. 559–582). CRC Press.

Dombovy, M. L. (2005). Rehabilitation management of neuropathies. In P. J. Dyck & P. K. Thomas (Eds.), *Peripheral neuropathy* (pp. 2621–2636). Elsevier Inc.

Doughty, C. T., & Seyedsadjadi, R. (2018). Approach to peripheral neuropathy for the primary care clinician. *The American Journal of Medicine, 131*(9), 1010–1016. https://doi.org/10.1016/j.amjmed.2017.12.042

Du, R., Auguste, K. I., Chin, C. T., Engstrom, J. W., & Weinstein, P. R. (2010). Magnetic resonance neurography for the evaluation of peripheral nerve, brachial plexus, and nerve root disorders. *Journal of Neurosurgery, 112*(2), 362–371. https://doi.org/10.3171/2009.7.JNS09414

Dyck, P. J., Oviatt, K. F., & Lambert, E. H. (1981). Intensive evaluation of referred unclassified neuropathies yields improved diagnosis. *Annals of Neurology, 10*(3), 222–226. https://doi.org/10.1002/ana.410100304

Eder, M., Schulte-Mattler, W., & Pöschl, P. (2017). Neurographic course of Wallerian degeneration after human peripheral nerve injury. *Muscle & Nerve, 56*(2), 247–252. https://doi.org/10.1002/mus.25489

England, J. D., & Asbury, A. K. (2004). Peripheral neuropathy. *Lancet (London, England), 363*(9427), 2151–2161. https://doi.org/10.1016/S0140-6736(04)16508-2

Esquenazi, Y., Park, S. H., Kline, D. G., & Kim, D. H. (2016). Surgical management and outcome of iatrogenic radial nerve injection injuries. *Clinical Neurology and Neurosurgery, 142*, 98–103. https://doi.org/10.1016/j.clineuro.2016.01.014

Gardner, E. D., Bunge & R. P. (2005). Gross anatomy of the peripheral nervous system. In P. J. Dyck & P. K. Thomas (Eds.), *Peripheral neuropathy* (pp. 11–34). Elsevier Inc.

Giannini, C. (2005). Peripheral nerve tumors. In P. J. Dyck & P. K. Thomas (Eds.), *Peripheral neuropathy* (pp. 2585–2606). Elsevier Inc.

Gonzalez, N. L., & Hobson-Webb, L. D. (2021). The Role of imaging for disorders of peripheral nerve. *Clinics in Geriatric Medicine, 37*(2), 223–239. https://doi.org/10.1016/j.cger.2021.01.001

Grant, I. A., & Benstead, T. J. (2005). Differential diagnosis of polyneuropathy. In P. J. Dyck & P. K. Thomas (Eds.), *Peripheral neuropathy* (pp. 1163–1180). Elsevier Inc.

Hamid, P., Malik, B. H., & Hussain, M. L. (2019). Noninvasive transcranial magnetic stimulation (TMS) in chronic refractory pain: A systematic review. *Cureus, 11*(10), e6019. https://doi.org/10.7759/cureus.6019

Haque, R., & Winfree, C. J. (2006). Spinal nerve root stimulation. *Neurosurgical Focus, 21*(6), e4. https://doi.org/10.3171/foc.2006.21.6.7

Harden, N., & Bruehl, S. P. (2010). Complex regional pain syndrome. In S. M. Fishman, J. C. Ballantyne & J. P. Rathmell (Eds.), *Bonica's management of pain* (4th ed., pp. 314–331). Lippincott Williams & Wilkins.

Herskovitz, S., Scelsa, S. N., & Schaumburg, H. H. (2010). *Peripheral neuropathies in clinical practice.* Oxford University Press.

Holzgrefe, R. E., Wagner, E. R., Singer, A. D., & Daly, C. A. (2019). Imaging of the peripheral nerve: Concepts and future direction of magnetic resonance neurography and ultrasound. *The Journal of Hand Surgery, 44*(12), 1066–1079. https://doi.org/10.1016/j.jhsa.2019.06.021

Hughes, R. A. C. (2005). Diseases of the fifth cranial nerve. In P. J. Dyck & P. K. Thomas (Eds.), *Peripheral neuropathy* (pp. 1207–1217). Elsevier Inc.

Italian General Practitioner Study Group (IGPSG). (1995). Chronic symmetric symptomatic polyneuropathy in the elderly: a field screening investigation in two Italian regions, I: Prevalence and general characteristics of the sample. *Neurology, 45*(10), 1832–1836.

Katona, I., & Weis, J. (2017). Diseases of the peripheral nerves. *Handbook of Clinical Neurology, 145*, 453–474. https://doi.org/10.1016/B978-0-12-802395-2.00031-6

Khdour, M. R. (2020). Treatment of diabetic peripheral neuropathy: A review. *The Journal of Pharmacy and Pharmacology, 72*(7), 863–872. https://doi.org/10.1111/jphp.13241

Kim, D. H., Cho, Y. J., Tiel, R. L., & Kline, D. G. (2003). Outcomes of surgery in 1019 brachial plexus lesions treated at Louisiana state university health sciences center. *Journal of Neurosurgery, 98*(5), 1005–1016. https://doi.org/10.3171/jns.2003.98.5.1005

Klein, M. K. (2005). Diseases of the seventh cranial nerve. In P. J. Dyck & P. K. Thomas (Eds.), *Peripheral neuropathy* (pp. 1219–1252). Elsevier Inc.

Kline, D. G., Kim, D., Midha, R., Harsh, C., & Tiel, R. (1998). Management and results of sciatic nerve injuries: A 24-year experience. *Journal of Neurosurgery, 89*(1), 13–23. https://doi.org/10.3171/jns.1998.89.1.0013

Koulousakis, A., Kuchta, J., Bayarassou, A., & Sturm, V. (2007). Intrathecal opioids for intractable pain syndromes. *Acta Neurochirurgica: Supplement, 97*(Pt 1), 43–48. https://doi.org/10.1007/978-3-211-33079-1_5

Leavitt, J. A., & Younge, B. R. (2005). Diseases of cranial nerves. In P. J. Dyck & P. K. Thomas (Eds.), *Peripheral neuropathy* (pp. 1191–1206). Elsevier Inc.

Lee, A. W., & Pilitsis, J. G. (2006). Spinal cord stimulation: Indications and outcomes. *Neurosurgical Focus*, *21*(6), e3. https://doi.org/10.3171/foc.2006.21.6.6

Lefaucheur, J. P., Antal, A., Ahdab, R., Ciampi de Andrade, D., Fregni, F., Khedr, E. M., Nitsche, M., & Paulus, W. (2008). The use of repetitive transcranial magnetic stimulation (rTMS) and transcranial direct current stimulation (tDCS) to relieve pain. *Brain Stimulation*, *1*(4), 337–344. https://doi.org/10.1016/j.brs.2008.07.003

Marques M. J. Queiroz L. S. Atlas de neuroanatomia para patologistas. Cérebro do adulto. Nervos cranianos. [cited 2021 March 1]. Available from: http://anatpat.unicamp.br/bineucerebroext-nervos.html.

Martyn, C. N., & Hughes, R. A. (1997). Epidemiology of peripheral neuropathy. *Journal of Neurology, Neurosurgery, and Psychiatry*, *62*(4), 310–318. https://doi.org/10.1136/jnnp.62.4.310

Matsuda, M., Kobayashi, S., & Ugawa, Y. (2012). Role of skeletal muscle MRI in peripheral nerve disorders. In G. Hayat (Ed.), *Peripheral neuropathy: Advances in diagnostic and therapeutic approaches* (pp. 65–84). InTech.

Melzack, R., & Wall, P. D. (1965). Pain mechanisms: A new theory. *Science (New York, N.Y.)*, *150*(3699), 971–979. https://doi.org/10.1126/science.150.3699.971

Mihailoff, G. A., & Haines, D. E. (2018). The cell biology of neurons and glia. In D. E. Haines & G. A. Mihailoff (Eds.), *Fundamental neuroscience for basic and clinical applications* (5th ed., pp. 15–33). Elsevier.

National Institute of Neurological Disorders and Stroke. (n.d.). *Peripheral neuropathy fact sheet*. NINNDS. Retrieved July 4, 2022, from www.ninds.nih.gov/health-information/patient-caregiver-education/fact-sheets/peripheral-neuropathy-fact-sheet

Pindrik, J., & Belzberg, A. J. (2014). Peripheral nerve surgery: Primer for the imagers. *Neuroimaging Clinics of North America*, *24*(1), 193–210. https://doi.org/10.1016/j.nic.2013.03.034

Plow, E. B., Pascual-Leone, A., & Machado, A. (2012). Brain stimulation in the treatment of chronic neuropathic and non-cancerous pain. *Journal of Pain*, *13*(5), 411–424.

Rasulić, L., Savić, A., Vitošević, F., Samardžić, M., Živković, B., Mićović, M., Baščarević, V., Puzović, V., Joksimović, B., Novakovic, N., Lepić, M., & Mandić-Rajčević, S. (2017). Iatrogenic peripheral nerve injuries-surgical treatment and outcome: 10 years' experience. *World Neurosurgery*, *103*, 841–851, e6. https://doi.org/10.1016/j.wneu.2017.04.099

Richardson, J. K. (2002). Factors associated with falls in older patients with diffuse polyneuropathy. *Journal of the American Geriatrics Society*, *50*(11), 1767–1773. https://doi.org/10.1046/j.1532-5415.2002.50503.x

Roth, B., Schiro, D. B., & Ohlsson, B. (2021). Diseases which cause generalized peripheral neuropathy: A systematic review. *Scandinavian Journal of Gastroenterology*, *56*(9), 1000–1010. https://doi.org/10.1080/00365521.2021.1942542

Rueda-Lopes, F. (2021). The cranial nerves: Extensions of the central nervous system or components of the peripheral nervous system. *CBR Radiologia Brasileira*, *54*(3), V–VI.

Scott, K. R., Ahmed, A., Scott, L., & Kothari, M. J. (2013). Rehabilitation of brachial plexus and peripheral nerve disorders. *Handbook of Clinical Neurology*, *110*, 499–514. https://doi.org/10.1016/B978-0-444-52901-5.00042-3

Seddon, H. J. (1942). A classification of nerve injuries. *British Medical Journal*, *2*(4260), 237–239. https://doi.org/10.1136/bmj.2.4260.237

Seddon, H. J. (1943). Three types of nerve injuries. *Brain*, *4*(66), 237–288.

Shealy, C. N., Mortimer, J. T., & Reswick, J. B. (1967). Electrical inhibition of pain by stimulation of the dorsal columns: Preliminary clinical report. *Anesthesia and Analgesia*, *46*(4), 489–491.

Simon, N. G., Spinner, R. J., Kline, D. G., & Kliot, M. (2016). Advances in the neurological and neurosurgical management of peripheral nerve trauma. *Journal of Neurology, Neurosurgery, and Psychiatry*, *87*(2), 198–208. https://doi.org/10.1136/jnnp-2014-310175

Smith, B. H., Torrance, N., Bennett, M. I., & Lee, A. J. (2007). Health and quality of life associated with chronic pain of predominantly neuropathic origin in the community. *The Clinical Journal of Pain*, *23*(2), 143–149. https://doi.org/10.1097/01.ajp.0000210956.31997.89

Sommer, C., Geber, C., Young, P., Forst, R., Birklein, F., & Schoser, B. (2018). Polyneuropathies. *Deutsches Arzteblatt International*, *115*(6), 83–90. https://doi.org/10.3238/arztebl.2018.083

Spinner, R. J., & Kline, D. G. (2000). Surgery for peripheral nerve and brachial plexus injuries or other nerve lesions. *Muscle & Nerve*, *23*(5), 680–695. https://doi.org/10.1002/(sici)1097-4598(200005)23:5<680::aid-mus4>3.0.co;2-h

Stonner, M. M., Mackinnon, S. E., & Kaskutas, V. (2017). Predictors of disability and quality of life with an upper-extremity peripheral nerve disorder. *The American Journal of Occupational Therapy: Official Publication of the American Occupational Therapy Association, 71*(1), 7101190050p1–7101190050p8. https://doi.org/10.5014/ajot.2017.022988

Streckmann, F., Zopf, E. M., Lehmann, H. C., May, K., Rizza, J., Zimmer, P., Gollhofer, A., Bloch, W., & Baumann, F. T. (2014). Exercise intervention studies in patients with peripheral neuropathy: A systematic review. *Sports Medicine (Auckland, N.Z.), 44*(9), 1289–1304. https://doi.org/10.1007/s40279-014-0207-5

Stuart, R. M., & Winfree, C. J. (2009). Neurostimulation techniques for painful peripheral nerve disorders. *Neurosurgery Clinics of North America, 20*(1), 111, viii. https://doi.org/10.1016/j.nec.2008.07.027

Sunderlands, S. (1951). A classification of peripheral nerve injuries producing loss of function. *Brain: A Journal of Neurology, 74*(4), 491–516. https://doi.org/10.1093/brain/74.4.491

Thomas, P. K., & Mathias, C. J. (2005). Diseases of the ninth, tenth, eleventh, and twelfth cranial nerves. In P. J. Dyck & P. K. Thomas (Eds.), *Peripheral neuropathy* (pp. 1273–1293). Elsevier Inc.

Thompson, P. D., & Thomas, P. K. (2005). Differential diagnosis and epidemiology: Clinical patterns of peripheral neuropathy. In P. J. Dyck & P. K. Thomas (Eds.), *Peripheral neuropathy* (pp. 1137–1161). Elsevier Inc.

Vinik, A. I., Maser, R. E., Mitchell, B. D., & Freeman, R. (2003). Diabetic autonomic neuropathy. *Diabetes Care, 26*(5), 1553–1579. https://doi.org/10.2337/diacare.26.5.1553

Vujaskovic, Z. (1997). Structural and physiological properties of peripheral nerves after intraoperative irradiation. *Journal of the Peripheral Nervous System: JPNS, 2*(4), 343–349.

Waldman, D. W., Waldman, C. W., & Kidder, K. A. (2017). Evolution and treatment of peripheral neuropathies. In S. D. Waldman (Ed.), *Pain management* (2nd ed., pp. 260–267). Saunders.

Walk, D., & Backonja, M.-M. (2010). Painful neuropathies. In S. M. Fishman, J. C. Ballantyne, & J. P. Rathmell (Eds.), *Bonica's management of pain* (4th ed., pp. 303–313). Lippincott Williams & Wilkins.

Waller, A. (1851). Experiments on the section of the glosso-pharyngeal and hypoglossal nerves of the frog, and observations of the alterations produced thereby in the structure of their primitive fibres. *Edinburgh Medical and Surgical Journal, 76*(189), 369–376.

Watson, J. C., & Dyck, P. J. (2015). Peripheral neuropathy: A practical approach to diagnosis and symptom management. *Mayo Clinic Proceedings, 90*(7), 940–951. https://doi.org/10.1016/j.mayocp.2015.05.004

Wilbouorn, J. (2005). Brachial plexus lesions. In P. J. Dyck & P. K. Thomas (Eds.), *Peripheral neuropathy* (pp. 1339–1373). Elsevier Inc.

Winfree, C. J., & Kline, D. G. (2005). Intraoperative positioning nerve injuries. *Surgical Neurology, 63*(1), 5–18. https://doi.org/10.1016/j.surneu.2004.03.024

Wohlfart, G. (1957). Collateral regeneration from residual motor nerve fibers in amyotrophic lateral sclerosis. *Neurology, 7*(2), 124–134. https://doi.org/10.1212/wnl.7.2.124

Younger, D. S. (2004). Peripheral nerve disorders. *Primary Care, 31*(1), 67–83. https://doi.org/10.1016/S0095-4543(03)00116-7

15 Amputations

LeRoy Oddie and Danielle Melton

It can be challenging to fully comprehend how life-changing an amputation is for an amputee. Until a limb is lost, it is easy to take for granted how effortlessly one can walk or how simple it is to manipulate the hand and position the arm to perform thousands of tasks without conscious thought. There is a misperception that prostheses restore an amputee's lost function, and while they do to an extent, they are poor substitutes for an intact natural limb. Even when prostheses partially restore functional deficits, they introduce a whole new set of problems that the evaluee[1] never had to be concerned with before amputation. Perhaps the most unappreciated aspect of amputation is the psychosocial toll. Having a permanently altered body image is a psychological challenge that prostheses simply fail to resolve, regardless of how realistic their appearance may be.

Before creating a *life care plan* (LCP), it is worthwhile to review its overall objectives beyond reviewing the medical history and projecting lifetime needs. In addition to providing the necessary resources to restore maximum function, the LCP goals should also include minimizing secondary complications, minimizing long-term needs, providing family support, preventing unnecessary complications, and restoring mental health and body image. While the LCP is often driven by litigation, its use extends beyond legal resolution and should be written to serve as a dynamic future resource for not just the evaluee but also the family, case manager, clinical team, and/or financial trust.

While the etiology of amputations is diverse, this chapter focuses on traumatic amputations. Unlike amputations secondary to cardiovascular or diabetic complications, traumatic amputations are sudden, with several implications. Foremost is the significant psychological impact due to the rapid change in body image and loss of mobility and/or function. In traumatic amputations, the primary concern is often saving the evaluee's life or preserving one or more mangled limbs. Only once the vital systems have been stabilized and infection risks minimized can the surgical team consider optimizing the residual limb(s) for future function.

Clinical Team Approach

Pragmatically, amputation is too often simply considered the loss of a limb. However, amputation is much more complex than limb loss, and despite best efforts, the physical and psychological restoration will likely never achieve pre-injury status. To achieve maximal restoration, an extensive clinical team with diverse skills is essential to develop and implement a comprehensive rehabilitation program. The clinical team may include a case manager, orthopedic surgeon, plastic surgeon, neurosurgeon, physiatrist, physical therapist, occupational therapist, prosthetist, psychiatrist, psychologist, nutritionist, social worker, pediatrician, rehabilitation counselor, dermatologist, and pain management specialist (Keszler et al., 2020; Lannan & Meyerle, 2019). In

DOI: 10.4324/b23293-15

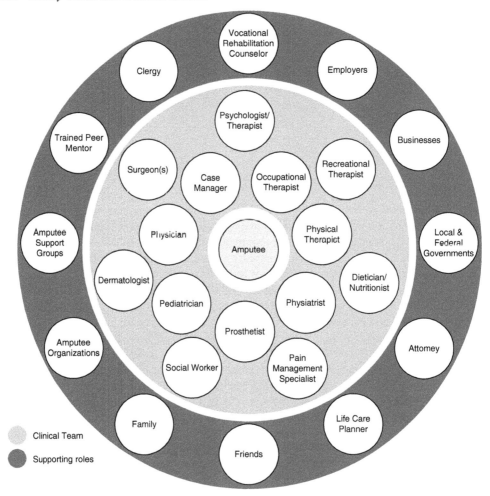

Figure 15.1 Supporting Role

cases with comorbidities such as *traumatic brain injury* (TBI) or *post-traumatic stress disorder* (PTSD), additional clinical experts may be needed. Furthermore, the functional loss, even after the provision of prostheses, may have a significant impact on vocational capacity, necessitating the expertise of a vocational rehabilitation specialist to evaluate future employment opportunities (Berens & Weed, 2018) (see Figure 15.1 regarding supporting roles).

Even if a life care planner has extensive experience with amputees, the expertise of both a physiatrist and a prosthetist should be consulted in all but the most simplistic cases.[2] The physiatrist is a key team member, as she or he will develop a comprehensive rehabilitation plan for the management of physical deficits, pain, and psychosocial issues. Specific to the LCP, the physiatrist can provide the time of *maximum medical improvement* (MMI); life expectancy; anticipated functional outcomes; type, quantity, and cost of rehabilitation services; needs and costs of adaptive equipment; necessary architectural modifications; hours and level of attendant care; psychosocial needs; vocational/avocational capacity and modifications; employment restrictions; future surgical and medical needs; and anticipated medical problems and their treatment options (Meier et al., 2013). In some regions, a physiatrist with extensive amputation experience may not be available locally. In such circumstances, regionally or nationally recognized *physical medicine and rehabilitation* (PM&R) physicians with extensive polytrauma amputation experience may be consulted. Note that *only a physiatrist or another physician is qualified to provide the medical foundation* for many aspects of an LCP, with the former often more knowledgeable and experienced with amputee rehabilitation.

While the physiatrist has a broad understanding of prosthetic components, there are simply too many options commercially available for the physiatrist to have a deep understanding of their functions and specific indications/contradictions. For instance, if a transfemoral amputee's body weight is above a specific weight, she or he will be contraindicated for a specific prosthetic component. However, the weight ratings vary from manufacturer to manufacturer, not by prosthetic component or amputee functional level classifications. The knowledge and experience of the prosthetist are essential for finalizing the prosthetic prescription. While a prosthetist legally is not authorized to prescribe prostheses, the physiatrist or physician in most situations will rely on the prosthetist to develop the final prosthetic prescription due to the complexity of selecting individual prosthetic components. In addition to assisting with the selection of the most appropriate prosthetic components, the prosthetist can provide the life care planner with their cost and replacement frequency. The former is particularly important as the methodology of determining the cost of prosthetic needs differs significantly from the methodology used in other aspects of the LCP. Thus, unless a life care planner has experience in both prosthetic billing practices and prosthetic clinical care, she or he should consult with a prosthetist in all amputation cases. Frequently, the cost of lifetime prosthetic components in amputation LCPs will account for a significant or majority portion of the LCP and will come under significant scrutiny by the opposing counsel. It is worth noting that the scope of practice of the prosthetist is limited to the prosthetic needs section of the LCP, even though the evaluee may have other needs (e.g., ambulatory aids, skincare products) associated with the use of a prosthesis.

For many life care planners, projecting the cost of prosthetic components is not within their scope of practice. If a life care planner fails to consult with a prosthetist while the opposing counsel retains a prosthetic expert, it will not be difficult for the opposing prosthetist to find flaws in the projected cost for prostheses, potentially eroding the credibility of the life care planner. Similarly, in some states, one can practice as a prosthetist without educational or credentialing requirements, while in the remaining states, prosthetist credentialing requirements are not as robust as other rehabilitation disciplines. Most prosthetists are unaware of or inexperienced regarding life care planning or do not have knowledge of the legal process and requirements. Thus, when developing an amputation LCP, the life care planner is strongly advised to select a consulting certified prosthetist versed in life care planning and the legal process (see Figure 15.2 regarding the amputation life care planning team).

Amputation Continuum of Care

In life care planning, often the evaluee is already an amputee by the time the life care planner becomes involved, and the rehabilitation process will have already commenced. However, in some cases, the evaluee will not yet be an amputee, yet elective amputation may be anticipated in the immediate future. Regardless, amputation rehabilitation should commence as quickly as possible and does not end when an amputee receives a prosthesis and completes gait retraining or functional rehabilitation. Rather, the continuum of care extends throughout the lifespan of an amputee with changing needs, depending on her or his life stage. Amputation rehabilitation may be divided into seven major phases discussed next (Esquenazi & DiGiacomo, 2001).

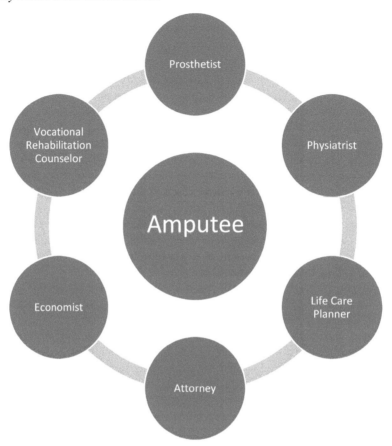

Figure 15.2 Amputation Life Care Planning Team

Preoperative Considerations

In cases of severe limb trauma, amputation is not always the first consideration. Due to significant advances in medicine, other options now exist such as limb allotransplantation and limb preservation, although the former is not yet considered a standard of care (Alolabi et al., 2017; Swanson et al., 2015). Once the evaluee's acute condition has stabilized, the surgical team can explore the best treatment plan, whether it is limb preservation or ultimately preparing the residual limb for use of a prosthesis.

Local and national media frequently provide coverage of highly successful amputees, while corporate commercials glorify amputees due to their inspiring achievements, and films depict amputees as heroes and heroines (Abernethy et al., 2017). While this has a positive impact on the acceptance of amputees socially and illustrates that amputation does not have to become a permanent disability, it also has potentially negative consequences. There is often a focus on the prosthetic technology, rather than the extensive rehabilitation therapy required, leading to the impression that prostheses effortlessly and completely restore lost function. Combined with the fantasy of science fiction in which prostheses may enhance human potential, the expectations of commercially available prostheses are often overly optimistic and unrealistic. As much as prosthetic technology has advanced, it still falls significantly short of the natural intact limb, particularly regarding function, cosmesis, body temperature regulation, durability, fluidity/

preciseness of movement, and energy efficiency. Thus, if the evaluee is not yet an amputee and is contemplating elective amputation, it is essential for the clinical team and the life care planner to communicate realistic expectations of what outcomes prosthetic technology can achieve and fully disclose their disadvantages and limitations. Conversely, there are other circumstances in which limb preservation fails to meet the expected prognosis after numerous surgical revisions, and the evaluee may have an improved outcome with an elective amputation and the use of a prosthesis (Fioravanti et al., 2018; Potter & Bosse, 2021).

Reconstructive surgeons view amputation as the beginning of a new phase of life rather than being the final step of a failed treatment plan (Azoury et al., 2020). If a prosthesis is ultimately indicated, multiple surgical techniques should be considered to maximize potential outcomes. In rehabilitation, the goal should be to restore the maximum function while simultaneously minimizing secondary complications.

Amputation permanently disrupts the skeletal function of weight-bearing and efficient limb movement via rigid skeletal levers. The most common intervention has been to interface the prosthesis to the residual limb with a prosthetic socket. The socket is only moderately effective, as it fails to restore the rigid load-bearing skeletal structure. While the objective of the socket is to restore function, it comes at the cost of a host of potential and common secondary complications including residual limb pain, soft tissue breakdown, poor body heat/moisture dissipation, and increased fall risk (Paternò et al., 2018). Furthermore, the socket has further disadvantages of poor accommodation of body weight changes, compromised limb range of motion, difficulty donning and doffing, altered proprioception, decreased stability regarding mobility, increased energy expenditure, poor sitting comfort, unrealistic aesthetics, and increased bulk. Thus, it is important to consider that the prosthetic socket introduces problems that did not exist before amputation.

Fortunately, the socket is no longer necessary for use of a prosthesis. Osseointegration (also referred to as *bone-anchored* or *osseous integration*) is a reconstructive surgical technique that restores the rigid skeletal structure, connecting prosthetic components directly to residual limb bone via a *fixture* or *press-fit* implant. While osseointegration has been in research and development for decades, it is now a standard of care for transfemoral amputees as a Food and Drug Administration (FDA) Class III approved device.[3] For other amputation levels, osseointegration may be available via alternative pathways such as the *humanitarian device exemption* (HDE), *custom device exemption* (CDE), or an *investigational device exemption* (IDE) (Van Norman, 2018). While amputees used to travel overseas for osseointegration, it is now available at numerous hospitals throughout the United States. Given the historical and frequent secondary complications of prosthetic sockets, osseointegration should be considered as an intervention when socket complications are experienced or anticipated. As many amputees are contraindicated for osseointegration, the evaluee's surgical and rehabilitation team must determine osseointegration candidacy with a comprehensive evaluation, including blood assessment and skeletal imaging. Osseointegration will require periodic future treatment due to the risks of superficial soft tissue infections, deep osseous infections, and/or implant loosening or failure (Atallah et al., 2018). Furthermore, it is worth noting that rehabilitation protocols for osseointegration require more extensive physical therapy due to the slow progression of weight bearing, which should be accounted for in the LCP. Should an evaluee be contraindicated for osseointegration, other surgical reconstructive techniques to maximize the potential outcomes with a prosthesis should be given consideration.

Several surgical reconstructive techniques may significantly improve the functional outcome with a prosthesis. If a residual limb is very short, the residual bone may be lengthened with the Ilizarov technique or a cadaver allograft. To enhance distal residual limb weight bearing, osteo-myoplastic reconstruction (also known as the *Ertl* procedure) bridges the tibia and fibula in transtibial amputees, increasing the surface area of the skeletal interface for distal weight bearing (Kahle et al., 2017). *Targeted muscle reinnervation* (TMR), the transfer of residual peripheral

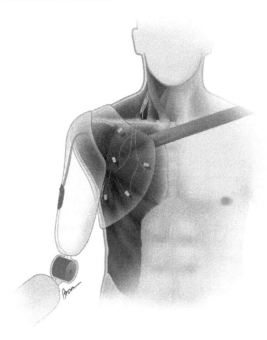

Figure 15.3 Targeted Muscle Reinnervation (TMR)

nerves, muscle motor nerves, improves upper limb prosthesis control and is an effective intervention for the prevention and treatment of symptomatic neuroma and *phantom limb pain* (PLP) (Bowen et al., 2017; Valerio et al., 2019). Surgeons may also employ myoplasty, myodesis, and muscle contouring techniques to enhance the efficacy of prosthetic socket use (see Figure 15.3 regarding Targeted Muscle Reinnervation).

In addition to identifying the optimal surgical solutions, the preoperative phase offers the opportunity for therapists to prepare the amputee for prosthesis use, increasing muscle strength and endurance while improving joint *range of motion* (ROM). An aerobic conditioning program and smoking cessation program will likely accelerate postoperative recovery if medically indicated. This period also offers an opportunity to educate the evaluee on prosthetic options; establish realistic expectations for functional recovery with a prosthesis; and provide postoperative self-care techniques such as joint contracture prevention, edema management, fall prevention, and desensitization of the residual limb.

Postoperative Management

Once the amputation and associated surgical revisions are complete, the acute focus is on healing. The clinical team manages post-surgical pain, incision site healing, and edema (Parnell & Urton, 2021). Education of safety is paramount to preventing falls for lower limb amputees. As amputees are not yet ambulatory, daily ROM exercises are essential to prevent the development of joint contractures from extended time in bed and/or wheelchairs.

Pre-prosthetic Therapy

Once the surgical sutures have been removed, the residual limb may be prepared for use with a prosthesis with desensitization exercises and residual limb volume reduction and shaping.

Overall strength and endurance conditioning may begin, as well as a discussion of prosthetic options and expectations of the rehabilitation plan. As this is a period of significant psychosocial change, it is an opportune time for the amputee to receive trained peer visitor support from successfully rehabilitated amputees concerning what to expect in the immediate and long-term future.

Prosthesis Prescription

It is often assumed that an evaluee should receive a prosthesis. However, while infrequent, the evaluee may achieve MMI without the use of prostheses. For example, due to the length of litigation timelines and lack of other prosthetic resources, the upper limb amputee may rapidly adapt to unilateral arm use, even for bilateral tasks, and may reject a prosthesis before the LCP is developed, litigation is resolved, or other available resources are identified. Thus, the first step in developing an LCP for amputations is to determine if the evaluee will benefit from the use of prostheses. This further reinforces the consideration for the life care planner to rely on the expertise of an experienced clinical team, particularly the physiatrist, and when prostheses are utilized, the prosthetist.

In developing a prosthesis prescription, the primary consideration is identifying the functional deficits and selecting the most appropriate prosthetic components to restore lost function. Additionally, as each evaluee is unique, her or his individual goals, activities, living environments, and vocational demands should also be considered.

The needs of lower limb amputees are vastly different from those of upper limb amputees. Lower limb amputees require mobility and stability, while upper limb amputees are challenged by activities of daily living (ADLs) and instrumental activities of daily living (IADLs), such as self-hygiene, grooming, meal preparation, and household chores. For evaluees with multiple amputations, both mobility and ADLs/IADLs may be compromised, necessitating increased care in other areas of the LCP such as increased caregiver support. Given the vast functional deficit differences between upper limb and lower limb amputees, this chapter discusses them individually when appropriate.

The restoration of mobility for lower limb amputees is dependent upon the level of functional deficits. Surgeons make their best efforts to preserve as many joints as possible, as prosthetic joints[4] are not as functional as anatomical joints. The loss of neurological control of the knee joint is particularly significant for mobility. As more anatomical joints are removed, the more challenging mobility becomes. Factors to consider when developing a prosthesis prescription for lower limb amputees include the life stage of the amputee, cardiovascular capacity, residual limb health, existing comorbidities, stability, balance, and the ability to negotiate uneven terrain, stairs, and ramps.

In selecting prosthetic components for lower limb amputees, the mobility potential of the amputee is first identified using the *Medicare Functional Classification Levels* (MFCLs).[5] The MFCLs range from basic mobility, such as transfers, to high-impact activities, such as running. The MFCL may be low initially if the amputee has not yet completed rehabilitation and achieved MMI. Once the evaluee's MFCL is identified, prosthetic components designed for the identified functional deficit level may be selected. Throughout a lifetime, the amputee's MFCL may change due to aging and decreased activities, and thus the prosthesis prescription should also change accordingly as the evaluee ages (see Table 15.1 regarding MFCLs).

Medicare and private insurance payors may have strict policies regarding what prosthetic components may be prescribed for a given MFCL. However, if developing an LCP, these policies should not always be applied to a prosthetic component prescription, as they do not always align with best clinical practices and may compromise safety and efficacy. For example,

Table 15.1 Medicare Functional Classification Levels (MFCLs)

	K Level	Description
	0	Does not have the ability or potential to ambulate or transfer safely with or without assistance and a prosthesis does not enhance their quality of life or mobility.
	1	Has the ability or potential to use a prosthesis for transfers or ambulation on level surfaces at a fixed cadence, typical of the limited and unlimited household ambulator.
	2	Has the ability or potential for ambulation with the ability to transverse low-level environmental barriers such as curbs, stairs, or uneven surfaces. This level is typical of the limited community ambulator.
	3	Has the ability or potential for ambulation with variable cadence, typical of the community ambulator who can transverse most environmental barriers and may have vocational, therapeutic, or exercise activity that demands prosthetic utilization beyond simple locomotion.
	4	Has the ability or potential for prosthetic ambulation that exceeds the basic ambulation skills, exhibiting high impact, stress, or energy levels typical of the prosthetic demands of the child, active adult, or athlete.

microprocessor knees may provide the most benefit for amputees with the least mobility due to their inherent stability and the increased stability deficits of this population. However, many payors will not provide coverage for microprocessor knees for amputees with lower MFCLs, likely due to their significant cost. If developing an LCP, these payor restrictions do not apply, as the primary objective is to restore the evaluee to her or his prior functional level rather than prosthetic components solely based upon their cost. Thus, it may be appropriate to prescribe a microprocessor knee in an LCP for an evaluee with a lower MFCL, even though it may not be typically reimbursed.

The cost of prosthetic components can vary greatly. For example, the cost of a prosthetic knee may vary from less than $1000 to more than USD 80,000. However, there is not a direct positive correlation between the cost of prosthetic components and their performance or benefits. Thus, selecting the costliest prosthetic components should not be considered unless those components are the best option for restoring the evaluee's functional deficits and achieving her or his individual goals. In an amputation LCP, it is not uncommon for the cost of prosthetic components to be a significant or major portion of the overall costs of life needs.

Prostheses are generally composed of modular components, most of which are compatible or interchangeable even though they may have differing manufacturers. With dozens and even hundreds of commercially available options for each component type, a prosthetist can effectively provide many thousands of possible combinations of prosthetic components. The physiatrist provides a prosthesis prescription from a high level, and the prosthetist may identify the most appropriate specific prosthetic components within the broader functional categories. There are many factors to consider in the selection of prosthetic components including functional capability, weight, compatibility, audible noise, stability features, environmental limitations (temperature extremes, soil, and water resistance), cosmesis, durability, body weight limitations, warranty period, extended warranty options, cognitive demand, biocompatibility, energy efficiency, power limitations, and build height requirements. Given the preceding unlimited options and complexity, it would be unwise for the life care planner to project a treatment plan without extensive knowledge of component indications/contraindications and/or consultation with a physiatrist and prosthetist.

Expanding on the preceding paragraph would fill an entire volume and is beyond the scope of this chapter. However, a brief discussion of core prosthetic components is warranted, as each element will usually be included in the prosthetic section of an LCP.

The vast functions, protective properties, aesthetics, and self-healing capability of intact human limbs are a marvel compared to artificial limbs. The design of prosthetic components is an exercise of compromise. Some prosthetic components may excel in one function while performing poorly in another. A single prosthesis may not be sufficient for the evaluee to restore her or him to a functional life, particularly if she or he engages in specific sports or recreational activities (Matthews et al., 2014). Thus, the evaluee may need more than one type of prosthesis to achieve her or his functional goals.

A primary prosthesis is used for mobility, ADLs, and IADLs in the home, social, and vocational environments. Other prostheses may have specific functional requirements such as waterproof components for boating activities or a high-energy return foot for jogging or running. Often a secondary "water leg" is included in the LCP for wet environments. However, not all amputees may benefit from a "water leg" and thus may not use one, as they may not find it to be practical in many situations such as swimming or showering. Showering with a prosthesis is not recommended since the socket must be removed to clean the residual limb and standing in a shower increases the fall risk. Rather, a safer option is the use of a shower bench and handheld shower for lower limb amputees, who are socket users, and suction sponges and a body dryer for upper limb amputees. Osseointegration amputees may benefit from a water leg with an anti-slip base for standing in the shower but should be cautioned about slip and fall risks. Additionally, a water leg may inhibit swimming for exercise, yet may provide stability for playing in a pool with children. Thus, is it important to evaluate the amputee in her or his environment before generically prescribing a water leg to ensure it is of benefit and need, particularly as many prosthetic components are now available with varying levels of water resistance or are waterproof, potentially eliminating the need for a dedicated water leg.[6] Each prosthesis requires a means of suspension to retain a connection with the residual limb. In osseointegration recipients, a solid connection is made with an abutment or dual cone adapter, the component which attaches to the residual bone and protrudes from the residual limb via the skin penetration site or stoma. In prostheses with sockets, the suspension is maintained via passive suction, elevated vacuum, liners with pin locks, and/or soft tissue compression proximal to osseous protuberances. Each of these socket methods of suspension, unlike osseointegration, is not completely rigid and results in a 'pistoning' motion of the residual limb soft tissue, potentially resulting in pain and/or skin breakdown.

During ambulation, the forces on the residual limb frequently exceed the force of body weight. For prostheses with sockets, an interface is necessary to absorb the shear and *ground reaction forces* (GRFs) of locomotion. The interface is typically a prosthetic liner composed of urethane gel or silicone, which the amputee rolls onto the residual limb before donning the prosthesis. The interface may be a direct skin fit and/or include socks, flexible/adjustable socket walls, and/or various medical-grade foam materials. When prosthetic liners and/or socks are used as the interface, they will need replacement on an annual or maintenance schedule determined by medical necessity and thus may be considered prosthetic supplies. It is not uncommon for the interface to also provide suspension. For osseointegration recipients, an interface is unnecessary due to the direct skeletal connection (see Figure 15.4 regarding Osseointegration).

For osseointegration recipients, protection of the residual bone in the event of falls is paramount to prevent secondary complications such as fractures and potential subsequent loss of residual bone length. Osseointegration prosthetic components may include a fail-safe mechanism that is designed to absorb excessive forces in one or more planes (e.g., sagittal flexion, traverse axial rotation) to protect the osseous anchor in the event of a fall. Some fail-safe mechanisms may be reset by the amputee after release, and thus such incidents do not affect the LCP. However, other fail-safe mechanisms require a visit to the providing physician, and thus the cost of replacement fail-safe components and associated service fees should be accounted for in the LCP.

For lower limb amputees, prosthetic ankle, knee, and hip joints are provided for varying degrees of mobility and stability, depending on the level of functional deficits. Advanced prosthetic joints include microprocessor control to enhance functional diversity,[7] increase variable cadence capability, and provide stability for uneven terrain, stairs, and ramps (Hahn et al., 2021). Externally powered joints increase function and decrease energy expenditure, but come at the

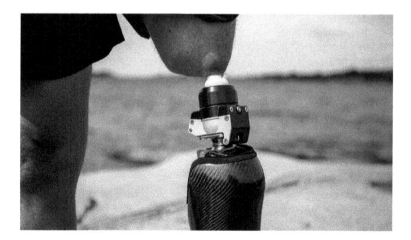

Figure 15.4 OPRA Transfemoral Osseointegration With Axor II Failsafe Mechanism (Integrum AB)

cost of significant weight, limited power, noise, and bulk; thus, their disadvantages often outweigh their advantages (Windrich et al., 2016). Due to their significant cost, advanced microprocessor-controlled lower limb components often are available with extended manufacturer warranties at the time of purchase and may be considered in the LCP whenever available (Hsu & Warych, 2017).

There are hundreds of prosthetic feet available to accommodate various levels of activities. They may be broadly grouped into the categories of basic feet, *energy storing and return* (ESAR), hydraulic ankles,[8] microprocessor-controlled, and activity-specific feet.[9] Basic feet are appropriate for lower-level ambulators who simply transfer or are limited household ambulators. ESAR feet are composed of composites with the intent of minimizing energy expenditure. Hydraulic ankles adapt well to uneven terrain, stairs, and ramps. Microprocessor-controlled feet use sensors to detect the intended function and employ algorithms to adapt the function to the desired activity. Activity-specific feet are diverse and may be suited for running, rock climbing, scuba diving, or other sport or recreational activities (Bragaru et al., 2012). Some feet may include multiple characteristics, such as having a microprocessor-controlled ankle with an ESAR keel. If an amputee engages in a diverse range of activities, multiple foot types with interchangeable couplers and/or multiple prostheses may be prescribed.

Restoration of body image is essential for the mental health of some amputees. Thus, there are several options to improve the aesthetics of functional prostheses. At the most basic level, protective covers for the preservation of the functional prosthetic components are available. These covers only offer moderate cosmetic restoration such as filling out pants or shirts. When body image is a primary concern, lifelike aesthetic restoration with silicone is possible with skin tone matching, artificial hair, skin texture, and simulated veins. As it is difficult to deceive the human eye, many amputees elect to forego a cosmesis altogether. Aesthetic restoration prostheses are often passive but generally not durable and may inhibit prosthetic component function, such as the movement of prosthetic knees during locomotion or fingers for gripping objects. Aesthetic prosthetic covers provide an alternative to a lifelike cosmesis, with a personalized visual aesthetic that may be preferred to the appearance of bare mechanical components (see Figure 15.5 regarding aesthetic prosthetic covers).

Some prosthetic components improve function for amputees but do not have anatomical equivalents. For example, for lower limb amputees, quick-disconnect components allow rapid interchange of different prosthetic components such as feet. Rotators allow amputees to position

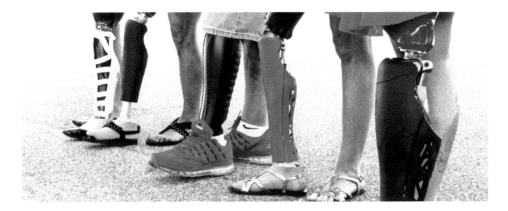

Figure 15.5 Aesthetic Prosthetic Cover (UNYQ)

the knee axially at any position, exceeding anatomical ROM. For upper limb amputees, many interchangeable terminal devices are available for very specific functional tasks, and myoelectric prostheses may have separate environmental proximity chips to enable rapid switching of functional hand modes.

Upper Limb Prosthesis Prescription

As the overall incidence of upper limb amputations is much less than lower limb, it is a specialized market with significantly fewer prosthetic component options. The number of *degrees of freedom* (DoF) in the arm and hand is much greater than in the lower limb with the capability of many grasps and gestures for ADLs/IADLs, while the lower limb is primarily used for standing and mobility. However, the number of control inputs for the upper limb is very limited, and subsequently, the restoration of upper limb functional deficits is much less than the lower limb when prostheses are used. As the restored function of upper limb prosthetic components often falls short of expectations, upper limb prosthesis abandonment is common (Salminger et al., 2020). It is essential to fit an upper limb prosthesis as quickly as possible post-amputation to prevent adaption without the use of a prosthesis, which may lead to premature overuse injuries.

Upper limb prostheses may be divided into several broad categories including *externally powered*,[10] *body-powered*,[11] *hybrid* (a combination of the previous two), *activity-specific*, or *passive*,[12] as illustrated in Figure 15.6 (Melton, 2017; Uellendahl & Uellendahl, 2006). Like lower limb prostheses, upper limb components have limited function, and thus an amputee may require more than one prosthesis to achieve as much functional restoration as feasible. Upper limb prostheses

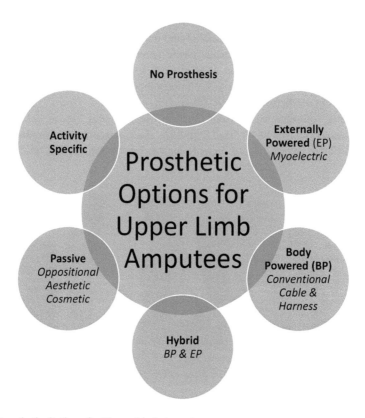

Figure 15.6 Prosthetic Options for Upper Limb Amputees

share several of the same components as lower limb, possibly including a socket, an interface, and a suspension. Additionally, when the hand has been amputated, a terminal device in the form of a hand, hook, or mechanical grasp is provided. Osseointegration is an option for finger, thumb, transradial, and transhumeral amputations, eliminating the need for a socket and its complications. As ADLs/IADLs are vast and specific in comparison to lower limb mobility requirements, many interchangeable task-specific terminal devices are available, particularly for recreational and sports activities. Unlike lower limb prosthetic components, many upper limb components may not be compatible or interchangeable, especially if electronic and from differing manufacturers. Due to the preceding limitations, the complexity, and the lower incidence, upper limb amputations may be considered a sub-specialty within prosthetics. Thus, in cases of upper limb amputation, the life care planner should consult with a certified prosthetist with upper limb expertise.

Rehabilitation

Therapy is essential for restoring mobility and/or ADLs/IADLs, whether an amputee receives a prosthesis or not. Therapy may resume on an outpatient basis, even if a prosthesis has not yet been provided, continuing with limb desensitization and strength, endurance, and ROM exercises. Once a prosthesis has been provided, specific training may commence and continues until the amputee can achieve the desired functional outcomes. Prosthesis training therapy should commence as soon as possible, particularly for upper limb amputees. Malone described the first month after amputation as the "Golden Period", a short window of opportunity in which the amputee is most likely to accept a prosthesis and establish a foundation for ideal outcomes (Malone et al., 1984).

While the loss of a limb presents many challenges, several are particularly relevant to therapy. First, most prosthetic components are passive or are controlled by muscles that are not used to control an intact limb. Thus, new neuromotor muscle patterns must be established to effectively control a prosthesis. Second, the functions of prosthetic components vary by design. The therapist must understand each prosthetic component's function to ensure biomechanical safety and efficacy, which comes from extensive experience training amputees.

The duration of therapy will vary depending on the amputee's overall health, motivation, amputation level, affected side (dominant vs. non-dominant), prior functional level, and presence of comorbidities (Meier, III, 2019). The initial therapy progress may be negatively impeded by numerous factors such as pain, acceptance, and rapid residual limb volume changes. For unilateral upper limb amputations in which the dominant side is affected, the duration of the therapy will likely be longer to permit hand dominance transfer to the non-dominant side. Many insurance payors cap the maximum allowable therapy visits annually, but these policies should not influence the therapy requirements of an amputation LCP, particularly for osseointegration recipients or in complex cases with multiple amputations which necessitate extensive therapy.

Further therapy may be needed periodically throughout the amputee's life. If prosthetic components are changed to differing designs, gait or functional retraining may be necessary. Additionally, if further future surgical procedures are anticipated, appropriate therapy should also be projected.

Community Reintegration

Perhaps the most challenging phase of amputation rehabilitation is community reintegration. The medical clinical team often excels in addressing the acute and immediate challenges in the preceding phases, from amputation, to proving a prosthesis, to prosthesis training. However, the medical team is not solely responsible for community reintegration and relies upon support from the community, including immediate family/household co-inhabitants, friends, social workers, trained peer visitors, employers, businesses, clergy, local governments, and the federal government (Meier & Atkins, 2004). Unfortunately, many of these individuals or organizations are not educated, experienced, or equipped to provide support for a smooth transition back into society. While it is easy to focus on the vocational environment of community reintegration, a comprehensive approach is required that also includes the household (housing other than home), commercial (businesses and retail shopping), health services, recreation, and social (restaurants, bars, hotels, theaters) and education environments (Hordacre et al., 2015). Research indicates that improvements in community reintegration improve both amputee function and *quality of life* (QoL) (Hawkins et al., 2016).

Lifelong Care

Whether an amputee receives a prosthesis or not, lifelong care will be necessary, particularly as amputation accelerates the aging process. If a prosthesis is provided, the lifelong care phase commences once the amputee has completed the prosthesis training and is stable at the desired functional level. The amputee should visit a physiatrist at regular intervals to ensure problems do not escalate. If problems develop due to the use of a prosthesis, the amputee should visit the prosthetist immediately for resolution. Amputees should also periodically visit a prosthetist at regular intervals, even if problems do not develop. Like preventative medicine, such periodic prosthetist visits ensure that undiscovered problems do not exacerbate and develop into complications. Furthermore, many prosthetic components require periodic inspection, maintenance, and/or servicing to ensure safety and maintain warranty standings. Such prosthetist visits are often already accounted for in the initial cost of the prosthesis due to the reimbursement system used for prosthetic components, based upon the Healthcare Common Procedure Coding System (HCPCS) L-Codes.

Lifelong care should not be limited to physiological needs and prosthetic components. The psychosocial adaptation to amputation is challenging and may never occur. Thus, long-term mental health may be periodically assessed to ensure the amputee can maintain the desired functional level and community integration (see Figure 15.7 regarding amputation levels).

Lower Limb Amputations

Toe and Partial Foot

While the functional impact of a toe or partial foot amputation may not be as significant as higher-level lower limb amputations, prostheses and possibly shoe modifications should be provided, as they may not only improve gait function but also prevent pathomechanic complications. Partial foot amputations may be classified as transmetatarsal, Lisfranc, or Chopart and are managed with custom orthoses, cosmetic silicone, slipper sockets, toe fillers, ankle-foot orthoses (AFOs), or clamshell-type prostheses (Crowe et al., 2019; Dillon et al., 2007). For some amputees, shoe modifications may be necessary to facilitate smooth biomechanical stance phase rollover or to equalize a leg length discrepancy due to the additional build height of the prosthesis (contralateral shoe build-up) or a plantar flexion contracture.

Ankle Disarticulation (Syme's)

An ankle disarticulation has the advantage of biomechanical gait efficiency compared to transtibial amputations and usually permits distal end bearing with and without a prosthesis, yet at the cost of a bulbous ankle region and limited selection of prosthetic feet. Prosthetic feet specifically designed for use with an ankle disarticulation prosthesis are available.

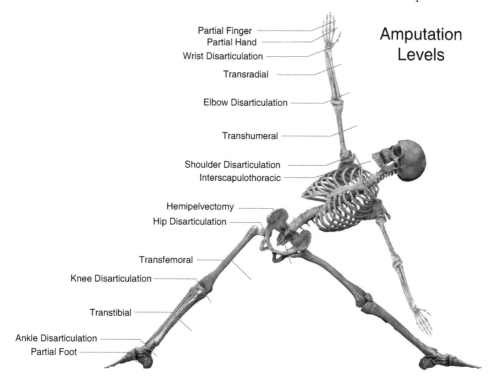

Figure 15.7 Amputation Levels

Transtibial

As transtibial amputation is the most common lower limb amputation, there are a plethora of prosthetic component options available. The prognosis for returning to a highly satisfying life-style is promising for both traditional socket and osseointegration prostheses. For highly active transtibial amputees, the potential benefits associated with eliminating the socket may not out-weigh the risks of complications secondary to osseointegration (e.g., implant failure, superficial infections, and deep osseous infections).

Transfemoral and Knee Disarticulation

The impact of losing the knee joint is much more significant than may be anticipated. As ambu-lation with the lower limb is composed of three primary joints (hip, knee, and ankle), the trans-femoral or knee disarticulation amputee loses two of three mobility joints and only can maintain control of the three ipsilateral joints via hip motion. This contributes to inefficient gait, which compromises mobility endurance, while basic mobility such as stair and ramp ascent/descent becomes particularly challenging. Furthermore, the risk of falls is elevated, and thus micro-processor knees may be considered to prevent associated secondary complications if deemed appropriate by the clinical team.

Hip Disarticulation and Hemipelvectomy

Hip disarticulation and hemipelvectomy amputations are very difficult to treat prosthetically. As all three primary lower limb joints have been lost, control of the ipsilateral prosthesis requires exaggerated pelvic motion. Gait efficiency, standing, ambulatory safety, and the development of secondary premature complications are of utmost concern. Many amputees at this level may elect to forego a prosthesis or only use one for transfers and cosmetic reasons, preferring a wheelchair for mobility. If a prosthesis is provided, the amputee is advised to receive care from a prosthetist who frequently treats these amputation levels. At this amputation level, when not wearing a prosthesis, customized wheelchair cushions or prosthetic seat sockets may be provided to maintain a healthy spine. While amputees at these levels may adapt to hopping on the sound limb, such ambulation should be discouraged due to the high stress incurred by the sound limb. This population in particular may benefit from an upper-body strength conditioning program due to the stresses placed on the upper limb joints, whether using crutches or a manual wheelchair, to prevent or minimize overuse syndromes such as rotator cuff pathology and carpal tunnel syndrome in both upper limbs.

Upper Limb Amputations

Prosthetic Components

Upper prostheses are composed of various prosthetic components including hands, terminal devices (e.g., hooks or task-specific), joints (wrist, elbows, shoulder), suspension (e.g., harness), and sockets. Ancillary components include electromyography (EMG) sensors, batteries, microprocessor controllers, and fail-safe mechanisms (exclusive to osseointegration recipients) as appropriate.

The prescription options for upper limb amputees fall into six categories (Melton, 2017; Uellendahl & Uellendahl, 2006):

1. No prosthesis provided.
2. Passive (oppositional, semi-prehensible).
3. Body powered (conventional, cable and harness, cable-driven).
4. Externally powered (myoelectric).
5. Hybrid (body-powered and externally powered).
6. Activity specific (e.g., for adaptive sports).

Depending on the vocational and avocational needs, the amputee may require more than one type of prosthetic device to restore functional deficits. Passive (oppositional) prostheses may provide aesthetic restoration of limb loss for body image and community reintegration, particularly in the first couple of years after traumatic amputation. Such prostheses aid with opposition for grasping and enabling bimanual tasks. Body-powered prostheses are durable, offer good proprioception, and rely on proximal body movement with a harness for prosthetic joint articulation. Externally powered prostheses are heavier, less durable, and less proprioceptive, yet may be a preferred solution when a harness is undesirable and/or for higher-level amputations or when a more lifelike restoration of the limb is desired. Hybrid prostheses provide both body-powered control and external power and may offer the best compromise when neither body-powered nor externally powered prostheses are ideal. An activity-specific prosthesis may be provided to achieve specific vocational tasks or recreational activities.

Control strategies for externally powered prosthetic components are challenging, as the availability of control inputs (residual muscles for control) is often limited. Pattern recognition systems increase the number of possible inputs with an EMG sensor array and offer more nuanced control of prosthetic joints. However, control for multiple prosthetics joints for all systems is still limited to sequential rather than simultaneous function. Thus, externally powered (myoelectric) prostheses may be rejected by amputees due to increased cognitive load and increased task time in addition to increased weight and decreased durability.

Osseointegration is particularly advantageous for upper limb amputees. Suspension of an upper limb prosthesis can be challenging or uncomfortable when a harness is required. A harness further compromises ROM, particularly for activities in which the arm is elevated. The sloppy interface of a prosthetic socket compromises the accurate positioning of the arm and hand in three-dimensional space. Prostheses offer little proprioception, which is essential for many functional tasks. Osseointegration significantly mitigates or eliminates the preceding problems and is available for transhumeral, transradial, thumb, and finger amputations.[13]

Finger and Partial Hand

Partial hand and finger amputations are some of the most challenging amputations to manage with prostheses; however, a variety of prosthetic components are available. In the past decade, technological innovation has led to the development of prostheses that utilize proximal joint motion (e.g., carpometacarpal [CMC] and metacarpophalangeal [MCP] joints) to permit the active mechanical function of distal prosthetic joints (see Figure 15.6) (Treadwell et al., 2020). Additionally, externally powered prostheses are available for partial hand amputations, utilizing surface-mounted EMG sensors to provide input for microprocessor control. While not as functional as other prosthesis types, passive cosmetic prostheses restore body image and provide digit opposition and object stabilization (see Figure 15.8 regarding MCP drivers).

Wrist Disarticulation and Transradial

It is particularly challenging to restore the lost functions of the human hand. As compensation, wrist disarticulation and transradial prostheses may be equipped with a quick-disconnect wrist, which allows for interchangeability of prosthetic hands, hooks, mechanical grippers, and various task-specific terminal devices.

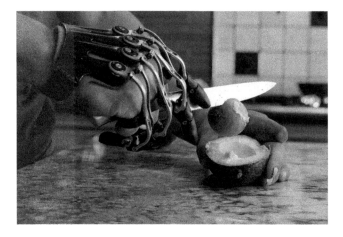

Figure 15.8 MCP Driver (Naked Prosthetics)

Elbow Disarticulation and Transhumeral

The loss of the forearm necessitates a prosthetic elbow, which may be body powered or externally powered. Regardless, the elbow must be first positioned to the desired angle before the hand, wrist, or terminal device may be used (sequential operation). Subsequently, the control of an elbow disarticulation/transhumeral prosthesis is significantly more challenging than more distal amputations, and the amputee with more proximal amputations may benefit to see an upper limb prosthetic specialist and therapists experienced with these amputation levels.

Interscapular-Thoracic and Shoulder Disarticulation

At the most severe upper amputation levels, prosthetic shoulder joints are available. However, they are passive and must be pre-positioned before the desired task. For unilateral high-level amputees, both the presence and absence of prosthesis weight are a concern, as the former decreases comfort, while the latter may result in postural complications due to uneven distribution of torso mass. An alternative is to provide an endoskeletal prosthetic design to balance posture and provide minimal function and cosmetic restoration. Bilateral high-level upper limb amputees will be severely impacted in the ability to perform the most basic ADLs/IADLs and may require attendant care. A custom rack will help facilitate donning and doffing if or when assistance is not available.

Complications

As there are many possible complications following amputation, the amputee will likely experience several sequelae throughout a lifetime. Unfortunately, acute and chronic pain is highly prevalent among amputations, yet the expertise needed to resolve the root causes requires the expertise of an extensive clinical team. Potential complications are discussed here and may be divided into the broader categories of neurological, dermatological, musculoskeletal, postural/gait disturbances, mental health, overall health, and residual limb revision surgeries.

Neurological Complications

Neurological complications include neuromas and PLP. Neuromas are common if a residual nerve is simply resected instead of reinnervated at the time of amputation. While some neuromas may be resolved with prosthetic socket modifications or medication, debilitating neuromas may require surgical excision.

PLP is a common symptom in amputees, not to be confused with phantom limb sensation (PLS). While there are many modalities for PLP, the efficacy is generally poor, and thus the clinical team may trial various pharmacological, non-pharmacological, and/or surgical treatments. Pharmacological treatments include opioids, anticonvulsants, anti-inflammatory medications, local anesthetics, antidepressants, calcitonin, botulinum neurotoxins, N-methyl-D-aspartate (NMDA) receptor antagonists, Mu opioid receptor norepinephrine reuptake inhibition (MOR-NRI) analgesics, and cannabinoids (Hall & Eldabe, 2018; McCormick et al., 2014; Richardson & Kulkarni, 2017). Non-pharmacological treatments include mirror box therapy, hypnotic imagery, *transcutaneous electrical nerve stimulation* (TENS), residual limb repositioning, residual limb massage, muscular electrostimulation, acupuncture, biofeedback, *electroconvulsive therapy* (ECT), repetitive transcranial magnetic stimulation, virtual reality therapy, augmented reality therapy, mental imagery, magnetic stimulation, vibration therapy, music, and use of a prosthesis (Batsford et al., 2017; Hyung & Wiseman-Hakes, 2021; Richardson & Kulkarni; Yaputra & Widyadharma, 2018). Surgical interventions for PLP include TMR (Dumanian et al., 2019; Kang, et al., 2022; Peters et al., 2020), rhizotomy, neurectomy, cordotomy, sympathectomy, myelotomy, and dorsal root entry zone lesioning. However, the efficacy of surgical treatments, excluding TMR, has yet to be determined (Richardson & Kulkarni).

Dermatological Complications

Only the intact hand palms and foot soles are intended to absorb the repetitive loading and shear forces. However, a prosthetic socket loads soft tissues not designed for the demands of mobility and ADLs/IADLs. Thus, it is not surprising that dermatological complications are common with prosthetic socket use. Dermatologic complications include adherent skin grafts, invaginated epidermis, scar tissue, allergic dermatitis/eczema, epidermoid cysts, folliculitis, boils, abscesses, cellulitis, fungal infections, blisters, and ulcers. Many of the preceding complications can be resolved with early treatment of proper hygiene (epidermis and prosthetic interfaces) and prosthetic socket adjustments. If chronic complications persist due to prosthetic socket use, osseointegration may be given consideration.

Musculoskeletal Complications

Skeletal complications include *heterotopic ossification* (HO), bony overgrowth (spurs), and osteopenia. HO and bony overgrowth may require surgical intervention if prosthetic socket accommodations do not resolve. The prevalence of disuse osteopenia in the residual limb of lower limb amputees utilizing prostheses with sockets is high due to the lack of direct skeletal connection to the prosthesis. Osseointegration may be an alternative intervention if deemed medically appropriate by the treating physician, as it directly loads the residual skeleton (Tillander et al., 2017).

Muscle and soft tissue complications include joint contractures, muscle spasms, low back pain, neck pain, disuse atrophy, and acquired scoliosis or abnormal biomechanics of the musculoskeletal system (Gailey et al., 2008). Treatment varies depending on the etiology but includes prosthetic alignment/height adjustments, gait retraining therapy, muscle strength training, or elimination of related complications such as a poorly fitting prosthetic socket.

The possible development of joint contractures is an immediate concern post-amputation, particularly in lower limb amputees (Ghazali et al., 2018). During the acute healing phase, the amputee may be bedridden with minimal ambulation and/or extensively use a wheelchair and subsequently sit for prolonged periods with the hip and/or knee in flexion. Unless managed, contractures may develop and compromise the future capacity to utilize a prosthesis safely and efficiently. Severe contractures may require surgical management and, in extreme cases, may result in a more proximal amputation with subsequent loss of the affected joint. Contractures may be prevented with education, therapy, and a regularly assigned exercise schedule. Once an amputee is fitted with a prosthesis and has completed gait therapy, the likelihood of developing contractures is greatly diminished.

As prostheses are not an adequate substitute for the intact limb, many amputees adapt biomechanical movements that favor the intact limbs and/or joints. Consequently, accelerated degenerative complications should be expected such as hip/knee/ankle arthritis, rotator cuff injury, and carpal tunnel syndrome.

Postural/Gait Disturbances

Due to the previously mentioned abnormal biomechanical movements, decreased proprioception, and leg length discrepancies, postural and gait disturbances are common (Gaunaurd et al., 2011). These may lead to falls and the aforementioned accelerated degeneration (Hendershot & Nussbaum, 2013).

Mental Health

Amputation has a profound effect on the mental health of the amputee, particularly due to the rapid transformation experienced in traumatic amputations. Complications include mood disorder, anxiety disorder, cognitive disorder, depressive disorder, substance dependence, and psychological impact on the immediate family/household (Jensen et al., 2011). Treatment modalities include counseling, pharmacological regimens, and recreational therapy.

Overall Health

The overall health of an amputee post-amputation may be impacted by numerous complications, particularly due to the likelihood of decreased physical and social activity and subsequent sequelae, such as hypertension or body weight fluctuation.

Due to the higher energy expenditure of ambulating with a prosthesis, many amputees are not as active as they were before their amputation. While locomotion is effortless for most healthy intact individuals, it may require intense effort for lower limb amputees, particularly with more proximal amputations. The high prevalence of pain among amputees, particularly that incurred by the socket or altered biomechanics, further reduces activity levels, as the natural tendency is to avoid or minimize pain-inducing behavior. Furthermore, if the amputee experiences depression or other psychosocial issues as a result of limb loss, changes in appetite may occur. Maintaining the same caloric intake as before the amputation in conjunction with the decreased activity level that most amputees have can cause weight gain or an increase in body mass index. Thus, unless the amputee adopts other strategies such as positively modifying dietary habits and/or adopting alternative exercises, she or he is likely to gain body weight. As a prophylactic measure, an evaluation with a nutritionist might be considered in the LCP to educate the amputee about the potential for undesirable weight gain and to ensure she or he can adopt nutritional and/or exercise strategies to prevent it.

Weight gain is likely to incur volume changes of the residual limb, which often affects the prosthetic socket fit. Prosthetists can adopt several strategies to account for residual limb changes with volume-adjustable sockets, flexible walls, inflatable bladders, and/or adding or removing prosthetic socks. However, generally, the socket must be replaced once an amputee's residual limb volume increases by 5% or decreases by 10% (Fernie & Holliday, 1982). The cost of replacement sockets is often a significant portion of the cost of a prosthesis. Furthermore, replacing sockets is not a trivial task for the prosthetist or amputee, as it takes time and possibly several iterations to create a socket that achieves a proper fit for the residual limb. As osseointegration eliminates the need for a prosthetic socket, the challenges of accommodating weight changes are also eliminated.

Residual Limb Revision Surgeries

An amputated limb is not an optimal design for accommodating the various forces an amputee may encounter. Thus, complications can develop, many of which have already been described, necessitating further intervention beyond the amputation. For a prosthesis with a socket, if the prosthetist is unable to resolve complications with socket modifications and/or replacement sockets, surgical revision may be necessary. Such revisions may be performed to resolve painful scarring, adherent or invaginated skin, chronic skin conditions, myodesis failure, redundant soft tissue, neuromas, skin graft problems, and osseous structures (e.g., bony prominences, bony spurs, bone contouring, and HO) (Bourke et al., 2011; Forbes et al., 2021).

For evaluees with osseointegration, surgical revisions may also be necessary for various complications. If osteomyelitis is not successfully resolved with oral or parenteral antibiotics or if the implant is damaged, then it may require surgical removal. However, with some osseointegration implants, it is possible to insert a replacement without loss of residual bone length.

LCP Categories of Need

As the needs of each evaluee are unique and the level of amputations is complex, it is not possible to provide an exhaustive discussion of every LCP category of need for various scenarios. However, a brief discussion of guiding principles and factors to consider is warranted and is briefly discussed here.

Projected Evaluations

At a minimum, periodic evaluation by the physiatrist and regular assessment by the prosthetist should be expected. As the sequelae of amputations are diverse, additional projected evaluations may be indicated including neurological, physical therapy, occupational therapy, speech therapy, and dietary. Electrical injuries often affect internal organs and result in related complications including cardiac scarring, arrhythmias, and premature cataracts. Depending on the mechanism of injury and the organs affected, evaluation by specialists such as audiology, cardiology, and ophthalmology may be warranted, particularly if there is a concern for undetected or delayed onset of complications (Bae et al., 2013; Wesner & Hickie, 2013).

Projected Therapeutic Modalities

Both long-term and short-term anticipated interventions should be included, whether regular or periodic. Such modalities may include individual and family counseling (Fossey & Hacker Hughes, 2014), sexual therapy, speech therapy, recreational therapy, physical therapy, and occupational therapy. The replacement of prostheses or sockets may result in a biomechanical change, particularly if new prosthetic components are selected (e.g., prosthetic foot, knee). If the preceding occurs or there are anatomical changes, the evaluee may require physical and/or occupational therapy to appropriately adapt to the changes.

Diagnostic Testing

Due to the increased risk of premature skeletal complications, periodic spinal imaging for back pain or scoliosis and/or periodic residual limb imaging for bone spurs, HO, and neuromas might be warranted if deemed related by the medical treating team. For osseointegration recipients, periodic imaging may be required if complications such as a periprosthetic fracture (Hoellwarth et al., 2020), implant failure, stress shielding (osseous resorption), and/or presence of deep osseous infection occur. If diagnostic testing is completed as part of a *projected evaluation*, it should not be included in this section of the LCP.

Wheelchair Needs

Wheelchair requirements are dependent on the anticipated mode of mobility. If the amputee ambulates well with a prosthesis, an ultralight manual wheelchair as a backup or for long-distance use may be needed. The mobility potential is correlated to the level of amputation, with more proximal or bilateral lower limb amputations having a higher impact. For such amputees, the wheelchair may be the primary mode of mobility. Another factor to consider is the anticipation of reduced mobility due to natural and premature aging. Amputees currently using a prosthesis for mobility may eventually transition to a wheelchair as they age.

Wheelchair Accessories and Maintenance

Depending on the extent of use, wheelchair accessories such as bags, seat cushions, gloves, etc., may be beneficial. For bilateral amputees, the lack of lower limb mass disrupts the *center of mass* (CoM), and if the wheel axis cannot be shifted posterior to the CoM, then anti-tip accessories should be added to prevent rearward wheelchair tip-over (Weed & Sluis, 1990).

Wheelchair maintenance requirements are directly dependent on the anticipated use. For example, if wheelchair use is only for long distances when prosthesis endurance is insufficient, then the wheelchair maintenance cost and replacement frequency should be reduced accordingly.

Aids for Independent Function

There are a few aids that provide an increased independent function for lower limb amputees and enhance safety. For lower limb amputees, changing shoes on prosthetic feet can be challenging, as the prosthetic foot shells are quite rigid. Lower limb amputees benefit from an extra-long, heavy-duty shoehorn designed specifically for the purpose. If the wheelchair is the primary mode of transportation, a reaching aid may be beneficial. Socket users should use a shower bench and a handheld showerhead to allow cleaning of the residual limb in a seated position. Amputees with osseointegration may use a water prosthesis with an anti-slip base of support and care given to prevent falls in the shower, which can be slippery, increasing the fall risk and subsequent complications. An elevated toilet seat may facilitate sit-to-stand transfers for some amputees, particularly in their elder years.

Upper limb amputees, depending on the level of functional deficits and dominance of the affected side, may benefit from a large variety of assistive devices to facilitate ADLs and IADLs, such as food preparation, grooming, dressing, household chores, and recreational activities (Author unknown, 2015). A custom rack for bilateral upper limb amputees will aid with donning and doffing prostheses. To determine the appropriate assistive devices, the life care planner should inspect the home environment, interview the evaluee, and if necessary, consult with an occupational therapist, as there are many available options. The requirements for unilateral amputees who are affected by the loss of the dominant arm or hand or are bilateral will have increased needs for functional aids. Overuse syndrome can be prevented by the use of assistive devices that minimize the contralateral or proximal joints. These may include an ergonomically structured desk and voice-activated software.

Orthotics and Prosthetics

Unless comorbidities exist, generally amputees will not require orthotics. However, lower limb amputees, particularly unilateral transfemoral amputees, may benefit from prophylactic foot orthoses for the contralateral intact foot to mitigate overuse injuries. Many prosthetists are certified orthotists and can provide guidance for orthoses along with the physiatrist.

In addition to the prosthesis, the amputee will also need ongoing prosthetic supplies. Typical supplies include shrinkers for edema management, various ply socks for accommodating residual limb volume changes, and if used, prosthetic liners for suspension/epidermal protection. The consulting or treating prosthetist can provide the cost of the prosthetic supplies. Other supplies related to the residual limb such as lotions may be accounted for in the drug/supply needs section of the LCP.

Excluding prostheses and prosthetic supplies, occasionally other needs will be required, depending on the unique situation of the evaluee. For example, a very active amputee may prematurely wear out the prosthetic foot shell, necessitating a higher rate of replacement than the prosthesis.

Home Furnishings and Accessories

Amputees may benefit from several home furnishings and accessories. An electronic personal assistant (e.g., Amazon Alexa, Apple Siri, Google Assistant) can automate and simplify tasks.

Drug/Supply Needs

Medications related to the amputation should be considered part of the LCP if recommended by the treating healthcare providers. These categories often include medications for pain, depression, sleep difficulty, or periodic complications such as infection or hyperhidrosis.

Home/Care Facility

Most amputees can live an independent life, so nursing or facility care is rarely required. Evaluees with multiple amputations may need assistance with ADLs/IADLs. While the need will increase with age, particularly due to the early onset of degenerative disease, assistance may be provided at early ages to delay accelerated aging. If or when an amputee uses a wheelchair as the primary mode of mobility, the need for assistance with basic chores increases, particularly household maintenance.

Future Medical Care—Routine

Routine medical care may vary and will become evident from the evaluation of the amputee, current medical providers, and review of the medical records. Such care may be associated with the development of secondary complications or the presence of comorbidities.

Transportation

The evaluee should have a driving evaluation to determine individual needs if she or he plans to drive a vehicle. Many unilateral amputees may be able to drive without any vehicle modifications. Other evaluees may need a steering ring(s)/spinner knob, hand controls, and automatic features (brakes, transmission) if currently using a manual vehicle or custom modifications. On occasion, a wheelchair-compatible vehicle such as a van may be required.

If the evaluee is not able to receive required specialized care locally, transportation costs for periodic treatment to a regional/national center of excellence should be considered. For evaluees attending national annual amputee events such as recreational camps and/or national conferences, transportation and lodging costs may be considered depending on the individual situation.

Health and Strength Maintenance

Amputees should be encouraged to engage in regular exercise, particularly aerobic exercise. An exercise program may help maintain body weight for prosthetic socket use, prevent early degenerative onset, improve or maintain a cardiovascular reserve for mobility endurance, and improve overall well-being and mental health. Exercise may be maintained in the home with personal gym equipment or with a local gym and/or pool memberships. The economic costs of an exercise program versus health benefits may be one of the best economic investments of the LCP.

Architecture Renovations

Architecture renovations improve function in the home and are essential for safety. If wheelchair use is anticipated, accessibility renovations are required such as widened doorways, halls, and ramps. Permanent wheelchair ramps are important for wheelchair use to facilitate community mobility. Bathroom modifications such as handrails, handheld showerheads, and walk-in/roll-in showers/bathtubs are particularly relevant for lower limb amputees. If the home is multilevel, a stairlift should be considered when compromised mobility/stability is anticipated. Other home modifications such as a body dryer, bidet, and level doorknobs can reduce dependence on caregivers and improve independent functioning.

Potential Complications

This chapter includes an extensive discussion of potential complications of amputations, organized by category (see the "Complications" section). In the LCP, potential complications may be pragmatically listed in the order of probable occurrence. Whenever possible, other sections of the LCP should include interventions to prevent potential complications, particularly if such complications are more probable than not, as the cost of prevention is typically less than the cost of treatment. While their costs may not be included, the life care planner should exercise due diligence to include all potential complications to ensure all parties understand the comprehensive challenges the evaluee will face and the impact on overall health and QoL.

Vocational/Educational Plan

If vocational changes are anticipated due to the extent of the evaluee's injuries, vocational coaching and job coaching/placement may be included in the vocational plan depending on the individual situation. Educational costs of tuition, books, fees, labs, and supplies may be included if education is a vocational plan component. Ergonomic considerations such as a custom workstation for vocation or education use may also be considered. If the life care planner is not a vocational rehabilitation expert, she or he is highly encouraged to enlist the services of one to prepare this portion of the LCP, particularly as the potentially large costs of lost income will draw significant legal scrutiny.

Future Medical Care—Surgical Intervention or Aggressive Treatment

Beyond the initial rehabilitation phase, there may be an infrequent need for aggressive treatment or surgical intervention. Examples include skin grafts and surgical removal of bony overgrowths or neuromas. In osseointegration recipients, treatment of deep osseous infection may necessitate implant removal and possible reinsertion (Hoellwarth et al., 2020). The individual situation needs to be assessed by the treating healthcare team, and often these interventions are potential needs and not probable.

Orthopedic Equipment Needs

Ergonomic crutches, hands-free cutches (e.g., iWalkFree 3.0), and/or a rolling walker improve safety whenever it is inconvenient to temporarily don a prosthesis, such as going to the bathroom during the night. Portable wheelchair ramps are important for facilitating community mobility for wheelchair users. Canes and/or walkers may be anticipated in elder years. For osseointegration recipients, bilateral crutches and canes are essential during therapy to aid progressive loading to the bone-anchored implant.

Additional Amputation LCP Considerations

Pre-Injury Status

While the future is impossible to predict, the past may serve as a guide for what is the most probable prognosis for an amputee. Thus, in addition to an in-person evaluation, the life care planner should carefully review the lifestyle, hobbies, recreational activities, and vocational requirements of the evaluee to determine future needs. It is insufficient to simply quantify the prosthetic needs in LCP tables. Rather, it is incumbent for the life care planner to set the stage for future needs in narrative form by painting a picture of where the amputee has been. Should a case proceed to trial, the jury can fully appreciate the list of lifetime needs if they visualize the evaluee's life before amputation and how the itemized needs are essential for returning to a sense of normalcy.

Current Status

Due to the delayed healing and extensive therapy timelines, often MMI has not yet been achieved at the time the LCP is created. The life care planner must capture the current status in narrative, images, and videos to illustrate the importance of the projected needs.

Prosthesis Replacement Rates

Unlike intact limbs, prosthetic components eventually wear out and must be replaced. The replacement rates of prostheses are directly dependent on the activity and impact level of the amputee. The more active the amputee, the more frequent prosthetic components must be replaced. For lower limb amputees, prosthetic components are generally rated for 3 million cycles (steps) over three years, with approximately 1 million steps per year. However, amputees generally are not as active as non-amputees and may also employ other modes of mobility, such as wheelchair use for long-distance activities. Thus, it is not uncommon for prostheses to last well beyond their warranty period. Some manufacturers offer extended warranties at the time of purchase, minimizing the prosthetic component cost over its useful life and decreasing the replacement frequency (Hsu & Warych, 2017). Repair costs should be included in the LCP in years in which the prosthetic component warranties have expired. As prosthetic components are modular, individual components may be repaired and replaced, without the need to replace the entire prosthesis. Except for prosthetic sockets, lower limb prosthetic components should be replaced approximately every five years with normal use in accordance with the CMS *Reasonable Useful Lifetime* (RUL) rule (Berry, 2020).[14] The RUL serves as a prosthesis replacement rate baseline and may be amended accordingly based on individual factors such as amputee activity level, impact level, living/vocational/recreational environments, life phase, etc.

In determining replacement rates, the life cycle of an amputee must be given consideration. Amputees progress through three phases over their life expectancy. The first phase may be described as the healing phase, the first 12–24 months after amputation, in which the residual limb experiences rapid changes in shape and volume due to atrophy of residual disused musculature and the soft tissue adaption to weight bearing (Eckard et al., 2015). During the healing phase, the socket will require more frequent replacement as the shape of the residual limb evolves (Berry, 2020).

The next phase of the amputee may be regarded as the mature phase. During this phase, the residual limb remains relatively stable. However, prosthetic sockets must be replaced once the amputee's residual limb volume cannot be accommodated by the socket or prosthetic sock management. Socket replacements should also be anticipated for wear and tear and resolution of fit problems such as residual limb volume changes or accommodation of bone spurs or neuromas. The anticipated replacement frequency for prosthetic sockets is approximately 24–30 months (Berry, 2020). As a new prosthetic socket is included with a replacement prosthesis, a line item in the LCP for replacement sockets is only needed approximately every 48–60 months in alternation with replacement prostheses.

The final phase of the amputee's life cycle may be regarded as the geriatric phase. While the exact age will differ from amputee to amputee, the activity generally will begin to decline near the age of 65 (Meier, III, 2019). Due to the decreased activity, the prosthesis and replacement socket may not need as frequent replacement as in the earlier phases.

Prosthetic Component Weight Ratings

Due to liability and durability concerns, prosthetic component manufacturers typically specify a maximum body weight rating. As many prosthetic components are developed internationally in countries where body weight averages may be lower than in the Unites States, the maximum body weight rating for many prosthetic components is relatively low in comparison to U.S. population body weights. In other words, prosthetic components may have a maximum body weight rating that is much lower than clinical standards for overweight or obese individuals. Thus, amputees with higher body weights have a limited selection of prosthetic components and may require bariatric or 'heavy-duty' rated components, which incur additional costs (Kulkarni et al., 2015). The maximum body weight ratings not only vary from manufacturer to manufacturer but also among components from the same manufacturer.

Comorbidities

While the focus of this chapter is on amputations, some evaluees may also have comorbidities that must be considered in the LCP if also a result of the catastrophic injury. For example, in blast injuries, TBI and/or PTSD are not uncommon and may not yet be diagnosed. Amputees with burn injuries may have compromised dermis in other areas of the body than the residual limb. Such comorbidities may be more severe than the amputation or impact the potential outcomes of prosthesis use. In such complex cases, the life care planner should consult with other specialized medical experts as appropriate.

Pediatric Amputees

The care of pediatric amputees is a sub-specialty within prosthetics and has its complexities that are beyond the scope of this chapter. The most common causes are congenital anomalies and malignancy. From the earliest ages of infants, there is debate as to when to initially provide prostheses and when to provide functional components. Surprisingly the child amputee adapts very well to the use of a prosthesis, although some fail to communicate initial fit problems until they become problematic. A challenge for the child amputee is adapting the prosthesis to growth, particularly during periods of rapid growth spurts. Annual replacement of a prosthesis is to be expected through to maturity. Another challenge is maintenance, as pediatric amputees frequently stress prosthetic components to the point of failure. Unlike the options for adults, the availability of pediatric prosthetics is generally limited to very basic components, with very limited selection. While the child amputee is very accepting of their situation, parents can present challenges, as their expectations of functional outcomes may not align with the functionality of pediatric prosthetic components. Some congenital upper limb amputees become so adapted to the use of their residual limbs, they find prostheses to become cumbersome and thus reject them. However, as the amputee ages, prosthetic solutions may become advantageous, and thus rejection at an early age may not ultimately preclude future use of prostheses, particularly as technological and surgical advances continue to develop. While osseointegration offers a significant improvement of the prosthetic socket for adults, it is contraindicated until an amputee is skeletally mature. In cases of pediatric amputation, the life care planner is advised to consult with physiatrists and prosthetists who frequently care for this population. For further information on pediatric amputations, the reader is recommended to consult authoritative texts dedicated to the topic (Meier, III, 2011; Meier & Atkins, 2004).

Amputee Evaluation

To fully assess the lifetime care needs of an amputee, the life care planner, physiatrist, and prosthetist should conduct evaluations (Malchow & Clark, 1984). Whenever possible, the life care planner's assessment should be conducted in the evaluee's living environment and include immediate family members and/or household co-inhabitants. If the life care planner is employed by the defense, the plaintiff's legal team may not permit access for an evaluation, yet attempts should be made. If a consulting physiatrist and/or prosthetist are employed and they are not the evaluee's treating providers, access should be made for them to also conduct an in-person evaluation whenever possible. In the evaluations, the interviewer should not focus just on information gathering but be prepared to educate the evaluee on available options and their advantages and disadvantages to ensure decisions regarding future care are fully informed. For example, it would be inappropriate to project myoelectric upper limb prostheses for an amputee who has already rejected them or is unwilling to use them given possible disadvantages. Photos and videos of the home environment should be obtained during the evaluation to provide a foundation for various categories of the LCP, particularly architectural modifications.

Conclusion

In cases of major catastrophic events, each type of traumatic injury presents unique and often significant challenges. However, perhaps no other injury results in such a broad range of functional outcomes as does traumatic amputations, ranging from the partial loss of an insignificant digit to the loss of three or four major limbs. Due to the extreme diversity and potential complexity of traumatic amputations, the life care planner is advised to seek the support of an experienced clinical team to develop an effective LCP for the evaluee with limb loss. Such a team should, at a minimum, include a physiatrist to determine an overall rehabilitation plan and provide a medical foundation, a vocational rehabilitation specialist for vocational evaluation (when appropriate), and a certified prosthetist to provide a detailed prosthetic component plan and associated costs.

Notes

1 In this chapter, the terms *evaluee, amputee, individual with limb loss*, and *individual with congenital limb deficiency* are synonymous.
2 It is no coincidence this chapter is the collaboration of a physiatrist and prosthetist.
3 At the time of this publication, the OPRA system (Integrum, AB) has received FDA Pre-Market Approval (PMA) for use in transfemoral amputees.
4 Prosthetic joints may be internal or external. This chapter exclusively discusses external prosthetic joints.
5 Also commonly referred to as *b*.
6 Standardized ingress protection (IP) ratings determine the degree of water resistance.
7 Microprocessor components may include alternative programmable functional modes for specific activities such as golf.
8 Generally, prosthetic ankles and feet are combined into one prosthetic component.
9 E.g., to accommodate high heel footwear, dedicated prosthetic feet are available.
10 Also referred to as *myoelectric*.
11 Also referred to as *cable and harness*.
12 Also referred to as *oppositional, cosmetic*, or *aesthetic restoration*.
13 At the time of this publication, these levels of amputation do not have FDA-approved implants available.
14 Centers for Medicare and Medicaid Services, 42 CFR § 414.210(f)(1).

References

Abernethy, L., Duncan, J. C., & Childers, W. L. (2017). A content analysis on the media portrayal of characters with limb loss. *JPO: Journal of Prosthetics and Orthotics, 29*(4), 170–176. https://doi.org/10.1097/JPO.0000000000000143

Alolabi, N., Augustine, H., & Thoma, A. (2017). Hand transplantation: Current challenges and future prospects. *Transplant Research and Risk Management, 9*, 23–29. https://doi.org/10.2147/TRRM.S94298

Atallah, R., Leijendekkers, R. A., Hoogeboom, T. J., & Frölke, J. P. (2018). Complications of bone-anchored prostheses for individuals with an extremity amputation: A systematic review. *PloS One, 13*(8), e0201821. https://doi.org/10.1371/journal.pone.0201821

Author unknown. (2015). *Daily living aids*. The War Amps. www.waramps.ca/pdf/english-site/ways-we-help/living-with-amputation/daily-living-aids.pdf

Azoury, S. C., Bauder, A., Souza, J. M., Stranix, J. T., Othman, S., McAndrew, C., Tintle, S. M., Kovach, S. J., & Levin, L. S. (2020). Expanding the top rungs of the extremity reconstructive ladder: Targeted muscle reinnervation, osseointegration, and vascularized composite allotransplantation. *Plastic and Aesthetic Research, 7*, 4. https://doi.org/10.20517/2347-9264.2019.44

Bae, E. J., Hong, I. H., Park, S. P., Kim, H. K., Lee, K. W., & Han, J. R. (2013). Overview of ocular complications in patients with electrical burns: An analysis of 102 cases across a 7-year period. *Burns: Journal of the International Society for Burn Injuries, 39*(7), 1380–1385. https://doi.org/10.1016/j.burns.2013.03.023

Batsford, S., Ryan, C. G., & Martin, D. J. (2017). Non-pharmacological conservative therapy for phantom limb pain: A systematic review of randomized controlled trials. *Physiotherapy Theory and Practice, 33*(3), 173–183. https://doi.org/10.1080/09593985.2017.1288283

Berens, D. E., & Weed, R. O. (2018). The role of the vocational rehabilitation counselor in life care planning. In *Life care planning and case management handbook* (4th ed., pp. 41–60). Routledge.

Berry, D. (2020). Prosthetic criteria and considerations for life care planning. *Journal of Nurse Life Care Planning, 20*(2), 21–30.

Bourke, H. E., Yelden, K. C., Robinson, K. P., Sooriakumaran, S., & Ward, D. A. (2011). Is revision surgery following lower-limb amputation a worthwhile procedure? A retrospective review of 71 cases. *Injury, 42*(7), 660–666. https://doi.org/10.1016/j.injury.2010.09.035

Bowen, J. B., Wee, C. E., Kalik, J., & Valerio, I. L. (2017). Targeted muscle reinnervation to improve pain, prosthetic tolerance, and bioprosthetic outcomes in the amputee. *Advances in Wound Care, 6*(8), 261–267. https://doi.org/10.1089/wound.2016.0717

Bragaru, M., Dekker, R., & Geertzen, J. H. (2012). Sport prostheses and prosthetic adaptations for the upper and lower limb amputees: An overview of peer-reviewed literature. *Prosthetics and Orthotics International, 36*(3), 290–296. https://doi.org/10.1177/0309364612447093

Crowe, C. S., Impastato, K. A., Donaghy, A. C., Earl, C., Friedly, J. L., & Keys, K. A. (2019). Prosthetic and orthotic options for lower-extremity amputation and reconstruction. *Plastic and Aesthetic Research, 6*, 4. https://doi.org/10.20517/2347-9264.2018.70

Dillon, M., Fatone, S., & Hodge, M. (2007). Biomechanics of ambulation after partial foot amputation: A systematic literature review. *JPO: Journal of Prosthetics and Orthotics, 19*, P2–P61. https://doi.org/10.1097/JPO.0b013e3180ca8694

Dumanian, G. A., Potter, B. K., Mioton, L. M., Ko, J. H., Cheesborough, J. E., Souza, J. M., Ertl, W. J., Tintle, S. M., Nanos, G. P., Valerio, I. L., Kuiken, T. A., Apkarian, A. V., Porter, K., & Jordan, S. W. (2019). Targeted muscle reinnervation treats neuroma and phantom pain in major limb amputees: A randomized clinical trial. *Annals of Surgery, 270*(2), 238–246. https://doi.org/10.1097/SLA.0000000000003088

Eckard, C. S., Pruziner, A. L., Sanchez, A. D., & Andrews, A. M. (2015). Metabolic and body composition changes in the first year following traumatic amputation. *Journal of Rehabilitation Research & Development, 52*(5), 553–564. https://doi.org/10.1682/JRRD.2014.02.0044

Esquenazi, A., & DiGiacomo, R. (2001). Rehabilitation after amputation. *Journal of the American Podiatric Medical Association, 91*(1), 13–22. https://doi.org/10.7547/87507315-91-1-13

Fernie, G. R., & Holliday, P. J. (1982). Volume fluctuations in the residual limbs of lower limb amputees. *Archives of Physical Medicine and Rehabilitation, 63*(4), 162–165.

Fioravanti, M., Maman, P., Curvale, G., Rochwerger, A., & Mattei, J. (2018). Amputation versus conservative treatment in severe open lower-limb fracture: A functional and quality-of-life study. *Orthopaedics & Traumatology: Surgery & Research, 104*. https://doi.org/10.1016/j.otsr.2017.12.013

Forbes, M. K. E., Cobb, M. W., Jeevaratnam, M. J., King, M. I., & Cubison, L. C. T. (2021). Amputation Revision Surgery—Refining the surgical approach. Ten years of experience and 250 cases, impressions, outcomes, and thoughts for the future. *Injury, 52*(11), 3293–3298. https://doi.org/10.1016/j.injury.2021.02.016

Fossey, M., & Hacker Hughes, J. (2014). *Traumatic limb loss and the needs of the family*. Blesma. Retrieved from https://www. researchgate. net/profile/Matt_ Fossey/publication/308617252_Traumatic_Limb_ Loss_and_the_Needs_of_the_ Family/links/57e8edcd08ae9e5e455946e3/Traumatic-Limb-Loss-and-the-Needsof-the-Family. pdf

Gailey, R., Allen, K., Castles, J., Kucharik, J., & Roeder, M. (2008). Review of secondary physical conditions associated with lower-limb amputation and long-term prosthesis use. *Journal of Rehabilitation Research and Development, 45*(1), 15–29. https://doi.org/10.1682/jrrd.2006.11.0147

Gaunaurd, I., Gailey, R., Hafner, B. J., Gomez-Marin, O., & Kirk-Sanchez, N. (2011). Postural asymmetries in transfemoral amputees. *Prosthetics and Orthotics International, 35*(2), 171–180. https://doi.org/10.1177/0309364611407676

Ghazali, M. F., Abd Razak, N. A., Abu Osman, N. A., & Gholizadeh, H. (2018). Awareness, potential factors, and post-amputation care of stump flexion contractures among transtibial amputees. *Turkish Journal of Physical Medicine and Rehabilitation, 64*(3), 268–276. https://doi.org/10.5606/tftrd.2018.1668

Hahn, A., Bueschges, S., Prager, M., & Kannenberg, A. (2021). The effect of microprocessor-controlled exo-prosthetic knees on limited community ambulators: Systematic review and meta-analysis. *Disability and Rehabilitation*, 1–19. https://doi.org/10.1080/09638288.2021.1989504

Hall, N., & Eldabe, S. (2018). Phantom limb pain: A review of pharmacological management. *British Journal of Pain, 12*(4), 202–207. https://doi.org/10.1177/2049463717747307

Hawkins, A. T., Pallangyo, A. J., Herman, A. M., Schaumeier, M. J., Smith, A. D., Hevelone, N. D., Crandell, D., & Nguyen, L. L. (2016). The effect of social integration on outcomes after major lower extremity amputation. *Journal of Vascular Surgery, 63*(1), 154–162.

Hendershot, B. D., & Nussbaum, M. A. (2013). Persons with lower-limb amputation have impaired trunk postural control while maintaining seated balance. *Gait & Posture, 38*(3), 438–442. https://doi.org/10.1016/j.gaitpost.2013.01.008

Hoellwarth, J. S., Tetsworth, K., Kendrew, J., Kang, N. V., van Waes, O., Al-Maawi, Q., Roberts, C., & Al Muderis, M. (2020). Periprosthetic osseointegration fractures are infrequent and management is familiar. *The Bone & Joint Journal, 102-B*(2), 162–169. https://doi.org/10.1302/0301-620X.102B2. BJJ-2019-0697.R2

Hordacre, B., Barr, C., & Crotty, M. (2015). Community activity and participation are reduced in transtibial amputee fallers: A wearable technology study. *BMJ Innovations, 1*, 10–16. https://doi.org/10.1136/bmjinnov-2014-000014

Hsu, J. C., & Warych, B. (2017). Upper Limb Prosthetic Rehabilitation and Life Care Planning Considerations. *Journal of Nurse Life Care Planning, 17*(4), 22–28.

Hyung, B., & Wiseman-Hakes, C. (2021). A scoping review of current non-pharmacological treatment modalities for phantom limb pain in limb amputees. *Disability and Rehabilitation*, 1–22. https://doi.org/10.1080/09638288.2021.1948116

Jensen, M. P., Moore, M. R., Bockow, T. B., Ehde, D. M., & Engel, J. M. (2011). Psychosocial factors and adjustment to chronic pain in persons with physical disabilities: A systematic review. *Archives of Physical Medicine and Rehabilitation, 92*(1), 146–160. https://doi.org/10.1016/j.apmr.2010.09.021

Kahle, J. T., Highsmith, M. J., Kenney, J., Ruth, T., Lunseth, P. A., & Ertl, J. (2017). The effectiveness of the bone bridge transtibial amputation technique: A systematic review of high-quality evidence. *Prosthetics and Orthotics International, 41*(3), 219–226. https://doi.org/10.1177/0309364616679318

Kang, N. V., Woollard, A., Michno, D. A., Al-Ajam, Y., Tan, J., & Hansen, E. (2022). A consecutive series of targeted muscle reinnervation (TMR) cases for relief of neuroma and phantom limb pain: UK perspective. *Journal of Plastic, Reconstructive & Aesthetic Surgery, 75*(3), 960–969.

Keszler, M. S., Wright, K. S., Miranda, A., & Hopkins, M. S. (2020). Multidisciplinary amputation team management of individuals with limb loss. *Current Physical Medicine and Rehabilitation Reports, 8*(3), 118–126. https://doi.org/10.1007/s40141-020-00282-4

Kulkarni, J., Hannett, D. P., & Purcell, S. (2015). Bariatric amputee: A growing problem? *Prosthetics and Orthotics International, 39*(3), 226–231. https://doi.org/10.1177/0309364614525186

Lannan, F. M., & Meyerle, J. H. (2019). The dermatologist's role in amputee skincare. *Cutis, 103*(2), 86–90.

Malchow, D., & Clark, J. (1984). Interviewing the amputee—a step toward rehabilitation. *Orthopaedic Review, 13*(11), 47–56.

Malone, J. M., Fleming, L. L., Roberson, J., Whitesides, T. E., Leal, J. M., Poole, J. U., & Grodin, R. S. (1984). Immediate, early, and late postsurgical management of upper-limb amputation. *Journal of Rehabilitation Research and Development, 21*(1), 33–41.

Matthews, D., Sukeik, M., & Haddad, F. (2014). Return to sport following amputation. *The Journal of Sports Medicine and Physical Fitness, 54*(4), 481–486.

McCormick, Z., Chang-Chien, G., Marshall, B., Huang, M., & Harden, R. N. (2014). Phantom limb pain: A systematic neuroanatomical-based review of pharmacologic treatment. *Pain Medicine, 15*(2), 292–305. https://doi.org/10.1111/pme.12283

Meier, III, R. H. (2011). Life care planning for the child with amputation. In *Pediatric life care planning and case management* (2nd ed., pp. 591–620). Routledge & CRC Press. www.routledge.com/Pediatric-Life-Care-Planning-and-Case-Management/Riddick-Grisham-Deming/p/book/9781439803585

Meier, III, R. H. (2019). Life care planning for the amputee. In *Life care planning and case management handbook* (4th ed., pp. 335–365). Routledge.

Meier, R. H., & Atkins, D. J. (2004). *Functional restoration of adults and children with upper extremity amputation*. Demos Medical Publishing, Inc.

Meier, R. H., Choppa, A. J., & Johnson, C. B. (2013). The person with amputation and their life care plan. *Physical Medicine and Rehabilitation Clinics of North America, 24*(3), 467–489. https://doi.org/10.1016/j.pmr.2013.03.004

Melton, D. (2017). Physiatrist perspective on upper-limb prosthetic options: Using practice guidelines to promote patient education in the selection and the prescription process. *Journal of Prosthetics and Orthotics, 29*, 40–44. https://doi.org/10.1097/JPO.0000000000000157

Parnell, B., & Urton, M. (2021). Rehabilitation nursing challenges for patients with lower limb amputation. *Rehabilitation Nursing: The Official Journal of the Association of Rehabilitation Nurses, 46*(3), 179–184. https://doi.org/10.1097/RNJ.0000000000000289

Paternò, L., Ibrahimi, M., Gruppioni, E., Menciassi, A., & Ricotti, L. (2018). Sockets for limb prostheses: A review of existing technologies and open challenges. *IEEE Transactions on Biomedical Engineering, 65*(9), 1996–2010. https://doi.org/10.1109/TBME.2017.2775100

Peters, B. R., Russo, S. A., West, J. M., Moore, A. M., & Schulz, S. A. (2020). Targeted muscle reinnervation for the management of pain in the setting of major limb amputation. *SAGE Open Medicine, 8*, 2050312120959180. https://doi.org/10.1177/2050312120959180

Potter, C. B. K., & Bosse, M. J. (2021). American academy of orthopaedic surgeons clinical practice guideline summary for limb salvage or early amputation. *The Journal of the American Academy of Orthopaedic Surgeons, 29*(13), e628–e634. https://doi.org/10.5435/JAAOS-D-20-00188

Richardson, C., & Kulkarni, J. (2017). A review of the management of phantom limb pain: Challenges and solutions. *Journal of Pain Research, 10*, 1861–1870. https://doi.org/10.2147/JPR.S124664

Salminger, S., Stino, H., Pichler, L. H., Gstoettner, C., Sturma, A., Mayer, J. A., Szivak, M., & Aszmann, O. C. (2020). Current rates of prosthetic usage in upper-limb amputees—Have innovations had an impact on device acceptance? *Disability and Rehabilitation*, 1–12. https://doi.org/10.1080/0963828 8.2020.1866684

Swanson, E., Cheng, H.-T., Lough, D., Lee, W., Shores, J., & Brandacher, G. (2015). Lower extremity allotransplantation: Are we ready for prime time? *Vascularized Composite Allotransplantation, 2*, 37–46. https://doi.org/10.1080/23723505.2015.1123798

Tillander, J., Hagberg, K., Berlin, Ö., Hagberg, L., & Brånemark, R. (2017). Osteomyelitis risk in patients with transfemoral amputations treated with osseointegration prostheses. *Clinical Orthopaedics and Related Research, 475*(12), 3100–3108. https://doi.org/10.1007/s11999-017-5507-2

Treadwell, K., Rock, D., & Wyatt, A. (2020). Novel mechanical finger prostheses. *Journal of Nurse Life Care Planning, 20*(2), 53–57.

Uellendahl, J. E., & Uellendahl, E. N. (2006). Body-powered upper limb prosthetic designs. In *Prosthetics and patient management: A comprehensive clinical approach* (pp. 141–153). SLACK Incorporated.

Valerio, I. L., Dumanian, G. A., Jordan, S. W., Mioton, L. M., Bowen, J. B., West, J. M., Porter, K., Ko, J. H., Souza, J. M., & Potter, B. K. (2019). Preemptive treatment of phantom and residual limb pain with targeted muscle reinnervation at the time of major limb amputation. *Journal of the American College of Surgeons, 228*(3), 217–226. https://doi.org/10.1016/j.jamcollsurg.2018.12.015

Van Norman, G. A. (2018). Expanded patient access to investigational new devices. *JACC: Basic to Translational Science, 3*(4), 533–544. https://doi.org/10.1016/j.jacbts.2018.06.006

Weed, R. O., & Sluis, A. (1990). *Life care planning for the amputee: A step-by-step guide* (1st ed.). CRC Press.

Wesner, M. L., & Hickie, J. (2013). Long-term sequelae of electrical injury. *Canadian Family Physician, 59*(9), 935–939.

Windrich, M., Grimmer, M., Christ, O., Rinderknecht, S., & Beckerle, P. (2016). Active lower limb prosthetics: A systematic review of design issues and solutions. *Biomedical Engineering Online, 15*(3), 5–19.

Yaputra, F., & Widyadharma, I. P. E. (2018). management of phantom limb pain: A review. *International Journal of Medical Reviews and Case Reports, 2*(2), 29–32.

16 Pain Medicine and Life Care Planning

Richard Bowman

The International Association for the Study of Pain defines pain as "An unpleasant sensory and emotional experience associated with actual or potential tissue damage or described in terms of such damage" (Merskey & Bogduk, 1994, Part III—Pain Terms, p. 211). The experience of pain requires input, awareness, and interpretation at the brain level. For this reason, pain is often characterized as being a subjective sensation. While there is a general understanding of the mechanism of pain signal transmission and the organization of neural pathways in the nervous system, the means needed to qualify and quantify pain remain elusive. The transmitted nerve signals that travel via neural transmission create the characteristic, intensity, duration, and perceived location of an individual pain experience; however, it remains challenging to qualify and quantify pain in a manner that would permit the experience of pain to be measured in units that can be compared between individuals. Physical function and disability associated with pain conditions are frequently used as a measurable method for qualifying and quantifying the impact of pain on an individual's physical condition.

Pain delivers a psychological and emotional impact on individuals suffering its presence. There is a limited understanding of the specific neural input necessary to yield long-term or short-term deleterious emotional or psychological effects on an individual. Still, the experience of severe acute pain or severe chronic pain conditions correlates with a high rate of psychological sequelae, including depression and posttraumatic stress disorder (Giesecke et al., 2005; Morasco et al., 2013).

Pain Conditions and Contrasts

Chronic Versus Acute Pain

Acute pain may be defined as "pain that arises from actual or threatened damage to non-neural tissue and is due to the activation of nociceptors" (Grichnik & Ferrante, 1991, p. 1003). The definition of chronic pain is described as "pain that persists past normal healing time and hence lacks the acute warning function of physiological nociception" (Bonica, 1953; Treede et al., 2015, p. 1003). Chronic pain is distinctly differentiated from acute pain in the scientific literature in that its presence, nature, treatment, and prognosis often differ from acute pain derived from a similar pain generator (Treede et al., 2019). Historically, chronic pain was often defined as pain equal to or exceeding a three-month duration (Grichnik & Ferrante). The International Classification of Diseases (ICD)-11 further classifies chronic pain into chronic primary pain, chronic cancer pain, chronic postsurgical and posttraumatic pain, neuropathic pain, headache and orofacial pain, visceral pain, and musculoskeletal pain (Treede et al.). The prevalence of

DOI: 10.4324/b23293-16

chronic pain in a region of the body is 20% to 25% in the general population, and the majority of chronic widespread pain is 10% in the general population (McBeth & Jones, 2007).

Nociceptive Versus Neuropathic Pain

The type of pain experienced by an individual is often described in terms of the proposed nature of the pain. The nomenclature utilized often consists of the nociceptive and neuropathic pain descriptors. The conceptual use of this terminology can be helpful for the guidance of a treatment strategy. The generally accepted clinical understanding of the nociceptive pain versus neuropathic pain descriptors is that the two pain types exist on a continuum. While a pure chronic nociceptive pain condition or a pure chronic neuropathic pain condition may be of low prevalence, it is expected that a chronic pain condition may be characterized as being composed of primary nociceptive pain characteristics or primarily neuropathic pain characteristics.

Somatic Versus Sympathetic Pain

Somatic pain sources are modulated primarily through nerve pathways, with the initial pain signals originating in the periphery. The nerve signal travels from the peripheral to the spinal nerves in the somatic pathway and then through the spinal cord to the brain. Neural connections that provide input from the bodily nervous system to the sympathetic nervous system are also present. Sympathetic pain sources are modulated primarily through the sympathetic nervous system. Input into the sympathetic nervous system may occur via multiple pathways. Signals from the periphery may be received into the sympathetic nervous system. The sympathetic nervous system is organized into several control centers known as ganglia. The sympathetic ganglia are located along a chain situated in the anterior aspects of the vertebral bodies. The sympathetic nervous system may also send signals via neural pathways to both the spinal cord (central nervous system) and the periphery. The relationship between the somatic and sympathetic nervous system is primarily believed to play an integral role in perpetuating certain neuropathic pain conditions such as complex regional pain syndrome (CRPS) type I.

Central Versus Peripheral Pain

Central pain syndromes are typically defined as syndromes where the etiology of pain is associated with damage to or pathology of the central nervous system. Painful brain and spinal cord disorders may include some individuals suffering from cerebrovascular accidents (stroke), multiple sclerosis, traumatic brain injury, and thalamic pain syndrome. Peripheral pain is typically classified as pain originating in the periphery and usually includes spinal pain conditions that induce pain in the adjacent nerve roots; cause pain in the spinal joints, discs, vertebral bodies, paraspinal muscles, dermatomes, or myotomes; or are associated with spine pathology distal to the conus medullaris.

Treatment of Chronic Pain

The treatment of chronic pain associated with one or more pain generators involves a complicated approach, often utilizing multiple modalities to achieve optimal pain control. Typical treatment of chronic pain requires identification of the pain generator or generators through history, examination, and diagnostic testing. A pain generator is typically defined as an underlying structural source from which pain is derived. Referral for further consultation to assist with diagnosis confirmation may be necessary. Following identification of the proposed mechanism or mechanisms causing the ongoing pain, a treatment plan is initiated. In the case of confirming a diagnosis via exclusion of other plausible sources, a treatment plan would then also be created. At times, the initial step or steps in a treatment plan may involve procedures that provide diagnostic information to confirm or exclude a diagnosis. Such procedures may offer additional therapeutic benefits. The typical approach for determining a treatment plan involves assessing the risk-versus-benefit analysis for the available treatments used for a given condition or conditions. Standard of care, supportive scientific literature, clinician background, clinician education, and clinician experience are usually utilized to complete the risk-to-benefit analysis.

Several approaches to managing chronic pain may be used individually or in combination. The medical pain management approach generally consists of the utilization of medications for pain control. Typical drugs used may include anti-inflammatory drugs, topical pain solutions, neuropathic pain medications such as neuroleptics, psychotropic medications, muscle relaxers, and opioids. Multiple medications are often utilized. Compliance monitoring with the utilization of controlled substances is recommended as described in the *CDC Guidelines for Prescribing Opioids for Chronic Pain* (Dowell et al., 2016). Typical mitigation measures used for compliance monitoring are frequent office visits, assessment of aberrant drug use behavior, urine drug screening, random pill counts, pharmacy utilization monitoring, and a narcotic agreement between the patient and provider. Many of these measures are required and strongly recommended by the medical provider by federal or local government, the state board of medicine agencies, and professional medical societies.

Alternative or holistic medicine is often utilized for the management of chronic pain. The National Institutes of Health (NIH) defines many commonly used modalities as alternative medicine. Several alternative medication treatment classifications have scientific literature to support their effective utilization for specific pain conditions. Acupuncture and electro-acupuncture are commonly used to reduce pain from various conditions. Ultrasound, iontophoresis, phonophoresis, diathermy, and fluidotherapy are examples of modalities used by practitioners such as physical therapists and occupational therapists to reduce pain. Chiropractors commonly use manipulation and laser therapies for pain reduction. Herbal supplements are often prescribed by providers such as holistic practitioners to treat chronic pain.

Multidisciplinary pain programs play a role in the management of chronic pain conditions. The combined utilization of medical pain management and psychological treatment and physical, occupational, and speech-language pathology therapies is typically used to address the reduction of pain with an emphasis on restoring physical function. Additional emphasis is typically placed on the identification and management of psychological factors that may be associated with the perpetuation of chronic pain in an individual. Intense care plans of durations consisting of several weeks are routinely employed to complete a multidisciplinary pain program. Emphasis on the reduction and/or elimination of controlled substances used for the management of pain is a common approach in many interdisciplinary pain programs.

Interventional pain medicine is an approach to the treatment of chronic pain conditions following the failure of conservative measures usually and typically utilized for the given situation. The process of attempting to identify the underlying cause or causes of chronic pain is imperative in the interventional pain medicine treatment approach. Diagnostic testing, consultation, history, and examination are utilized to determine proposed pain generators. Interventional pain medicine procedures will sometimes confirm or exclude pain conditions based on patient response to treatment (*Interventional Pain Medicine*, 2012). The interventional pain medicine approach involves the treatment of both spinal and peripheral sources of pain. The pain treatment approach may vary between individual patients with similar conditions based on factors including patient presentation, patient-reported pain severity, provider training, provider experience, patient response to treatment, and patient consent.

Peripheral Pain Conditions and Treatment

The variety of conditions that may result in chronic pain is voluminous but may be reduced to several causative categories. Muscular chronic pain conditions may be localized in one or more areas or may be found widespread in various regions of the body. Interventional pain medicine treatment of localized muscular pain may include trigger point injections to tender muscles and/ or trigger points. The *Oxford Dictionary* defines a trigger point as "a sensitive area of the body, stimulation or irritation of which causes a specific effect in another part, especially a tender area in a muscle that causes generalized musculoskeletal pain when overstimulated."

A trigger point injection typically consists of solutions of medications that may contain anesthetics and corticosteroids. One or more injections may be required to achieve pain control. If a tender area of a muscle reveals chronic spasm consistent with dystonia and if the pain from the dystonic muscle is relieved for a limited duration of time with trigger point injections, chemodenervation with botulinum toxin injection of the muscle may be employed to provide relief of the dystonia and associated pain for a typical duration of three months. Longer-acting toxins have been developed to give durations on chemodenervation exceeding three months for cases where an increased time of relief of dystonia and pain is desirable. Physical modalities such as stretching, kinetic exercise, and myofascial release may also be employed to accentuate pain relief provided by trigger point injections or chemodenervation.

Rheumatological conditions may result in peripheral pain. Rheumatological pain conditions may be further broken down into categories of pain affecting an individual joint versus pain affecting several joints. Both types may additionally present with localized or widespread muscular pain. Systemic rheumatological pain conditions include diseases affecting multiple joints, such as rheumatoid arthritis, lupus, Sjogren's syndrome, and polymyalgia rheumatica. Infections inducing autoimmune responses or direct pathology of joints may cause similar symptomatology and should be considered during diagnostic testing. Lyme's disease and rheumatic fever are infectious processes that may cause widespread chronic joint pain. The management of chronic pain associated with systemic rheumatological conditions typically involves consultation and medical management of a rheumatologist, but may also affect the direct treatment of one or more individual joints with interventional pain medicine techniques to reduce pain not adequately controlled with rheumatological medical management.

Treatment of individual peripheral joint pain with interventional pain medicine techniques requires an accurate diagnosis of the joint-related source of pain. Care should be taken to assess for infection of the painful joint. Consultation with orthopedic surgery is sometimes required to determine if surgery is recommended before initiating interventional pain treatments. Intraarticular injection of a peripheral joint with a local anesthetic may confirm or exclude an individual joint as a pain generator based on the pain response within the active duration of the injected anesthetic agent. Injection of a non-infected joint with a corticosteroid may provide prolonged pain relief but may require sequential injections to reduce pain intensity and adequate duration of pain relief. Most peripheral joints can be injected if suspected to be inflamed and the cause of joint-related pain. Injection guidance may include anatomical landmarks, ultrasound guidance, fluoroscopic guidance, or computed tomography (CT) scan guidance. In joints where pain relief duration with corticosteroid is lacking, where corticosteroid is medically contraindicated, or where corticosteroid is otherwise undesirable, visco-supplementation may be considered. Visco-supplementation has not been studied extensively on all joints. Still, the scientific literature has supported its approval for use in the knee joint for pain associated with arthritis where adequate articular cartilage persists and no contraindications to injection of visco-supplementation are present. Modalities of lower risk have failed to offer substantial and durable relief of pain. Depending on the type utilized, visco-supplementation injections may be required in sequence or a single dose. Visco-supplementation injections may provide pain relief for several months and may be repeated when the pain returns if medically appropriate.

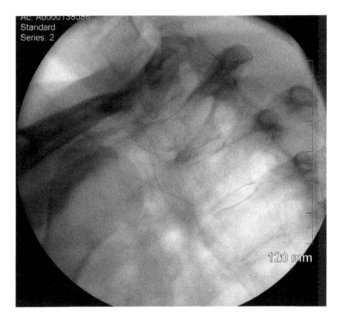

Figure 16.1 Intraarticular Shoulder Joint Injection (Needle Placement Without Contrast Shown)

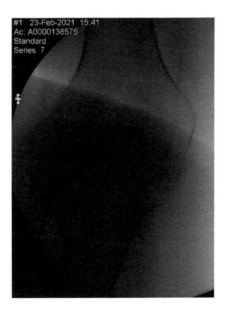

Figure 16.2 Intraarticular Knee Joint Injection (Needle Placement Without Contrast Shown)

Peripheral nerve blocks of certain peripheral joints may provide pain relief from chronic joint pain. In cases where the intraarticular injection is undesirable, contraindicated, or has previously failed to yield pain relief, joints with identifiable sensory nerves innervating the joint may be treated with nerve blocks. If nerve blocks of the sensory nerves of a painful joint have been shown in the medical literature to yield safe and effective relief of pain, this treatment approach may be considered. The genicular nerves of the knee are examples of sensory nerves of joints typically blocked to yield relief of chronic pain.

The superior medial, inferior medial, and superior lateral genicular nerves are often blocked with injected anesthetic under fluoroscopic guidance. One or more sequential genicular nerve block injections at these sites may provide short-term and/or long-term relief of pain. Future genicular blocks may be performed if the pain is later exacerbated or recurs.

In cases where genicular nerve block treatments have successfully relieved knee region pain but the duration of pain relief has been less than six months, radiofrequency ablation of the described genicular nerves may be performed. The duration of pain relief of six months following genicular nerve radiofrequency ablation has been defined (Konya et al., 2020). Radiofrequency ablation can be repeated to restore pain relief if the knee pain returns after the nerves have regenerated. Repeat radiofrequency ablation of the genicular nerves after the return of pain between 6 and 18 months following a prior radiofrequency ablation does not necessarily necessitate repeat diagnostic blocks preceding an additional radiofrequency ablation based on the current standard of care, but repeat radiofrequency ablation of the genicular nerves more than 18 months' duration following a prior radiofrequency ablation may necessitate repeat genicular nerve blocks potentially preceding an additional genicular radiofrequency ablation. Radiofrequency of sensory nerves of other peripheral joints has also been studied. Some practitioners have published promising successful results with radiofrequency ablation of the sensory nerves innervating the hip joint and sensory nerves innervating the glenohumeral joint.

Treatment of injury to a named peripheral nerve associated with pain may involve injection along the damaged nerve with local anesthetic with or without corticosteroid. One or multiple injections may be required to achieve pain relief. If long-term pain relief fails to occur with injections, then additional treatment for pain associated with peripheral nerve damage may be required. Treatment of refractory neuropathic pain of individual nerves in the periphery may involve neuromodulation. Neuromodulation may be considered to treat pain from damaged peripheral nerves when less invasive modalities have failed and when the location of the pain remains within the dermatomal distribution of the named peripheral nerve. Permanent placement of a peripheral nerve stimulator device along a painful named peripheral nerve may be performed as a last resort for pain control (Pope et al., 2012). A trial placement of the stimulator lead or leads usually precedes the permanent placement of the stimulator device. A peripheral nerve stimulator lead may be surgically implanted along the location of the damaged nerve. The power source for the lead contacts may be implanted in some systems or located externally in other systems.

Treatment of chronic refractory peripheral pain in a region may be necessary. CRPS is a condition resulting in refractory pain in a region. The diagnostic criteria for CRPS have been standardized and simplified through a list of criteria known as the Budapest Criteria. The Budapest Criteria for CRPS were validated following a study published in 2010 (Harden et al., 2010). The criteria have a 99% sensitivity and a 68% specificity for the diagnosis. The diagnosis of CRPS remains a diagnosis of exclusion. The typical treatment regimen involves initiating treatment early in the course of the syndrome. If a high index of suspicion for CRPS exists, therapy with physical therapy or occupational therapy with a focus on desensitization training is recommended. The prescription of one or more medications typically used to treat neuropathic pain conditions is often performed if appropriate. If consistent progress toward resolution of the syndrome or suspected syndrome does not occur, then the addition of interventional pain medicine techniques is recommended. For CRPS of the periphery, sympathetic blockade of the affected upper extremity or lower extremity is recommended. One of two techniques is usually utilized for the upper extremity to perform sympathetic blockade. A Bier block can be performed by exsanguinating an extremity via compression or gravity and isolating the circulation of the extremity from the central circulation by a tourniquet, followed by venous injection with a local anesthetic. A second technique providing sympathetic nervous system blockade of the upper extremity is known as a stellate ganglion blockade. An injection into the stellate ganglion via anatomic landmarks or fluoroscopic visualization can be performed. The ganglion is typically injected at the C6 or C7 level at its anatomical location anterior to the cervical vertebral bodies. The needle is usually placed from an anterior approach. Local anesthetic with or without corticosteroid is often injected. This ganglion controls sympathetic nerve flow from the ipsilateral upper extremity and ipsilateral lower face. In the lower extremity, the sympathetic nervous system blockade typically involves injection at the lumbar sympathetic ganglion. Ipsilateral injection of this ganglion, which is located anterior to the L2, L3, and L4 vertebral bodies, is performed to block sympathetic nerve flow to the affected lower extremity. Local anesthetic with or without corticosteroid is often injected.

One or more sympathetic nerve blocks are usually performed to help reduce pain from CRPS. Therapy with desensitization and neuropathic pain medications are often continued between sympathetic blocks. If functional improvement, pain reduction, and regression of CRPS findings occur with the addition of sympathetic blocks to the treatment regimen, then multiple blocks may be warranted. If functional improvement, pain reduction, and regression of CRPS findings do not occur or if progress plateaus with treatment, then higher-risk treatment options for CRPS are often considered. Ketamine infusions are sometimes considered for the treatment of CRPS, and this modality requires monitoring via anesthesia. Spinal cord stimulation with trial implantation and permanent system implantation is a Food and Drug Administration (FDA)–approved modality for long-term use as a last resort for treating chronic neuropathic pain of the extremities, such as the pain experienced with CRPS. This modality is often used for refractory neuropathic pain of the limb or limbs associated with CRPS. Intrathecal pump infusion systems are another modality of last resort that may be utilized to treat chronic neuropathic pain of the extremities, such as the pain experienced with CRPS. Morphine and octreotide are two types of intrathecally administered medicines that are FDA approved to be utilized in this device. Both medications have been studied for use, and octreotide is commonly used for the treatment of CRPS refractory to other modalities. In addition to the risks associated with the surgical implantation and management of the intrathecal pump infusion system device and the risks associated with the intrathecal medication itself, there are additional considerations for the device, including the need for needle-based intrathecal infusion system medication refills performed by a professional and adjustments of the intrathecal infusion system pump rate via computer performed by a professional.

CRPS is a syndrome typically resulting in pain and functional deficits experienced through the end of life. There are cases where the pain and disability associated with the syndrome improve or resolve. The resolution of the condition is reported to occur most often when an early suspected diagnosis followed by prompt and thorough treatment is pursued. There are also cases where the function, pain, and atrophy associated with CRPS worsen. Furthermore, this syndrome tends to migrate or spread to other extremities, where similar findings may require a comprehensive treatment regimen on the newly affected extremity or extremities.

Spasticity in the extremities causes reduced mobility and function but may also be a significant source of pain. Whereas spasticity is a process manifested in the central nervous system, the impact of spasticity is most often realized in the periphery. Treatment of spasticity of the periphery may involve therapy, bracing, oral medications, surgical tendon lengthening or transfers, and intrathecal medications. Intramuscular administration of botulinum toxin is a procedure often utilized by interventionalists to reduce muscle spasticity. The technique involves the injection of the botulinum toxin into the muscle or muscles identified. Several serotypes and subsequent preparations of botulinum toxin are available commercially to be injected to treat spasticity. Electrodiagnosis may be used to guide needle placement to determine the appropriate placement into the muscle and identify the parts of the muscle having the greatest spasticity. Botulinum toxin works by irreversibly binding to the presynaptic cholinergic nerve terminals. This action subsequently inhibits acetylcholine release. The duration of effect is limited by the time necessary for the body to regenerate new nerve terminals, restoring function and resulting in the recurrence of spasticity in the muscle fibers innervated by the nerve associated with the terminal. For this reason, repeated injections with botulinum toxin are typically performed at durations of three months to six months, depending on the toxin preparation utilized and the clinical duration of reduced spasticity exhibited on examination.

Neuropathic conditions affecting the peripheral nervous system may be associated with the development of chronic pain. Conditions such as idiopathic brachial plexopathy (Parsonage-Turner syndrome), peripheral neuropathy, acute and chronic inflammatory demyelinating polyneuropathy, polyradiculopathies associated with various causes, and lumbar plexopathy are examples of neuropathic conditions that may cause chronic pain. These conditions may result in pain refractory to relief with medications, therapy modalities, and injection therapies. If the standard-of-care interventional pain medicine–recommended treatments and procedural techniques generally considered to be of lower risk than neuromodulation have failed, spinal cord stimulation may be employed to reduce pain in the periphery caused by nerve damage. Implantation of a stimulator lead or leads with electrodes positioned in the epidural space powered by a generator is an FDA-approved surgical technique for last resort use in chronic neuropathic pain of the trunk or limbs.

Spinal Pain Conditions

Spinal pain from the cervical, thoracic, and lumbar sources is highly prevalent and accounts for most interventional pain medicine techniques performed to treat chronic pain. Lumbar pain alone has a lifetime prevalence of 50% to 80% in adults (Rubin, 2007). There are many available options for interventional pain treatment for refractory spinal pain. Successful treatment typically requires accurately determining the type of spinal pathology causing the pain. Identification of the proposed cause or causes of spinal pain permits the conclusion of an optimal treatment plan to minimize or eliminate pain from spinal sources. There are distinct differences in spinal anatomy and function that necessitate differences in interventional techniques based on the anatomy of the treated area.

Noninvasive Treatments of Spinal Pain

The cervical, thoracic, lumbar, sacral, and coccygeal areas of the spine may be amenable to the treatment of pain with noninvasive modalities, assuming the cause of the pain does not necessitate immediate surgery, does not require spinal immobilization, is not due to infection, and is not prohibitive due to the location or type of malignancy. Some types of noninvasive treatment may or may not be tolerable due to pain. Just as with pain of the periphery, physical therapy, occupational therapy, chiropractic therapy, and acupuncture are frequently utilized as first-line treatments for pain of spinal origin. Numerous holistic therapies may be considered. Non-opioid classes of medications commonly used for pain control include muscle relaxers, anti-inflammatory pain medications, topical agents, and antidepressant medications. Neuroleptic pain medications are widely utilized but may be controlled similarly to opioids or classified as opioids in some locations. Opioid pain medications are often used acutely and are less often used chronically since changes in recommendations for the use of and regulations for prescribing these medications have changed in many locations following the publishing of the *CDC Guidelines for Prescribing Opioids for Chronic Pain* and subsequent changes in law and/or standards of care in many states or regions of the United States (Dowell et al., 2016). The use of opiates for the management of chronic non-malignant pain as it applies to life care planning is described in the section titled "Chronic Management of Opioids." The concept of undergoing a reasonable course of conservative treatment before considering interventional pain medicine procedures to relieve benign and tolerable pain is preferred. Multiple modalities may be utilized individually or simultaneously. Even if interventional pain medicine techniques are necessary to achieve pain control, so long as conservative modalities are effective, they may be continued or stopped briefly in conjunction with most interventional pain medicine treatments to accentuate pain relief.

Cervical Spine

Anatomy

The cervical spine consists of seven vertebral bodies. The first and second cervical vertebral bodies have anatomy that varies significantly from the third through seventh vertebral bodies. The first vertebral body is also known as the atlas. It interfaces superiorly with the occiput. The right and left occipital-atlanto facet joints provide movable interfaces between this segment and the occiput. The spinal cord passes anterior and medial to these joints. The vertebral arteries pass lateral to these joints, and the dens (a superior portion of C2) pass posterior to the most medial and anterior aspects of the atlas. The C1 nerve roots exit lateral and inferior to the occipital-atlanto facet joints. The second cervical vertebral body is also known as the axis. The right and left interfaces of the atlas and axis are known as the atlantoaxial facet joints. These joints lie anterior to the cervical spinal cord, and the right and left vertebral arteries pass just lateral to these joints. There is no intervertebral disc between the skull and atlas or between the atlas and axis. The C2 nerve roots exit inferior and lateral to the atlantoaxial facet joints but superior to the C2–C3 disc. The C2 and C3 vertebral bodies interface posterior to the spinal cord at the right and left zygapophyseal (facet) joints. The spinal cord is medial and anterior to the C2–C3 joints, and the most superior intervertebral disc is located between C2 and C3. The C3 nerve roots exit the spine through the C2–C3 foramina situated laterally to the C2–C3 disc. The C3 and C4 vertebral bodies interface posterior to the spinal cord. The C3–C4 facet joints are located posterior to the spinal cord, and the spinal cord remains anterior and medial to the C3–C4 facet joints. The C3–C4 disc separates the C3 and C4 vertebral bodies, and the C4 nerve roots exit the spine through the C3–C4 foramina located laterally to the C3–C4 disc. Uncovertebral joints are present along with the anterior-lateral aspects of the inferior C3 and superior C4 vertebral bodies and provide a minor interface between the vertebral bodies. The anatomy between C4 and C5, C5 and C6, and C6 and C7 is analogous to C3 and C4. The respective vertebral interfaces posterior to the spinal cord occur at the right and left facet joints. The spinal cord remains anterior and medial to the facet joints at these levels. An intervertebral disc separates the vertebral bodies at these levels, and the respective nerve roots that exit the spine through the adjacent foramina are located laterally to the individual disc at each level. Uncovertebral joints are located along with the anterior-lateral aspects of the vertebral bodies and provide a minor interface between the vertebral bodies at each of these individual levels.

The anatomy between the C7 and T1 vertebral bodies differs. T1 is the most superior thoracic vertebral body and is flanked by the right and left first ribs. The spinal cord remains anterior and medial to the C7–T1 facet joints, and the C7–T1 intervertebral disc separates the C7 and T1 vertebral bodies. The nerve roots exiting through the foramina located laterally to the C7–T1 disc are numbered as C8. There are typically no uncovertebral joints located between C7 and T1.

Interventional Pain Procedures Performed

The cervical facet joints are a common cause of cervical pain. Inflammation from both traumatic and non-traumatic causes can account for the pain of these joints. Cervical facet joint pain is most often suspected when the mechanical movement of the neck induces axial pain. Axial loading of the facet joints, where extension, rotation, and automatic axial loading of the joints are simultaneously applied, is a common maneuver used to identify potential cervical facet joint pain from the mid and lower cervical spine facet joints. Pain from the occipital-atlanto or atlantoaxial facet joints is more often suspected with painful head rotation inducing pain in the posterior-superior cervical spine and occiput. Treatment of pain from the cervical facet joints may involve the intra-articular injection of joints. Medications used in the injections often include a local anesthetic and corticosteroid. Fluoroscopy is typically used for guidance of needle placement. One or more sequential injections into the painful joints may be needed to achieve desired pain control. If the desired magnitude and duration of pain relief are achieved, future cervical facet joint injections may be considered for pain recurrences. A similar technique used to relieve pain from cervical facet joints involves injecting medicine along the nerves innervating the respective facet joint. This technique is typically described as a cervical facet medial branch block/injection. The occipital-atlanto and atlantoaxial facet joints are not managed with this technique due to their unique anatomy. Intra-articular joint injections are the typical treatment for interventional management of occipito-atlanto and atlantoaxial facet joint pain. The C2–C3 facet joints receive a dual innervation from the ipsilateral third occipital nerve and an articular branch from the posterior ramus of C3. The C3–C4 joints are innervated from the medial branch of C3 and C4. The C4–C5, C5–C6, and C6–C7 facet joints are also innervated by the medial branches reflective of the nomenclature for the joint at the individual level (example: C6 and C7 medial branches innervate C6–C7). The C7–T1 joints receive innervation from the medial branches of C7 and C8 (Bogduk, 1982). Relief of pain when the joint or joints are anesthetized or the medial branch nerves innervating the joint or joints are anesthetized has been determined by Dr. Bogduk to be the optimal way to identify the joint or joints as pain generators positively. Temporary relief of pain identified via anesthesia of the cervical facet joint and medial branches that are replicable yet yield an inadequate duration of pain relief is the usual and typical indication for consideration of radiofrequency ablation of the nerve innervation of the painful facet joint or joints.

Radiofrequency ablation is typically performed to relieve the pain of cervical joints from C2–C through C7–T1. Continuous radiofrequency ablation is often not considered for treatment of the occipito-atlanto and atlantoaxial facets joints due to the technical difficulties associated with the unique anatomies at C1 and C2. Radiofrequency ablation is a process where heating of the nerve is performed via a probe inserted through a specialized needle. The needle is placed adjacent to the nerve to be ablated. The probe is placed through the needle with the probe's tip adjacent to the nerve. The probe is powered at its proximal end by a radiofrequency generator.

Destruction of the cervical facet medial branch nerves with continuous radiofrequency ablation at standard temperature and duration typically yields pain relief for approximately 12 months. Still, the technique may need to be repeated as frequently as every six months if nerve regeneration clinically appears to have occurred based on symptom recurrence (MacVicar et al., 2012). The return of pain associated with regeneration of the nerves is due primarily to nerve resprouting (regrowth). The duration for regeneration has variability between individuals, which could account for individual differences in the duration of pain relief experienced.

The cervical nerve roots are a typical structure associated with acute and chronic cervical pain. The pain of the cervical nerve roots may commonly occur due to disc protrusion, spinal instability, cervical vertebral body fracture, epidural fibrosis, or post-herpetic neuralgia. Inflammation and pain of the nerve roots associated with lack of space and friction present with neuroforaminal stenosis and central spinal stenosis are other common causes of nerve root pain. There is a multitude of less common causes of cervical nerve root pain. Most common structural causes of cervical root pain may occur or develop and become symptomatic in the absence of trauma, may be exacerbated and become more symptomatic due to trauma, may have been asymptomatic if not for the occurrence of trauma, or may have developed exclusively due to a given trauma. Cervical nerve root pain is often treated with interventional techniques following the failure of conservative treatment and lack of ability to tolerate the pain associated with traditional modalities such as physical therapy.

It should be noted that neurosurgical or orthopedic surgical consultation or intervention may be prioritized instead of interventional pain techniques if the cause of the cervical root pain necessitates prompt surgical intervention. A cervical epidural steroid injection is the typical interventional technique initially performed. If the affected patient lacks contraindications for performing one or more cervical epidural steroid injections, an injection with guidance is typically ordered.

Sterile technique in an operating room or procedural suite with guidance such as fluoroscopy is usually utilized. The most common type of cervical epidural injection performed is the interlaminar injection. An interlaminar cervical epidural injection is when the needle enters the epidural space at or near the posterior anatomical midline and passes through the ligamentum flavum. The medicine is delivered into the epidural space, which is the potential space located between the ligamentum flavum and the dura at the posterior midline. The location for injection is typically performed at C7–T1 or C6–C7 since there is often a larger potential anatomic space for safe needle placement at C7–T1 or C6–C7 than is present in the more cephalad cervical segments. A review of a relatively recent advanced imaging study of the cervical spine preceding the performance of cervical epidural steroid injections is preferable whenever such a study is feasible to obtain. One or more sequential cervical epidural steroid injections may be performed to achieve the desired magnitude and duration of pain relief. Three or fewer epidural injections performed two or more weeks apart is not an atypical interventional pain medicine treatment approach.

Another technique for cervical epidural medication delivery involves intraforaminal delivery of medication. This technique may be preferred in some instances and requires needle placement into the lateral epidural space in the foraminal space where the nerve root exits the spine. Recommendations regarding the patient positioning, fluoroscopic imaging positioning, medication type and quantity, and imaging modality for the performance of this procedural technique are noted to vary in the medical literature. This technique continues to be utilized by some practitioners for diagnostic purposes, such as assisting neurosurgery in determining which anatomical levels may benefit from surgical decompression. Some practitioners use this technique routinely for therapeutic relief of cervical root pain from various sources.

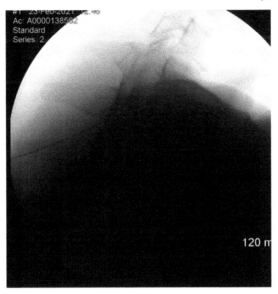

Figure 16.3 Cervical Interlaminar Epidural Steroid Injection (Lateral View Needle Placement With Contrast Shown)

In cases where cervical epidural steroid injections provide sufficient efficacy and sufficient duration of pain relief but symptoms occur months to years following one or more cervical epidural injections, an additional cervical epidural injection or series of injections may be considered. In cases where relevant non-interventional treatment techniques and cervical epidural steroid injections have not yielded sufficient magnitude or duration of pain relief, neurosurgical or orthopedic spine consultation for consideration of elective surgical intervention may be considered. Suppose cervical nerve root pain persists following treatment with relevant non-interventional treatment techniques, treatment with relevant interventional pain medicine injection techniques, and neurosurgical or orthopedic spine surgical intervention or there is a determination by neurosurgery or orthopedic spine surgery that surgery should not be performed. In that case, consideration of a trial spinal cord stimulator for pain control may be considered. Cervical spinal cord stimulation has been an effective means of pain management for conditions including cervical radiculopathy (Deer et al., 2013). If a spinal cord stimulator trial provides adequate relief of pain and improves function and/or quality of life, then a permanent spinal cord stimulator system may be implanted. With stimulator implantation in the periphery of the spine, sedation may be used for the trial procedure, but an overnight stay is typically not needed for a trial procedure. With permanent stimulator implantation in the periphery of the spine, sedation is generally required. With spinal cord stimulator permanent implantation, a laminectomy lead placed by a neurosurgeon or orthopedic spine surgeon requires a laminotomy to permit lead placement. This technique often requires general anesthesia and somatosensory evoked potential monitoring and typically requires an overnight stay. An advanced imaging study of the spine region where the laminotomy will be performed, such as magnetic resonance imaging (MRI) or a CT myelogram, is usually necessary before the laminectomy lead placement. Less invasive placement of percutaneous leads in a permanent stimulator system usually requires sedation, may occasionally require an overnight stay, and may require an advanced imaging study of the location of lead placement before the permanent stimulator surgery. As with spinal cord stimulator systems used for other conditions, the permanent stimulator system requires some ongoing medical management. Reprogramming the system is necessary when the system appears functional but desirable pain relief is not being achieved. This technique is often needed multiple times in year one and then approximately once or more yearly. The spinal cord stimulator generator requires surgical removal and replacement when no longer functional. Modern systems may last for nine years but can also fail to function for two years when high current demands are necessary to achieve pain relief. A typical range for replacing modern spinal cord stimulator generators may be estimated at three to seven years. It will vary considerably based on programming changes that may occur over time, the implantation of rechargeable versus non-rechargeable generators, and alterations in epidural impedance that may occur over time. Furthermore, trauma such as falls may result in damage requiring premature surgical replacement of the spinal cord stimulator or damage of spinal cord stimulator leads. Intrathecal pump infusion systems remain an additional last resort modality for severe cervical pain that has not responded to and is not amendable to other relevant treatment modalities. Intrathecal pump infusion system placement is typically preceded by one or more single-shot epidural or intrathecal injection "trials" or may be preceded by a tunneled epidural trial of medications to determine if a permanent intrathecal pump infusion system is likely to provide beneficial pain relief. Irrespective of the spinal catheter placement location, in permanent intrathecal pump infusion system surgical placement, the surgery is typically preceded by an advanced imaging study of the area where the catheter will be placed. The surgery typically requires sedation and may be followed by an overnight stay.

Thoracic Spine

Anatomy

The thoracic spine is composed of 12 vertebral body segments numbered T1 through T12. Each segment is flanked left and right by ribs numbered 1 through 12. Their vertebral levels interface posteriorly at the right and left zygapophyseal joints. The joints are oriented approximately 60 degrees to the transverse plane and 20 degrees to the frontal plane. The spinal cord is located anterior to the zygapophyseal joints. The costovertebral joint located along the posterior-lateral superior vertebral body is where the rib interfaces with the spine. It is also notable that the transverse process also interfaces with the adjacent rib forming a costal facet. The neural foramen where the adjacent spinal nerve root exits lie inferior and slightly posterior to the costovertebral joint. The vertebral bodies are located anteriorly and are separated by an intervertebral disc named by the vertebral body above and below it (example: the T2–T3 disc is situated between T2 and T3). The thoracic spine has less mobility than the cervical or lumbar spine. Disc protrusion, zygapophyseal joint arthropathy, spinal stenosis, and neuroforaminal stenosis occur at frequencies lower than expected in the cervical and lumbar regions.

Interventional Pain Procedures Performed

The thoracic zygapophyseal joints are a potential cause of thoracic pain. Rotation plus axial loading of the thoracic spine typically causes axial pain along and inferior to the symptomatic thoracic facet joint or joints. As with zygapophyseal joint pain or the cervical or lumbar spine, associated muscular tenderness of the adjacent paraspinal muscles is commonly present. Mechanical movement-type activities often provoke thoracic zygapophyseal joint pain. The treatment of zygapophyseal joint pain involves one or more sequential intraarticular joint injections of the symptomatic joints or may involve two or more sequential thoracic facet medial branch blocks preceding a potential radiofrequency ablation procedure. As with the cervical facet joint injections and lumbar facet joint injections, repeat thoracic zygapophyseal injections may be repeated for future pain recurrences if the desired magnitude and duration of pain are achieved. If only a short period of pain relief is achieved with thoracic zygapophyseal injections or radiofrequency ablation is the preferred treatment modality, then radiofrequency ablation may follow successful temporary relief of thoracic pain with each of (typically) two thoracic facet medial branch block injections. As with the cervical and lumbar spine, repeat radiofrequency ablation may be performed upon the recurrence of pain. The duration of pain relief typically correlates with the median length of time required for the nerves to regenerate. This duration is normally 12 months but could be as short as 6 months or longer than 12 months.

Thoracic epidural steroid injections are typically performed for conditions not requiring immediate neurosurgical or orthopedic surgical intervention but causing nerve root inflammation and thoracic radicular pain. As is the case in the cervical and lumbar spine, thoracic root pain is frequently caused by disc protrusion, central canal stenosis, neuroforaminal stenosis, post-herpetic neuralgia, and epidural fibrosis. The interlaminar epidural technique (as described in the cervical spine section) is the most frequent technique performed. In the absence of any anatomical variances, space-occupying pathologies, or other contraindications, an interlaminar epidural steroid injection could be delivered at any thoracic interlaminar location, and the area that can be feasibly accessed and is closest to the suspected pain generator is typically the interlaminar space of choice.

One or more sequential injections may yield durable relief of pain. If successful pain relief is achieved, future recurrences of pain may be treated with additional thoracic epidural steroid injections. Suppose an insufficient magnitude or duration of pain relief is achieved and other relevant noninvasive or minimally invasive treatment modalities have failed. In that case, neurosurgical or orthopedic spine consultation may be considered. As is the case in the cervical and lumbar spine, spinal radicular pain that fails relevant treatment modalities and is resolved with neurosurgical or orthopedic spine surgery or is not amendable to neurosurgical or orthopedic spine intervention may be appropriate for consideration for neuromodulation therapy. Neuromodulation is less frequently utilized to manage thoracic radicular pain than its more frequent usage for the management of lumbar radicular pain and cervical radicular pain. Still, there are clinical studies documenting its successful application. Dr. Kapural described the successful use of spinal cord stimulation for neuropathic pain of abdominal structures innervated by thoracic nerve roots (Kapural et al., 2020). The upper thoracic spine is the typical neuromodulation electrode target for many thoracic radicular pain conditions. In contrast, the lower thoracic spine is the common neuromodulation electrode target for many lumbar radicular pain conditions. Intrathecal pump infusion systems are a modality of last resort for severe thoracic pain that has not responded to and is not amendable to other relevant treatment modalities. The use of the intrathecal pump infusion system modality for intractable last resort thoracic pain has traditionally been more prevalent than spinal cord stimulation in many parts of the United States.

Lumbar Spine

Anatomy

The lumbar spine is composed of five vertebral bodies. The lumbar spine is flanked superiorly by T12 and inferiorly by the sacrum. The presence of anomalies is not uncommon, and a sixth lumbar vertebral body, also described as L6, may be present and may include an intervertebral

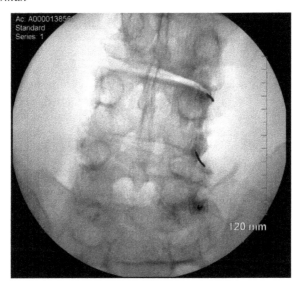

Figure 16.4 Lumbar Facet Medial Branch Blocks (AP View Needle Placement Shown)

disc between the vertebral body and the sacrum. This relatively common anomaly is present when the S1 segment of the sacrum develops as a separate and movable structure. Other partially fused S1 segments, described as transitional segments, comprise a prevalent anomaly seen in the lumbar spine. Each specific lumbar vertebral segment has right and left zygapophyseal joints located posteriorly that interface with superior and inferior segments. The spinal canal is located anterior to the zygapophyseal joints. Still, since the spinal cord terminates at the conus medullaris located at approximately L1 (T12–L3), it is the bundle of spinal roots known as the cauda equina that passes through the majority of the lumbar spinal canal. The vertebral bodies are located anterior to the spinal canal and are separated from both the inferior and superior vertebral bodies by an intervertebral disc. The disc is named by the two segments it separates, except for the disc between L5 and the sacrum. This disc is named L5–S1, with S1 designating the first portion of the fused sacral bone. The right and left lumbar nerve roots exit out of the intervertebral foramina located laterally at each level. The lumbar spine is a mobile part of the spine and is subject to exception loads. This factor makes the lumbar spine particularly susceptible to injury requiring interventional pain treatments.

Interventions

The lumbar zygapophyseal joints are subject to significant mechanical forces with routine repetitive movements and trauma. Treatment of pain of the lumbar zygapophyseal joints remains one of the most frequent reasons patients undergo interventional pain medicine procedures. Data quantifying the number of lumbar zygapophyseal joint injections performed in the United States in 2016 estimates that over 800,000 injection sessions were performed. The same database estimates that over 360,000 lumbar radiofrequency procedures were performed in the United States in 2016 (Starr et al., 2019). A suspected diagnosis of pain derived from the zygapophyseal joints may occur when rotation plus axial loading of the painful area of the lumbar spine causes replication of the axial pain and replicates symptomatic lumbar complaints. Associated muscular

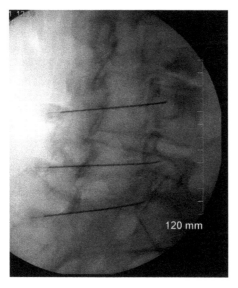

Figure 16.5 Lumbar Facet Medial Branch Blocks (Oblique View Needle Placement Shown)

tenderness of the adjacent paraspinal muscles often coincides with pain and inflammation of the lumbar zygapophyseal joints. Intervention pain medicine treatments are typically considered for the lumbar zygapophyseal joints following the failure of tolerable conservative measures such as physical therapy, chiropractic therapy, a home exercise program, or holistic treatments. Medications such as muscle relaxers and anti-inflammatories may have also been tried and failed to yield long-term pain relief. Treatment and confirmation of the diagnosis of lumbar zygapophyseal joint pain typically require one or more sequential lumbar facet medial branch blocks or lumbar facet intraarticular joint injections of the symptomatic joints. If the pain significantly improves or resolves for a sustained period with lumbar facet intra-articular joint medial branch block procedures and each of at least two separate procedures yields significant pain relief of limited duration, then radiofrequency ablation of the respective lumbar facet medial branches may be considered with the intent to deliver sustained pain relief. As with radiofrequency ablation in the cervical or thoracic spine, pain may return once the medial branch nerves regenerate. Although the nerves may regenerate, prompting the return of pain as soon as 6 months, the typical time necessary for nerve regeneration is approximately 12 months. Once the nerves regenerate, pain may be experienced from these joints. From that time forward, repeat radiofrequency ablation may become necessary. If the pain relief duration following radiofrequency ablation exceeds the usual and typical time of expected relief, such as greater than 18 months, repeating the lumbar facet medial branch block procedures before moving forward with radiofrequency ablation might become necessary.

Inflammation of lumbar nerve roots is widespread. In cases where appropriate types and durations of tolerable conservative treatment have failed and where emergency surgical intervention is not medically necessary, lumbar epidural steroid injections may be performed provided there is no absolute contraindication for the procedure and there is evidence on history, physical examination, and diagnostic testing that supports this modality. Common conditions that may result in the eventual need for lumbar epidural steroid injections include lumbar disc protrusion, lumbar compression fracture, lumbar central spinal stenosis, lumbar neuroforaminal stenosis, and post-herpetic neuralgia of lumbar nerve roots. Different epidural injection techniques may be employed by the treating practitioner. The interlaminar epidural process (described in the cervical section) involves placing a needle at or near the posterior midline with medication delivery between the ligamentum flavum and the dura. This procedure may be performed at any lumbar interlaminar space from T12–L1 to L5–S1. An additional epidural technique used with prevalence in the lumbar spine is the transforaminal technique. Unlike the cervical spine, this technique is performed from a posterior approach with needle placement guided by imaging such as fluoroscopy. Needle placement begins lateral to the midline as the needle is guided toward the desired neuroforamen with imaging assistance.

Medication is delivered into the epidural space after confirming appropriate needle placement in the foramen. This technique shares some similarities with the transforaminal approach in the thoracic spine. The lumbar locations for potential delivery of medication via the transforaminal approach include the L1–L5 levels right and left. Another commonly utilized method of epidural delivery of drugs to treat lumbar radicular pain is the caudal epidural approach. This approach involves the placement of medication into the epidural space via the sacral hiatus. The sacral hiatus is located along the sacrum's inferior aspect, several centimeters from the L5 level. It is generally understood that injection of a sufficient volume of medication via a caudal epidural injection may yield an adequate spread of the drug far enough cephalad to treat lower lumbar radicular pain appropriately. Regardless of the epidural technique utilized, one or more sequential epidural injections may be required to achieve sufficient durable pain relief. If pain improves significantly or resolves, repeat epidural injections may be considered if future pain recurrence develops.

Multiple minimally invasive procedural techniques have been developed for use both by interventional pain practitioners and surgeons to more aggressively treat conditions such as lumbar disc protrusion and spinal stenosis. The discussion of such procedures is addressed in the "Other Spinal Procedures" section. In cases where appropriate conservative treatment measures and appropriate interventional pain procedures have failed to yield resolution of lumbar radicular pain or surgical intervention is not deemed feasible for the resolution of this condition, last resort measures such as spinal cord stimulation or intrathecal pump infusion system implantation may be considered. Spinal cord stimulation in the lumbar spine begins with a trial stimulator procedure to determine the optimal lead placement location and the hardware configuration needed for the permanent device. The trial remains helpful in determining the efficacy of both pain relief and physical function improvement that may be expected if permanent spinal cord stimulator implantation is pursued. The neural structures targeted for electrode placement to yield pain relief for lumbar radicular pain include dorsal epidural locations in the mid and lower thoracic spine and dorsal root ganglion locations in the lumbar spine. As described in greater detail in the "Cervical Spine" section, the permanent stimulator placement may involve percutaneous or laminectomy leads. Appropriate preoperative and intraoperative diagnostic testing costs should be considered. The future costs associated with long-term management of the spinal cord stimulator system, such as generator reprogramming, generator replacement, and potential replacement of damaged/fractured leads, should be considered.

Intrathecal pump infusion system placement is also an option of last resort for the pain of the lumbar spine, whether radicular or non-radicular. As described in the "Cervical Spine" section, permanent placement of an intrathecal pump infusion system is typically preceded by a trial. The future costs of managing permanent intrathecal pump infusion systems include the costs associated with pump refills by a skilled medical provider, surgical replacement of the pump reservoir upon loss of battery life, and potential pump complications involving the catheter or reservoir. Pump complications may result in the future need for pump side port studies, surgical catheter revisions, or surgical reservoir replacements. The costs of intrathecal medications utilized for pump refills should additionally be considered.

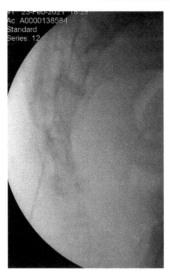

Figure 16.6 Caudal Epidural Injection (Lateral View Needle Placement With Contrast Shown)

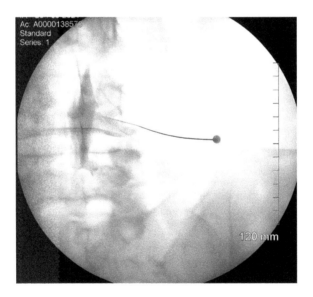

Figure 16.7 Lumbar Transforaminal Epidural Steroid Injection (AP View Needle Placement With Contrast Shown)

Sacral and Coccygeal Spine

Anatomy

The sacrum is a triangular, wedge-shaped bone flanked by the lumbar spine, inferiorly by the coccyx and to the right and left by the iliac bones. The sacrum houses five right and five left sacral nerves. There is an identifiable anterior and posterior neuroforamina where dorsal and ventral roots exit the spine. Located anterior-superior to the sacrum is the L5–S1 intervertebral disc that connects the sacrum to the L5 vertebral body. Located posterior-superior to the sacrum are the right and left L5–S1 zygapophyseal joints. The spinal canal enters the sacrum between the posterior zygapophyseal joints and the anterior L5–S1 disc. The canal continues in a caudad direction ending at the sacral hiatus. The sacral hiatus is located along the inferior-posterior midline of the sacrum. The sacral hiatus marks the most caudal end of the spinal canal and is the needle entry point into the canal for a caudal epidural injection. The sacrum's lateral aspects form movable joints and the adjacent iliac bones called the sacroiliac joints. The sacrococcygeal symphysis connects the sacrum to the coccyx. Anterior to the sacrococcygeal symphysis lies the ganglion impar. It is the most caudad sympathetic chain ganglion. The coccyx is the most caudal segment of the spine. It is composed of three to five fused bony segments. The fifth sacral nerve exits the sacral hiatus, and the sacral hiatus is flanked inferiorly by the coccygeal cornua.

Interventions

Joint pain of the right or left sacroiliac joint is a common condition requiring intervention if failed conservative treatment such as physical therapy fails to resolve the pain symptoms. Intra-articular injection of the sacroiliac joint is typically performed with image guidance such as fluoroscopy. The needle placement typically involves a posterior-to-anterior, medial-to-lateral trajectory with final placement into the lower posterior one third of the joint. One or more sequential injections may yield short-term or long-term pain relief.

If only short-term pain relief is achieved with injections, consideration for radiofrequency ablation of the sensory nerves innervating the joint may be considered. The sensory nerves providing innervation to the joint that may be ablated include an inferior branch of the ipsilateral L5 dorsal ramus and the lateral branches of the ipsilateral sacral nerves of S1, S2, S3, and S4. The Cleveland Clinic Department of Pain Management, Society of Interventional Radiology reports that consensus in the medical literature suggests that successful radiofrequency ablation of these nerves typically provides temporary relief of sacroiliac joint pain for 6 to 12 months. It should also be noted that some practitioners may choose to perform one or more nerve blocks of the sensory nerves as a diagnostic test or tests before performing radiofrequency ablation. An additional alternative to radiofrequency ablation is the surgical fusion of the sacroiliac joint. This outpatient surgery may be performed by a neurosurgeon, an orthopedic spine surgeon, or an interventional pain medicine physician. This outpatient surgery is usually only required to be performed once over a lifetime. It is served with image-guided assistance and with sedation via anesthesia.

Transforaminal epidural steroid injections may address sacral radicular pain upon failure of appropriate conservative treatment. Conditions including L5–S1 disc protrusions frequently inflame the S1 nerve. Sacral radiculitis is also caused by trauma with or without sacral fracture. Other less common causes of sacral radiculitis include Tarlov cysts of the sacrum and epidural fibrosis. A transforaminal epidural injection in the sacrum involves the posterior placement of the needle into the desired foramen. Image guidance is routinely utilized.

One or more sequential transforaminal epidural injections may be performed to achieve desired pain relief. Future epidural injections may be considered if future pain recurrence develops. Caudal epidural steroid injections performed through the sacral hiatus may be utilized to reduce sacral radicular pain. This technique is further described in the "Lumbar Spine" section. If sacral radiculitis fails to resolve with appropriate conservative treatment and interventional pain procedures and if neurosurgical or orthopedic spine surgical options either fail or are not feasible to pursue, then last resort treatment options may be considered. Stimulation for relief of sacral radiculitis may involve dorsal column stimulation, with typical placement performed in the lower thoracic spine, or peripheral nerve placement along with the sacral roots, with leads placed through the sacral foramina. Regardless of the lead placement location, the same future cost considerations as detailed in the lumbar and cervical spine sections should be considered if a permanent system is placed. Sympathetically mediated pain of the lower sacral nerve root distribution areas such as the rectum may be addressed with an injection of the ganglion impar. The technique typically involves steering the needle from just lateral to the sacrococcygeal symphysis to the anterior surface of the distal sacrum. One or more injections may yield pain relief from sympathetically mediated pain modulated through this ganglion. As with other spinal regions, refractory pain of the sacral or coccygeal spine may be amendable to intrathecal pump infusion system implantation for pain management. Cost considerations are detailed in the "Lumbar Spine" section.

Other Spinal Procedures

While many less frequently performed interventional pain spinal procedures may be encountered in life care planning, several should be discussed to ensure familiarity. Percutaneous removal of disc material may be performed utilizing various hardware kits to remove portions of disc protrusions. These procedures are typically performed with fluoroscopic guidance and usually do not require an overnight stay. Intervertebral spacers may be implanted between the lumbar spinous processes to reduce lumbar extension at a given segment. This treatment may be used for treatment in some instances of symptomatic lumbar spinal stenosis. Intervertebral implant procedures are typically performed with fluoroscopic guidance and usually do not require an overnight stay. Vertebral compression fractures or sacral insufficiency fractures may be treated with the placement of bone cement into the fractured bone. These techniques may involve using a variety of hardware kits, may require guidance such as fluoroscopy, and may involve elevation or height restoration of the fractured vertebral segment. These fracture stabilization techniques usually require light sedation and only sometimes need an overnight stay.

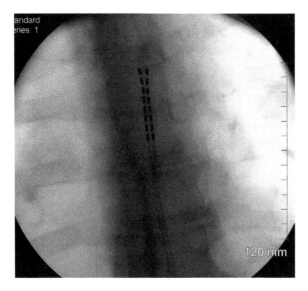

Figure 16.8 Spinal Cord Stimulator Lead Placement (Two Leads in the Thoracic Epidural Space Are Shown)

Additional sympathetic nervous system control centers such as the splanchnic nerves or celiac plexus ganglion at the thoracic level may be injected or ablated for upper abdominal neuropathic pain control. The hypogastric plexus ganglion at the lower lumbar level may be injected to achieve management of lower abdominal or pelvic neuropathic pain. A discogram is a diagnostic technique used to identify or exclude the presence of pain caused by a disc and involves intradiscal injection and interpretation of induced symptoms and imaging findings. Discograms may be performed on cervical, thoracic, or lumbar discs. Intradiscal injection of stem cells may be performed to regenerate a disc with reduced disc height.

Therapeutic Modalities

Following successful resolution or reduction of a chronic pain condition, the importance of restoration of physical function cannot be understated. Once pain is better controlled, physical therapy and occupational therapy modalities may be much easier to tolerate and potentially more effective. Building core strength of the muscles supporting a spinal region, building peripheral strength of the muscles supporting a peripheral joint, and improving flexibility of muscles stabilizing the spine or periphery are potential benefits of therapy. Chiropractic treatments and massage also provide similar potential benefits to flexibility and well-being. Home exercise programs, aqua aerobics, and yoga offer additional restorative benefits. When appropriate for the patient and conditions, any or all of these modalities may aid in the restoration of physical function. Improved core strength or peripheral strength and flexibility may reduce the likelihood of pain recurrences with many conditions. Providers commonly employ intermittent repeat therapy regimens to reduce the rate of progressive decline in physical functioning that may occur in association with deconditioning. Deconditioning is a frequent complication of reduced physical activity associated with chronic pain symptoms.

Continuity of Care

Following the development of chronic pain conditions, costs associated with continuity of care with providers for the management of these conditions should be considered for life care planning. If interventional pain medicine techniques are utilized to achieve pain control, future visits with the interventional pain medicine provider will typically be needed. At least one annual visit for continuity in the absence of active treatment is typical, and additional pre-procedural and post-procedural office visits during active treatment should be expected. Other visits with the treating pain provider or primary care provider may be needed for medical management, electrodiagnostic testing, or laboratory testing. Imaging studies may be required to monitor conditions that may progressively worsen with time, such as disc protrusions, spondylolisthesis, or traumatically injured joints. Office visits for implanted equipment management such as spinal cord stimulator reprogramming or intrathecal pump infusion system dose adjustments should also be considered.

Treating physician office visits should also be considered for preventative management of conditions often associated with chronic pain disorders, such as reduced gait and reduced balance. Gait assistive devices, adaptive equipment for fall prevention within the home, and home structural modification costs should be considered. These needs commonly associated with chronic pain conditions may be prescribed or recommended by providers to prevent recurrences or worsening of chronic pain conditions. Treating physician office visits may be required for assessment and prescription of home support services because of chronic pain conditions related to disability. Referrals to consultants may be made by treating physicians as appropriate.

Chronic Management of Opioids

The management of opioids for chronic non-malignant pain is regulated at the federal and state levels. States and state boards of medicine provide regulations for providers that vary between states. In addition to following all regulatory requirements, the provider must provide care that is within the standard of care acceptable for their specialty and their region of the country. The salient points to consider in life care planning include the frequency of office visits, the frequency and types of laboratory tests, and the costs of the medications. Highly regulated opioid or non-opioid medications in Schedules II or III will usually necessitate monthly office visits for monitoring. Less regulated opioids or other controlled substances may require monitoring four times yearly in some areas or monthly in other regions. Urine drug screen testing will be required intermittently. It is not uncommon for practices to require a monthly point-of-care urine drug testing and random comprehensive urine drug screening. The comprehensive drug tests, which include techniques such as gas chromatography and mass spectrometry, clarify the appropriate use of the prescribed agent and may exclude or identify a multitude of illicit drugs and controlled prescription drugs not detectable or discernable by basic urine drug screening evaluation. Costly comprehensive drug screening is typically performed on a randomized basis and may be performed more frequently in high-risk patients and less frequently in low-risk patients. Three tests yearly are a typical average number of comprehensive urine drug screens performed randomly in a low or moderate risk-stratified pain patient treated regularly with opioids. Medication costs differ by type, dose, preparation, and location or region obtained. These factors should be considered when estimating the medication cost.

References

Bogduk, N. (1982). The clinical anatomy of the cervical dorsal rami. *Spine, 7*(4), 319–330. https://doi-org.proxy.library.vcu.edu/10.1097/00007632-198207000-00001

Bonica, J. J. (1953). *The management of pain.* Lea & Febiger.

Deer, T., Skaribas, I., Haider, N., Salmon, J., Kim, C., Nelson, C., Tracy, J., Espinet, A., Lininger, T., Tiso, R., M Archacki, M., & Washburn, S. (2014). Effectiveness of cervical spinal cord stimulation for the management of chronic pain. *Neuromodulation, 17*(3), 265–271. https://doi.org/10.1111/ner.12119. Epub 2013 September 24.

Dowell, D., Haegerich, T., & Chou, R. (2016). CDC Guideline for prescribing opioids for chronic pain—United States, 2016., *Morbidity and Mortality Weekly Report, 65*(1), 1–49. Centers for Disease Control and Prevention.

Giesecke, T., Gracely, R., Williams, D., Geisser, M., Petzke, F., & Clauw, D. (2005). The relationship between depression, clinical pain, and experimental pain in a chronic pain cohort. *Arthritis & Rheumatism, 52*(5), 1577–1584. https://doi.org 10.1002/art.21008, American College of Rheumatology.

Grichnik, K. P., & Ferrante, F. M. (1991). The difference between acute and chronic pain. *The Mount Sinai Journal of Medicine, 58*(3), 217–220.

Harden, R., Bruehl, S., Perez, R., Birklein, F., Marinus, J., Maihofner, C., Lubenow, T., Buvanendran, A., Mackey, S., Graciosa, J., Mogilevski, M., Ramsden, C., Chont, M., & Vatine, J. J. (2010). Validation of proposed diagnostic criteria (The "Budapest Criteria") for complex regional pain syndrome. *Pain, 150*(2), 268–274.

Kapural, L., Gupta, M., Paicius, R., Strodtbeck, W., Vorenkamp, K. E., Gilmore, C., Gliner, B., Rotte, A., Subbaroyan, J., & Province-Azalde, R. (2020). Treatment of chronic abdominal pain with 10-kHz spinal cord stimulation: Safety and efficacy results from a 12-month prospective, multicenter, feasibility study. *Clinical and Translational Gastroenterology, 11*(2), e00133. https://doi-org.proxy.library.vcu.edu/10.14309/ctg.0000000000000133

Konya, Z., Takmaz, S., Başar, H., Baltaci, B., & Babaoğlu, G. (2020). Results of genicular nerve ablation by radiofrequency in osteoarthritis-related chronic refractory knee pain *Turkish Journal of Medical Sciences, 50*(1), 86–95. https://doi.org/10.3906/sag-1906-91

MacVicar, J., Borowczyk, J. M., MacVicar, A. M., Loughnan, B. M., & Bogduk, N. (2012). Cervical medial branch radiofrequency neurotomy in New Zealand. *Pain Medicine (Malden, Mass.), 13*(5), 647–654. https://doi-org.proxy.library.vcu.edu/10.1111/j.1526-4637.2012.01351.x

McBeth, J., & Jones, K. (2007). Epidemiology of chronic musculoskeletal pain. *Best Practice and Research in Clinical Rheumatology*, *21*(3), 403–425. https://doi.org/10.1016/j.berh.2007.03.003.

Merskey, H., & Bogduk, N. (1994). *Classification of chronic pain* (2nd ed.). IASP Task Force on Taxonomy. IASP Press. www.iasp-pain.org/Education/content.aspx?ItemNumber=1698

Morasco, B., Lovejoy, T., Lu, M., Turk, D., Lewis, L., & Dobscha, S. (2013). The relationship between PTSD and chronic pain: Mediating role of coping strategies and depression. *Pain*, *154*(4), 609–616. https://doi.org: 10.1016/j.pain.2013.01.001

Pope, J., Bowman, R., & Deer, T. (2012). Spinal cord stimulation. In A. Gupta (Ed.), *Interventional pain medicine*. Oxford University Press.

Rubin, D. I. (2007). Epidemiology and risk factors for spine pain. *Neurology Clinics*, *25*(2), 353–371.

Starr, J., Gold, L., McCormick, Z., Suri, P., & Friedly, J. (2019). Trends in lumbar radiofrequency ablation utilization from 2007 to 2016. *Clinical Study*, *19*(6), 1019–1028. https://doi.org/10.1016/j.spinee.2019.01.00

Treede, R. D., Rief, W., Barke, A., Aziz, Q., Bennett, M. I., Benoliel, R., Cohen, M., Evers, S., Finnerup, N. B., First, M. B., Giamberardino, M. A., Kaasa, S., Korwisi, B., Kosek, E., Lavand'homme, P., Nicholas, M., Perrot, S., Scholz, J., Schug, S., Smith, B. H., Svensson, P., Vlaeyen, J., & Wang, S. J. (2019). Chronic pain as a symptom or a disease: The IASP Classification of Chronic Pain for the International Classification of Diseases (ICD-11). *Pain*, *160*(1), 19–27. https://doi.org/10.1097/j.pain.0000000000001384

Treede, R. D., Rief, W., Barke, A., Aziz, Q, Bennett, M., Benoliel, R., Cohen, M., Evers, S., Finnerup, N. B., First, M. B., Giamberardino, M., Kaasa, S., Kosek, E., Lavand'homme, P., Nicholas, M., Perrot, S., Scholz, J., Schug, S., Smith, B., Svensson, P., Vlaeyen, J., & Wang, S.-J. (2015). A classification of chronic pain for ICD-11. *PAIN*, *156*(6), 1003–1007. https://doi.org/10.1097/j.pain.0000000000000160

17 Burn Trauma and Plastic and Reconstructive Surgery

Gerard Mosiello

The Skin

The skin is the major organ that is exposed to external elements and excess temperature. The skin is composed of two different layers: the epidermis and dermis. The two main layers of the skin are the stratum corneum and the stratum germinativum. The stratum germinativum is the deepest layer of the epidermis and produces new skin cells. The cells contain the pigment melanin, which is responsible for skin color. These pigment cells migrate upward into the stratum corneum. The stratum corneum is the most superficial layer composed of tough, dry cells that die and slough off.

The dermis consists of mostly connective tissue rich in capillaries, collagen fibers, and elastin fibers. Within the dermis are skin appendages, mainly hair follicles, sweat glands, and sebaceous glands. Therefore, if only the epidermis is lost, a new epidermis can form. If the epidermis, dermis, and glands are lost, no new skin can form. Thus, scar tissue remains as seen in burn injury. Beneath the dermis is the subcutaneous layer with loose connective tissue, fat cells, muscle, tendon, and bone. Nerve endings sensitive to pain are in the epidermis, dermis, and subcutaneous layers.

Mechanism of Burn

The major causes of burns are thermal, such as flame, chemical, and electrical burns. The burn wound consists of three zones. The central area is called the zone of coagulation and is composed of non-viable tissue. Surrounding the central area is the zone of stasis. Initially, blood flow is present here, but over the first 24 hours ischemia will prevail, and part of this area becomes the zone of coagulation. Surrounding the zone of stasis is the outer zone of hyperemia, which contains viable tissue. The depth of the burn is the primary determinant of mortality following burn injury. Wound depth is also a major determinant of a patient's long-term esthetic outcome and function after a burn.

Evaluation of a Burn Patient

It is important to remember that burn patients are trauma patients and require thorough evaluation so effective treatment can be rendered. Airway, breathing, and circulation must be assessed immediately, and additional injuries, particularly life-threatening injuries, must be assessed. A thorough history of the burn etiology is necessary to formulate a treatment plan. The patient's existing comorbidities will also need to be assessed.

DOI: 10.4324/b23293-17

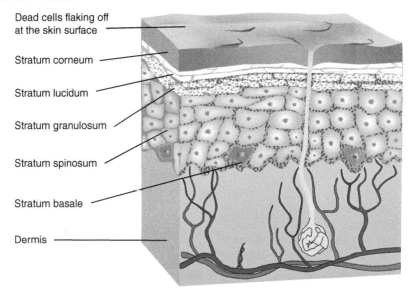

Anatomy of the Epidermis

Figure 17.1 Skin Anatomy

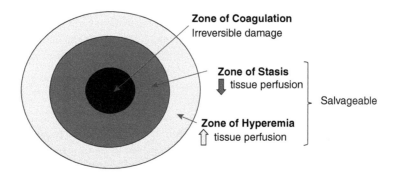

Figure 17.2 Burn Zones of Injury

Burn Classification

Burns are classified according to the depth at which the tissue was injured. First-degree burns involve the epidermis only and are superficial. There is redness, edema, and pain, which does not require hospitalization. This type of burn usually heals in three to five days.

Partial-thickness burns involve the epidermis and a portion of the dermis. They are further divided into superficial and deep partial-thickness burns. Superficial and deep partial-thickness burns differ in appearance and the need for surgical treatment such as skin grafts. Superficial partial-thickness burns are typically moist, pink, and painful with blisters. These burns will heal within two weeks and generally will not result in scarring.

Treatment includes anti-microbial topical agents such as Silvadene. Deep partial-thickness burns involve the epidermis and deep reticular portion of the dermis. There are typically dry and

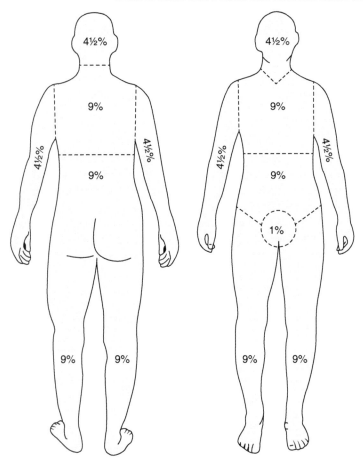

Figure 17.3 The "Rules of Nines" for Estimating Total Body Surface Area

mottled with a pink/white appearance. They may heal in five to eight weeks with scarring and contracture. If there is no epithelialization in three to four weeks, then excision and skin grafts are recommended.

Full-thickness burns involve the epidermis and entire dermis. They may extend into the fat, fascia, muscle, and even bone. These wounds can be brown or black and insensate. These are best treated by excision and skin grafting.

The extent and depth of the burn wounds are established following admission. The total body surface area (TBSA) involved is calculated using many techniques. The Rule of Nines is the best-known method of determining burn extent. Superficial burns are not included in the TBSA calculation; however, partial- and full-thickness burns are included.

The American Burn Association has identified those burn cases that should be referred to a burn center. These include the following:

- Second- and third-degree burns greater than 10% TBSA in patients less than 10 or greater than 50 years old.
- Second- and third-degree burns greater than 20% TBSA in patients in other age groups.

- Third-degree burns greater than 5% in any age group.
- Second- and third-degree burns involving the face, hand, genitals, perineum, and major joints.
- Electrical burns, including lightning injury.
- Chemical burns with a serious threat to a function or cosmetic impairment.
- Burn injury in patients with preexisting medical problems that can complicate management.

Initial Management

The goal of therapy is to replace the fluid sequestered because of the burn injury. The best guideline for adequacy of resuscitation in the first 24 to 48 hours is the hourly urine output. Crystalloid in the form of lactated Ringer's solution is utilized. Several formulations are used to resuscitate burn patients. The Parkland formula is generally recommended, which calls for lactated Ringer's 4 cc/kg/TBSA burn in the first 24 hours. Half the fluid should be given in the first 8 hours and the other half of the fluid given in the next 16 hours. A urine output of 0.5 cc/kg/hr indicates adequate tissue perfusion.

Burn Complications

Major acute complications of burn injury are smoke inhalation, infection, gastrointestinal disorders, and thrombophlebitis.

Inhalation Injury. The inhalation of products of combustion can lead to devastating pulmonary injury. Inhalation injury significantly increases burn mortality. The gold standard for the diagnosis of inhalation injury is bronchoscopy. Management of inhalation injury is usually supportive. Patients with suspected inhalation injury with worsening of their respiratory status may require mechanical ventilation.

Infection. Infection is the leading cause of death in burn patients. Susceptibility to infection increases with the extent of burn injury, especially with greater than 30% TBSA. debridement of the burn wound and the use of topical anti-microbials such as Silvadene can prevent burn wound sepsis.

Gastrointestinal Disorders. Gastrointestinal disturbances such as stress ulcers are a common complication following burn injury. The best protocol against stress ulcers is feeding the patient and the use of protein pump inhibitors.

Deep Vein Thrombosis. Patients who sustained burn injuries have multiple risk factors for deep vein thrombosis. Prolonged bed rest with an indwelling catheter can increase the risk of deep vein thrombosis. Therefore, prophylaxis is required in burn patients who are hospitalized and unable to ambulate.

Late effects of a burn injury can include complications such as acute kidney injury (AKI), peripheral nerve compression of the lower extremities, hypertrophic scarring, Marjolijn's ulcers, and heterotrophic ossification (You et al., 2022; Wu et al., 2013).

Surgical Management

The surgical goal of acute burn care is to remove eschar caused by burn trauma. Early burn excision and skin grafting have become the standard of care for full-thickness burn wounds. This method has shown increased survival, decreased infection rates, decreased hospital stay, and decreased risk of hypertrophic scarring.

The surgery should begin on post-burn day 3 for major burns and spaced out two to three days apart until all the eschar is removed and the burn wound is covered. The skin graft begins revascularization 48 hours after placement. In addition to revascularization, the organization phase begins in which the skin graft integrates with the wound bed.

Skin grafts are classified according to their thickness as either split-thickness or full-thickness. The split-thickness grafts generally have only a portion of the dermis within it, and the full-thickness graft incorporates all the layers of the dermis. Skin grafts can also be meshed or unmeshed. Skin grafts that are not meshed generally have a better cosmetic result than meshed grafts. Split-thickness skin grafts contract more than full-thickness skin grafts. Therefore, full-thickness skin grafts should be on anatomical areas such as the face, hands, and forearms to enhance the cosmetic appearance.

Skin graft dressings can include Xeroform bolsters to aid in adherence and, more recently, the use of vacuum-assisted closure (wound VAC) to apply negative pressure to prevent shearing and skin graft movement. Hansbrough et al. (1995) demonstrated the efficacy of Xeroform as an adherence agent for skin grafts in their study of 142 split-thickness skin grafts on 100 patients. They found that on postoperative day 5 evaluations, the mean skin graft take in all patients was 98.54% +/- 0.72%. Hansbrough et al. concluded that Xeroform and coarse-mesh gauze dressings used to cover split-thickness skin grafts and left intact for 5 days until the initial dressing change resulted in highly successful graft outcomes, with minimal postoperative nursing care compared with other dressing methods for skin grafts.

Burn Rehabilitation

Physical and occupational therapy play an essential role in the acute management of all burn-injured patients. Rehabilitation care plans and goals should be devised with a multidisciplinary burn team, the patient, and the patient's family. The short-term rehabilitation goal is the preservation of the patient's range of motion and functional capacities. Long-term goals are to return the patient to independent living and retrain the patient to compensate for any functional loss. The rehabilitation phase can begin as early as two weeks or may not start until two to three months after burn injury.

Acute rehabilitation with physical and occupational therapy focuses on the prevention of deformity and scar contractures. The performance of a passive, active, and active-assisted range of motion should be utilized. Exercises should be started on the first day after admission when the patient has been stabilized and should be performed daily until full range of motion is achieved and maintained. Bed mobility, transfers, and ambulation should be encouraged as early as possible.

Patient positioning is designed to reduce extremity edema, provide proper body alignment, and prevent contracture positions. Anti-contracture positioning can be achieved by splinting, traction strapping, and serial casting. Splints are indicated to prevent scar deformities, protect exposed joints and tendons, and aid in controlling edema and inflammation. When burns are healing, pressure garments are employed to minimize scarring.

Plastic Surgery Burn Reconstruction

Secondary reconstruction of the burn wound poses one of the greatest challenges to plastic and reconstructive surgeons. Early excision and grafting have improved outcomes from a burn injury, yet an overwhelmingly large number of patients fail to return to their previous professional or personal pre-injury level of function. This type of reconstructive surgery is deferred until skin graft scar maturation is complete and the maximal benefits of physical therapy have been realized. Multiple operations are often required and frequently take place over a period of many years. This requires a well-functioning support system including nurses, therapists, social

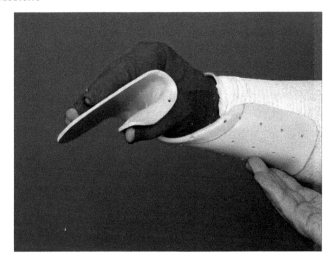

Figure 17.4 Hand Splint to Prevent Scar Contracture

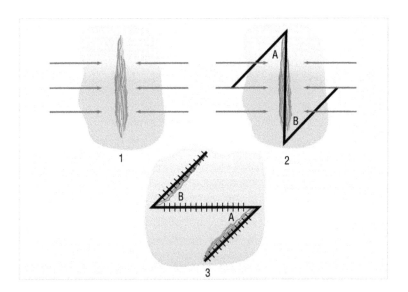

Figure 17.5 Z-Plasty Flap for Burn Scar Contracture

workers, psychologists, and a supportive family environment. All these factors affect the outcome of surgery. Some modalities for burn reconstruction include scar revision with Z-plasty, surgical flaps, tissue expansion, and laser therapy.

Subsequent reconstructive procedures commonly employ the use of pressure garments to decrease the recurrence of hypertrophic scarring and contracture. Pressure garments are typically worn 24 hours per day for up to a period of two years. Since the garments last approximately three to four months, refitting is required. Therefore, the costs can be expensive and should be included in life care plan.

Burn Vocational Rehabilitation and Life Care Planning

Burn injury often results in significant barriers to returning to work, which can include scar contracture deformities, loss of self-esteem, anxiety, and depression. Predictors for return to work include the timing of the injury, TBSA, surgical procedures including skin grafting, and response to treatment.

Vocational planning should include mental health consultation to allow the patient to have a support system in place to handle psychological and emotional issues. This may enhance the probability of employment success. Research suggests that 28% of all burn patients never return to any form of employment. Yet those who return have a 93% retention rate and an average of 24 days from injury to return to work.

Work-related accommodations may be beneficial due to burn-patient limitations. Examples include parking close to the work site, accessible entrances, accessible break rooms and restrooms, and reducing worksite temperature for burn patients experiencing heat and cold sensitivity.

Life care planning for the burn-injured patient should focus on maintaining range of motion, skilled nursing for any ongoing wound problems, assistance for daily dressing and grooming, physical and occupational therapy to prevent contractures and maximize function, mental health services, and transportation services. Assistive devices for daily living should also be considered in the life care plan due to the multidimensional nature of the burn-injured patient. A burn survivor is followed on a long-term basis by a physiatrist who is skilled in burn management and a plastic surgeon who specializes in the treatment of burns and their sequelae.

References

Hansbrough, W., Doré, C., & Hansbrough, J. F. (1995). Management of skin-grafted burn wounds with Xeroform and layers of dry coarse-mesh gauze dressing results in excellent graft take and minimal nursing time. *The Journal of Burn Care & Rehabilitation*, *16*(5), 531–534. https://doi-org.proxy.library.vcu.edu/10.1097/00004630-199509000-00012

Wu, C., Calvert, C. T., Cairns, B. A., & Hultman, C. S. (2013). Lower extremity nerve decompression in burn patients. *Annals of plastic surgery*, *70*(5), 563–567. https://doi-org.proxy.library.vcu.edu/10.1097/SAP.0b013e31827aef9c

You, B., Yang, Z., Zhang, Y., Chen, Y., Gong, Y., Chen, Y., Chen, J., Yuan, L., Luo, G., Peng, Y., & Yuan, Z. (2022). Late-onset acute kidney injury is a poor prognostic sign for severe burn patients. *Frontiers in Surgery*, *9*, 842999. https://doi-org.proxy.library.vcu.edu/10.3389/fsurg.2022.842999

18 Canadian Life Care Planning and Cost Projection Analysis

A Comparison of Process and Application

Claudia von Zweck and Dana Weldon

A life care plan is a document that identifies the level of trauma and outlines the lifelong needs of an individual following a catastrophic injury or chronic illness. The development of a plan involves a systematic process, based on published standards of practice that includes comprehensive assessment and integrated analysis of data obtained through consultation and research (International Association of Rehabilitation Professionals, 2015). In Canada, several terms may be used interchangeably to describe a life care plan, including *future cost of care analysis, future needs analysis*, or *future care cost assessment*. Despite the terminology used, the resulting document serves as a roadmap that identifies and prices an individual's current and future needs stemming from impairments sustained from an injury or illness. Such needs may relate to medical or rehabilitation treatments or any other necessary services or support to allow an individual to enjoy the same quality of life as if the injury or illness had not occurred.

In life care planning, a holistic perspective is used to consider an individual's needs. The plan addresses a broad range of issues that optimize independence and function, promote health stability, prevent future complications, and provide assistance for activities an individual can no longer perform.

Use of Life Care Plans Legal System

Life care plans are most often initiated to assist with the settlement of personal injury claims within the legal system. Such claims frequently arise from motor vehicle collisions, work accidents, medical negligence, or property or product liability. Examples of liability claims include slips and falls occurring on public or private property, or injuries sustained from malfunctioning or defective equipment. Life care plans may also be used in other types of legal action where costing is required regarding the long-term needs of an individual, such as divorce proceedings or estate disputes.

In adjudicating legal action, the court is concerned that an individual receives reasonable future care, based on the impact of an injury or illness for participation in gainful employment and other important daily activities. As the determination of reasonableness is individually based, expert opinion is often required through reports and testimony. Life care plans are therefore used as an objective tool by either the plaintiff (affected individual) or defense to promote understanding of the scope and impact of an individual's injury or illness-related impairment, as well as the costs necessary for reasonable future care and services.

DOI: 10.4324/b23293-18

Individuals and Caregivers

A life care plan provides a blueprint for individuals affected by injury or illness for recommended intervention and support to optimally achieve life goals and priorities. The life care plan is designed to promote wellness and stability of health while respecting individual needs and goals. Used as a case management tool, the plan provides education regarding the long-term impact of an injury or illness, and assists evaluees and their caregivers to make informed decisions regarding future rehabilitation and care. The plan may serve to identify options and entitlements not previously considered and promote the realistic and timely organization to ensure required products and services are available when needed throughout the individual's lifetime. In some circumstances, life care plans may define alternatives for care and rehabilitation that may be considered as an individual progresses through life, for example, to identify and cost different options for housing for a young adult when living with immediate family is no longer feasible or desired. Settlements may be structured to timelines outlined in the life care plan to ensure funding is available for accessing identified supports and services as required.

Society

Life care plans ensure that individuals impacted by injuries or illness have the necessary resources to allow them to engage as productively as possible in their community. This vital support reduces strain on publicly funded programs and services while promoting optimal individual contributions to society.

Life care plans also provide a mechanism for determining the optimal use of available funds by evaluating the cost and benefit of alternate approaches to rehabilitation. For example, Morrison and associates demonstrated the cost and benefit of locomotor training for individuals with an incomplete spinal cord injury by comparing the life care plan costs for equipment, home renovations, and transportation after receiving or not receiving the intervention (Morrison et al., 2012).

Life Care Planning Education and Certification

To qualify for certification as a Certified Canadian Life Care Planner (CCLCP), a potential candidate must satisfy the definition of a *qualified health care professional*. The International Commission on Health Care Certification (ICHCC), the certifying body, defines *qualified health care professional* guidelines as follows:

> The designation of a health care professional must be specific to the care, treatment, and/or rehabilitation of individuals with significant disabilities and does not include such professions as an attorney, generic educators, general administrators, etc., but does include such professions as counseling and special education with appropriate qualifications. This designation of qualified health care professional is based on a background of education, training, and practice qualifications. A background of only experience and/or designated job title is not accepted as defining qualified health care professionals. Completion of training in the respective credential's focus area, experience, or being qualified in the court system as an expert witness do not necessarily meet the definition of qualified health care professional under the ICHCC standards. This definition can only be met when all educational, training, and practice qualification components are reviewed and met.
> (The International Commission on Health Care Certification, 2021, p. 11)

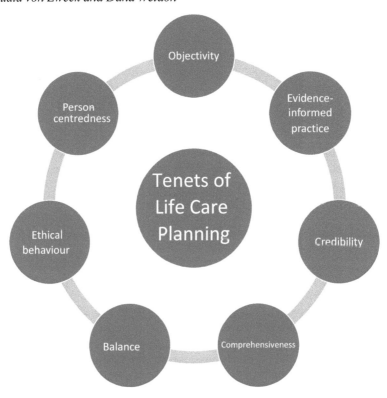

Figure 18.1 Tenets of Life Care Planning

In addition to recognition as a qualified health care provider, an applicant must have 120 hours of training from an ICHCC-approved training program. A listing of training programs can be found on the ICHCC website at www.ichcc.org. Of the required 120 hours, 16 must be dedicated to orientation, methodology and standards of practice in life care planning.

Tenets of Life Care Planning

Tenets for life care planning are outlined in Figure 18.1. The tenets are interconnected and, when considered together, form a solid basis for the development of life care plans.

Objectivity

Regarding the development of a life care plan, the life care planner is expected to act objectively and impartially. Any perception of bias in the opinion of the life care planner impacts the acceptability of the life care plan and the potential use of the findings. The life care planner, therefore, does not advocate on behalf of any party and works without influence in providing a fair evaluation of the impact of an individual's impairment and determination of future care requirements. Professional judgment is solely used by the life care planner to assess information that is collected from multiple sources for decision-making for the life care plan, with the interests of the referring party having no bearing on recommendations regarding future care needs.

Evidence-Informed Practice

The evidence-informed practice promotes the acceptability of the life care plan by the evaluee and the court. The evidence-informed practice process requires life care planners to dedicate time and use critical thinking skills to consider evidence that is obtained from expert opinion and peer-reviewed published research and assessed within the context of objective evaluation data regarding the needs, goals, and priorities of the evaluee.

Credibility

Factors influencing the credibility of a life care plan include the probability, justifiability, feasibility, and reasonableness of the report recommendations. Recommendations address only needs that are considered probable, meaning that there is a more than fifty percent likelihood that the costs are necessary and will be incurred in the future. The costs must be related to needs stemming from the injury or illness and based on what is in the best interests of the individual, as justified by the evidence presented. Implementation of the recommendations must be feasible for the individual given time, financial, and other resource implications, for example, the ability of the individual to attend multiple therapy visits despite low energy reserves. Costs for goods or services must be consistent with the individual's pre-injury or pre-illness lifestyle to be accepted as reasonable. Canadian accepted standards of reasonableness are based on optimal care and may be more generous than available from public-funded programs. The court must be assured, however, that claims do not enhance an individual's prior quality of life or result in the squandering of funds.

Comprehensiveness

The development of a life care plan requires a comprehensive understanding of the impact of an injury or illness for the functional skills and abilities of the evaluee to engage in needed or desired activities. All recommendations of the life care plan must be based on a thorough understanding of the needs and priorities of the evaluee. Although recommendations of the life care plan may be limited to particular areas of need for the evaluee, the evaluation process used by the life care planner is never compromised so as to interfere with the comprehensive understanding needed for the development of valid recommendations.

Balance

Life care planning requires the consideration of evidence received from multiple sources. Such evidence may be conflicting in nature, reflecting differing opinions and perspectives regarding the cause, nature, and impact of an individual's impairments. The life care planner must use professional judgment to appraise and integrate the evidence to obtain a balanced understanding of the future care needs of the individual. The life care planner uses an iterative process to objectively review and assess each piece of evidence in the context of what is known regarding the evaluee to formulate and test a theory regarding the expected life course and future needs of the individual.

Ethical Behaviour

To become a life care planner in Canada certified by the International Health Care Commission, an individual must be a qualified health care provider, with membership in a professional regulatory organization. Life care planners are therefore expected to uphold the code of ethics prescribed by their regulatory organization. Ethical considerations outlined in such documents include:

- Avoidance of conflicts of interest and detrimental or exploitive relationships
- Respect for the integrity and welfare of individuals and groups involved in the life care planning process, with a primary obligation to the evaluee
- Objectivity for provision of service without bias
- Competency and commitment to professional development
- Adherence to confidentiality and consent procedures to safeguard information privacy

Person-Centredness

Life care planners work collaboratively with evaluees in the development of life care plans. The life care planner has a responsibility to ensure the plan is compatible with the evaluee's future life vision. Information from individual evaluees and caregivers is therefore used to identify goals, values, and beliefs that must be considered in the plan. The life care planner seeks to understand how an illness or injury impacts the ability of individuals to engage in activities that provide value and meaning for them; this understanding requires respect and openness for the social and cultural preferences and choices of the individual. Difficult discussions may, however, be necessary with the evaluee and caregivers regarding what is realistic and can be justified within the confines of the life care plan.

Life Care Planning Process

The development of a life care plan involves several steps, as outlined in Figure 18.2. While development usually follows a sequential order, work may occur concurrently in several steps.

Referral

The life care planning process is initiated when a referral is received. Before accepting the referral, the life care planner conducts a review of information received from the referring party to ensure a clear understanding of report expectations and timelines. Often life care plans are commissioned for settlement negotiations or court proceedings, involving inflexible timelines that the life care planner must be prepared to meet. Life care planners must also ascertain they

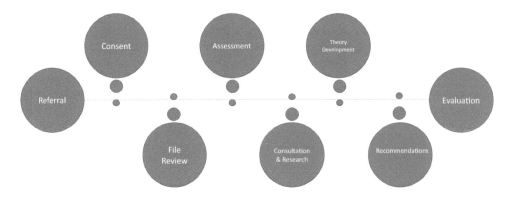

Figure 18.2 Life Care Planning Process

have the required competency and expertise to accept the referral. The expected life care planning process is then communicated to the referring party to ensure a mutual understanding of time, activities, and costs.

Consent

After accepting the referral, the evaluee is contacted to obtain consent for the development of the life care plan. Before asking for consent, it is necessary to ensure the evaluee has a full understanding of the purpose of the plan and the process that will be used to complete the report. Discussions relating to the consent process also address risks, benefits, and alternatives to the life care plan to ensure the evaluee is fully informed before agreeing for the report to proceed.

File Review

Before meeting with the evaluee, the life care planner reviews relevant background material that is provided by the referring party. The material outlines the history of the evaluee's injury or illness, including reports from hospitals and physicians, documentation from rehabilitation team members, and other relevant information such as independent evaluation reports. The information is reviewed to determine the impairments the evaluee sustained as a result of the injury or illness, intervention received, future prognosis, and recommendations for future care and support. Information regarding the evaluee's premorbid history is also examined to gain an understanding of the impact of any pre-existing health issues on the individual's ability to engage in daily activities.

Assessment

To promote ease and comfort of the evaluee with the evaluation process, life care planning assessments are usually conducted in the home. Evaluations in the home environment provide valuable information to the life care planner regarding the social and cultural context of evaluees, as well as their roles, interests, and lifestyle. In addition, direct observations can be made regarding the physical accessibility of the home and the availability of adaptive equipment required by the individual, if allowed by the scope of practice of the life care planner, for example, by planners who are occupational therapists.

Initially in the assessment, the evaluee is interviewed regarding the types of medical and rehabilitation interventions that are received. Consent for the release of information is sought from the evaluee for the life care planner to communicate with treatment team members regarding future care needs. Information is also sought from evaluees regarding their symptoms and their past and current activities in personal care, housekeeping, home maintenance, work, and leisure. Evaluees are also asked to share their expectations for their future, for example, plans to return to work or intentions regarding housing. The self-report provides essential information regarding an evaluee's resilience and ability to adapt to changes in functional performance. The interview also offers an opportunity for the life care planner to make clinical observations regarding the evaluee's physical, cognitive, and emotional function, for example, to note pain behaviors or difficulties with memory.

During the assessment, the life care planner often seeks collateral information from family or other caregivers, particularly if the evaluee is a child or severely cognitively impaired. Helpful information can be gained from caregivers regarding the type and frequency of assistance required by the evaluee. The life care planner obtains information from caregivers both in the presence of the evaluee and separately to ensure an accurate understanding of the assistance required.

To supplement the interview data, performance-based tests are undertaken during the assessment where appropriate within the scope of practice of the life care planner. Such tests may be administered to evaluate physical capacity in areas such as joint range of motion, muscle strength, fitness and endurance, mobility, and hand dexterity. If concerns are suspected regarding cognition, standardized tests may be administered to assess mental functions such as memory, planning, problem-solving, and abstract reasoning. Screening tests may also evaluate psychological symptoms such as anxiety or low mood. Administration of standardized tests helps provide normative data regarding the function of the evaluee compared to peer group performance.

In addition to standardized tests, evaluees are evaluated on the performance of functional tasks during the home assessment. Assessment tasks involve observation of self-care and productive activities discussed during the interview to determine how an impairment affects the individual's functional skills. The life care planner looks for consistency between findings of reports examined during the file review, the impairments observed during standardized testing, the self-report of function provided by the evaluee in the interview, and the performance of functional activities. If such assessments are not within the scope of practice of the life care planner, observations made during the evaluation are recorded for discussion with the treatment team at a later time.

Using information from multiple sources for the life care plan is necessary to assess the sincerity of effort during the evaluation tasks and explain discrepancies between assessment findings. For example, an evaluee with poor insight into cognitive dysfunction as a result of a traumatic brain injury may underreport impairments during the interview and in self-report questionnaires; the true impact of impairment for planning and executing activities may only become evident through discussions with a caregiver or observations of the evaluee during a multistep functional task, such as a preparing meal from a recipe.

Consultation and Research

By completing the file review and evaluee assessment, the life care planner gains insight into the evaluee's needs and priorities. A review of the research literature may be necessary to supplement this data collection, for example, to understand the expected course of the evaluee's impairment over time or identify effective treatment approaches. In addition, expert opinion or research evidence must be obtained to address the needs of the evaluee that fall outside the scope of practice of the life care planner. As an example, in Canada, only medical doctors and nurse practitioners can prescribe medications in most jurisdictions. Consultation with the evaluee's doctor or nurse practitioner is therefore necessary to justify the inclusion of prescription medications in the life care plan.

The life care planner usually solicits expert opinion through meeting with the other health professionals or sending a life care planning questionnaire for their completion. Information sought by the life care planner includes the types of services or products required by evaluees as a result of their injury or illness and the expected frequency and duration of need for the service or product throughout the evaluee's lifetime. If the health professional is interviewed, a reiteration letter is sent by the life care planner to confirm the information received that will be included in the life care plan. Written documentation of expert opinion is often requested during legal proceedings to justify recommendations made in the life care plan.

Theory Development

The data gained through consultation and research is reviewed in the context of the evaluee's needs and priorities. Through a reflective process, a theory is developed regarding the most probable life course of the evaluee. The theory considers changes in the function of the evaluee over time, with particular attention to the effects of the individual's impairment on the development of complications. Many individuals with early onset of a disability may experience a decline in abilities due to overuse injuries and secondary conditions such as osteoarthritis.

The life care plan theory serves as a basis for formulating the life care plan. Assumptions regarding the evaluee's life course to support this theory are stated in the life care plan report. All recommendations for future care for the evaluee are aligned with the life care plan theory to be consistent with the diagnosis, expected prognosis, and functional limitations of the individual.

Recommendations

Recommendations outlined in the life care plan are broadly categorized in several areas, as summarized in Table 18.1. The recommendations are based on appropriate care for the evaluee and outline needs of the individual to maintain or restore function impaired as a result of the injury or illness or to replace services the evaluee is no longer able to perform due to injury or illness-related impairment. Recommendations include both a comprehensive narrative description of each required product or service and a table that outlines the associated costs of the future care needs.

For each recommendation, a rationale is provided that outlines the evidence available from expert opinion or the research literature to justify the need for the product or service for the evaluee. The recommendations assume success; it is not reasonable, for example, to make a recommendation for the lifelong provision of regular physiotherapy intervention, as it is expected

Table 18.1 Life Care Plan Recommendation Areas

Area	Examples
Medical services	Costs for medical or surgical consultations or procedures that are not covered by government health insurance programs, for example, cosmetic surgery
Medications	Prescription medicines
	Over-the-counter medications recommended by health practitioners
Supplies	Medical or health-related supplies such as incontinence products or wound dressings
Health professional evaluations and interventions	Assessments and interventions recommended by health professionals, for example, occupational therapy, physiotherapy, and psychology
Adaptive equipment	Assistive devices and other equipment recommended by health professionals, for example, home exercise equipment and mobility aids
Architectural renovations	Modifications needed to improve accessibility to the home or work environment of the evaluee
Housekeeping and home maintenance support	Services required by the evaluee such as home handyman assistance, house cleaning, outdoor maintenance, and contractors
Health maintenance	Services needed to promote the health and well-being of the evaluee, such as membership in a fitness program
Vocational	Supports needed to promote the evaluee's involvement in productive activities, such as tuition costs for a retraining program
Avocational	Supports needed to promote the evaluee's involvement in leisure and recreation activities, such as costs for trialling a new hobby or interest
Other goods and services	Other services and products needed to support the evaluee in life activities, for example, services of an accountant for an individual no longer able to complete an annual tax return
Transportation	Costs incurred by the evaluee to travel for medical or rehabilitation intervention

the service will no longer be required when the treatment is successful. Recommendations are therefore often staged according to phases an individual may encounter over time when living with an impairment. The life care plan clearly outlines the start and end dates, as well as the frequency for the provision of the required services and products. Overprogramming or duplication of services is avoided to ensure recommendations are both reasonable and feasible.

The costing of the recommendations is based on average pricing received from different local sources and includes maintenance and replacement fees. Costs are not included for items considered to be in general use by Canadians, for example, smartphones, or services provided free through government programs, such as medical consultations and hospital care. Extraordinary care that is voluntarily provided by family and other caregivers is costed according to the market value of the services.

Evaluation

The quality of a life care plan is integral to the overall credibility, acceptance, and usefulness of the document. The quality of the life care plan also impacts the reputation of the creator of the report and, potentially, future work and viability of the career of the life care planner. Adopting a continuous quality improvement approach allows life care planners to evaluate their work on an ongoing basis to learn from their experiences in developing life care plans and implement practices that promote quality and value in the services they provide.

Quality is a multidimensional concept, with many factors that may be measured when evaluating the work of a planner in the development of a life care plan. The Quality Evaluation Strategy Tool (QUEST) outlines a framework with core indicators that measure seven dimensions of quality (World Federation of Occupational Therapists, 2020). Quality dimensions evaluated by QUEST include appropriateness, sustainability, accessibility, efficiency, effectiveness, person-centredness, and safety, as outlined in Table 18.2. By reviewing the performance of the life care planner relating to these dimensions, a comprehensive perspective of the quality of service is provided.

Appropriateness

Appropriateness refers to the provision of the 'right' service, to the 'right' person, at the 'right' place and time that is dependent upon the competency of the life care planner. Competency can be measured by whether the life care planner is qualified to prepare life care plans, as evidenced

Table 18.2 QUEST Quality Dimensions

Quality Dimension	Definition
Appropriateness	Competency to deliver the right services, at the right time, to the right person, in the right place.
Sustainability	The ability to extend services into the future by using resources today without compromising the health of current or future generations.
Accessibility	The ease of obtaining services from a physical, financial, or social perspective.
Efficiency	The optimal use of resources in service delivery to yield maximum benefits.
Effectiveness	The degree of achieving desired outcomes is reliant on the provision of evidence-informed services to those who could benefit.
Person-centredness	The ability to meet legitimate expectations of people receiving services.
Safety	The degree to which reduction of risk and avoidance of harm is considered in the provision of services.

by certification as a life care planner with the ICHCC. Assessing competence also involves reflection on knowledge gaps and new learning gained during the life care plan preparation. Such reflection helps to identify and prioritize needs for future professional development.

Sustainability

This measures the degree to which access to services and resources is possible without compromising future availability. Life care plans need to address the long-term needs of evaluees; attention is required to ensure services and resources are available not only for initial rehabilitation needs but throughout the life course of the evaluee. Appropriate support is needed to ensure the evaluee can participate in the required and desired activities outlined in the life care plan. Consideration is also necessary whether the life care plan addresses sustainable economic, social, and environmental outcomes, for example, by reviewing the origin, production, and sustainability of recommended equipment and services to choose local or low-carbon alternatives.

Accessibility

Accessibility relates to the ease of obtaining services from a physical, financial, or social perspective. Measures of accessibility of life care planning services include the ability of the life care planner to meet agreed-upon timelines for the development of the life care report, charge fees consistent with market prices, and be flexible for required meetings with the evaluee and treatment team members.

Efficiency

This quality dimension evaluates the degree to which time and other resources of the life care planner are used optimally to yield maximum benefits. Efficiency can be measured by the number of hours required by the life care planner to complete the life care plan report. Although the time required varies with the complexity of the report, the measure should closely approximate the estimate provided to the referring party.

Effectiveness

This is dependent upon the use of evidence to inform the life care plan. Evidence from expert opinion or peer-reviewed research, assessed within the context of evaluee priorities, should underlie all recommendations of the life care plan.

Person-Centredness

This addresses the ability of the life care planner to meet the legitimate needs of the evaluee. Person-centredness is present when the life care plan considers the unique requirements and priorities of the evaluee to develop feasible and credible recommendations.

Safety

Safety considers the degree to which reduction of risk and avoidance of harm are considered by the life care planner. The evaluation examines how risks identified for the safety of the evaluee are addressed in the life care plan, for example, to avoid the onset of complications and promote health and well-being.

Critiquing Life Care Plans

There are instances where life care planners are called upon to critique the report of another life care planner. The purpose of the critique is to understand weaknesses in the reviewed life care plan. A critique focuses on the degree to which the report meets the goal of life care planning in terms of identifying what goods and services are needed and their associated costs, based on the evaluee's injury or impairment. For example, in conducting the review, items may be found to be missing, excessive, or minimized. Comments of the critique are limited to the quality of the life care plan and should not be used to attack the personal integrity of the report author. Table 18.3 identifies areas and questions that may be considered when conducting the critique.

Vocational Rehabilitation Considerations in the Life Care Plan

Dr. Paul Deutsch, widely known in the field of rehabilitation for his founding work in life care planning, noted that

> For most, work is a fundamental aspect of an adult's identity, sense of purpose, social interaction, and sense of community. In addition to recognizing the important psychosocial aspect of work, a vocational analysis is a critical component of a comprehensive assessment of the economic damages in both catastrophic and non-catastrophic cases.
>
> (Deutsch, 2012)

According to Human Resources and Skills Development Canada (2012), work is among the indicators of well-being in Canada, with employment being "the main source of income for most Canadians and their families, enabling them to satisfy basic needs and pursue other interests. Individuals may derive a sense of purpose and accomplishment from their work" (Work—Overview Indicators of Well-being in Canada, 2012). In a working paper series from the University of British Columbia (Helliwell, 2002), being unemployed rather than working is said to lower one's subjective well-being, or measure of how a person experiences their quality of life which, in turn, is evidenced to be mutually influential on good health (Diener & Chan, 2011).

Exploration and support of an individual's vocational rehabilitation are considered a warranted component of successful rehabilitation and future care costs that may need to be included in the life care plan. Fundamental questions require consideration, such as: Is the individual medically capable of a return to work in some capacity? Or does the severity of the injury preclude a return to work? Examples of some possible vocational entries in a life care plan are outlined in Table 18.4.

Vocational rehabilitation can enable a person with an impairment or disability to assume a role as a worker, most often with very specific services and resources in place. Examples of service recommendations could include transferable skills analysis, vocational assessment, career exploration, job skills and job search training, job coaching, job placement assistance, vocational counseling, and labor market research. These services can occur individually on a standalone basis or in various combinations as the vocational consultant deems appropriate for the individual's needs.

In most cases, the vocational recommendations are provided through the case manager or certified rehabilitation counselor (CRC) for the costs to be included in the plan. In some cases, a vocational assessment has already been conducted.

Damages for loss of future earning capacity are identified when an individual's injuries result in permanent physical or mental disabilities or if there is a real or substantial possibility that the individual will suffer a loss of income-earning capacity in the future as a result of injuries sustained in the accident.

Table 18.3 Critique Areas of Review

Area	Questions
File review	• Have all available and relevant records describing the evaluee both before and after the injury been noted in the report?[1] • Given the scope of the review and the age of the information reviewed, was the current functioning of the evaluee reflected in the planner's summary profile? • If baseline data describing evaluee functioning was incomplete, did the planner request additional evaluations, for example, neuro-cognitive testing, auditory processing evaluations, another sensory testing, neuro-ophthalmological testing?
Plan structure and accuracy	• Did the planner accurately summarize the evaluee's current health status and abilities, as well as tasks that required the help of another person? • Did the planner accurately differentiate between deficits in function attributable solely to the disabling injury and areas of function that had no relationship to the disabling injury? • Were the planner's assertions about evaluee functioning consistent with opinions available in file records? • Does the file review developed by the planner identify the past medical needs as documented in available records? • Does the life care plan include recommendations with a narrative explanation, as well as cost tables?
Evaluation methods	• Did the planner demonstrate a comprehensive understanding of the evaluee's skill levels and ability to participate in functional activities? • As a result of this development of this understanding, could the planner definitively identify the appropriate amount of time and staffing levels needed to keep the evaluee safe, risk-free, and healthy? • Did the planner determine the effect of the disability on the evaluee's psychological functioning? • Did the planner collect information about the caregiver's emotional and health status to determine the extent of potential caregiver burn-out?
Foundation	• Were qualified health care practitioners consulted about the resources recommended in the report to ensure technical consultation was received in areas outside of the planner's area of expertise? • Were providers asked to opine on the future need for resources dictated by the processes of life transitions, changes in living arrangements, and aging? • Did the planner's file contain a record of all questions or correspondence directed to each provider as well as proof of answers given by the provider? • Did the planner identify sources of information for recommendations?
Costing	• Was each resource adequately supported by the file review, assessment findings, collaboration with the medical and rehabilitation team, or the expertise of the planner? • Were the costs identified for an appropriate level of care, for example, was a companion rather than a personal care worker considered? • Was each resource recommended described with sufficient detail? Are there large allowances with no breakdown? • Were the cost calculations provided by the planner correct? • Were there any cost overlaps? • Were the costs based on provincial averages rather than by geographical region? • Did the planner *include* every resource the evaluee needed? • Did the planner *exclude* resources that the evaluee needed?

Table 18.4 Sample of Vocational Entries in a Life Care Plan

Item/Service	Recommended By	Used For	Unit Cost	Replacement Frequency	Duration
Vocational Assessment	Vocational Consultant	Identification of interests, abilities, and aptitudes for retraining to secure employment	$2,500.00	One Time	3–6 hours
Career Exploration/Job Search Training	Vocational Consultant	Choosing a realistic employment goal and preparing for re-entry to the job market.	$2,500.00	One Time	25-hour program over 6–8 weeks.
Office Administration at Community	Vocational Consultant	If chooses an administrative type of occupation she will require basic skills.	$1,965.30	One Time	Three months—some courses available online
Driver Assessment and Rehabilitation Program	Vocational Consultant	If chooses a job driving a school bus or a type of disabled transportation vehicle, she will receive specific training from the company. However, a driving desensitization program would be advisable, as she expressed a certain amount of anxiety about driving since her accident.	On-Road Assessment $300–$1,000 In-vehicle lessons from $60–$150 per lesson. Timing and number of lessons to be determined by OT following assessment.	One Time	To be determined
Vocational Case Management	Vocational Consultant	Ongoing guidance and assistance throughout the job search process. Suggest ways to overcome employment barriers and how to maximize the potential for obtaining employment.	$2,000–$2,500 This represents 20–25 hours for $100 per hour. Transportation and HST would be additional.	One Time	Four to five months while she searches for employment.

Expert Witness Testimony

An expert has been defined as "a person with the status of an authority (in a subject) because of special skill, training or knowledge; a specialist" (Oxford English Dictionary). An "expert" in a legal case is someone who has special skill, knowledge, training, or experience, such that their observations and opinions will assist the ultimate decision-maker (a judge or jury) in adjudicating a legal case.

Duties of the Expert Witness

Canadian courts have accepted the duty of experts as set out in a 1993 decision by Cresswell, a British judge, in a case known as The Ikarian Reefer. Acting as an expert is an important role and one that should provide the court with the specialist and impartial input to be able to decide a case. It is not for experts to be advocates or make decisions that are the preserve of the court, but to maintain an independent professional advisory role at all times (What Expert Witnesses Can Learn from Judgements . . . ., 2019).

Justice Moore of the Ontario Superior Court of Justice in 2010 summarized the duties of experts as follows:

1. Expert evidence (2019) presented to the Court should be, and should be seen to be, the independent product of the expert uninfluenced as to form or content by the exigencies of litigation . . .
2. An expert witness should provide independent assistance to the Court by way of objective unbiased opinion about matters within his [or her] expertise. . .. An expert witness . . . should never assume the role of an advocate.
3. An expert witness should state the facts or assumptions upon which his [or her] opinion is based. He [or she] should not omit to consider material facts which could detract from his [or her] concluded opinion.
4. An expert witness should make it clear when a particular question or issue falls outside his [or her] expertise.
5. If an expert's opinion is not properly researched because he [or she] considers [there to be] . . . insufficient data . . . available, then this must be stated with an indication that the opinion is no more than a provisional one. . .. In cases where an expert witness who has prepared a report could not assert that the report contained the truth, the whole truth and nothing but the truth without some qualification, that qualification should be stated in the report. (Frazer v. Haukioja, 2008 CanLII 42207 (ON SC), 2008)

Duties of the Life Care Planner as an Expert

Life care planners are considered to be experts as they have special skills, training, and experience to produce life care plans. When serving as an expert, the duty of a planner is to the court and limited to providing an opinion within the area of expertise of life care planning. Experts must rely on what is written in their report at trial and cannot testify outside their expertise area. For example, a life care planner cannot make a diagnosis or provide a prognosis. As noted by Justice Moore in the Expert Witness Issues in *Frazer v. Haukioja* (Frazer v. Haukioja, 2008 CanLII 42207 (ON SC), 2008).

[162] The life care planner "was brought forward to opine on G's care needs and associated costs. Her proposed evidence gave rise to a concern regarding its impartiality and also whether she is qualified to give evidence as an expert at all. The court ruled that she was not qualified to speak to care needs beyond her particular area of expertise.

[163] The court should not need to take the time to review the proposed evidence of any expert to determine whether the witness is qualified to offer the evidence. That is a function of the role of the expert. The court expects the expert to know his or her professional limitations and expects the expert to decline to speak to matters beyond them.

[164] Although much of the evidence that she proposed to give was not received, it must be said of the proposed care needs and costs that she assembled referencing treatments, therapies, goods, and services, not one of the medical experts at trial stated that any listed need was either reasonable or necessary and in G's best interests. There was no evidence either to explain why the itemized list had not been presented to and funding claimed from G's health care or motorcycle insurers over the past seven years. The objectivity of the author of such a summary in the context of the medical evidence at the trial of this action must be questioned."

The life care planner in this case ventured out of her area of expertise, and as a consequence of that, her evidence was not accepted.

Vallance v. Vallance [1994] B.C.J. No. 3288 (S.C.) is a British Columbia case that also illustrates the principle that experts must stay within their area of expertise or risk having their opinions ruled inadmissible. The expert described himself as an expert in "orthopaedic and spinal surgery". The following passage was ruled inadmissible because the life care planner ventured into the area of vocational expertise.

No harm or damage would accrue should she choose to return to her former work as a barmaid/waitress. However, she may find this work uncomfortable and may wish to consider alternative vocations requiring less lifting. Clearly, she is not totally disabled and many vocations are available in the guideline stated above. Vocational counseling may be helpful should she choose not to return to work in her former capacity.

All provinces in Canada without exception have rules regarding the duties and responsibilities of expert witnesses. The Ontario Rule 4.1.01 entitled "Duty of Expert" provides as follows:

4.1.01 (1) It is the duty of every expert engaged by or on behalf of a party to provide evidence concerning a proceeding under these rules, (a) to provide opinion evidence that is fair, objective, and non-partisan; (b) to provide opinion evidence that is related only to matters that are within the expert's area of expertise and (c) to provide such additional assistance as the court may reasonably require to determine a matter in issue.

Similar rules for experts can be found in Alberta Rules of Court, Rules 5.34–5.40 and Form 25; British Columbia Supreme Court Civil Rules, Rule 11–2; Nova Scotia Civil Procedure Rules, Rule 55.04; and Prince Edward Island Rules of Civil Procedure, Rule 53.03 and Form 53E. The Quebec Code of Civil Procedure, Art. 416–41816 is unique among provincial provisions relating to the duties of experts. All experts must swear to "perform [their] duties faithfully and impartially".[2]

When providing testimony at trial, the objective is to assist the trier of fact in deciding the facts based on testimony. In this role, the expert witness is providing facts that are pertinent to the case at hand without being an advocate for one side or the other. Life care planners do not advocate on behalf of any party involved in the court process and maintain the highest level of objectivity and professional integrity at all times. Practical recommendations outlined by DeMaio-Feldman (1987) for providing expert witness testimony are outlined in Table 18.5.

Table 18.5 Recommendations for Expert Witness Testimony

- Prepare all basic exhibits and outlines of testimony carefully, arranging them in an orderly sequence before taking the witness stand.
- Speak loud enough for all to hear and do not talk too fast. Endeavor to obtain and hold the interest of the judge or jury.
- Avoid unnecessary conversation with the judge or opposing counsel. Be courteous, fair, and frank. Keep calm and even-tempered, even in trying circumstances.
- State [your] qualifications fully, but without "puffing" or indulgence in the trivial. Do not be flattered by offers to concede qualifications; for this may be a ploy to prevent the judge or jury from learning important details.
- After reviewing [your] qualifications, state [your] results and opinions. Follow with a clear and adequate explanation of [the] methods employed in reaching [your] conclusions.
- Present testimony as you would wish to have it presented if you were the judge. Observe any doubts which may appear to arise in the judge['s] or jury's mind, and try to assist in resolving them. This, after all, is a primary function of an expert witness.
- Hold to the essentials of the testimony. Develop a sense of proportion. Avoid unimportant detail.
- Avoid the appearance of being an incorrigible partisan. Face up to the strong points which may be presented by opposing witnesses. Endeavor to demonstrate that, while those points should be given consideration, they must be viewed in the context of the total picture.
- If not prepared to answer a question, be honest enough to say so. A bluffer is easily detected, and then a cloud is cast over the entire testimony.
- Be concise. After a point is made, stop talking.

Summary

Life care plans serve as an integral tool for understanding the future services and products required by an individual following a serious injury or illness. Life care plans are designed to reduce disability, promote participation in productive activity, and ensure the best use of available funding and other resources needed for optimal quality of life following an injury or illness. The reports are useful for the affected individuals and their caregivers, as well as for the courts to ensure required services and products are available as needed over time and throughout the life span.

Life care plans in Canada are prepared by Certified Life Care Planners who meet competency standards established by the ICHCC. A multiple-step process is followed to develop life care plans, grounded in fundamental tenets, such as the need for objectivity, evidence-informed practice, credibility, comprehensiveness, ethical behaviour, and person-centredness. The process culminates in a series of recommendations that address a broad range of issues to enhance independence and function, promote health and prevent future complications, and provide assistance for activities an individual can no longer manage as a result of injury or illness. An evaluation of the quality of services of the life care planner is the final step of the life care planning process. The evaluation promotes learning and continuous improvement needed to advance professional development and ensure the maintenance of standards of practice within the life care planning profession.

Notes

1 Records can include vocational rehabilitation records, school records, home health records, medical records of care received prior to the accident, medical records of all care received after the accident from any provider, employment records prior to and after the accident, psychological testing prior to and after the accident, neuro-cognitive testing, school records prior to and after the accident, recent records of community providers, and any applications for benefits in those records.
2 www.canlii.org/en/#search/text=expert%20witness%20rules%20in%20canadian%20provinces

References

DeMaio-Feldman, D. (1987). The occupational therapist as an expert witness. *The American Occupational Therapy Journal*, *47*(9), 590–596.

Deutsch, P. M. (n.d.). *Vocational analysis* (2012). Paul M. Deutsch & Associates, PA. n.p. www.paulm-deutsch.com/services-vocational-analysis.htm

Diener, E., & Chan, M. Y. (2011). Happy people live longer: Subjective well-being contributes to health and longevity. *Applied Psychology: Health and Well-Being, 3*(1), 1–43. https://doi.org/10.1111/j.1758-0854.2010.01045.x

Expert Evidence. (2019). *What expert witnesses can learn from judgments*. Expert Evidence. expert-evidence.com

Frazer v. Haukioja. (2008). CanLII 42207 (ON SC), paragraph 141, <https://canlii.ca/t/20hfp>. Retrieved June 28, 2022, from www.canlii.org/en/on/onsc/doc/2008/2008canlii42207/2008canlii42207.html?resultIndex=1

Helliwell, J. F. (2002, July). How's life? Combining individual and national variables to explain subjective well-being. *NBER Working Paper Series*. National Bureau of Economic Research. Print.

Human Resources and Skills Development Canada. *Work—overview*. *Indicators of Well-being in Canada*. HRSDC. Updated June 10, 2012. Web. June 10, 2012.

International Association of Rehabilitation Professionals (IARP). (2015). *Standards of practice for life care planners* (3rd ed.). International Academy of Life Care Planners, IARP.

Morrison, S. A., Pomeranz, J. L., Yu, N., Read, M. S., Sisto, S. A., & Behrman, A. L. (2012). Life care planning projections for individuals with motor incomplete spinal cord injury before and after locomotor training intervention: A case series. *Journal of Neurologic Physical Therapy: JNPT*, *36*(3), 144–153. https://doi-org.proxy.library.vcu.edu/10.1097/NPT.0b013e318262e5abwww.ichcc.org/images/PDFs/Practice-Standards-and-Guidelines-2020.pdf Oxford English Dictionary

The International Commission on Health Care Certification. (2021). Qualified health care professional. *Practice Standards and Guidelines*, *21*, 11. https://ichcc.org/images/PDFs/Standards_and_Guidelines.pdf

World Federation of Occupational Therapists. (2020). *Quality evaluation strategy tool*. WFOT.

19 Functional Capacity Evaluation

Process, Utility, and Life Care Planning and Case Management Applications

Virgil Robert May III

Life care planners and case managers are challenged daily with providing appropriate service implementation and making decisions in the best interest of their clients, whether clients are defined as being health care benefit providers who pay for services or the disabled individual in question (Matkin & May, 1981). Life care planners are charged with evaluating the medical services and rehabilitative services and to determine the independent living potential and needs for the disabled individual (Busch, 2017). The life care plan offered by life care planners is considered a "comprehensive document that objectively identifies the residual medical conditions and ongoing care requirements of ill/injured individuals; Individuals with requisite, medically-related goods and services throughout probable durations of care" (Gonzales, 2017, p. 13).

Life care planners should not assume the role of a case manager, as there may evolve an ethical conflict of service provision should a life care planner agree to provide case management services to the disabled individual of whom she or he wrote and prepared a life care plan. Such a conflict could be challenged by an opposing counsel that could result in the nullification of the life care plan. The provision of case management services could place the life care planner in an advocacy role to benefit the disabled person, and his or her testimony could be challenged as being biased by opposing counsel.

Simply put, life care planners cannot serve as advocates for either their referral source (i.e., insurance benefit provider, defense counsel), who may be their client by definition, or the disabled person in question, who may have been referred by the attending physician, hospital, or independent medical facility without imbursement obligations for services. The obligation of the life care planner is to present a thorough, unbiased life care plan to the referral source that is evidenced-based and well documented regarding the need for medical services and supplies, rehabilitative services, and home health services that may address home modifications for a more barrier-free environment. The International Commission on Health Care Certification (ICHCC), the certifying body for health care professionals of varying health care–related training and formal academic degrees in the United States and Canada, noted in its Principles and Associated Rules that certificants shall serve as *advocates* for fair and balanced reporting regardless of the referral source, with the health, care, and safety of people with disabilities not to be compromised as a result of a submitted respective report. Rule 3.1 of the ICHCC's Principles reads:

> The ICHCC certificants shall further use his or her specialized knowledge and skills to do no harm to the "disabled" individual with regards to the summary and conclusions of reporting, regardless of the referral source.

(p. 30)

DOI: 10.4324/b23293-19

Regarding case managers, advocacy for disabled clients is acceptable and expected. The Commission on Certified Case Managers (CCMC) mandates in the CCMC Code of Professional Conduct that the case manager is an "advocate" for the disabled client, ensuring that a comprehensive assessment will identify the client's needs, options for necessary services will be provided to the client, and clients are provided with access to resources to meet individual needs. The reality of the case management position in rehabilitation is that it has obligations to many individuals outside of the recipient of services that may include but not be limited to the injured/disabled person's family, medical professionals, treating physicians, therapists, attorneys (plaintiff and/or defense), the employer, community resources, and in most cases, a claims adjuster or nurse case manager from the insurance company (Pressman, 2007).

One pressing challenge added to the compendium of service delivery challenges is the case manager's ability to balance clinical services and post-rehabilitative discharge services (i.e., return-to-work services) with that of cost (Carr, 2005). To satisfy this balance, the case manager often engages the use of evidence-based criteria in all rehabilitative-related decisions (Carr). Similarly, life care planners are encouraged to consider the usual, customary, and reasonable (UCR) price for services in order to effectively project the monetary value of future services and care within a life care plan (Busch, 2017). More third-party health care insurance benefit providers are demanding of life care planners as well as of case managers that evidence-based management processes be implemented in life care plans and case management paradigms. The goal-oriented results are that life care planners and case managers can validate appropriate care with quality indicators, checklists, reporting, alignment of case management protocols with the Centers for Medicare & Medicaid Services (CMS) guidelines, improve quality of case management service delivery with more time for patient care, and drive appropriate care with rule-based, patient-specific decision support using evidence-based medicine.

The continuum of care for individual cases may include the hospital (emergency room [ER], intensive care unit [ICU[, and acute care), rehabilitation hospital (inpatient), home health services, and outpatient therapy center (physiotherapy, occupational therapy, or combination of therapies) (Tigerman, 2012). One valuable evidence-based service available to the life care planners and case managers is the functional capacity evaluation (FCE), designed to be used in various rehabilitative settings, such as in therapy clinics for documentation of rehabilitation goal achievement, in work hardening programs for progress documentation of work activity stressors and physical tolerances, and in litigation resulting from work injury or personal injury. The FCE offers the life care planner and case manager a means for determining the injured client's propensity to achieve their rehabilitative program goals, their capability for independent functioning and activities of daily living skills retention, their feasibility for returning to the competitive labor market as well as their most suitable occupational category, and the overall effect their injuries may have on disability and impairment (Cheng & Cheng, 2010; King et al., 1998; Matheson, 2003; Roy, 2003; Streibelt et al., 2009). The primary benefit of the FCE to life care planners is that their life care plans can address residual income losses/gains and determine the potential for the disabled individual to live independently as well as determine the quality of one's executive functions.

Definition and Historical Perspective

An FCE is defined as a systematic method of measuring one's ability to perform meaningful tasks on a safe and dependable basis, with an emphasis on "safe" (Harper, 2010; Matheson, 2003). Dr. Lynn Matheson developed the protocols in the 1970s for the FCEs that are administered in today's health care environment, and his definition, as noted earlier, does not specify an application to the essential functions of work only, but leaves it open to include an assessment of one's activities of daily living. Regarding the essential functions of work, Dabatos et al. (2000) defined the FCE as a systematic, comprehensive, and objective measurement of an individual's maximum work abilities. They added that the FCE addresses the physical demands of work given that the FCE provides a detailed evaluation of an individual's functional level and performance abilities. Abdel-Moty (as cited in Roy, 2003) is more explicit in his interpretation of FCEs and supports Matheson's premise that FCEs have strong applications outside of essential job function capabilities.

Roy (2003) noted that physical, physiological, and functional measures are translated into performance potential for activities of daily living as well as work tasks.

Deconstructing the term "functional capacity evaluation" allows the life care planner and case manager a better understanding of the definition of FCE as well as comprehending its applications to various settings. The term *function* refers to the performance of a task that has a deliberate, meaningful, or useful goal with a beginning and end that has a result that can be measured (Isernhagen, 2009; Jahn et al., 2004; Matheson, 2003). For example, an examinee is requested to engage in the Work Evaluation Systems Technology (WEST) lift system due to the fact that the examinee's job requires that she or he access a vertical work plane from floor level to at least 78 inches from the floor while lifting between 10 and 35 pounds. The WEST incorporates a repeated lift cycle following a specific pattern (Ogden-Niemeyer, 1989).

The term *capacity* has a complex application to the FCE process and must be interpreted carefully by the life care planner and case manager while processing his or her client's test results. Simply put, capacity refers to the maximum lifting ability or capability of the examinee (Isernhagen, 2009). Capacity connotes that the individual engages in his or her maximum function in response to performing a task while demonstrating the ability to perform the task safely and efficiently. In essence, the thought of working to one's capacity requires one to work beyond their level of tolerance that is measured (Matheson, 2003). The life care planner and case manager should understand that capacity as applied to the FCE process is rarely achieved by an individual with an anatomical injury. An example of when capacity is achieved is best illustrated in athletic settings. Athletes, through their competitive nature and their desire to "make the team" or to win at a competitive sport, will function at maximum capacity more so than an individual who works over an 8- to 12-hour work day. Frequently, the functional capacity evaluator will state that the examinee performed at his or her maximum capacity as evident by the data result. In actuality, the life care planner and case manager should be aware that the examinee who gives his or her good or best effort actually gave his or her best or *maximum allowable effort*. This performance level is termed the examinee's tolerance for the demands of the task (Matheson, 2003). Thus, the maximum dependable ability of the examinee is usually less than his or her tolerance. What this means to the life care planner and case manager is that the individual's FCE performance with regard to one's capacity for physical work tasks may be at a lower performance level than his or her maximum dependable ability, which is lower than his or her tolerance, which ultimately is lower than his or her capacity. The determining factors of the worth of the FCE results as applied to one's capacity for safe functioning rests with the many uncontrolled factors that may influence one's demonstrated capacity within each of the FCE test components.

Evaluation as applied to the FCE process is a systematic approach used by the evaluator to gather test data designed to measure one's functional abilities (Matheson, 2003). This process requires the evaluator to administer standardized tests, collect data, and interpret data. More importantly, the evaluation requires the evaluator to present performance documentation in a report that the reader can understand and process, but more importantly, apply to the referral questions in an effort to achieve case management goals of that respective case. The evaluation process begins at the time the examinee enters the clinic waiting room, upon which the evaluator documents observed behaviors (i.e., pain, mechanical deficits in extremities, or postural discomfort behaviors). With the examinee set to engage in the actual test components, the evaluation requires the evaluator to document performance behaviors and achieved functional levels in manual muscle strength tests, collateral ratings, work-sample testing, materials handling and gait analysis, and simulated essential job function tasks. It is noteworthy that the life care planner and case manager can expect the evaluation process to include in its report not just the test scores but an outcome statement with functional applications identified, as well as objective criteria used to accept the test results as a valid representation of the examinee's true functional capabilities. The underlying benefit of the FCE to the life care planning and case management processes is that service providers now have access to evidence-based test protocols that can objectively address disabled individuals' abilities to function safely and competently in work settings and at home independently.

One must wonder: Why did such a comprehensive testing protocol that offers such detailed functional information about persons with different system injuries take so long to evolve for life care planners and case managers? Actually, the FCE evolved out of the post–World War II industrial development and the resulting increase in work-related injuries and disabilities (Dabatos et al., 2000). To accommodate the dramatic increase in work injuries and to ensure proper maintenance of health-appropriate behaviors, the American Medical Association (AMA) introduced the notion of systematic medical examinations in industry. At this time the U.S. Civil Service Commission was preparing a classification system of physically disabling conditions to be matched with compatible positions of employment available within the federal government. This was the first attempt to define work activities of the job that gave rise to the U.S. Department of Labor's *Dictionary of Occupational Titles*, a resource that is utilized and most valuable to today's FCE's protocols.

The AMA credits Dr. Bert Hanman with developing examination protocols for determining the physical capacity of injured workers in the latter 1950s (Dabatos et al., 2000; Jahn et al., 2004). He introduced the concepts of physical demands analysis (PDA) and functional capacity assessment (FCA) for physicians performing return-to-work examinations and implemented the concept of safety within the physician's physical work examination protocols (Hanman, 1958). A series of assessments evolved from the FCA that was designed to examine an individual's capacity to perform the physical tasks of the essential functions of work found in the PDA. Two components were addressed in this process that included the evaluation of medical fitness and the evaluation of work capacity (Dabatos et al.).

It was not until the late 1970s that the components of the FCE model practiced today evolved into the comprehensive objective test methodology that is accepted in state and federal courts and in damages negotiations (mediations) across the United States and courts in Canada, Australia, the Netherlands, and several European countries. Dr. Lynn Matheson, a vocational evaluator and rehabilitation counselor by training at the Rancho Los Amigos Hospital in Downey, California, at the time, researched and developed a work capacity evaluation protocol that evolved into the FCE that is offered today (Isernhagen, 2009; May & Martelli, 1999). Dr. Matheson continued his research and development at his training and research facility, the Employment and Rehabilitation Institute of California, where he eventually derived the FCE model that is practiced today (Matheson, 1984, 1987). Since Matheson's early developmental research of the FCE process, contributions to the FCE process have been made by occupational and physical therapists, as well as by vocational analysts and evaluators (Dabatos et al., 2000). Dr. Matheson provided training and residency programs for physical therapists, occupational therapists, and vocational evaluators interested in learning to administer FCEs through the Employment and

Rehabilitation Institute of California. By 1983 the first commercial FCE system became available, designed for physical and occupational therapists, and was called the Polinsky Functional Capacity Assessment (Isernhagen, 2009). Matheson's primary contribution was that he proved that work capacity could be measured, and as such FCE systems proliferated in the marketplace by the 1990s. It was this proliferation throughout the 1990s that saw FCE emerging as the objective test and measurement approach to matching physical abilities with critical job demands, targeting treatment goals to justify work-hardening therapy, identifying job modifications to enhance worker safety, and delineating functional capacities in cases of litigation and disability determination (Dabatos et al.). A listing of FCE commercial systems that evolved from the 1990s is illustrated in Table 19.1 (King et al., 1998).

FCE Utility

The term *utility* as applied to the FCE is the most important characteristic of a test measure, and it represents what value the test has to the referral source (Matheson, 2003). In essence, the referral source utilizes the FCE in an attempt to answer specific referral questions that may seek evidence of the injured worker's functional competency to tolerate the essential functions of jobs or to perform activities of daily living (Soer et al., 2009). These results may be utilized to address the client's functional capacity within a particular occupational category or in the general competitive labor market without concern for specific jobs and to determine the individual's competency for independent living with a focus on activities of daily living performance. FCE data can be used to establish functional baselines and therapeutic treatment goals and to monitor one's progress in a work-hardening or physical therapy program. The FCE can disclose one's propensity to magnify symptoms as well as determine the appropriate and inappropriate factors of one's overall non-physiological performance. Most importantly, however, is that the FCE can be used to determine the examinee's current ability to return to work safely and support the physician's assessment regarding maximum medical improvement (MMI) leading to the need for case closure (Dabatos et al., 2000).

Life care planners and case managers should understand that the utility of any FCE is predicated on the validity and reliability of the FCE multicomponent tests used by the evaluator (Matheson, 2003). Although several noted clinical authors documented the FCE as being that of a "systematic, comprehensive, and objective [process] (Dabatos et al., 2000; Hart et al., 1993; Jahn et al., 2004), the term "objective" only applies to the evaluation results if the FCE model components utilize tests that have peer-reviewed and published validity and reliability data. Without the utilization of validated test components, the FCE results have weak applications to the referral questions and, in fact, may not have any defensible application at all. The most serious threats to the utility of the FCE process for the life care planner and case manager refer to the reliability of the instrument that restricts the validity of its components for all applications. Validity is established when the test is determined to measure the properties that it purports to measure and thus can be used to make inferences regarding functional and worker trait factors (King et al., 1998). There are six validity types that include face validity, content validity, construct validity, criterion validity, concurrent validity, and predictive validity (Reneman et al., 2009). Each of these is presented in detailed description enumerated next as defined by Reneman et al.:

1. Face Validity: The apparent ability of an assessment to measure what it intends to measure via a seemingly plausible method of doing so (p. 402).
2. Content Validity: The degree to which test items represent the performance domain the test is intended to measure, i.e., ability to work (p. 402).

Table 19.1 Commercial FCE Systems

FCE System	Developer	No. of Years Available	Full or Module Format	Length of Assessment	Length of Report	Validity and Reliability	Peer-Reviewed Published Research	Standardized Instruction Manual
Blankenship	Keith Blankenship	18	Unknown	2.5–4 hr	30 min with software	Based on published medical research	No	No
IWS	Susan Isernhagen	15	Full format, modified available for specific requests	5h over 2d; modified—3h over 2-part period	20–45 min to dictate; software available	No	Yes	Yes
Ergo Science (PWPE)	Deborah Lechner	9	Both	3–4 h	30 min (less time with software)	Yes[10]	Yes	Yes
WEST-Epic (Cal-FCP	Leonard Matheson	9	Both	All 5 components = 2 h	Cal-FCP=5 min; WEST-Epic=15 min; Software available	Validity and reliability tests on lifting capacity only	Yes	Yes
WorkAbility Mark III	GC Heyde and J Shervinton	11	Both	2–4 h	2 h with software package	No	No	Yes
WorkHab	David Roberts and Sam Bradbury	5.5	Both	2–3.5 h	1.5–2 h; software available	No	No	Yes
AssessAbility	Michael Coupland	6	Both	2 h	...	Based on methods-time measurement standards and research	No	Yes
ARCON	Dana Rasch	15	Both	2h	...	No	Yes	Yes
ERGOS	Work Recovery Inc.	15	Both	4 h	40 min	Reliability and validity studies performed	Yes	Yes
Key	Glenda Key	17	Both	3.5–4 h	15–20 min with software	Yes	No	Yes

Source: Used with permission of the American Medical Association. King, P., Tuckwell, N., & Barrett, T. (1998). pp 852–866 ©Copyright American Medical Association (1998).

3. Construct Validity: The extent to which a test can be shown to measure a hypothetical construct. For example, an FCE may be considered to have some support for construct validity if it is able to differentiate between examinees who are able to lift safely and examinees who are not able to do so, when the construct being measured is "safe lifting ability." "Discriminate validity" is often referred to as this type of validity, when the test results successfully discriminate between groups, such as those persons with lumbar disc/vertebral body injuries vs. those persons with knee (ligament tears) injuries.

4. Criterion Validity: The systematic demonstration of the extent to which test performance is related to some other valued measure of performance or eternal criterion. For example, the grip strength measures using the JAMAR dynamometer refer to the strength output data of persons grouped by gender and age. Results offered by the JAMAR are based on the criterion of hand strength previously measured, thus assuring that the JAMAR dynamometer grip strength system has criterion-related validity. Criterion validity is composed of two other types of validity: concurrent and predictive validity. It is this validity that is considered to be the most practical approach to validity testing as well as being the most objective (p. 403).

5. Concurrent Validity: The correlation between two or more measures given to the same subject at approximately the same time, with both presumably reflecting the same ability or behavior.

6. Predictive Validity: The degree to which an examinee's performance at the initial time of testing accurately predicts performance obtained at a future date as measured by another highly valued performance-measured process or "gold standard." Regarding the FCE, the ability to predict the examinee's success in returning to work is a common and valued utility and criterion on which the FCE is valued.

Reliability refers to the extent to which repeated measurements of a single test in healthy persons produce similar results (Reneman et al., 2009). These test scores should be reproducible across evaluators and the date and time of test administration. Using the JAMAR dynamometer as an example, a single examinee should produce similar maximum grip strength output across all five handle positions at three test trials per handle position, with symmetrical strength curves between both hands. These results are expected to occur between two raters or evaluators (interrater reliability), over time (test-retest reliability), between more than one identical FCE session rated by the same evaluator (intrarater reliability), or between equivalent parts of the same test (internal consistency) (Reneman et al.). The two most important types of reliability include interrater reliability and test-retest reliability (King et al., 1998). However, from a practical application, the most utilized reliability test is the test-retest reliability. It is often that an examinee is evaluated long before his or her case comes to resolution, whether that resolution is in terms of the examinee returning to work or participating in litigation with scheduled mediation or trial. The examinee needs to be re-evaluated prior to a return-to-work case resolution due to the attending physician requiring an updated evaluation so that return-to-work criteria (restrictions) can be current before releasing the patient. From the litigation side, a re-examination is necessary to update the examinee's current functional status, and the same evaluator is asked often to rate the examinee a second time to ensure functional data are current and accurate as well as reliable. Thus, test-retest reliability is the key component for providing accurate functional data over extended periods of time. Bear in mind that reliability as applied to the FCE process identifies the effort of an individual to complete a test component. A less than "best" or maximum allowable effort may result in excessive variances among repeated test measurements, leading to unacceptable reliability coefficients. Such violations of the testing process negate the test's validity in that it is no longer measuring what it purports to measure due to the uncontrolled factors, which usually present with a false-negative result. Thus, the FCE with poor reliability resulting in indefensible validity negates the application of any test results in terms of one's work feasibility, work-related restrictions, MMI status, and disability benefits award.

Matheson (2003) documented that utility is very difficult to achieve and is threatened by many variables of which the life care planner and case manager should be aware. One significant tenet of FCE is that the testing protocol is a poor predictor of return to work, and normative values to which FCE results can be compared are non-existent (Cheng & Cheng, 2010, 2011; Gross & Battié, 2004, 2006; Gross et al., 2004; Harper, 2010; Streibelt et al., 2009). There have been studies to determine the predictive value of the FCE regarding one's ability to return to work as well as studies to establish normative values regarding FCE results. Cheng and Cheng (2010) studied the predictive ability of the job-specific FCE for 713 patients diagnosed with non-specific lower back pain. Their findings showed that the length of the patient's disability period (defined as from day of injury to FCE), plus the patient having a compensable injury that included medical and supplemental income benefits, and the higher the physical demand characteristic of the job to which the patient was to return significantly reduced the predictive ability of FCE. Gross et al. studied 114 patients with a diagnosis of a work-related lower back injury in an effort to predict return-to-work competency of those who successfully completed FCE. Their results showed that a good performance on the FCE was not a valid predictor of a faster recovery time. Only 5 patients passed all of the FCE tests, and yet 95% of the 114 participants had their temporary total disability benefits suspended; failing FCE functional components demonstrated no correlation with patients who failed the tests and perhaps required additional rehabilitative or medical management. There were 25 tasks assigned to the FCE model used in this study, and only one task, the floor to waist lift, appeared to predict a person's capability to return to work more so than all other 24 tests combined. Gross and Battié studied 224 patients with work-related lower back injuries regarding the predictive ability of the FCE readiness or the ability of these subjects to return safely to work. They concluded that the FCE performance as indicated by a lower number of failed FCE tasks was associated with higher risk of reinjury once temporary total disability benefits had been suspended and patients returned to their prior jobs. They further concluded that the validity of the FCE's purported ability to identify claimants who are deemed "safe" to return to work per their performance on the FCE is suspect at best. Cheng and Cheng (2011) had better success with their study of 194 examinees with the diagnosis of a distal radius fracture while evaluated using a job-specific FCE model. Their results showed that a job-specific FCE resulted in better predictive validity in relation to the return to work of patients with a specific injury than of patients with a non-specific injury. Similar to their earlier study, their later study concluded that a longer period from injury to FCE and compensable injury reduce the predictive ability of job-specific FCE. Regarding predicting one's ability to sustain employment once he or she returned post medical release, Streibelt et al. concluded that their study of 220 patients with chronic musculoskeletal disorders showed that the predictive ability of FCE models was poor, the predictive efficiency of models was low, and sustained return to work could not be proved.

Regarding the establishment of normative data for FCE, Soer et al. (2009) attempted to gain normative values for an FCE testing a sample of 701 healthy, non-injured, and non-disabled workers. Their study resulted in the establishment of norm values for materials handling, postural tolerance (overhead working and forward bending while standing), and repetitive coordination of the hands. However, they documented the limitations of the study and suggested that the normative values should be used as guides rather than as "rules" that are without direct application to work.

Life care planners and case managers should not avoid the utilization of FCEs in their practices because of what research has concluded about the predictability of FCEs and the lack of normative data applications for the total FCE results of a respective client. The FCE's utility is not subject to just predictability, but rather it has many other beneficial characteristics that may contribute to a timely resolution of a respective case as well as help the life care planner identify an item of need that may otherwise have gone overlooked. The FCE uses and applications may be applied to many case management goals for functional clients who need case closure who have experienced extended disability periods. Involving clients in FCE processes can prove beneficial to the life care planner providing a summary vocational/educational needs and the case manager, which include but are not limited to the following:

1. *Case Management Return-to-Work vs. Disability Case Goal Setting*: FCE testing can determine whether the respective injured client has the capability to perform essential job functions within the competitive labor market, or whether the client is absent of abilities to perform work-simulated activities involved in gainful employment, placing the client in a category of disability. The case manager can determine case goals earlier in the case management process with the early application of an FCE, determining whether case management protocols should focus on rehabilitation with eventual return-to-work or on acquiring an appropriate disability level (Isernhagen, 2009). Similarly, the life care planner can determine if a vocational category of need is necessary, and if it is, what vocational services/education is justifiable (i.e., supported employment, work shop, vocational technical training).
2. *Work Modifications*: The FCE can assist in determining appropriate work-site modifications that would allow the client access to the competitive labor market (Isernhagen, 2009; Roy, 2003). The FCE can match physical abilities with critical job demands and thus can be used in identifying work environmental and task modifications (Dabatos et al., 2000).
3. *Rehabilitation*: The FCE can determine the entry point for work-related rehabilitation, as in work-hardening program structuring and goal-setting (Isernhagen, 2009). More specifically, the FCE can assist the disabled individual and therapist to improve role performance through the identification of functional decrements so that they may be resolved through a work-structured physical therapy program or in a work-hardening therapy program (Harper, 2010; Matheson, 2003).
4. *Litigation:* The FCE provides data that assists in medicolegal consultations and negotiations among parties, with the life care planner's and case manager's role being that of a consultant (Roy, 2003). The FCE can determine the presence and, if present, the degree of disability so that bureaucratic entities (i.e., administrative law judges) can assign, apportion, or deny financial and medical disability benefits and circuit court judges and juries can award or deny monetary settlements received through tort actions (Matheson, 2003).

FCE Influencers

The FCE evaluator may use a reliable and valid FCE model, but there remains no guarantee a valid and reliable performance will result from the test session. The life care planner and case manager should be aware that there are many uncontrolled variables that may influence the validity of the client's FCE performance results outside of the FCE protocol. One source of error that can nullify FCE results is that of the evaluator. The life care planner and case manager must do his or her homework regarding the evaluators working in one's local area, particularly with reference to their background, education, experience, and most importantly, their training in the FCE process. This begs the question of what health care specialty groups are best suited to administer FCEs. Currently, physicians, occupational therapists, physical therapists, vocational evaluators, kinesiologists, psychologists, and exercise physiologists are known evaluators, with most of the evaluations being administered by physical and occupational therapists (Isernhagen, 2009; Matheson, 2003). The FCE concept evolved out of vocational rehabilitation and has since been embraced by occupational therapists, who are accustomed to vocational evaluation concepts and tests/work samples (Isernhagen). What distinguishes a clinical therapist, physician, or vocational evaluator from one who administers FCEs is the post-graduate training they have completed over their careers in the FCE process. There are several FCE training programs in today's marketplace, and these include the National Association of Disability Evaluation Professionals (NADEP) training, OccuPro FCE training, Roy Matheson FCE Training, JTECH FCE Training, and ERGO Science FCE Training. It is in the best interest of the case manager and the client that when choosing a program, the evaluator should have undergone training in one of these programs or at least in one that may be offered at a respective evaluator's professional annual conference.

Training in FCE does not guarantee that the evaluator is competent in the FCE model. The Council on Forensic Sciences, an affiliate of the American Chiropractic Association, identified that most FCE administrators are not sufficiently grounded in science, case law, and forensic issues (Jahn et al., 2004). The council cited such transgressions as involving evaluators misquoting standard journal articles and texts in their summaries, making false statements, providing "junk science" opinion and interpretations, and deliberately omitting important facts and knowledge in their reports. Although this is somewhat excessive maladaptive professional behavior, it behooves the life care planner and case manager to evaluate the reputation of the evaluating clinician who administers the FCE at any particular health care provider clinic or hospital in addition to reviewing the evaluator's post-graduate training in FCE.

The other significant threat to FCE reliability and validity is the disabled individual. Life care planners and case managers should understand that their clients' self-efficacy may be weak to a point that clients restrict themselves in functional tasks, whether those tasks are activities of daily living, functional test activities, or work activities. Self-efficacy is the belief and confidence an injured person has regarding his or her ability to perform a behavior or task (Asante et al., 2007). Efficacy expectations influence the degree of effort a patient with chronic pain or a chronic disability will expend in various activities (Kaplan et al., 1996). The life care planner and case manager, as well as the evaluator, should understand that the examinee more than likely has been told by their health care provider not to perform certain tasks or assume certain postures since their first post-injury examination. Thus, asking the client to perform tasks and assume postures they have not done or assumed since the day of their injury may have a devastating effect on their self-efficacy. The other component that may affect the examinee's performance is their perceived disability. Perceived disability refers to the level to which an individual believes his or her ability to perform a given task is limited due to a health condition such as back pain or joint pain in the extremities (Asante et al.). The difference between these two thought processes is that self-efficacy is a positive evaluation of oneself, while perceived disability is achieved through a negative evaluation (Asante et al.). Thus, both dimensions involve cognitive processing, assessment of the activity to be performed, awareness of physical health status, and previous experience with an activity or posture to be performed, as well as motivation (Asante et al.).

The life care planner and case manager need to consider other client factors that may contribute to an invalid performance outcome. The evaluator has responsibility for ensuring that a valid test is administered as well as that his or her evaluation skills are at acceptable and competent FCE levels. However, the client has the greatest potential to invalidate an FCE through a myriad of factors that may have evolved since the injury. Kaplan et al. (1996) identified depression, anxiety, and self-efficacy as significant threats to validity of the FCE performance outcomes. They studied 64 lower back patients and concluded that patients who gave less than their maximum allowable effort reported significantly more anxiety and self-reported disability. These patients demonstrated lower expectations for both their FCE performance and for returning to work, and they had a tendency to report more depressive symptomatology. Similarly, Cheng and Cheng (2010) studied 713 patients with diagnoses of non-specific low back pain in an attempt to predict a patient's return-to-work outcomes post medical and rehabilitative treatment. They discovered that perceptions of self-efficacy, fear of movement-related pain, cognitive coping, and anxiety on the performance of functional tasks had significant impact on the functional quality and activity of the patient.

Matheson (2003) concluded that the issue of reliability and validity threats are closer to the actual testing environment and include the examinee's test reactivity. He defined this concept as being the effect of the measurement process on the examinee's response to testing. He noted that this threat evolves from the reaction of the examinee to the test instrument, the test environment, and the symptom response patterns experienced during testing activities. The life care planner and case manager should realize that test reactivity from the examinee may not be a strategy on the examinee's part to enhance their disability appearance. Some reasons may be related to medically determined impairments that should be considered legitimate factors contributing to an invalid performance. However, fraudulent attempts by the examinee to circumvent the disability determination process should never be ruled out (Kaplan et al., 1996).

Life care planners and case managers with disabled individuals who have chronic pain disorders should not be surprised of these individuals' dysfunctional etiology and potential FCE deficit performance results. Gross and Battié (2005) studied 170 injured workers with low back injuries in an attempt to identify the primary influential factors in one's functional capabilities demonstrated in FCE. They found that self-perception of disability and pain significantly contributed to one's dysfunctional physical behaviors. De Jong et al. (2011) studied 186 patients diagnosed with chronic complex regional pain syndrome type I (CRPS Type I) in two separate studies. They researched the effects of pain on the physical functional capabilities of 79 patients with early onset of CRPS and 107 patients with chronic CRPS. The results showed that those persons with early onset of CRPS limited their functional capabilities as a result of pain severity vs. fear of movement (reinjury). The chronic CRPS group perceived harmfulness of activities as measured with pictorial assessment forms as significantly predicting functional limitations beyond and above the contribution of pain severity. The fear of movement and of reinjury was not a key factor in limiting one's function in this study, but rather the perceived harmfulness of the evaluation activity (FCE component).

Although the threats to validity and reliability are correlated with the evaluator's skill levels and the client's motivations, personal goals, and psychological well-being over the course of his or her disability period, there remains other conditions specific to the FCE process that must be met in order to ensure a valid FCE. King et al. (1998), Hart et al. (1993), and Matheson (2003) identified these conditions as follows:

1. *Safety*: The FCE procedure should not be expected to lead to injury. However, this may be out of the control of the evaluator based on the diagnosis and subsequent medical treatment of the injury, the examinee's success in rehabilitation, and the psychological well-being of the examinee in his or her disability process. In essence, the examinee could injure himself or herself in spite of the efforts of the evaluator to present a safe application of testing protocols and test environment.

2. *Reliability*: The scores derived from a respective test utilizing repeated-measure protocols should be dependable within test trials across evaluators and the date/time of test administration. Often, an examinee will be referred for an updated FCE as the date of a scheduled hearing or trial approaches. The repeat FCE utilizes the same tests applied in the same sequence, and thus should produce similar results to those of the initial FCE.
3. *Validity*: The decisions based on interpretations of the score derived from the FCE measures should reflect the examinee's true ability, provided most, if not all, of the threats to validity are controlled. The interpretation of the test scores should reflect, at best, the examinee's performance in the target work setting.
4. *Practicality:* The cost of administration, interpretation, and reporting of the FCE measures should be reasonable.
5. *Utility*: As noted earlier, this factor is the most important characteristic of a measure. It defines the usefulness of the FCE regarding the degree to which it meets the needs of the examinee, referrer, and payor. Regarding case management, the FCE should meet the case management objectives of the respective examinee, and FCE results should readily apply to the case objectives, leading to the meeting of the case management goals. Otherwise, the FCE has little to no purpose.

FCE Components, Types, and Applications

The FCE model remains fairly consistent in its structure across the many applications it has in rehabilitation and in tort law. The FCE protocol can be job specific, pathology specific, or a more generic protocol addressing one's competency to perform all defined activities of daily living (Soer et al., 2009). Maher (2006) noted that FCE falls under two categories: (a) job-specific FCE and (b) generic FCE. The category of "job-specific" FCE focuses on identifying specific jobs, if not the examinee's original job, and determines the most suitable occupational category if the original job is ruled out. The "generic" FCE is used primarily for case closure in terms of workers' compensation settlements, assignment of disability and damages for tort law trials, and determining rehabilitative progress as a result of therapeutic program participation.

Subsequent protocol adjustments to FCE models have led to the creation of FCEs designed for more specific referral question applications from the case manager that differ significantly from its early developmental purpose. For example, Hart et al. (1993) listed three types of FCE that included (a) baseline capacity evaluation, (b) job capacity evaluation, and (c) work capacity evaluation, and 16 years later Genovese and Isernhagen (2009) identified 11 FCE types and applications that are listed in Table 19.2.

The baseline capacity evaluation is an evaluation that quantifies workers' traits listed in the *Dictionary of Occupational Titles*. Its focus is to determine if any trait factors have significantly changed, such that the individual's worker trait profile as defined by the U.S. Department of Labor no longer matches those profiles that apply to jobs that the examinee has worked over his or her work history. This evaluation tests an individual's physical demands that include sitting, standing, walking, balancing, climbing, kneeling, stooping, crouching, reaching, lifting, carrying, pushing, pulling, motor coordination, fine dexterity, medium dexterity, grasping, and pinching.

The job capacity evaluation tests specific job demands of a particular job to which an examinee is scheduled to return. It matches the physical abilities of the worker to the demands of the job.

The work capacity evaluation assesses the examinee's tolerance potential to withstand the basic demands of competitive employment, such as full-day workplace tolerance and daily attendance. This FCE model applies work simulation activities that may require two or more

Table 19.2 Summary of FCE Purposes and Referral Criteria

Purpose of Functional Tests	Suggested Name	Referral Source	Length and Components
Injury Prevention			
Assess worker qualifications to perform specific job-related skills before job offer	**Pre-offer tests**	Employers	Short and job-specific
Assess worker qualifications to perform specific job-related skills before job offer	**Pre-offer tests**	Employers	Short and job-specific
Move employees within the work setting to accomplish a transfer of access if employee can perform essential functions of the job or worker (e.g., aging) has changed.	**Periodic screening (job placement) tests**	Employers	Short-to-moderate length; job specific
Assess if employee with non-work-related condition (generally with residuals) can return to former job or another available position; may be accompanied by medical evaluation; employee motivated to do well	**Fitness-to-duty FCE**	Employers	Short to moderate; job specificity dependent on context; should include clinical evaluation
Work-Related Injury or Illness Management (Early or Noncomplex)			
Job-specific physical progress evaluation performed in the context of ongoing treatment to reduce lost work-time or restricted time	**Early return-to-work testing**	Employers, medical providers	Short and job-specific
Physical progress evaluation with addition of tests to assess "sincerity of effort" (usually when patient showing evidence of "delayed recovery")	**Mini FCE**	Medical providers, insurers	Short; might or might not be job-specific; tests for consistency of effort
Assess if employees who continue to be symptomatic (usually at MMI) can return to work at own job or in any capacity, even if there are significant physical restrictions and employee does not want to return; (sincerity) of effort	**Return-to-work FCE**	Medical providers, employers, insurers, case managers	Moderate length; generic with or without job-specific components and inclusive of testing to assess sincerity of effort

(Continued)

Table 19.2 (Continued)

Purpose of Functional Tests	Suggested Name	Referral Source	Length and Components
Chronic Injury or Illness Management Provide objective information regarding whether employee can return to own job or to alternative position; if not at MMI, may be used in preparation of entrance to a work conditioning or work hardening program (to set treatment goals)	**Residual functional abilities assessment**	Medical providers, employers, insurers, case managers	Moderate length; job-(or work) specific or generic, depending on context; may be repeated
Ordered as a prelude to claim settlement to assess residual functional capacities, the level of effort, and the consistency of symptoms. Results are seen by IME physician and interpreted in the context of the medical record and his or her clinical evaluation.	**Disposition FCE with IME**	Case managers, lawyers, insurers, physicians	Moderate to long; usually generic; includes clinical evaluation and testing to assess "sincerity of effort"
Ordered as a prelude to claim settlement to assess residual functional capacities, the level of effort, and the consistency of symptoms. Results are seen by IME physician and interpreted in the context of the medical record and his or her clinical evaluation.	**Disposition FCE with IME**	Case managers, lawyers, insurers, physicians	Moderate to long; usually generic; includes clinical evaluation and testing to assess "sincerity of effort"
Also ordered to assess residual functional capacities as a prelude to claim settlement. Results are not interpreted by the IME physician, but by other third-party (depends on referral source).	**Dispositional FCE-stand alone**	Case managers, lawyers, insurers	As earlier, but long; should include comprehensive clinical evaluation
Assess work capacity in individuals with chronic medical illnesses such as chronic fatigue, multiple sclerosis, etc. Because many of these persons state that they are debilitated by their inability to sustain physical activity, this must be assessed as part of the FCE, preferably by ordering testing over several days.	**Special-purpose FCE**	Insurers, lawyers, medical providers	Long; usually generic (as earlier) with additional testing for aerobic capacity (endurance) and positional tolerance needed

days and is usually added to the baseline or job capacity evaluation. Genovese and Isernha-gen's (2009) FCE models easily fit into one of the three FCE models offered by Hart et al. (1993), and all models can be classified under Maher's (2006) two categories of job-specific FCE and generic. For example, the 11 FCE types detailed by Genovese and Isernhagen include (a) pre-offer tests, (b) post-offer tests, (c) periodic screening (job placement tests), (d) fitness for duty FCE, (e) early return-to-work testing, (f) return-to-work FCE, and (g) residual functional capacity evaluation. All of these can fit under the job-specific FCE category, while the more generic FCE models include (h) mini FCE, designed to test for one's consistency of effort; (i) dispositional FCE with independent medical evaluation (IME) that is usually ordered just before claim settlement and is designed to assess residual functional capacities, the level of effort, and the consistency of symptoms; (j) dispositional FCE – stand-alone, without IME or physician involvement; and (k) special-purpose FCE, used for persons with chronic debilitating medical conditions, focusing on aerobic capacity (endurance) and positional tolerance required of daily activities.

Matheson (2003) identified five types of FCE models among the existing compendium of FCE models practiced in the health care industry in the early 2000s. These types include the functional goal setting FCE, the disability rating FCE, the job matching FCE, the occupation matching FCE, and the work capacity evaluation. Each model is described as follows:

1. Functional Goal Setting: This model is most applicable in therapeutic settings during the planning stages of the rehabilitation program for the injured worker. The functional goal set-ting model measures the functional status of the anatomical components affected by impair-ment in order to set therapeutic goals. Additionally, this model can be used to measure one's progress through the therapy program with periodic measurements of strength, range of motion, or both, and compare such measurements to those collected during baseline func-tional capacity testing.

2. Disability Rating: This model is used frequently in tort law cases that involve personal injury resulting from the negligence of other persons. It frequently utilizes an impairment rating in conjunction with the functional capacity ratings using the *AMA Guides to the Evaluation of Permanent Impairment*, editions 5 or 6, depending on the state in which the alleged damages occurred. This method is used to determine the influence of one's physical, cognitive, and/or neurological damages on the examinee's lifetime earning capacity and overall resulting func-tional deficits. Life care plans are often used in conjunction with this FCE model to identify the categories of need and the medical and rehabilitative needs required to assist the injured person with maintaining as close of a lifestyle to which he or she has been accustomed in their lifetime.

3. Job Matching: This FCE model utilizes two sets of information: (a) information concern-ing the physical demands of a particular job and (b) information concerning the worker's impairment and medical status. The job matching FCE employs a standardized test battery to identify the presence of trait-factor deficits that may significantly influence the worker's worker trait profile that may not match that which is required of the particular job.

4. Occupation Matching: This model incorporates the physical demands of an occupation of which such information is obtained from sources such as the U.S. Department of Labor's *Dictionary of Occupational Titles* or the O*NET system. The FCE components are structured around the occupational group's physical demands that are identified in Table 19.3. These physical demands are applied to all jobs and the resulting conglomerate of occupational groups defined by the U.S. Department of Labor in the Dictionary of Occupational Titles.

5. Work Capacity Evaluation: This FCE model has a broad application since its focus is not on any one particular job, but rather the worker trait profile as a whole. This test model assesses

Table 19.3 Department of Labor Classification of Work Demands

Physical Demand Level	Occasional 0%–33% of the Workday	Frequent 34%–66% of the Workday	Constant 67%–100% of the Workday
Sedentary	10 lbs	Negligible	Negligible
Light	20 lbs	10 lbs and/or walk/stand/ push/pull of arm/leg controls	Negligible and/or push/ pull arm/leg controls while seated
Medium	20–50 lbs	10–25 lbs	10 lbs
Heavy	50–100 lbs	25–50 lbs	10–20 lbs
Very Heavy	Over 100 lbs	Over 50 lbs	Over 20 lbs

frequently encountered task demands and worker behaviors; behaviors are assessed through observation of performance in a simulated work environment. The work capacity evaluation model uses work simulations that are constructed based on descriptions found in published resources. This evaluation can last from one to two hours to multiple days depending on whether or not the individual can meet the basic criteria for work pace tolerance and sustained activity tolerance.

Overall, Gross and Reneman (2011) summed up the primary utility of the FCE process as being one that measures all required activities of daily living (ADLs) and work competencies and identifying the disabled individual's occupational performance capabilities. They noted specific applications to include:

1. Informing return-to-work decision making including whether or not an injured worker has sufficient functional ability to safely perform the essential functions of respective jobs.
2. Test results that are used to set activity limitations (temporary and permanent).
3. Identifying necessary prescriptions for accommodated work.
4. Guiding the development of rehabilitation and functional restoration programs.

FCE Components and Case Studies

The components of an FCE are fairly standard with some variance in component structures depending on the referral questions and other factors. For example, FCE systems/types may differ in the methodology they use to assess an examinee's cooperation and sincerity of effort, determination of the end points for stopping the FCE during the examinee's performance, degree of work simulation, initial lift-screening and materials handling protocols, results interpretation, and type of equipment used. However, the following components are standard in the FCE process regardless of these differences (King et al., 1998):

1. Medical records review
2. Clinical interview pertaining to specific injury events and rehabilitative chronology, activities of daily living competency, financial status (disability benefits insurance, stress with monthly financial obligations, etc.), family and social history, and educational/vocational histories
3. Questionnaires/profile sheets completion
4. Physical measures/musculoskeletal evaluation

5. Physiological evaluation
6. Functional measures (Galper, 2009; Isernhagen, 2009; King et al., 1998)

The model types identified earlier in this chapter utilize the previously listed components and some additional ones depending on the preferences, background, education, and training of the FCE evaluator. I practice the National Association of Disability Evaluating Professionals FCE model, or better known in the commercial marketplace as the NADEP FCE Protocol. This standardized model enlists all of the earlier FCE components and titles these components as follows:

1. Clinical interview/intake screening and patient profiling
2. Grip strength testing
3. Physical tolerance range of motion as applied to the vertical work plane, range of motion study, and manual muscle testing
4. Diagnosis-specific functional testing to include treadmill (gait analysis and endurance), and postural analysis (stooping, crouching, kneeling)
5. Materials handling/lifting evaluation
6. Domain testing

The NADEP FCE is a standardized method for testing one's functional capacity and for determining the effects of injury on one's worker's trait profile in addition to one's functional capabilities. The case manager should look for facilities that offer *standardized* FCE models that are research-based in their testing protocols. Standardization refers to the development of test administration procedures, the specific types of tests, and the sequence in which they are administered without any variation among evaluators and clinics (locations) offering such evaluative services. In short, *standardization* refers to a clearly defined set of procedures for administering and scoring tests (Genovese & Isernhagen, 2009; King et al., 1998). Clinically, standardization helps minimize threats to validity and reliability regarding the functional outcomes of the examinee, thus ensuring the results are a valid representation of the examinee's true functional capabilities.

The first component of any FCE, clinical interview/intake screening and patient profiling, is by far the most time-consuming component in a generic FCE protocol aside from the domain testing component. The evaluator is charged with reviewing all available medical documentation of injury and rehabilitation chart notes indicating the degree of the examinee's recovery up through the day of evaluation. Often, these records are not available to the evaluator for review at the time of the evaluation, requiring the evaluator to spend more time interviewing the examinee to ensure that all diagnoses are revealed and all rehabilitation modalities discussed. The evaluator is charged with reviewing all records, whether they are available before the evaluation or after the session, and to make changes in the clinical interview section of the report as necessary.

The patient profiling component is essential in helping the evaluator understand the mindset of the examinee that may involve significant self-efficacy issues, functional activity fears, elevated perceptions of disability, or the individual's tendency to magnify symptoms in response to activity or in response to sustained posturing during the interview. I use several profiling forms throughout the FCE evaluation period that provide some clarification and understanding of the functional results analyzed at the end of the evaluation. Case Studies 1 and 2 explain how forms are integrated in the evaluation process and are provided for the reader at the online reading room designed just for this chapter at www.ichcc.org/resources/research-publications.html.

Click on the file "profile charts" in each Case Study to gain a visual concept with interpretation as to what information these charts provide the evaluator. Case Studies 1 and 2 explain how forms are integrated in the evaluation process and are provided for the reader in Appendices 1 and 2.

The individual's grip strength is tested regardless of the diagnosis of the respective examinee. This test provides the evaluator an opportunity to observe testing behaviors that more than likely will continue throughout the testing period for all administered components. This test provides the evaluator a preview of the examinee's allowable effort applied during testing, as well the frequency or presence of overt pain behaviors in response to applied resistance testing. The reader is advised to go to Appendix 19A (on page 415) to review the grip strength test to see how these data are presented and the interpretation of the profile curves.

The physical tolerance range of motion as applied to the vertical work plane, range of motion study, and manual muscle testing component is designed to observe the individual's functional joint ranges passively and to determine sincerity of effort through the repeated measures protocol utilized in manual muscle testing. It is during this component that the examinee may demonstrate the first sign of functional deficits barring the results of the grip strength study. The evaluator is able to observe the individual's willingness to engage in resistance testing or to engage in applying pressure to a load-cell using joint motion and musculature that may be part of the diagnosis. Frequently the locus of pain complaints is not related to the diagnosis; rather, it is as a result of poor muscle sequencing such that muscular groups within the area of injury are affected by application. The reader is directed to Appendices 1 and 2 and to review either case study to gain a perspective of what motions, technique, mechanical applications, and test protocols are involved in this component.

The FCE is designed to evaluate one's tolerances and capacities required to access the full vertical work plane in all work settings and to demonstrate appropriate mechanical applications to postures required to access various vertical work plane levels. The fourth component involves treadmill exercises for gait analysis and endurance and stooping, crouching, and kneeling postures that typically are required to access the full vertical work plane. These postures are typical of the industrial and skilled occupations of which most of the examinees who are referred for FCE have worked their adult lives.

Regarding the gait analysis and postural analysis, we use video recordings to accentuate any gait antalgia or derangement and any mechanical instability or mechanical compensation in joints as well as pain behaviors in the postural analysis. The reader is directed to review the treadmill gait analysis summary and postural analysis summary that are included in the FCE reports in the appendices. Report summaries under each component reference the video clips to emphasize the points of discussion. It is an FCE standard of the NADEP FCE model that the report is sent to the referral source with video clips that can be found at www.ichcc.org/resources/research-publications.html, and these clips review mechanical joint compensation and any behavioral or functional anomaly.

The materials handling and lifting evaluation component involves dynamic lifting and handling activities of graduated weighted crates that are handled at floor level up to 78 inches from the floor. I use the WEST EPIC evaluation system for clinically controlled lifting through the full vertical work plane (Matheson, 1986), as well as the Progressive Isoinertial Lifting Evaluation (PILE) system with a lift and carry component to evaluate the examinee's lifting and carrying tolerances and capacity (Mayer et al., 1988). The evaluator does not administer both of these lift tests, but rather chooses the one that best fits the individual's functional capacity as demonstrated in the prior test components, as well as which system best addresses the referral questions.

The final component, domain testing, is applied based on the information requested in the referral question(s). Up to this point in the FCE the process has been categorized as "generic" while the domain testing component can evolve the FCE to that of a more job-specific test. For example, the referring party may wish to determine if the examinee is capable of working a specific job safely and dependably. The question may require the evaluator to address any specific trait-factor adjustments or losses with regard to work, and standardized work samples and specific job-function simulations may be incorporated to make this determination. Domain testing may focus on the impact of the disability on the individual's cognitive functioning, such as the effects of acquired brain injury sequelae on memory, spatial/form perception, eye/hand coordination, and motor coordination. Additional pencil/paper tests as well as work samples may be utilized to clarify the head trauma effects on these trait factors necessary for some jobs or for some activities of daily living.

Referring for FCE and Choosing the Evaluator

The life care planner and case manager must consider several aspects of their particular case before making the referral for an FCE. They must ask the question "Why?" and in doing so, they must ask if the referral is for injury prevention, for injury or illness management, or for client disposition in terms of case resolution or claim settlement (Genovese & Isernhagen, 2009). The life care planner and case manager must consider the maximum medical improvement status of their disabled individuals, and if this status has not been documented, this does not rule out the FCE. The FCE can be ordered as part of the individual's treatment plan used in monitoring one's rehabilitative progress. To the benefit of the claim's manager, the life care planner, and the case manager, it may be used as a dispositional tool toward resolving open claims issues associated with the case and bringing the case to a final resolution.

The training, skills, and interactive qualities of the FCE evaluator cannot be overemphasized and bear readdressing as a final thought. The FCE is only as good as the person conducting the evaluation. In other words, the FCE relies heavily on the evaluator's training and experience, requiring the evaluator to be aware of his or her personal bias and the limitations of the FCE protocol. Further, they should have training in clinical reasoning (Galper & Genovese, 2009). Bear in mind that the evaluator will be with the individual anywhere from two to four hours in most cases, and he or she is responsible within that time period for creating and maintaining a trust relationship, a safe testing environment, and engaging a compassionate approach to testing that communicates to the examinee that the evaluator understands his or her condition as well as any resulting functional deficits and/or injury sequelae. Aside from the examinee, the evaluator has an obligation to the life care planner and to the case manager and/or referral source to communicate well and to be available for questions and other communications. The evaluator is required to write a professional report that is clear and uncomplicated in terminology or statistical applications in the results section. Galper and Genovese offer the following outline that summarizes the attributes of a good evaluator:

1. Evaluator has knowledge of and expertise in clinical evaluation, functional testing, and the application of this testing to injury prevention, injury management, and medical legal settings. More specifically, the evaluation has knowledge of:

   a. The impact of injury and illness on function
   b. Clinical assessment methods (educational background in the musculoskeletal system, movement, and pathologies)
   c. Processes used to measure function
   d. The demands of occupation within the workplace environments
   e. Occupational analysis and workplace demands

2. Evaluator has expertise in functional testing methods
3. Evaluator is a reflective clinician

    a. Is aware of his or her personal bias
    b. Knows the limitations of the FCE instrument
    c. Has training in clinical reasoning

4. Evaluator is able to develop and maintain a good working relationship with the referral source and the examinee

    a. Is an effective verbal and written communicator
    b. Is responsive to questions (pp. 338–339)

Summary and Conclusions

Life care planners and case managers are finding that life care planning referral sources and case management administrators are mandating the application of evidence-based medical and rehabilitative services for all caseloads, particularly those that are in need of disposition or resolution. The FCE is a systematic method of measuring one's ability to perform meaningful tasks on a safe and dependable basis, and given the current research as applied to FCE methodologies, the FCE has evolved as an objective evidence-based evaluative tool for determining a client's work feasibility, documenting a client's rehabilitative and therapeutic goal achievement levels, and determining a client's progress in therapeutic rehabilitation programs and work-hardening therapeutic programs. The FCE identifies work activity stressors and physical tolerances, thus allowing the life care planner and case manager to offer recommendations for job site modifications and/or job function modifications. More importantly, the FCE helps the life care planner and case manager understand their disabled individual's mindset regarding returning to work or participating in rehabilitation programs and whether or not they have a propensity to achieve their rehabilitative program goals or to apply minimal effort toward getting well or returning to a productive lifestyle. Life care planners and case managers through FCE gain a better perspective of their clients' capabilities for independent functioning and ADL skills retention and the overall affect their injuries may have on disability and impairment when advising carriers and other referral sources on case resolution strategies.

The FCE is only as valid as the training, skills, and evaluation/communication qualities of the evaluator. The life care planner and case manager are charged with researching the background of the FCE evaluator before making the referral, as a poorly trained evaluator allows for a greater risk of invalid functional results or a mis-assignment of functional restrictions. Additionally, life care planners and case managers are charged with evaluating the FCE protocols that are used in their local health care communities, to ensure that their clients will benefit from a research-based protocol with established validity and reliability.

The FCE has a strong future given the emphasis in today's health care system to minimize and/or cut costs. The FCE is an evidence-based tool that can help the life care planner and case manager determine the benefit of continuing health care services for the client or to focus on case disposition through settlement recommendations.

Appendix 19A

Case Study 1

Richmond Functional Performance Lab

Functional Capacity/Work Disability

Evaluation Report

REPORT OF

_____, M.D.

Determinations based on the
AMA Guides to the Evaluation of Permanent Impairment, Fifth Edition,
and the National Association of Disability Evaluating Professionals Functional
Capacity Evaluation Protocols, Southern Illinois University

Certified Disability Examiner: Virgil Robert May III, Rh.D., CRP, CDE II

13801 Village Mill Drive ● Suite 103 ● Midlothian, Virginia 23114
Telephone: (804) 378–7273 ● Fax: (804) 378–7267

Functional Capacity/Work Disability

Evaluation Report

Virgil Robert May III, Rh.D., CRP, CDE II

<u>SUMMARY PAGE</u>

NAME: _____, M.D.

DATE OF BIRTH: CENSORED

DATE OF INJURY: 06/24/1988

DATE OF EVALUATION: 04/21/2015

DATE OF COMPLETED REPORT: 04/30/2015

TOTAL TIME (Interview/Testing/Physical Exam):   18.0 hrs

DIAGNOSIS: See Medical Summary

MMI: N/A

IMPAIRMENT RATING: N/A

PHYSICAL DEMAND LEVEL: Restricted Work Plane: SEDENTARY—LIGHT

                                    Unrestricted Work Plane: UNEMPLOYABLE

**COMPATIBLE CAREER OPTION: 189.167–010 CONSULTANT, MEDICAL
    (PROFESS. & KIN)**
Functional Capacity/Work Disability
Functional Capacity/Work Disability

Evaluation Report

Referring Party: _____ , Esq.

Evaluation Location: Richmond Functional Performance Lab, Inc.

13801 Village Mill Drive

Suite 103

Midlothian, VA 23114

Examinee: _____ , M.D.

D/Injury: 06/24/1988

D/Eval.:   04/21/2015

Medical Intake/History Review

I examined Dr. _____ in my office per the request of _____ , Esq. for the purpose of determining Dr. _____'s functional capacity with regards to work.

MEDICAL RECORDS PROVIDED BY: _____ , Esq.

_____

_____ Street

Charlottesville, VA _____

SUBJECTIVE AND RECORDED HISTORY OF PRESENT INJURY:

I had the pleasure of seeing Dr. _____ in my office for a functional examination in an attempt to determine her capacity to return to her customary and usual occupational position as an **INTERNIST (medical ser.) alternate titles: internal medicine specialist**. Dr. _____ was referred by her husband's divorce counsel, _____ , Esq. Dr. _____ reports today status post multiple orthopedic trauma resulting from a single car crash, with additional system disorders that have evolved over the 27 year period since her car crash.

Dr. _____ has an extensive medical history and this evaluator reviewed all records forwarded to this office by Mr. Kitzmann. A summary of her diagnoses include the following:

1. Status post cervical pain, uncontrolled
2. Status post cervical radiculitis, uncontrolled
3. Status post Cervical spondylosis without myelopathy, uncontrolled
4. Status post facet syndrome, uncontrolled
5. Status post nonallopathic lesion of the cervical region, uncontrolled
6. Status post laminectomy syndrome of the thoracic region, uncontrolled
7. Status post laminectomy syndrome of the cervical region, uncontrolled
8. Status post thoracic spondylosis without myelopathy, uncontrolled
9. Status post C5 through T1 fusion
10. Status post spastic quadriplegia
11. Status post central cord syndrome
12. Status post chronic neurogenic pain
13. Status post proximal rupture of artificial tendon
14. Status post urinary incontinence
15. Status post neurogenic bladder
16. Status post cervical regional myelopathy
17. Status post fibromyalgia
18. Status post narcolepsy and sleep disorder
19. Status post position dependent sleep apnea syndrome
20. Status post depression
21. Status post panic and anxiety disorder
22. Status post right thumb IP Joint fusion
23. Status post left thumb MP joint fusion
24. Status post bilateral stenosing tenosynovitis long and ring fingers
25. Status post hypothyroidism
26. Status post hypercholesterolemia

Her procedures over her medical history included:

1. Casper plating C6, C7 with corpectomy and iliac bone crest grafting, halo, and fusion with eventual diagnosis of nonunion
2. Anterior/posterior decompression and fusion bilaterally at C5–T1, resulting in nonunion and ongoing spinal cord pressure
3. Right hand IP joint ligamentous tenodesis 2nd—5th MP joints and extensor indices proprius transfer to right thumb
4. Left IP fusion of first finger, brachioradialis transfer to thumb with active Hunter rod, Stage 1
5. Right extensor tendon realignment and brachioradialis transfer to thumb with active Hunter rod, Stage 1 of right opponensplasty, brachioradialis transfer with active tendon for right thumb opposition. Pulley was palmaris longus and flexor carpi radialis tendon
6. Removal of hardware of left thumb MP joint and extensor tenolysis
7. Extensor tenolysis right index finger and right thumb, tendon transfer, right, IP joint fusion of the right thumb
8. Rupture of active Hunter rod while skiing
9. Reapproximation of tendon rod after proximal rupture of active tendon rod

10. Rupture active Hinter rod, status post combative patient altercation in ICU while intern
11. Tendon reconstruction of the right hand, free tendon graft from right ring finger
12. Multiple facet injections a C7 through T6; Multiple injections over many years involving her hands, neck, back, trigger points, and spine.

Dr. _____ practiced for 20 years (including residency) before having to terminate her practice and turn in her medical license due to her belief that she could no longer serve her patients sufficiently due to her illness sequelae. Dr. _____, osteopathic physician and pain management specialist, saw Dr. _____ on October 23, 2013, at which time he documented that she explained that she had issues related to her pain medication and recently notified the Virginia Commonwealth Board of Medicine that she felt that she was an impaired physician due to pain medication use. Additionally, Dr. _____ was terminated as a physician at her previous medical practice due to her pain and her multiple diagnostic sequelae and functional limitations. Dr. _____ has undergone pain treatments that included multiple facets injections at C6–7, C7–T1, T1–2, T2–3, T3–4, and T4–5. Additionally Dr. _____ has been fitted with an implantable intrathecal opioid delivery device for her pain management as a result of her excessive spinal stenosis that precluded the implantation of a spinal stimulator. Under Dr. _____'s care during the initial visit, she underwent two facet injects; one in C7 through T6, and the other in her left 1 through 5 ribs.

Current medical documentation reports that in 1988 Dr. _____ suffered multilevel burst fractures of her cervical spine resulting in an incomplete spastic quadriplegia with head injury. She underwent a bilateral cervical laminectomy and was diagnosed as having spinal arachnoid adhesions of the cervical spine, Syringoma, and myelitis of the cervical spine. She developed a neurogenic bladder condition with a sensory deficit with large bladder capacity, of which she self-treats with self-catheterization and occasional indwelling Foley catheter. She noted that she has lower extremity spasticity and has incurred gastroparesis due to her neurogenic disorder. She states that she has episodes of frequent vomiting and cannot tell when she's hungry. Dr. _____ states that she has had ulnar distribution neuropathic pain since 1988, that she has facet arthropathy of her cervical spine and upper thoracic spine. She noted that she experiences muscle spasms in her neck and has occasional lower extremity spasticity. She has incurred an autonomic disorder as a result of her spinal cord injury and has degenerative arthropathy.

Dr. _____ documented chronic, bilateral numbness in her arms and hands and has experienced a loss of hand intrinsic muscle function and use with atrophy since 1988 due to Central Cord Syndrome. She presented to this evaluator with a right claw-hand and she failed to make a complete fist with her right hand. She reported that she experiences bilateral hand pain, neuropathic since 1988. This evaluator observed her left hand as significantly more functional and controlled in terms of motor function and finger dexterity as compared to her right hand.

Dr. _____ documented that she experiences medication side-effects that are disabling, and her medication regimen is changed often. Her current medications include Cymbalta 120 mg; gabapentin (Neurontin) 300 morning; 900 mg at bedtime; Ibuprofen 200–800 mg 3x per day; Provigil 200 mg 1x extra 200 mg p.r.n.; valium 200 mg bed-time; 2 mg p.r.n.; Baclofen; Dilaudid (infusion with remote). Unrelated medications include Crestor 10 mg 1 x daily; Spironolactone 200 mg; Centroid 100 mcg; and Abilify 1 mg. Her medical care and monitoring of her medications is provided by _____, M.D., PCP, once per three months. She has been released from her cognitive behavioral therapist and has been released from pain management. She continues to see 3 specialists who include Dr. Robert Goldstein, pain management specialist, Dr. _____, psychiatrist, and Dr. _____, neurologist.

EFFECTS OF INJURY ON DAILY LIVING:

Dr. _____ is not independent in all of her activities of daily living. She uses adaptive household utensils when in the kitchen, and modified personal care items such as nail clippers. She has had to modify some of her activities of daily living, such as having food delivered and prepared, modifying her shower/bathtub in bathing as she has slipped in her shower. She employs a housekeeper and a personal care assistant. She wears non-shoe-laced shoes, or slip-on shoes and has difficulty with bending forward, kneeling, and crouching due to her Baclofen pump.

CURRENT COMPLAINTS AS PER PAIN DIAGRAM:

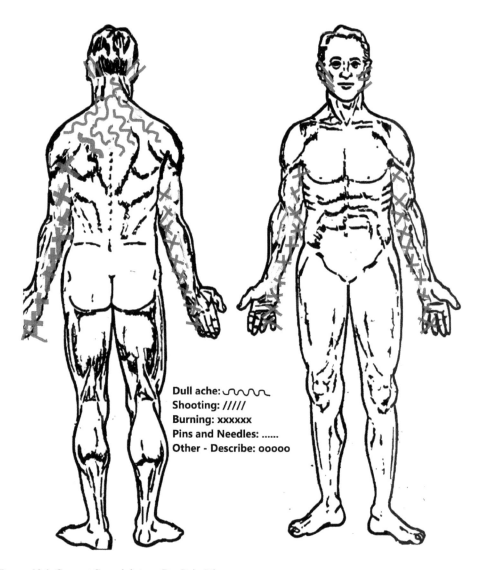

Figure 19.1 Current Complaints as Per Pain Diagram

Dr. _____ presents with a diagnosis-specific pain profile. She documented a significant amount of dull aching pain from C2 down into her mid-thoracic spinal region with reference into her bilateral scapulae. She documented ulnar neuropathy down the medial bilateral upper extremities to her 4th and 5th fingers. She documented sensitivity in both ears coupled with searing intense aching pain. She noted that it is related to wind or objects placed in her ear, such as stethoscopes or ear plugs. Her chief complaint is that of constant pain in her right upper extremity and cervical/thoracic spinal regions. She noted that the pain intensity/duration differs on occasion as some days are good for her while others she finds herself focusing on her pain.

Author's Note: The pain chart is used to identify anatomical areas (orthopedic in this case) where symptom response patterns are documented in accordance with the individual's daily function (activities of daily living performance). This chart provides the evaluator anatomical areas that may be more responsive than other areas to functional testing components of the FCE protocol, and what type of pain behaviors and functional tolerances can be expected during the testing period. This profile form provides the evaluator the opportunity to correlate the symptom responses to the examinee's medical and rehabilitative behavioral histories, and may suggest either inconsistence or consistency in her symptom response pattern reports.

PAST MEDICAL HISTORY:

Surgical History -	See Medical Summary
A) Past illnesses/injuries:	N/A
B) Prior on-the-job injuries:	N/A
C) Allergies:	N/A

FAMILY/SOCIAL HISTORY:

Dr. _____ is married with two children ages 10 and 12. She noted that her divorce is in progress at this writing, and that she has been involved in depositions. Her primary emotional support system has been her parents, as they are very active in her and her children's lives. She noted that although they live in Maryland, they visit frequently and stay anywhere from a week to two weeks at a time. Socially, she noted that she has close friends who have children her sons' ages. They get together weekly for play dates that include the parents as well as the children.

FINANCIAL INFORMATION:

Dr. _____ is receiving Social Security Disability Insurance benefits (SSDI). Additionally, she noted that she is receiving temporary alimony and doesn't know the outcome of her receiving any form of monetary support from her ex-husband at the final disposition of her divorce.

EDUCATIONAL/VOCATIONAL HISTORY:

Dr. _____ attended medical school in Philadelphia and did a residency at Vanderbilt Medical Center in internal medicine. She worked in internal medicine including a residency for 20 years before stepping down due to health complications.

Evaluation Protocol

The examination protocol used to determine Dr. _____'s capability to perform work was the NADEP protocol which is research-based out of Southern Illinois University. The scheduled components consisted of the initial intake screening, examinee profiling, physical range tolerance to specific work-related postures, grip strength, manual muscle testing, range of motion of affected joints, and domain tests. Given her questionable changes in motor control of her hands/fingers and her manual/finger dexterity, the Minnesota Rate of Manipulation Tests were used to document any upper extremity/hand functional deficits. The MRMT assesses physical tolerance to a sustained flexed posture similar to that which is required of desktop assembly and electronic workers, as well as other "production" type of workers. Given Dr. _____'s medical condition and neurological sequelae, it is a useful test in determining her functional manual/finger dexterity and motor coordination under stress in a timed test situation.

Please note that her performance summary follows this section. The Raw-Data section consists of a description of each test and her specific performance outcome for that test.

Summary and Conclusions

Dr. _____ completed all of the assigned test activities. She demonstrated a consistent effort throughout this evaluation as evidenced by the data output as applied to her repeated measure test activities detailed in the Raw Data Section. It is noteworthy that she demonstrated excessive variances in her repeated measures for cervical extension. Given that she participated in 44 repeated measure tests for this multicomponent functional capacity evaluation, one test with excessive variances is insignificant and not indicative of her feigning her effort for personal gain. She managed and controlled her symptom response patterns well, such that pain symptoms did not influence her functioning during the tests. Please note in Figure 19.2 that her pain sequelae actually decreased to a point to where by the end of this evaluation she was pain-free. Dr. _____ was requested to profile her response to physical activities as well as to document the degree of change in the performance of those respective activities. Her profiles are illustrated later.

Activity Ratings:

Activity Rating Chart

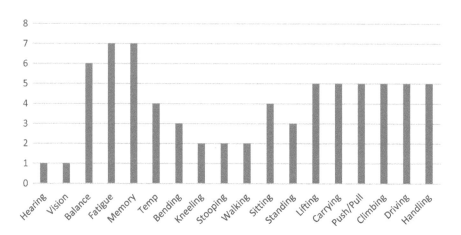

Figure 19.2 Activity Rating Chart

Dr. _____'s rating of the change in ability to perform the listed activities, where 0 indicates no change and 10 indicates a total loss of ability

Activity Ratings Comments:

Dr. _____ documented a diagnosis-specific profile as evidenced by her choices of sensory and physical trait factor changes. For example, she documented changes in her hearing due to what she noted to be tinnitus on occasion and pain in her auditory canal due to wind pressure, cold temperatures, and her stethoscope. She documented changes in her vision and attributed this to being age-related. She documented significant changes in her balance that are related to her lower extremity occasional spasticity such that her right leg will give away causing her to stumble and, at times, fall. She noted that fatigue and memory are significant problems in that she feels tired constantly regardless of how well she thinks she slept the night before, and she continues with short-term memory lapses. She noted that her short-term memory has become a significant problem. Dr. _____ documented changes in bending (lumbar flexion), stooping, kneeling, and crouching due to balance and strength deficits in her lower extremities as well as interference she experiences with her Baclofen intrathecal pump. She noted that she is capable of walking well on even, flat surfaces, but climbing stairs remains a challenge due to her tendency to "miss steps" coupled with balance issues. She noted that sitting and standing postures are good for short durations and lifting and carrying objects/materials are dependent on weight and size. She documented that she is capable of pushing a shopping cart, but cannot push a lawnmower and has difficulty walking down inclines. She noted that driving is good for short distances, and with long trips she requires frequent breaks due to her cervical pain that worsens over time in her car. Handling objects is a problem bimanually due to her lack of motor coordination and digit joint motion and control in her right hand. She noted that she has developed her own compensated mechanical approaches to handling and fingering objects, using her left hand as the primary hand and her right hand is used as a support structure. She noted that she has lost sensation along her bilateral ulnar distributions. Regarding temperature adjustments, she noted that she has incurred autonomic dysfunction and will perspire profusely with an increase in temperature, and she noted she is very intolerant to heat. It becomes more complicated when her bladder is full or her gastroparesis "acts up." She noted that her short-term memory is a big problem such that she has difficulty with "staying on task."

Author's Note: This profile form is unique in that it provides the evaluator a functional "picture" of the individual's physical capabilities and tolerances before participating in the physical test components of the FCE. Debriefing the examinee on this profile form allows the evaluator to learn and focus on areas the examinee has noted that have a tendency to put her or him at risk for fall and/or injury; Additionally, it indicates whether or not she or he will complete all test components of the FCE without accommodation or have to terminate the testing early before completing all test components.

Discomfort Rating:

Discomfort Activity Rating Chart

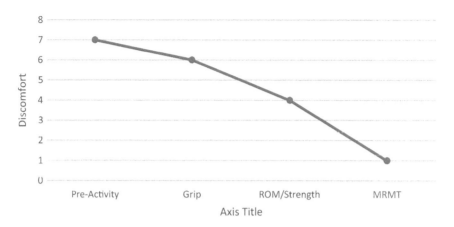

Figure 19.3 Discomfort Activity Rating Chart

Discomfort Activity Rating Comments:

Dr. _____ documented a decrease in her pain sequelae as she progressed in this study. However, as noted in the raw data section, her post-Minnesota Rate of Manipulation Test illness behavior was significant and was non-pain related. She rested on the floor until she felt she could trust her condition to assume a standing/sitting posture.

Author Note: This profile form tells the evaluator two pieces of very important information; 1) the degree of pain at the time of their arrival for the evaluation, and 2) the propensity for the pain to worsen with increased activity. The pain diagram in Figure 19.1 is somewhat rare to the extent that her pain decreased over time significantly. Pain does decrease in some individuals while in activity, but I have never seen it to this degree.

To summarize, Dr. _____ demonstrated excellent control over her pain but her symptom response patterns were fairly overt. However, she demonstrated an ability to negotiate her symptoms so that a higher level of task completion could be achieved such that she completed all assigned test components to her maximum allowed effort. She exhibited mechanical and strength deficits in range of motion and dynamic activities, particularly in bimanual and right unilateral manual dexterity when manipulating objects. Regarding the dynamic lifting study, this test was waived due to this evaluator's observance of her hand functional deficits in prior testing components suggesting that her manipulating a weighted crate over the full vertical work plane would pose a safety risk to her. Based on the medical records and her performance on this functional study, it is this evaluator's conclusion that Dr. _____ cannot function independently in the competitive labor market without accommodation and worksite modifications. Her physical functioning criteria for positioning are detailed in Table 19.1.1.

Table 19.1.1 Functional Capacity Summary and Recommendations

Activity	Demonstrated Output	Competitive Recommendations
BENDING	Demonstrated	Restricted to non-repetitive schedule
KNEELING	Demonstrated	Eliminate
STOOPING	Demonstrated	Not restricted
CROUCHING	N/A	Eliminate
REACHING	Demonstrated	Restricted to unilateral function—left upper extremity rather than right—avoid bimanual manipulation greater than 17 inches from center fulcrum and above shoulder height
SITTING	Greater than 60 minutes	Restricted—periodic adjustment as needed
STANDING	Greater than 60 minutes	Restricted—periodic adjustment as needed
WALKING	Demonstrated	Restricted—even terrain without walkway obstacles
CLIMBING	Demonstrated	Restricted to stairs with railing support—avoid ladders

Author Note: This form is completed based on the evaluator's review of all profile data and repeated test-trial outcomes. Once the functional performance foundation has been established through data review and functional behavioral observations, the evaluator uses clinical judgement to complete this Table. It is imperative that the examinee's work potential, sincerity of effort, maximum test-effort applications, and validity of functional output be determined with a review of all data and accompanying behavioral observations. Maximum voluntary effort, as well as sincerity of effort cannot be determined by the results of one test-component.

Vocational Implications:

Based on the U.S. Department of Labor definitions for **WORK** and accompanying physical exertion demand levels, it is this examiner's conclusion that the examinee qualifies for the **Light** work category within the ***restricted*** work plane, provided that the work criteria, as presented earlier, are integrated into any return-to-work considerations. When considering the competitive ***unrestricted*** vertical and horizontal work planes, the examinee remains unemployable.

    Work Place Considerations: Dr. _____ performed well in this study given her medical history and current residual sequelae and system disorders. She has multiple orthopedic mechanical and pain challenges that she has to address periodically during her day as well as in her evenings. This is not to rule out her returning to some form of gainful employment, although based on a part-time schedule at best. Her suggested restrictions as presented in Table 19.1.1 are significant, but due to her background, education, and medical experience, she is capable of working in the health care provider market. There are conditions that must be met, however, before this can be a feasible goal for her. First, she must be allowed to work at her own pace and to be provided the necessary time for medical reprieve on her part. Her consistency in terms of working a day and subsequent days in the week is guarded at best, and more than likely her work time will be interrupted for her to address medical condition sequelae. Secondly, she must be allowed to work on a part-time schedule; a schedule that is fitted to her medical needs as they arise, thus ruling out a full-time or a minimum of a 40-hour work week.

One of the first statements Dr. _____ made to this evaluator was that she wants to work in health care in some capacity. The Vocational Worksheet attached to this report identifies the best practice scenario for her and is a very achievable goal. In essence, she is relegated to that of a consultant's role in the health care field of her expertise; more specifically, working with catastrophically disabled individuals through her development of life care plans in workers' compensation and personal injury settings. As noted, this is further discussed in the Vocational Worksheet attached to this report.

Vitals Response:

Dr. _____'s blood pressure and heart rate were monitored continuously throughout the evaluation period. The purpose of such monitoring was to determine her effort when engaged in activity, thus revealing the level of effort Dr. _____ was willing to produce for each test. Studies by[1] Rubler and Bruzzone, and[2] Herkenhoff, Lima, Goncalves, Souza, Vasquez, and Mill, and[3] McCartney and McKelvie confirm increased changes in blood pressure and heart rate in response to stress, particularly in diastolic response. Dr. _____'s vital responses are illustrated in Vitals Response Chart (Figure 19.4).

Discussion:

Dr. _____ gave her maximum allowable effort to participate in this study as evidenced by her vitals response patterns across all test components. Please note the increase in heart rate from her initial pretest resting period following her grip strength study. Her heart rate increased as expected, and due to her deconditioning, her diastolic pressure increased with the heart rate as well. She became more relaxed during the range of motion study, but following the Minnesota Rate of Manipulation Test, she engaged in orthostatic hypotension as evidenced by the continued decrease in her diastolic pressure and the spike in her heart rate. She requested to lie down to where she placed herself on the floor until she felt she could resume a standing/upright position without fainting. After a rest her vitals returned to normal levels.

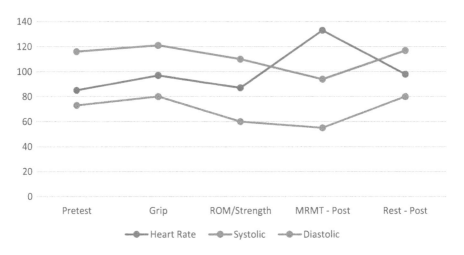

Figure 19.4 Vitals Response Chart

Author Note: This table contains vitals data collected over the course of the evaluation. It is a good source for determining sincerity of effort and maximum effort levels based upon the research on heart and diastolic profiles while the person is engaged in exercise. Vitals are used to support the evaluator's conclusions regarding the validity of the examinee's effort.

Thank you for allowing me to evaluate your client's ex-wife.
Sincerely yours,

Virgil Robert May III, Rh.D, CDE II, CRP
Certified Disability Evaluator

Raw Data and Test Results

GRIP Strength Study

Ms. _____ was tested for her grip strength utilizing the protocols developed by[4] Mathiowetz. These protocols quantify an individual's grip strength in one or more standard grip positions, and compare such strength to recognized population norms. The testing protocols used were identical to that which was used by[5] Niebuhr and Marion for determining sincerity of effort using the JAMAR dynamometer. Her grip patterns are detailed in the strength chart (Figure 19.5).

Discussion:

Dr. _____'s profile is atypical of that which was expected as researched by Mathiowetz et al. (1985). Please note that her grip strength peaked at handle position 4 rather than at handle positions 2 or 3. However, her strength profiles for each hand across all handle positions are symmetrical. Additionally, her variances among the repeated test trials are minimal and within the accepted ranges. Therefore this evaluator concludes that she gave her best allowable effort

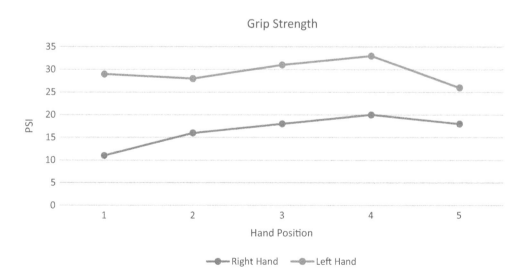

Figure 19.5 Grip Strength Chart

Table 19.1.2 Grip Strength

Individual Test Results		Strength Data		Normative Data		
TASK NAME	DATE	Average Force	Coefficient of Variation (CV)	Population Norm	Standard Deviation	Comparison to Norm
Position 1—Left	4/21/2015	29.0 lbs	6.9 %	n/a	n/a	n/a
Position 1—Right	4/21/2015	11.0 lbs	9.1 %	n/a	n/a	n/a
STANDARD— Left	4/21/2015	28.0 lbs	6.2 %	56.0	+/– 12.7	Below Norm
STANDARD— Right	4/21/2015	15.7 lbs	3.7 %	62.2	+/– 15.1	Below Norm
Position 3—Left	4/21/2015	30.7 lbs	1.9 %	n/a	n/a	n/a
Position 3—Right	4/21/2015	17.7 lbs	3.3 %	n/a	n/a	n/a
Position 4—Left	4/21/2015	33.0 lbs	8.0 %	n/a	n/a	n/a
Position 4—Right	4/21/2015	20.3 lbs	2.8 %	n/a	n/a	n/a
Position 5—Left	4/21/2015	26.0 lbs	3.8 %	n/a	n/a	n/a
Position 5—Right	4/21/2015	18.0 lbs	5.6 %	n/a	n/a	n/a

("**n/a**" indicates results that are not available or applicable for the listed task)

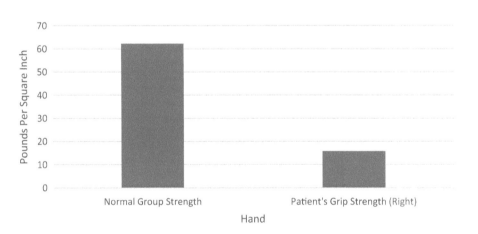

Figure 19.6 Comparison of Right-Hand Strength Deficit to Norm Group Strength Output

to participate in this study. Please note that her bilateral strength output at handle position 2 is below the normative standard. This suggests that she has significant strength loss in her bilateral hands, greater in the right dominant hand. This fact confirms she has lost digit functioning in the right hand as well as strength.

Dr. _____'s bilateral strength loss as compared to the normative average of her norm group is best illustrated in the two graphs (Figure 19.6 and Figure 19.7).

Dr. _____ requested if she could change her grip mechanic that would allow her to use both hands on the instrument. Her adjusted grips are illustrated in Figures 19.8 and 19.9. Additionally, she had difficulty with transferring the dynamometer from her left hand to her right and vice-versa.

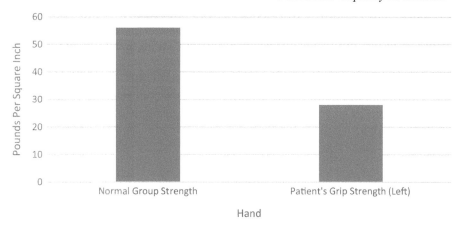

Figure 19.7 Comparison of Left-Hand Strength Deficit to Norm Group Strength Output

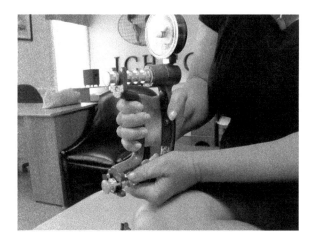

Figure 19.8 Compensated Right Mechanic Grip

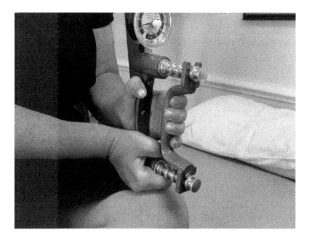

Figure 19.9 Compensated Left Mechanic Grip

Author Note: As noted earlier, grip strength testing provides the evaluator a lot of information regarding the examinee's test-behaviors while under stress, and with hand/injury cases or cases where nerve-pain affects hand function, strength deficits and the degree of strength loss can be easily identified. Given today's software technology, strength loss and gains (as modified FCEs are applied to rehabilitative therapy programs) can easily be graphed for better illustration of functional changes since injury and during rehabilitative programs.

Range of Motion

Dr. _____ underwent a range of motion study of her right fingers and cervical spine using the protocols established by the AMA and that are published in the[6] *AMA Guides to the Evaluation of Permanent Impairment*, 5th Edition. Her range data are presented in Table 19.1.3. Her ranges of motion are illustrated in Figures 19.10–19.22.

Table 19.1.3 Range of Motion

Joint	Pattern	Side	Average ROM	CV	Normative Data*
Cervical	Flexion		33.7 deg	8.6%	50 deg
Cervical	Extension		39.0 deg	**(16.8%)**	60 deg
Cervical	Lateral Flexion	Right	21.3 deg	5.4%	45 deg
Cervical	Lateral Flexion	Left	25.7 deg	4.5%	45 deg
Cervical	Rotation	Right	70.3 deg	2.2%	80 deg
Cervical	Rotation	Left	64.3 deg	4.5%	80 deg
Thumb	IP Joint Flexion	Right	69.0 deg	3.8%	80 deg
	MP Joint Flexion		Fused—30 deg	—	60 deg
2nd Finger	DIP Joint Flexion	Right	87.7 deg	5.0%	70 deg
	PIP Joint Flexion		102.6 deg	2.0%	100 deg
	MP Joint Flexion		45.0 deg	2.0%	90 deg
3rd Finger	DIP Joint Flexion	Right	84.6 deg	3.5%	70 deg
	PIP Joint Flexion		99.3 deg	3.3%	100 deg
	MP Joint Flexion		80.3 deg	4.3%	90 deg
4th Finger	DIP Joint Flexion	Right	68.3 deg	4.2%	70 deg
	PIP Joint Flexion		102.3 deg	1.4%	100 deg
	MP Joint Flexion		75.6 deg	4.6%	90 deg
5th Finger	DIP Joint Flexion	Right	73.3 deg	6.7%	70 deg
	PIP Joint Flexion		86.3 deg	3.7%	100 deg
	MP Joint Flexion		74.6 deg	2.0%	90 deg

* Indicates excessive variances among repeated measures

Table 19.1.4 Range of Motion—Digit Extension

Joint	Pattern	Side	Average ROM	CV	Normative Data*
Thumb	IP Joint Extension	Right	0.0 deg	—	80 deg
	MP Joint Extension		Fused—30 deg flexion	—	60 deg
2nd Finger	DIP Joint Extension	Right	38 deg	—	70 deg
	PIP Joint Extension		56 deg	—	100 deg
	MP Joint Extension		7.6 deg	7.5%	90 deg
3rd Finger	DIP Joint Extension	Right	6.0 deg	—	70 deg
	PIP Joint Extension		38.0 deg	—	100 deg
	MP Joint Extension		18.0 deg	—	90 deg
4th Finger	DIP Joint Extension	Right	34.0 deg flexion	—	70 deg
	PIP Joint Extension		8.0 deg	—	100 deg
	MP Joint Extension		4.0 deg	—	90 deg
5th Finger	DIP Joint Extension	Right	65.0 deg flexion	—	70 deg
	PIP Joint Extension		66.0 deg flexion	—	100 deg
	MP Joint Extension		10.0 deg	—	90 deg

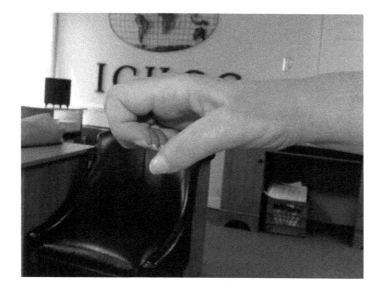

Figure 19.10 Digit Flexion

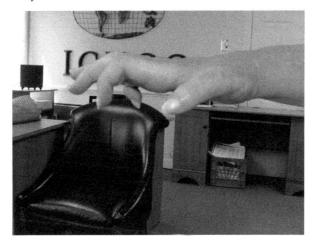

Figure 19.11 Digit Extension

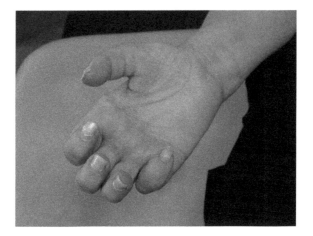

Figure 19.12 Claw Hand Relaxed

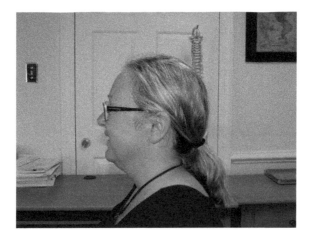

Figure 19.13 Extension (Neutral)

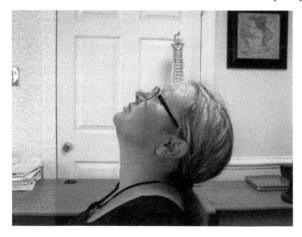

Figure 19.14 Extension

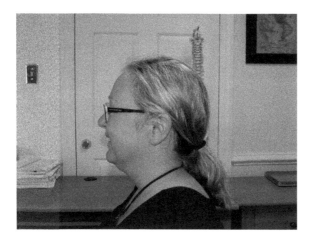

Figure 19.15 Flexion (Neutral)

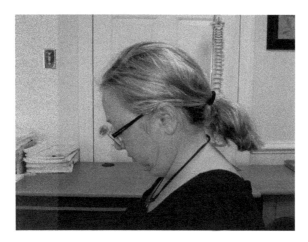

Figure 19.16 Flexion

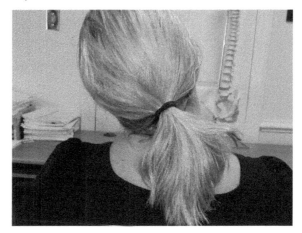

Figure 19.17 Lateral Flexion Left

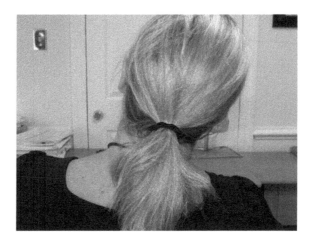

Figure 19.18 Lateral Flexion Right

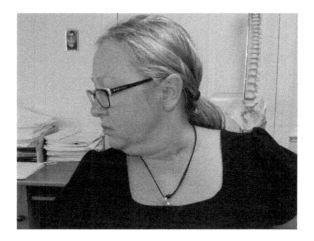

Figure 19.19 Cervical Rotation Right

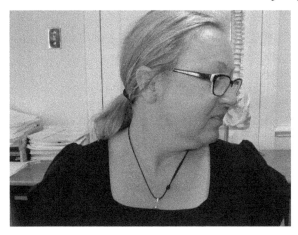

Figure 19.20 Cervical Rotation Left

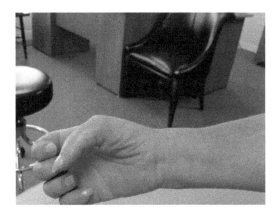

Figure 19.21 Maximum Thumb MP Flexion

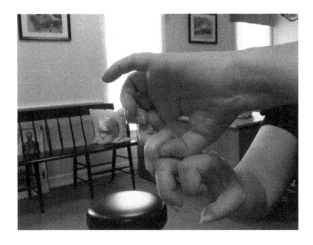

Figure 19.22 Mechanic Used to Measure Fourth-Finger PIP Joint Flexion

Discussion:

Dr. _____ had difficulty with measurements of some of her PIP and DIP joints given her contractures of those joints and her need to modify her mechanics so that measurements could be achieved and recorded. Her greatest range deficits were found to be in extension in her right fingers since her finger joints are contracted in flexed positions. Her greatest range of motion deficit was found in her 5th finger PIP and DIP joints for extension. Please note in Table 19.1.4 for extension that her 5th finger PIP and DIP joints were ankylosed at 65 and 66 degrees flexion respectively. The results of her range of motion test for both directions suggest the presence of significant hand impairment for the right hand. Her cervical spinal ranges of motion were with deficits as well when compared to her normative group; again, suggesting the presence of ratable impairment.

Author Note: The FCE evaluator should always measure ranges of motion for affected extremities and spinal joints. Such testing can identify motion deficits and instability when muscle sequencing is applied, usually resulting in excessive or elevated coefficients of variation for the respective joint tests. Please note in this case that the case manager or life care planner will see in table format that the examinee only demonstrated elevated variances in her repeated measure test for cervical extension. Pictures are important in that they illustrated any mechanical compensation for achieving measurement on the part of the examinee. Such a compromise in this case study was illustrated in Figure 19.22. Other illustrations of the hand pinpoint range deficits and ankylosed joints, which provides the case manager valuable information when determining the most suitable essentials functions of work for the examinee.

Minnesota Rate of Manipulation Test

The *Minnesota Rate of Manipulation Tests* (MRMT) is designed to measure manual dexterity with a direct application in functional capacity evaluations to assess work tolerance—i.e., how the individual will respond to sustained upper extremity motor activity in a stooped standing position. Performance on the MRMT can be used to predict success in jobs requiring arm-and-hand dexterity. For individuals undergoing rehabilitation, it is also useful in determining functional tolerance for standing, stooping, fingering and handling activities.

There are five separate tests in the MRMT. The Placing Test, the Turning Test, and the Two-Handed Turning and Placing test are the three most commonly used tests for gainful employment considerations. Each test is administered with a practice session that addresses any learning curve factors. Two additional trials are administered to assess reliability, and the ***test score*** is the total time required to complete the two test trials. Dr. _____'s results are illustrated in Table 19.1.5.[7]

Table 19.1.5 Minnesota Rate of Manipulation Tests

Subtest	Raw Score—Time	Percentile Ranking
Placing Test	159	0
Turning Test	142	0
Two Handed Turning/Placing Test	178	0

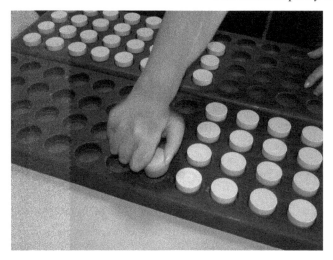

Figure 19.23 Hand Placing Test

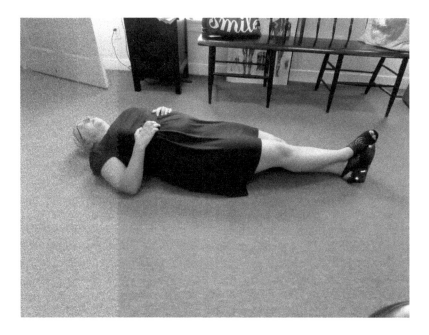

Figure 19.24 Examinee Response to Orthostatic Hypotension

Discussion:

Dr. _____ failed to register within any of the percentile ranges established for each of the three tests in which she participated. Her weakest performance was in the 2-Handed Turning and Placing Test due to her utilizing her left hand to manipulate the block back into the respective hole when the protocol called for only one hand was to be used to place the blocks into the board-holes. Such a compensated mechanic significantly slowed her time on task to where she accumulated extra time to finish the test-protocol. Additionally, her flexed fingers with a lack of extension in the right hand in addition to her manual and finger dexterity deficits resulted in excessive time-on-task for all three tests. Thus, she failed to register within any of the percentile rankings established for the Minnesota Rate of Manipulation Tests.

Author Note: The reader can clearly surmise the importance of illustrations as well as video capture of function in this particular case study just by viewing Figures 19.17 and 19.18. More importantly, video is provided that captured her hand function qualities while engaged in eye-hand coordination and applying gross motor skills as well as manual finger dexterity. The reader will note that her videos for this evaluation can be found online at www.ichcc.org/resources/research-publications.html.

Vocational Applications of Functional Data Results and Resulting Worker Trait Profile Adjustments

Author Note: This section is usually an optional section on most FCE reports. However, the life care planner and case manager may want to review this content to understand the applications of vocational data in a life care plan and in the practice of case management as well. This section is most beneficial to the life care planner and case manager in their justification of their decision regarding the examinee's employability potential, given the adjustments of the examinee's worker trait profile and the examinee's resulting transferability of skills. The transferability of skills determination is based on specific work skills that apply to the federal data base categories of directly transferable occupations, closely transferable occupations, generally transferable occupations, and unskilled occupations

Functional Capacity Levels and Criteria

Dr. _____ has incurred significant functional restrictions secondary to her cervical and spinal cord injuries and chronic pain conditions as well as bilateral upper extremity functional changes related to the car crash that occurred over 27 years ago. Subsequent upper extremity and hand surgeries with tendon releases and transfers have further impaired her motor coordination and manual/finger dexterity, in addition to her strength output deficits. Other sequelae have involved her responses to her head injury/spinal cord syndrome, orthostatic hypotension, chronic pain and neurogenic pain disorders, incontinence with intrathecal pump placement, neurogenic bladder, narcolepsy sleep disorder, sleep apnea, chronic fatigue and depression. These factors preclude her from performing the essential functions of her customary and usual job described below and titled as **INTERNIST (medical ser.) alternate titles: internal medicine specialist 070.101–026 (medical services).** Her recommended work restrictions are enumerated earlier and do not need repeating here. These restrictions are considered in the following worker trait profile adjustment analysis.

Worker Trait Profile Adjustments

Dr. _____'s primary vocational goal is to secure a job as a medical consultant as determined by the functional outcomes of this functional capacity evaluation. She was clear to this evaluator that she wants to work in some capacity within the medical field. As noted earlier in the **Summary and Conclusion** section of this report, Dr. _____ will have to function in a work setting and at a work schedule that allows her the flexibility to make periodic adjustments to her physical discomfort, to address fatigue and pain issues, as well as to step away from the work setting altogether for medical reprieve. Such a setting that meets these criteria is that of a *medical consultant*. The specific field for medical consultation is that of catastrophic injured/disabled individuals who require life care planning services to account for their future medical/rehabilitative, and habilitative needs. The specific occupational listing and description of her preinjury medical specialty group as defined by the U.S. Department of Labor is:

CODE: **070.101–042**
TITLE(s): **INTERNIST (medical ser.) alternate titles: internal medicine specialist**

Description (Essential Functions): Diagnoses and treats diseases and injuries of human internal organ systems: Examines patient for symptoms of organic or congenital disorders and determines nature and extent of injury or disorder, referring to diagnostic images and tests, and using medical instruments and equipment. Prescribes medication and recommends dietary and activity program, as indicated by diagnosis. Refers patient to medical specialist when indicated.

GOE: 02.03.01 STRENGTH: L GED: R6 M5 L6 SVP: 8 DLU: 87

Dr. _____'s preinjury, unadjusted worker trait profile as defined by the U.S. Department of Labor is listed in Table 19.1.6. Her required strength level, or physical demand characteristic, is rated at LIGHT, exerting a force up to 20 pounds occasionally or 10 pounds frequently, or negligible force constantly. This PDC level may involve significant stand/walk/push/pull trait factors. Her environmental trait factors are presented in Table 19.1.5.

These trait factors represent the minimal trait factor frequencies required when considering her worker trait profile of internal medical specialist (medical services). Her minimal aptitude percentile rankings for this position are presented in Table 19.1.8.

Table 19.1.6 Preinjury Physical Worker Trait Frequencies

Physical/Sensory Trait Factor	Duration
Reaching	Frequent
Handling	Frequent
Fingering	Frequent
Feeling	Occasional
Talking	Frequent
Hearing	Frequent
Near Acuity (Under 20 Inches)	Frequent
Accommodation (Focal Length Change)	Occasional
Color Vision	Occasional

Table 19.1.7 Preinjury Environmental Factors

Trait Factor	Duration/Level
Noise Intensity Level	Constant/Quiet

Table 19.1.8 Preinjury Minimal Aptitude Applications

Aptitudes	Percentile	Typical Performance Level
Intelligence	Over 89 Percentile	Superior
Verbal	Over 89 Percentile	Superior
Numerical	66% to 89%	Above Average
Spatial Perception	Over 89 Percentile	Superior
Form Perception	Over 89 Percentile	Superior
Clerical Perception	66% to 89%	Above Average
Motor Coordination	66% to 89%	Above Average
Finger Dexterity	Over 89 Percentile	Superior
Manual Dexterity	66% to 89%	Above Average
Eye/Hand/Foot Coordination	10% to 33%	Below Average
Color Discrimination	34% to 65%	Average

Adjustments

The following adjustments are based on Dr. _____'s functional output and competencies as determined in this functional capacity evaluation. These adjustments are as follows:

STRENGTH: This trait factor remains at **Light** due to her mechanical and strength deficits in her bilateral upper extremities and hands, particularly in her right dominant hand, her chronic fatigue patterns, residual sequela from her cord syndrome, her chronic pain and chronic neurogenic pain syndromes, her periodic adjustments in her intrathecal pump and personal hygiene, her occasional onset of orthostatic hypotension due to positioning and postural changes, and her questionable capability for sustained concentration as well as sustained physical engagement in work activity.

PHYSICAL DEMANDS: Ms. _____'s physical trait factors are adjusted as follows:

1. **Handling**—Bimanually, this is changed to "**Not-able-to-do**" rating as a result of her right-hand deficits in manual/finger dexterity and her lack of functional digits for fingering and grasping. Regarding bimanual applications, she remains at "**Not-able-to-do**," and regarding her left hand, or unilateral applications, given her left arm/hand medical history of tendon transfers and resulting sequelae, the frequency rating is changed to **Occasional**, or no more than 1/3 of the work day time period.
2. **Fingering**—This trait factor is similar to her "Handling" rating, and it is changed from her preinjury functional levels of frequent to that of "**Not-able-to-do**" when considering any bimanual applications to her work. When unilaterally engaging her left hand for handling purposes, her frequency is elevated to that of "**Occasional**,", or up to 1/3 of the workday.
3. **Kneeling**—Changed to **Occasional** due to her postural interferences with her intrathecal pump placement and lower extremity weakness and occasional spasticity.
4. **Crouching**—**Not-Able-to-Do** due to her postural interferences with her intrathecal pump placement, as well as her lower extremity weakness.
5. **Crawling**—Not-Able-to-Do.
6. **Stooping**—Occasional.
7. **Balancing**—Occasional due to instability in the lower extremities given weakness and pain, and spasticity.

ENVIRONMENTAL CONDITIONS (To which the worker is exposed): No Change

APTITUDES: Dr. _____ has incurred significant changes in a few of her aptitudes required of an internal medicine specialist. Her aptitude changes are presented in red text in Table 19.1.9.

Discussion:

Given the worker trait profile adjustments, Dr. _____ has incurred a significant loss of access to the competitive labor market. It is the conclusion of this evaluator that Dr. _____ should consider a secondary occupational option given that her adjusted worker trait profile does not match nor support her required worker trait profile for full-time work as a physician in any field; general or specialized. Based on the restrictions cited in the **Summary and Conclusion** section of this report and her worker trait profile adjustments, Dr. _____ has incurred a significant loss of access to the competitive labor market, detailed in Table 19.1.10.

Table 19.1.9 Post-Injury Minimal Aptitude Adjustments

Aptitudes	Percentile	Typical Performance Level
Intelligence	Over 89 Percentile	Superior
Verbal	Over 89 Percentile	Superior
Numerical	66% to 89%	Above Average
Spatial Perception	Over 89 Percentile	Superior
Form Perception	Over 89 Percentile	Superior
Clerical Perception	**10% to 33%**	**Nonfunctional Application**
Motor Coordination	**10% to 33%**	**Nonfunctional Application**
Finger Dexterity	**Not Present**	**Avoid Bimanual Application**
Manual Dexterity	**Not Present**	**Avoid Bimanual Application**
Eye/Hand/Foot Coordination	10% to 33%	Below Average
Color Discrimination	34% to 65%	Average

TEMPERAMENT INCOMPATIBILITIES: No Change

Table 19.1.10 Labor Market Access Loss

	Pre-Injury	Post-Injury	Percentage of Loss
Directly Transferable Occupations	18	0	100%
Closely Transferable Occupations	0	0	100%
Generally Transferable occupations	127	0	100%
Unskilled Occupations	2675	0	100%

Discussion and Occupational Access Recommendations

Dr. _____ indicated to this evaluator her desire to work in the healthcare field. She noted that she wants to contribute in some way to persons with debilitating conditions, but is not clear as to what role she could be successful. After discussing her areas of interests and options before and during this evaluation, it was clear to this evaluator that she is well informed, well trained, and most knowledgeable in medicine; it is the field of medicine where she should concentrate her occupational pursuits.

There is no doubt that Dr. _____ is no longer functionally competent to work in her chosen field of internal medicine, nor in any medical field as a practicing physician with a patient load. However, it is the conclusion of this evaluator that she could function as a medical consultant; specifically, as a medical consultant for catastrophically injured persons. The DOT does not have a listing or a definition for the occupational title of "Medical Consultant" but includes medical consulting applications in its definition of "Consultant." The DOT lists this occupation and documents its definition as follows:

CODE: **189.167–010**
TITLE(s): **CONSULTANT (profess. & kin.)**

Description (Essential Functions): Consults with client to define need or problem, conducts studies and surveys to obtain data, and analyzes data to advise on or recommend solution, utilizing knowledge of theory, principles, or technology of specific discipline or field of specialization: Consults with client to ascertain and define need or problem area, and determine scope of investigation required to obtain solution. Conducts study or survey on need or problem to obtain data required for solution. Analyzes data to determine solution, such as installation of alternate methods and procedures, changes in processing methods and practices, modification of machines or equipment, or redesign of products or services. Advises client on alternate methods of solving need or problem, or recommends specific solution. May negotiate contract for consulting service. May specialize in providing consulting service to government in field of specialization. May be designated according to field of specialization such as engineering or science discipline, economics, education, labor, or in **specialized field of work as health services**, social services, or investment services.

GOE: 11.01.02 STRENGTH: S GED: R5 M5 L5 SVP: 8

The "consultant" worker trait profile as defined earlier is compatible with her post-injury worker trait profile with adjustments. Her job description would be of one who consults directly with legal counsel or insurance benefit case managers in either a defense or plaintiff setting regarding the needs of a catastrophically injured/disabled individual. Additionally, her peers could refer to her their patients who would benefit from a documentation of their future medical, rehabilitative, and personal-life needs. She would be required to meet with the medical team staffing the case as well as the rehabilitation service providers involved. She would be responsible for detailing the patient's medical, medication, surgical, rehabilitative, home modification, specialized equipment, transportation, and personal care needs through the patient's remaining life span. Additionally, she would detail the potential complications based on the diagnose(s) and provide her findings in a life care planning report with categories of need charts. She has a wealth of training, medical knowledge and expertise to offer this highly specialized service delivery system and those medical providers who participate. This specialized service delivery system has the potential to generate a very compatible income to insure her functional independence both physically and emotionally. There are parameters that must be followed for Dr. _____ to be able establish an independent consulting practice in her field of medicine. These are enumerated as follows:

1. **Independent Practice**: Dr. _____ will have to be independent and self-employed rather than work for an established life care planning company.
2. **Support Staff**: Dr. _____ will have to have a transcriptionist as well as a driver for transportation to appointments, client staffings, and other meetings pertaining to her cases given her difficulty with driving for long durations, as well as transcribing her reports given her lack of bimanual motor coordination and manual/finger dexterity.
3. **Medical Reprieve**: Dr. _____ will need to step out of her work role at any given time during the day to address her pain, her intrathecal pump and personal hygiene, and any other condition that may cause her such discomfort that she cannot concentrate or remain on task. Thus, her need for independence in the work-force through self-employment is vital.

Dr. _____ is employable given the listed restrictions and work scenario. She has a lot to offer this particular field of consultative medicine given her background, specialty area of medicine, and her expertise and knowledge. Additionally, she would be well received by many life care planning companies for her review of cases and offering medical opinions on cases where access to the medical providers/rehabilitation service providers is difficult at best.

Notes

1 Rubler, S., & Bruzzone, C. (1985). Blood pressure and heart rate responses during 24-hour ambulatory monitoring and exercise in men with diabetes mellitus. *American Journal of Cardiology, 55*(6), 801–806.
2 Herkenhoff, F., Lima, E., Goncalves, R., Souza, A., Vasquez, E., & Mill, J. Doppler echocardiographic indexes and 24-hour ambulatory blood pressure data in sedentary middle-aged men presenting exaggerated blood pressure response during dynamical exercise test. *Clinical Experimental Hypertension, 19*(7), 1101–1116.
3 McCartney, B., & McKelvie, R. (1996). Circulatory responses to weight lifting, walking, and stair climbing in older males. *Journal of American Geriatric Society, 44*(2), 121–125.
4 Mathiowetz, V., Kashman, N., Volland, G., Weber, K., Dowe, M., & Rogers, S. (1985). Grip and pinch strength: Normative data for adults. *Archives of Physical Medicine and Rehabilitation, 66*, 69–72.
5 Niebuhr, B., & Marion, R. (1987). Detecting sincerity of effort when measuring grip strength. *American Journal of Physical Medicine, 66*(1), 16–24.
6 Normative data taken from the AMA Guidelines 5th Edition
7 From *The Minnesota Rate of Manipulation Tests*, American Guidance Service, Inc., Publisher's Building, Circle Pines, Minn., 1969.

References

Asante, A., Brintnell, E., & Gross, D. (2007). Functional self-efficacy beliefs influence functional capacity evaluation. *Journal of Occupational Rehabilitation, 17*, 73–82.

Busch, R. (2017). The notion of UCR in a life care plan. *Journal of Life Care Planning, 15*(3), 3–44.

Carr, D. (2005). The case manager's role in optimizing acute rehabilitation services. *Case Management, 10*(4), 190–200.

Cheng, A., & Cheng, S. (2010). The predictive validity of job-specific functional capacity evaluation on employment status of patients with non-specific low back pain. *Journal of Occupational and Environmental Medicine, 52*(7), 719–724.

Cheng, A., & Cheng, S. (2011). Use of job specific functional capacity evaluation to predict the return to work of patients with a distal radius fracture. *Journal of Occupational Therapy, 65*(4), 445–452.

Dabatos, G., Rondinelli, R., & Cook, M. (2000). Functional capacity evaluation for impairment rating and disability evaluation. In R. Rondinelli & R. Katz (Eds.), *Impairment rating and disability evaluation* (pp. 73–94). W. B. Saunders.

De Jong, J., Vlaeyen, J., Gelder, J., & Patijn, J. (2011). Pain-related fear, perceived harmfulness of activities, and functional limitations in complex regional pain syndrome type I. *The Journal of Pain, 12*(12), 1209–1218.

Galper, J. (2009). Baseline functional capacity evaluation components. In E. Genovese & J. Galper (Eds.), *American Medical Association guide to the evaluation of functional ability* (pp. 53–60). American Medical Association.

Galper, J., & Genovese, E. (2009). Choosing a functional capacity evaluation evaluator. In E. Genovese & J. Galper (Eds.), *American Medical Association guide to the evaluation of functional ability* (pp. 335–342). American Medical Association.

Genovese, E., & Isernhagen, S. (2009). Approach to requesting a functional evaluation. In E. Genovese & J. Galper (Eds.), *American Medical Association guide to the evaluation of functional ability* (pp. 19–40). American Medical Association.

Gonzales, J. (2017). *A physician's guide to life care planning.* American Academy of Physician Life Care Planners.

Gross, D., & Battié, M. (2004). The prognostic value of functional capacity evaluation in patients with chronic low back pain—part 2. *Spine, 29*(8), 920–928.

Gross, D., & Battié, M. (2005). Factors influencing results of functional capacity evaluations in workers compensation claimants with low back pain. *Physical Therapy, 85*, 315–322.

Gross, D., & Battié, M. (2006). Does functional capacity evaluation predict recovery in workers' compensation claimants with upper extremity disorders? *Occupational and Environmental Medicine, 63*(6), 404–410.

Gross, D., Battié, M., & Cassidy, D. (2004). The prognostic value of functional capacity evaluation in patients with chronic low back pain—part 1. *Spine, 29*(8), 914–919.

Gross, D., & Reneman, M. (2011). Functional capacity evaluation in return-to-work decision making. In J. Talmage, J. Melhorn, & M. Hyman (Eds.), *AMA guides to the evaluation of work ability and return to work* (2nd ed., pp. 87–98). American Medical Association.

Hanman, B. (1958). The evaluation of physical ability. *New England Journal of Medicine, 258*(20), 986–993.

Harper, J. (2010). Is functional capacity evaluation useful in preplacement examinations? *Journal of Occupational and Environmental Medicine, 52*(5), 567–568.

Hart, D., Isernhagen, S., & Matheson, L. (1993). Guidelines for functional capacity evaluation of people with medical conditions. *Journal of Orthopaedic and Sports Physical Therapy, 18*(6), 682–686.

Isernhagen, S. (2009). Introduction to functional capacity evaluation. In E. Genovese & J. Galper (Eds.), *American Medical Association guide to the evaluation of functional ability* (pp. 1–18). American Medical Association.

Jahn, W., Cupon, L., & Steinbaugh, J. (2004). Functional and work capacity evaluation issues. *Journal of Chiropractic Medicine, 1*(3), 1–5.

Kaplan, G., Wurtele, S., & Gillis, D. (1996). Maximal effort during functional capacity evaluations: An examination of psychological factors. *Archives of Physical Medicine and Rehabilitation, 77*(2), 161–164.

King, P., Tuckwell, N., & Barrett, T. (1998). A critical review of functional capacity evaluations. *Physical Therapy, 78*, 852–866.

Maher, H. (2006). The functional capacity evaluation. *Workplace Health and Safety (formerly American Association of Occupational Health Nurses Journal), 54*(9), 420.

Matheson, L. (1984). *Work capacity evaluation: Interdisciplinary approach to industrial rehabilitation.* Employment Rehabilitation Institute of California.

Matheson, L. (1986). Evaluation of lifting & lowering capacity. *Vocational Evaluation and Work Adjustment Bulletin, 19*, 107–111.

Matheson, L. (1987). *Work capacity evaluation: Systematic approach to industrial rehabilitation.* Employment Rehabilitation Institute of California.

Matheson, L. (2003). The functional capacity evaluation. In G. Andersson, S. Demeter, & G. Smith (Eds.), *Disability evaluation* (2nd ed., pp. 748–768). Mosby Yearbook.

Mathiowetz, V., Kashman, N., Volland, G., Weber, K., Dowe, M., & Rogers, S., (1985). Grip and Pinch Strength: Normative Data for Adults. *Arch Phys Med Rehabil, 66*, 69–72.

Matkin, R. E., & May, V. R. (1981). Potential conflicts of interest in private rehabilitation: Identification and resolution strategies. *Journal of Applied Rehabilitation Counseling, 12*, 15–18.

May, V., & Martelli, M. (1999). *The NADEP guide to functional capacity evaluation with impairment rating applications* (Chapter 4, pp. 4–52). NADEP Publications.

Mayer, T., Barnes, D., Kishino, N., Nichols, G., Gatchel, R., Mayer, H., & Mooney, V. (1988). Progressive isoinertial lifting evaluation. I. A standardized protocol and normative database. *Spine, 13*(9), 993–997.

Ogden-Niemeyer, L. (1989). *Procedure guidelines for the WEST standard evaluation*. Employment Rehabilitation Institute of California.

Pressman, H. (2007). Traumatic brain injury rehabilitation: Case management and insurance-related issues. *Physical Medicine and Rehabilitation Clinics of North America, 18*(1), 165–174.

Reneman, M., Wittink, H., & Gross, D. (2009). The scientific status of functional capacity evaluation. In E. Genovese & J. Galper (Eds.), *American Medical Association guide to the evaluation of functional ability* (pp. 393–420). American Medical Association.

Roy, E. (2003). Functional capacity evaluation and the use of validity testing. *The Case Manager, 14*(2), 64–69.

Soer, R., van der Schans, C., Geertzen, J., Groothoff, J., Brouwer, S., Dijkstra, P., & Reneman, M. (2009). Normative values for a functional capacity evaluation. *Archives of Physical Medicine and Rehabilitation, 90*, 1785–1794.

Streibelt, M., Blume, C., Karsten, T., Reneman, M., & Mueller-Fahrnow, W. (2009). Value of functional capacity evaluation information in a clinical setting for predicting return to work. *Archives of Physical Medicine and Rehabilitation, 90*, 429–434.

20 The Medical Cost Projection

Reva Payne

Some things in life are intuitive or deductive. For instance, you don't have to fracture your leg or fall on a flight of stairs to know both would be painful. It's a given. When driving down any street and observing a curb lined with overflowing trash cans, no one has to tell you it is trash pickup day. Likewise, it would be easy to surmise that a medical cost projection is a *projection* of medical costs. The definition is in the title. However, intuition and deductive reasoning will only take you so far when defining the medical cost projection. While facts and rules are essential in constructing a medical cost projection, patterns and trends are equally as important. A medical cost projection *is* a projection of medical cost, but much more. The medical cost projection balances facts, rules, patterns, and trends through a multifaceted approach to achieve the best and most accurate outcomes possible.

A medical cost projection is not an anomaly. However, pinpointing its exact origin may not be possible. It is not a stretch to suggest it was invented around the kitchen table. Just imagine a cluttered tabletop, a person frantically placing receipts into designated piles. The calculator sputters, pencils break, as the ensuing head-scratching, bewilderment, and surprise mount as the totals climb. Estimating medical costs are typically at the top of the list for those with ongoing medical concerns, chronic conditions, families with children, older adults, and those considering retirement. Knowing the current and future medical costs is an integral part of any family budget. In addition, when injuries or illness result from an individual's employment, accident, or even medical malpractice, the medical cost projection can be a salient component of the entire claims and legal process. Whether medical cost projections are used by individuals, families, government, or industries, their importance should never be underestimated.

Health care coverage and spending in 2019 in the United States alone accounted for 16.8% of the nation's gross domestic product (U.S. Health Care Coverage and Spending, 2022). According to this report, most of the spending was for hospital care, physician, and professional services. Health consumption expenditures (HCEs) have been increasing about 10% annually since 1960. In the United States, the study further emphasized that Medicare, a federal health insurance program, had an estimated 58 million individuals (18.1% of the U.S. population) enrolled in the program in 2019. In addition, this study noted that employer-sponsored insurance and non-group health insurance covered an estimated 221 million individuals combined in the United States in 2019. Out-of-pocket spending for HCE totaled $407 billion in 2019.

The National Health Expenditure Projections for 2020 through 2027 estimated national health spending growth at an average of 5.7%. It will reach nearly $6.0 trillion by 2027 (Sisko et al., 2019). With an expected gross domestic product (GDP) growth of only 4.6%, health spending as a percentage of GDP will likely be more than 10.4% by 2027. In addition, the report estimates utilization growth higher over 2020–2027 for Medicare beneficiaries and private health insurance. With statistics and predictions like these, getting a handle on health care spending

DOI: 10.4324/b23293-20

is essential and a necessity. Health care costs impact everyone whether you have health care concerns or not, and statistically, at some point, you will. Need proof? According to the Centers for Disease Control and Prevention (CDC), 6 in 10 adults in the United States have a chronic disease and 4 in 10 have two or more (National Center for Chronic Disease Prevention and Health Promotion, 2022). The report identifies the United States' leading causes of death and disability as heart disease, cancer, chronic lung disease, stroke, Alzheimer's disease, diabetes, and chronic kidney disease. The CDC points out that smoking, poor nutrition, lack of physical activity, and excessive alcohol use are contributing factors. However, the ever-rising health care costs are inescapable for individuals, employers, and the government alike. A medical cost projection can undoubtedly be a helpful tool in identifying, budgeting, and planning for future medical and related costs.

What Is a Medical Cost Projection?

A medical cost projection is a condensed, simplified, abstract document that summarizes the medical costs associated with an injury, illness, or treatment. It can also be completed to estimate a single elective procedure or surgery. The medical cost projection is used to estimate the medical services, therapies, goods, and related services required throughout an ill/injured individual's life expectancy, a specified timeframe, or a single event. Medical cost projections are typically based on the most recent two years of records, pharmacy histories, payment records, bills, invoices, and all pertinent information necessary to complete the estimate of medical treatment, therapies, goods, and related services. However, the most recent two years of records are a general rule but vary depending on the situation. For example, complex injuries may require a review of more records, and less complicated or more recent injuries may require less documentation.

Generally speaking, the industry standard for report completion is approximately three weeks from the date of the last record received. More time may be needed to complete the report based on the case's complexity and if contact with the parties is requested. A medical cost projection can be constructed on a rush basis, but most professionals would not recommend this. A three-week turnaround time is sufficient time to complete the assignment and would allow for a thorough review and a more accurate report in most cases.

Who Completes a Medical Cost Projection?

Medical cost projections are completed by a wide variety of professionals across a varied landscape, both public and private. When we think of a medical cost projection, we may conclude that a medical professional would be the only type capable of producing an accurate medical cost projection. It is not the case. Indeed, physicians, nurses, and related health care professionals have insight into the field of medicine; however, the ability to estimate medical costs is not confined to the health care industry. Medical cost projecting is used in law, insurance, and government to estimate medical expenses for various reasons. Estimating future medical costs can be completed by attorneys, case managers, rehabilitation specialists, and other human services professionals as the needs arise. However, there is a distinction: a comprehensive and professional medical cost projection is most often a report completed by an individual with particular experience, training, and certification.

Currently, there are four recognized certifications through the International Commission on Healthcare Certification (ICHCC) that would include medical cost projections as an area of focus and advanced training (The International Commission on Health Care Certification,

2021): a Certified Medical Cost Projection Specialist (CMCPS), a Certified Life Care Planner (CLCP), a Canadian Certified Life Care Planner (CCLCP), and the Medicare Set-aside Certified Consultant (MSCC). A CMCPS is an individual who meets minimum educational and professional experience qualifications as defined by the ICHCC. Every CMCPS not holding a certification as a CLCP or CCLCP must complete a 45-hour training course, receive a passing score on the certification examination, and submit a sample medical cost projection for peer review. The work sample is carefully scrutinized and must meet rigorous professional standards. The CMCPS must maintain a level of competency in medical cost projection through continuing education units with 80 required hours every five years.

The CLCP and CCLCP hold a minimum of a master's degree in a health-related field. In the absence of a master's degree, either must maintain certification or licensure in rehabilitation counseling, case management, counseling, special education, or social work. There is a requirement of a minimum of three years of field experience. According to the ICHCC, a *certified* life care planner has completed a minimum of 120 hours of post-graduate or post-specialty degree training in life care planning. In addition, they have received a passing score on the certification examination. They must submit for peer review a sample life care plan. Likewise, the work sample undergoes a comprehensive inspection and must meet all the professional standards as defined by the ICHCC. In addition, every life care planner must maintain competency in life care planning (which includes the medical cost projection) through continuing education units with 80 required hours every five years.

Tenet, Basis, and Methodology of a Professional Medical Cost Projection

Merriam-Webster defines a tenet as a principle, belief, or doctrine generally held to be accurate, especially one held in common by members of an organization, movement, or profession (Tenet, n.d.). The foundational principle that guides the process of a medical cost projection and the professional is a code of ethics that emphasizes integrity, objectivity, professional competence, confidentiality, and professional behavior (Hayes, 2022). For serious professionals, ethical guidance will be a cornerstone of the practice and the product. An experienced professional and their work will be judged by how consistently they follow their specific code of ethics. Hence, the medical cost projection is constructed with an adherence to ethical principles. The report is objective, impartial, fair, and evenhanded with an approach to activities without bias and external influence. The medical cost projection is completed by a professional who can perform their duties with a practical skill base and acceptable quality.

A working definition for the word "basis" includes the underlying support or foundation for an idea, the argument, or process; the system of principles to which an activity or process is carried out (a starting point); and the justification for or reasoning behind something (i.e., support, base, footing, rationale) (Basis, n.d.). The basis or foundation for a medical cost projection is to determine what the future medical care will be based on a review of the records provided and price those treatments, services, and related items using generally acceptable pricing resources. At this point, the medical cost projection can anticipate the associated medical and related costs over a designated timeframe. The projection then can be used to help claims professionals set appropriate reserves, increase reserves, position a file for settlement, and aid in planning and budgeting. They can also use it to price optional treatments or surgical procedures as recommended by a treating physician. Thus, the medical cost projection may be used in various ways. Still, the foundational aspect of medical cost projection is to determine the cost of future medical care and related services as outlined in the medical and associated records provided for review.

When you think of *methodology* as it applies to a medical cost projection, you should think of a *plan or course of action*. This is the method of operation, or the series of steps taken to complete a medical cost projection—the scheme of the process. The methodology is the *contextual framework* for the report and the overall process. For our purposes, the methods for medical cost reporting will involve a step-by-step process that will enhance the understanding of a particular assignment and all of its content. There is no *required* order. However, the process must address the *method of operation* for each activity. Each step will cohesively build on the last. The contextual framework takes shape. The projection is being constructed step-by-step; this is foundational. The process of medical cost projecting promotes a certain level of uniformity without detracting from the individual factors present in every medical cost projection. For example, even though two lumbar spine medical cost projections may have similarities, they are distinctly different reports in content. The mechanism of injury, the extent of injury, the diagnoses, the treatments provided, the prognosis, and the eventual outcomes can be distinctively different. However, a consistent step-by-step process brings a level of focus and promotes consistency.

As defined, a medical cost projection relies on a thorough review of the medical and related information provided. The step-by-step process is listed as follows:

1. A formal request for a medical cost projection is the first step in the process. The referral for service provides demographic information and identifies the specifics of the injury or illness and the basic expectations for the assignment. The referral will determine (or should) the purpose of the medical cost projection.
2. The professional communicates directly with the referral source. Communication can be by email. However, there is no substitute for discussing the assignment by phone or even video-conferencing. It can be quite a departure for those of is whose first-line and preferred communication methods are email and texting. Although emails and texts have the advantage of being a written record, personal contact helps develop a relationship with the referral source and facilitates a better understanding of the file and the purpose of the assignment.
3. The records are requested based on the condition or injury information provided in the referral form and any special considerations or instructions that may be outlined, keeping in mind that the complexity and status of the injury can impact what is requested for review.
4. Once the records have been received, we will conduct a cursory inspection of the information. Any missing documents will be requested.
5. The records and ancillary information are carefully and thoroughly reviewed, and the narrative portion of the medical cost projection is completed.
6. The professional conducts medical research while reviewing the information provided and while writing the report narrative. This research will support the components of the report as/ if needed. Therefore, the narrative portion of the report is adjusted as appropriate.
7. Pricing is completed based on the referral request. Medical cost projections can utilize a variety of pricing resources depending on the specific use of the report. These include workers' compensation fee schedules, usual and customary pricing, usage of payment and pharmacy histories, and even Medicare pricing. At this point, the itemized and total costs of the medial cost projection are compiled and placed in a spreadsheet format.
8. The professional may contact the referral source to let them know the medical cost projection has been completed. The report is converted to a PDF or similar format and is delivered typically by email.
9. After the report is delivered, the professionals are available to answer any questions or concerns the referral source may have.

Reviews can include bills, invoices, payment histories, pharmacy histories, court orders, settlement documents, and medical and surgical reports. Additionally, the examination can include case management reports, vocational evaluation reports, durable equipment estimates, and a wide variety of miscellaneous information. A medical cost projection is dependent on a professional's ability to conduct a *systematic* investigation of the records provided and their ability to perform supportive research. Therefore, the professional's process of discovering and uncovering the status of the file and the recommended and anticipated future direction of the treatment are critical to the overall usefulness of a medical cost projection.

Have you ever been involved in a conversation with a colleague where they referred to their source of important information as "they": they said, reported, or recommended? As you listen intently, you wonder who "they" are. Once the source is identified, you find it is frequently not a source of credible information or, at the very least, is not exceptionally reliable. Consequently, decisions are often made on sources and resources that are quickly challenged or disqualified. It is crucial for medical cost projections to rely upon and identify credible, reliable, and generally accepted sources and resources to complete the medical cost projection. A credentialed professional has explicitly been trained to approach research in a systematic and investigative manner through collecting data, documentation of critical information, and analysis and interpretation of the information they have collected. Frequently, not all the data needed to complete the medical cost projection can be identified within the information provided for review. In addition, treating professionals can be very inconsistent when outlining treatment recommendations. Some physicians state future treatment is needed and fail to identify the specific type or duration of the treatment. At the same time, others specify a particular treatment type but forget to set the length for treatment and vice versa. Finally, of course, some make no recommendations at all. In these cases, additional medical and pricing research must be performed to determine the practice guidelines and standard of care for the condition being treated. These standards and policies frequently will provide a recommended duration for the treatment as well.

A professional medical cost projection relies first on the recommendations outlined by the treating professionals. Secondarily, through credible medical resources, when a lack of direction or specificity is provided by treating physicians, specialists, or related providers. The professional completing the report, even if a licensed practicing physician or knowledgeable credentialed professional in medical cost projecting and life care planning, cannot offer their own *opinion* as fact within the medical cost projection. They would be practicing outside of their area of expertise (as the report author). Medical cost projections are supported by reliable and credible resources, not personal opinion or wishful thinking. Assertions regarding future medical needs are supported by a *rationale* or explanation of why they are included or excluded from the medical cost projection. Additionally, further support is provided when treating medical professionals make their recommendations for treatments and related services.

By providing rationales, the medical cost projection can be further supported, strengthening the foundation. But again, a medical cost projection must represent the treatment recommendations and, in the absence of treatment recommendations, must be supported by credible, reliable, and generally accepted resources. For instance, an orthopedic surgeon treating an individual for an ankle injury may conclude future medical treatment in the form of either an ankle fusion or ankle replacement will be likely within the remaining life expectancy.

The physician bases the recommendation on a current diagnosis of post-traumatic arthritis that is progressive. The professional has a decision to make: include a fusion or an ankle replacement. The present research reveals either procedure may be an acceptable treatment for the diagnosis. The professional will need to research and determine both approaches' risks, benefits, and potential outcomes when applying the particulars within the medical records reviewed. They will support their inclusion with their rationale and the credible medical research that supports their assertion.

Medical cost projections are also completed using a set of rules, sometimes referred to as *handling protocols*. Protocols may be specific or generalized relative to each assignment and often include expectational directives from referral sources. For instance, a referral source may request a particular pricing resource for every referral. In addition, they may ask for a rated age on all their referrals as the basis for determining life expectancy (Sage Settlement Consulting, n.d.). They may even specify a directive to provide a medical cost projection that includes *and* exclude a possible surgery when a surgical recommendation is present. Whatever the handling protocols include, generally speaking, these rules/protocols provide additional consistency to developing a medical cost projection from each referral source (individual or corporate). Once a thorough review and interpretation of the information have been completed, the medical cost projection narrative can be compiled.

The Components of a Medical Cost Projection

A medical cost projection estimates future medical expenses irrespective of whether these costs would be covered or not by Medicare. Although there are many ways to present the information within the medical cost projection, at a minimum, there will be a demographic section. This section outlines identifying information such as names, dates, claim numbers, life expectancy used, etc. Generally, this information is positioned at the top of the medical cost projection report. It can provide a variety of identifying information. There is no required format for presenting this information, and there are many designs that exist in the marketplace today. The sample illustrated in Table 20.1 is one possible format.

A description of the accident, injury, or illness often follows the demographic information. It will include the mechanism of injury or exposure. Some medical cost projections will provide a brief history of the initial treatment provided, especially if the injury date was years before the date of the records provided for review. The report will identify all the conditions related to the injury or illness and those pre-existing if appropriate. The information will give synapses on the medical and related services documented in the records provided for review. The synapses are presented chronologically, or *tell the story* format, which includes the most recent medical treatment for the related conditions and injuries (Kenton, n.d.). There can be a section dedicated to the current treatment plans and physician recommendations, independent or second opinion recommendations, and recommendations by other providers of medically related goods and services. Or a more popular presentation of this information is a narrative-style description of each item included in the report. This information becomes the recommendation section of the medical cost projection. Each line item may consist of a rationale to support the inclusion in the medical cost projection. Again, there are no required formats, and there are many styles

Table 20.1 Demographic Information in Medical Cost Projection

Claimant Name:	**Claim #:**
Date of Birth:	**DOI:**
Actual Age:	**Jurisdiction:**
Rated Age:	**Pricing Method:**
Life Expectancy:	**Medicare & SSDI Status:**
Life Table Used:	**Records Reviewed: (date range)**
Report Prepared By:	**Total Medical Cost Projection:**

likely encountered to present this information. However, a narrative line-item depiction of all the necessary medical and related needs is prevalent in the marketplace today. A sample format is presented next.

Medical Cost Projection

1. *Physician visits*: the record supported ongoing follow-up with Dr. Smith and Dr. Jones quarterly for condition and medication management. Therefore, quarterly visits are included for both treating physicians and are outlined through life expectancy.
2. *Laboratory testing*: a provision for laboratory testing is included due to the continued use of prescriptive medications monitoring the impact on bodily systems. The inclusion is consistent with the standards of care.
3. *Diagnostic testing*: a provision for additional left ankle x-rays and MRIs is included to monitor the conditions and due to persistent pain complaints. The inclusion of further diagnostic testing is consistent with the standards of care.
4. *Medication*: the medications are outlined based on the pharmacy history provided for review and represent the most recent physician recommendations and refill history.
5. *Emergency Room Visits*: based on a review of the medical records, a provision for additional ER visits is included. The documents demonstrated an annual visit was needed to address pain flares. Dr. Jones indicated this was likely to continue for the foreseeable future.
6. *Equipment*: a provision for additional TENS units and TENS supplies are included based on the recommendations for continued use by Dr. Jones and generally accepted replacement intervals. The invoice and payment history were utilized for pricing per referral instructions.
7. *Surgery/Outpatient Procedures*: a provision for a right ankle fusion included per Dr. Jones. The procedure was documented as likely within the remaining life expectancy due to the development of traumatic arthritis.
8. *Therapy*: a provision for physical therapy to address pain flares and or exacerbations is outlined based on the recommendation by Dr. Smith. Additional postoperative physical therapy was included due to the inclusion of a left ankle fusion.
9. *Injections*: a provision for additional left ankle joint injections is included based on the previous benefit of joint injections. As well, Dr. Jones indicated more injections might be required in the future.
10. *Home Care/Attendant Care*: at this juncture has not been reported as ongoing. Therefore, no home health or attendant care costs are included going forward.
11. *Miscellaneous Costs*: Dr. Jones has recommended a one-year gym membership at the local YMCA. Therefore, a provision for this is included.

The inclusion of the items in the medical cost projection by line-item narrative can vary depending on the treatment recommendations, standards of care, and medical research performed in the absence of formal recommendations by treating providers.

A medical cost will include a *References, Resources, and Bibliography* section to identify the resource used for pricing. In addition, references, bibliographies, and even websites used as the basis for the report, a summary section (or recap) of the information presented is frequently included. At some point in the medical cost projection, the purpose of the report is documented. Once the narrative portion of the report is completed, a medical cost projection worksheet, or the itemized and total costs associated with each narrative description, will be presented. The worksheet will identify the narrative item, rate, frequency of need, and number of years needed and provide the total and annual cost through life expectancy. The entire medical expense will

Table 20.2 Line-Item Example in Medical Cost Projection; Life Expectancy 17 Years

Physician Visits	Rate	Frequency	Total # Years	Annual Cost	Physician Total Costs
Orthopedic Surgeon (99215)	$206.18	1	17	$206.18	$3,505.06
MD Totals				**$206.18**	**$3.505.06**

Laboratory Testing	Rate	Frequency	Total # Years	Annual Cost	Physician Total Costs
Blood work (85025/80053/36415)	$69.05	1	17	$69.05	$1,173.85
MD Totals				**$69.05**	**$1,173.85**

Diagnostic Testing	Rate	Frequency	Total # Years	Annual Cost	Physician Total Costs
X-rays, Lumbar Spine (72110)	$124.43	1	5	$36.60	$622.15
MD Totals				**$36.60**	**$622.15**

Table 20.3 Summary of Costs in Medical Cost Projection

Category Totals	Annual Costs	LE Costs
Physician Visits	$206.18	$3,505.06
Laboratory Testing	$69.05	$1,173.85
Diagnostic Testing	$36.60	$622.15
Medications	$0.00	$0.00
ER Visits	$0.00	$0.00
Equipment	$0.00	$0.00
Surgery/Outpatient Procedures	$0.00	$0.00
Therapy	$0.00	$0.00
Injections	$0.00	$0.00
Home Care/Attendant Care	$0.00	$0.00
Misc. Costs	$0.00	$0.00
Projection Totals	**$311.83**	**$5,301.06**

be summarized in a separate table representing each line item to be included in the medical cost projection. A line-item medical cost projection is illustrated in Tables 20.2 and 20.3.

In some instances, a medical cost projection may include a section outlining any identified issues during the review process. For example, it may suggest the presence of inconsistencies, overlapping services, or problems that need further clarification. In addition, the professional may include a section identifying potential cost savings measures. A claims specialist may request this information at the time of the referral; however, frequently, the professional will recognize these as part of their overall medical cost projection services. An example of an issue may include noting the individual was non-compliant with treatment plans. A case manager may be beneficial for monitoring physician visits and recovery. A recommendation for second opinion evaluations or other types of independent assessments to assist with defining diagnoses or treatment options may be outlined when there may be some disagreement between treating professionals. For example, a cost-savings measure may document the continued use of brand-name medications. However, there may be acceptable alternative medications or generic formulations that might offer a significant cost savings opportunity when approved by the prescribing physician. Sometimes, multiple drugs prescribed may represent a therapeutic duplication (i.e., two anti-inflammatory medications), which can be discussed with the prescribers. By outlining potential issues and concerns and cost savings opportunities, the medical cost projection can assist the claims specialist in managing the claim more effectively. It may also improve the outcome of a specific claim.

Why Are Medical Cost Projections Needed?

A primary reason a medical cost projection is requested is to set *reserves*. Reserves are also referred to as *claim reserves* and are funds set aside to pay for future claim-related[1] obligations. For example, when an insured person has been injured or becomes ill and files a claim, the reserve gives the insurance company sufficient funds to pay the claim. These funds are required by law. In addition, the reserve represents the overall exposure of the individual claim and, considering all accounts, can be a barometer of the company's financial well-being. Therefore, there is an urgency to set the file's reserves quickly and as accurately as possible. In these cases, when needed, the claims specialist can request a medical cost projection. Likewise, when there are changes in treatment, a request for an update to the medical cost projection is requested. In some cases, the estimates are simple. The claims specialist can complete them without a need for an outside referral. Medical cost projections can also be an effective tool for planning and budgeting. A claims specialist may request them for these reasons.

Without getting into the specific legal perspectives, a medical cost projection can be requested when the file is positioned for settlement negotiations (or mediation) (LegalVision, n.d.). The negotiation and mediation activities generally occur before court hearings and proceedings. Still, they can begin at any point in time in the life of the claim. Sometimes a medical cost projection is requested to price a potential or recommended surgery. The claims specialist may need this price to increase the reserves on a file. A single cost component such as medication or durable medical equipment may represent a task assignment in the form of a medical cost projection. Often, task assignments are used when costs for a particular component represent a large percentage of the overall medical cost projection. By isolating a single part, the claims specialist may better understand the costs that are driving the claim. This information can be used to actively address any issues within the control of the claims process. In these types of assignments, the professional's recommendations are often solicited.

The Differences and Similarities: Medical Cost Projection or Life Care Plan

The most obvious similarity is that the medical cost projection and the life care plan estimate medical costs. They both require a review of the medical records and ancillary documentation to complete a report. Both will require medical and pricing research. Both life care plans and medical cost projections can be considered a guide to cost-effective management. Both processes calculate costs annually and throughout a lifetime. The life care plan and the medical cost projection follow nationally accepted standards of care which provide another level of foundational support to the report. The timing for the reports is different. A life care plan occurs toward the end of active treatment. A medical cost projection can occur at any point in the treatment process. Although the medical cost projection can become part of the legal process (generally as a subpoena), the life care plan is the definitive report used for litigation and testimony. Therefore, it is considered a legal document for *active* litigation. The level of medical research conducted on the life care plan is much more extensive than a medical cost projection. Although the medical cost projection requires medical research, it often covers only a portion of the care. The life care plan will include an interview with the ill/injured party and communication with the treatment team. The medical cost projection can consist of a visit with the ill/injured party and contact with the primary treatment provider; however, both are optional. A life care plan is reactive because it is usually completed at the end of the treatment once the individual stabilizes. At the same time, the medical cost projection can be considered proactive in some respects, as it is completed at any time during the treatment. The life care plan is also used for more catastrophic cases such as traumatic brain injury, amputations, burns, blindness, ventilator-dependent, transplants, AIDS, etc. The medical cost projection is utilized for less severe injuries and, as stated previously, may involve a request for a limited or even a task-specific assignment.

Finally, the life care plan is highly comprehensive in scope. It involves medical costs and potential complications the ill/injured individual may face throughout life expectancy. In addition, it manages non-medical expenses such as vocational training, home modifications, and transportation costs. A comprehensive life care plan will require a significant amount of additional time to complete than a medical cost projection. The medical cost projection is more limited in scope. It typically will not include any non-medical costs, complications, or an implementation strategy.

Identifying the Market for the Medical Cost Projection

Medical cost projections are utilized in a variety of markets. As previously mentioned, insurance companies specializing in workers' compensation use medical cost projections for setting reserves, revising reserves, planning, budgeting, and positioning claims for settlement negotiations (mediations) Kagan, 2022). They are used in personal injury cases, including motor vehicle accidents, slips and falls, medical malpractice, dog bites, assault/battery, other intentional injuries, and injuries resulting from product liability (Goguen, n.d.; Products Liability, n.d.). Finally, they are used by both plaintiff and defense attorneys to assist with settlement negotiations and mediation and to determine the potential settlement value or exposure of a claim (Legal Help, Advice, Legal Forms, and Lawyers (n.d.).

A virtually untapped market for medical cost projection can include estate planning and retirement planning. A significant concern for those retiring is the potentially high health care costs, including health insurance, after one retires. In addition, many retired workers go back to work in some capacity because they cannot afford medical costs or lack medical coverage (Silvestrini, 2022). Thus, it presents an opportunity to use a medical cost projection to assist individuals and their financial planning professionals in identifying medical costs throughout the life expectancy after retirement.

Summary

A medical cost projection can be a versatile tool for estimating future medical costs. The report can be used at the beginning of a claim for setting reserves when treatment changes or as the need arises for planning, budgeting, or settlement purposes. The report can function as a resource and guide when completed by a well-trained, well-versed, certified professional. It can provide each user with a higher level of confidence, allowing for a more accurate allocation of monetary resources. It may improve the management and delivery of medically related goods and services.

The professional medical cost projection derives its strong foundation from applying a code of ethics. In addition, the ICHCC monitors the profession to maintain the highest level of professional standards and adherence to practice guidelines. The medical cost projection uses a step-by-step multifaceted approach focusing on reviewing, collecting, analyzing, and interpreting data. A systematic process to conduct credible and reliable medical and pricing research. The professional's ability to appropriately document and effectively communicate the results of a comprehensive review and analysis of the information provided for review clearly and concisely is required and expected.

A medical cost projection is presented in a narrative and cost summary format. It identifies the future medical costs for an ill or injured individual and most often is projected annually and through life expectancy. It is essential to recognize that the medical cost projection is a condensed, simplified, abstract document that summarizes the future medical costs associated with an injury, illness, or treatment. It is not a life care plan. Although the medical cost projection can be used in a variety of situations, it has its limitations. For example, the medical cost projection can be used early in treatment and does not address potential complications or non-medical items. In addition, the individual may not be stable and or may be actively involved in treatment. These factors make it less likely to be the product used in active litigation or as a lifelong guide to managing medical and related service needs.

The medical cost projection has become a go-to product in the workers' compensation industry for setting accurate reserves and beginning settlement negotiations. In addition, it has a significant presence in personal injury and product liability claims. The process of budgeting and planning medical costs for those retiring is yet another role where the medical cost projection can be adopted and become a helpful guide and tool. There is every indication the medical cost projection has proven to be a valuable asset to the business community at large. It is here to stay.

Note

1   A chronology presents the medical information in date order. A tell-the-story style is more narrative and works well with medical treatment provided by a small number of providers and more routine care.

References

Basis. (n.d.). In *Merriam-Webster's collegiate dictionary*. Basis Definition & Meaning—Merriam-Webster.

Goguen, D. (n.d.). *Common kinds of personal injury cases*. AllLaw. www.alllaw.com/articles/nolo/personal-injury/kinds-of-cases.html

Hayes, A. (2022). *Code of ethics*. Investopedia. www.investopedia.com/terms/c/code-of-ethics.asp

Kagan, J. (2022). *What is workers' compensation*. Investopedia. www.investopedia.com/terms/w/-workers-compensation.asp#:~:text=Workers'%20compensation%20is%20a%20form,sue%20their%20employer%20for%20damages.

Kenton, W. (n.d.). *Balance sheet reserves*. Investopedia. www.investopedia.com/terms/b/balance-sheet-reserves.asp

Legal help, advice, legal forms, and lawyers. (n.d.). TheLaw.com. www.thelaw.com/

LegalVision. (n.d.). *What are settlement negotiations?* LegalVision. https://legalvision.com.au/settlement-negotiations/

National Center for Chronic Disease Prevention and Health Promotion (NCCDPHP). (2022). *Chronic diseases in America*. Centers for Disease Control and Prevention. Chronic Diseases in America | CDC.

Products liability. (n.d.). *Legal information institute, Cornell law school*. www.law.cornell.edu/wex/products_liability

Sage Settlement Consulting. (n.d.). *Rated ages can the key to saving your client money*. www.sagesettlements.com/blog/2018/december/rated-ages-can-be-the-key-to-saving-your-client-/

Silvestrini, E. (2022). *Health care costs in retirement.* Annuity.org. www.annuity.org/retirement/health-care-costs/

Sisko, A. M., Keehan, S. P., Poisal, J. A., Cuckler, G. A., Smith, S. D., Madison, A. J., Rennie, K. E., & Hardesty, J. C. (2019). National health expenditure projections, 2018–27: Economic and demographic trends drive spending and enrollment growth. *Health Affairs (Project Hope), 38*(3), 491–501. https://doi.org/10.1377/hlthaff.2018.05499

Tenet. (n.d.). In *Merriam-Webster's collegiate dictionary.* Tenet Definition & Meaning—Merriam-Webster.

The International Commission on Health Care Certification Practice Standards and Guidelines. (2021). *The international commission on health care certification.* https://ichcc.org/images/PDFs/Standards_and_Guidelines.pdf

U.S. Health Care Coverage and Spending. (2022). *Congressional research service.* IF10830 (congress.gov).

21 Expert Witness Testimony

Legal, Practical, and Ethical Considerations

Alex Karras and Jennifer Lambert

While there are certainly those in the scientific and clinical disciplines who enter their profession with the purpose of participating in the legal process, the decision to testify as an expert witness is often not an initial consideration for most. The evolution of a clinical practitioner into a legal expert is often unplanned and typically occurs gradually—with one toe dipped into the courtroom "water" at some point during a career in medicine or another helping profession. The result of these initial forays may result in an ongoing and potentially lucrative adjunct to one's clinical practice or even a focused practice where most of the work done by the professional is at the request of attorneys or in service of a legal or administrative body. That there is plenty of demand for experts in the courtroom is indisputable—a 1991 study found that experts appeared in 86% of trials and that there were on average 3.3 experts per trial. More recent studies show that number increasing to 4.31 experts per trial (Imwinkelried, 2020). A survey of federal judges published in 2002 indicated that medical and mental health experts constituted more than 40% of the total number of testifying experts. Medical evidence is a common element in product liability suits, workers' compensation disputes, medical malpractice suits, and personal injury cases (Wong et al., 2011). Another recent survey of pain clinicians indicated that approximately 72% of them had engaged in forensic work within the past year (Kulich et al., 2003).

When transitioning into the courtroom, scientists and clinicians will find themselves on an unusual footing—respected for their expertise, yet still demanded to prove themselves. To do so, they must tailor and present that expertise—in the form of opinion testimony—according to legal standards with which they may be entirely unfamiliar. This chapter will present an overview of aspects of the American legal system, both substantive and procedural, as well as an outline of the "rules of the road" for expert testimony—from meeting the *Daubert* standard to ethical considerations. It is important to note that there have been millions of pages written on the subject of expert testimony—this chapter is by no means an exhaustive review of the subject, nor is it meant to provide specific advice or guidance on how to manage the demands of forensic work. Rather, the main purpose of this chapter is to provide a primer for those considering expanding their practice and a set of useful reminders and relevant updates for those who already engage in legal work.

The American Court System

In the United States, the organization of the judiciary evolves from our federalist structure. This results in 51 court systems in the country—one federal court system and the court systems of each of the 50 states. Having numerous court systems means having diverse court hierarchies, as well as differences in procedural and substantive law across jurisdictions. States may, and often do, seek guidance or choose to adopt federal law, rules, and procedures, but there is nothing

DOI: 10.4324/b23293-21

compelling them to do so (Calvi, 2017). Therefore, when serving as an expert witness, it is important to understand the venue of the case, as that will determine the applicable laws and procedures.

At the federal level, there exist constitutional and legislative courts. Constitutional courts are those specifically authorized by Article III of the Constitution and include U.S. District Courts, U.S. Courts of Appeal, and the Supreme Court, as well as specialized courts such as the Foreign Intelligence Surveillance (FISA) court. Cases are generally brought in one of 94 federal district courts, and litigants typically are allowed to appeal a district court's final decision to one of the 13 regional courts of appeal. The U.S. Supreme Court may then, at its discretion, exercise appellate jurisdiction over decisions from the U.S. Court of Appeals or from a state appeals court (Nolan & Thompson, 2014).

The Constitution also grants to Congress the power to create "inferior courts". The Supreme Court has recognized that Congress has the discretion to create legislative tribunals and to assign the task of adjudicating cases (*Freytag v. Commissioner*, 1991). These legislative courts, or "Article I courts", may exercise similar authority as Article III courts, such as entering their own judgments. Examples of "Article I" legislative courts include the U.S. Tax Court and the Court of Federal Claims. Other legislative courts, the so-called "adjunct courts", may also have similar adjudicative functions, but are considered subordinate to, and subject to review by, Article III courts. These "adjunct" legislative courts include administrative agencies such as the Social Security Administration (Nolan & Thompson, 2014).

A case or controversy will originate in federal or state court based on rules of jurisdiction. Federal courts are courts of limited jurisdiction, meaning they can only hear cases authorized by the Constitution or federal statutes. For a case to be heard in federal court, it must involve a federal question (i.e., violation of the Constitution or federal law), or, in the case of a civil matter that would otherwise be governed by state law, a federal court may hear the case under diversity jurisdiction. Diversity jurisdiction applies when the litigants are residents of two different states and the dispute involves damages in excess of $75,000 (Calvi, 2017).

Each of the 50 states has its own set of courts. The major trial courts of the states are referred to as courts of general jurisdiction, meaning they deal with criminal matters, civil matters, and matters pertaining to the state constitution. Each state has the authority to hear cases that come up within its geographic territory. As with federal courts, states have various levels of courts, each designed to resolve different types of questions. Trial courts, appellate courts, and supreme courts can be found in all states, with the rules regarding the role of each defined by that state's constitution and laws (Calvi, 2017). States also have courts of limited jurisdiction (i.e., municipal courts) and administrative agencies with their own adjudicatory bodies, operating as permitted by the constitution or law of each state.

Legislative courts are created by Congress. Congress has the power to regulate certain activities that affect our lives on a daily basis. This authority is delegated to specialized bodies and agencies within the executive branch of the government. Those agencies promulgate rules and regulations by which citizens and businesses "live" their lives. Many administrative agencies have quasi-judicial functions. Take, for example, the Veterans Administration or the Social Security Administration. These agencies make an initial determination of whether a person is eligible for benefits, based on the submission of an application. If a person is denied benefits, there are procedures in place to appeal that decision. These adjudicatory procedures are put in place to prevent arbitrary and capricious action at the hands of an anonymous agency (Calvi, 2017). Although the decisions of these agencies were historically accepted without much questioning by applicants, there has been an explosion in appeals of adverse decisions in recent years. Each administrative agency has levels to its appeal process, much like the structure of federal and state courts. Ultimately, applicants whose benefits have been denied may choose to appeal the decision to a federal district court.

Substantive and Procedural Law

Aside from the "where" of a case—federal or state court—the "why" and "how" are typically the major concerns for the law. The "why" refers to substantive law—why the litigants are in the courtroom in the first place. "Law" in the United States refers generally to civil and criminal law. Both criminal and civil law have their origins in English common law. Criminal law deals with activities that are proscribed by the government—the case involves "the people" vs. the criminal. Civil law governs the relationship between individuals in the course of their private affairs. This includes torts—a dispute that arises between two people when one is injured. While both seek to deter bad behavior, criminal law focuses on the punishment of the wrongdoer, and civil law focuses on the compensation of the victim (Calvi, 2017). Administrative law is another key area of substantive law, having similarities to both criminal and civil law.

Criminal Law

Modern criminal law is driven entirely by the state or federal penal code. Specific statutes are promulgated by Congress or the state legislatures identifying crimes, defining the elements of crimes, and prescribing punishment for the crimes. With regard to criminal procedure, each element of a crime, as defined by statute, must be proven in order to convict an individual of that crime. Only the government can initiate proceedings in a criminal matter. A crime is considered as a transgression against the "state", rather than against a particular individual. One person may file a criminal complaint against another person, but only the government can charge an individual and initiate the legal proceedings designed to hold that individual responsible. Because the punishment when a person is convicted of a crime may include incarceration and/or loss of other constitutionally guaranteed rights, the burden of proof in criminal matters is higher than that of civil matters—the state bears the burden of demonstrating all elements of a crime "beyond a reasonable doubt". Moreover, criminal matters, unlike civil matters, cannot be resolved between the parties. Even plea deals must be approved by a judge and can be rejected for a variety of reasons (Erstad, 2018).

When prosecuting a criminal matter, the government generally seeks to demonstrate two necessary elements—the "*actus reus*" and the presence of "*mens rea*". In order to be convicted of a crime, a defendant must have committed an *actus reus*, or criminal act. Although generally defined as a positive act in most criminal statutes, the *actus reus* may in some circumstances be an omission or failure to act. For example, the crime of burglary may be defined as "the breaking and entering into someone else's dwelling at night with the intent of committing a felony". Therefore, if a defendant is on trial for burglary, the prosecution will have to prove that the defendant broke into another person's dwelling, that he entered the dwelling, that he did so at night, and that he intended to commit a felony therein. If the prosecution fails to prove even one of these elements, the defendant will be acquitted. Although a failure to act is less frequently a basis for a criminal prosecution, there are circumstances under which an individual is obligated to act, and failure to do so may result in criminal proceedings (*Commonwealth v. Pestinkas,* 1992). "*Mens rea*" refers to the state of mind statutorily required in order to convict a particular defendant of a particular crime (*Staples v. United States*, 1994). In order to be guilty of most crimes, the defendant must have had the *mens rea* required for the crime he was committing at the time he committed the criminal act. As with the *actus reus*, there is no single *mens rea* that is required for all crimes. Rather, it will be different for each specific crime. Although *mens rea* may vary by offenses, it is a necessary element for all crimes (*United States v. Aguilar*, 1995). Expert testimony in criminal cases may address both the *actus reus* (i.e., did the defendant commit the act, proved via DNA analysis) and whether the defendant possessed the necessary *mens rea* (i.e., expert testimony regarding state of mind, or affirmative defenses such as insanity) to be convicted.

Civil Law

Civil law, on the other hand, is not bound to statutes or codes in its application. The American system is a "common law" system, which relies upon court precedent, or case law when determining the outcome of a case. Even in civil cases where a code or statute is at issue, judicial determinations in earlier court cases are applied to the matter at hand. This is called precedent and provides predictability when it comes to the rule of law, even though the application of the rule will vary depending on the facts of the individual case (Calvi, 2017). Civil law carries a lesser burden of proof than criminal law—typically a "preponderance of the evidence" or "clear and convincing" standard. A judgment in a civil matter typically results in a financial reward/penalty or an order to change behavior. Civil suits are often settled outside the courtroom—either as a result of negotiation and agreement between the parties and their attorneys or via alternative dispute methods, such as mediation (Erstad, 2018).

When it comes to civil law, most people are probably familiar with the classic tort law case of negligence. Tort law is a body of law that provides redress between individuals, and negligence is a typical theory of a tort law case, in which an injured person alleges that the negligence of another is the cause of their injuries and that the individual should be held responsible, typically by paying monetary damages. Negligence has four elements that must be proven in order to prevail in a civil suit: (a) duty—a defendant must owe a duty to the plaintiff; (b) breach—the defendant must have breached the duty owed to the plaintiff; (c) causation—the breach must be the legal cause of the plaintiff's injuries; and (d) damages—the plaintiff must have suffered some measurable damage as a result of their injuries (Calvi, 2017).

As a prosecutor must prove all the elements of a crime, so must a plaintiff prove all the elements of a negligence claim. Case law in each jurisdiction provides guidance on how to prove each element of the claim, and it is the job of the attorney to muster the necessary proofs, including via the use of expert testimony. With regard to the duty owed, the standard most often used is that of the "ordinary, reasonable prudent person". This *reasonable person* is a creation of the law and is defined as a "hypothetical person who sensibly exercises qualities of attention, knowledge, intelligence, and judgment" (*Unified Judicial System of Pennsylvania*, 2020). Alternatively, the law may provide that duty is established by a special relationship, such as a doctor to their patient. In which case, the duty owed is that of the reasonable physician to his patient (Calvi, 2017). Having established the duty, the plaintiff must then demonstrate that the defendant breached that duty, which in turn was the direct or proximate cause of the plaintiff's injuries. Causation may be mitigated by other factors, such as intervening events, negligence on the part of the plaintiff, or an assumption of the risk (*Rabutino v. Freedom State Realty Company, Inc.*, 2002). Finally, the plaintiff must demonstrate damages—bodily harm, pain and suffering, property damage, etc. Damages are ultimately measured by a jury's award of monetary recovery, often in the millions of dollars. In a civil law negligence case, expert witness testimony may be required to address issues related to breach of duty, causation, and damages.

Administrative Law

Three things have contributed to the evolution of administrative law in the United States: the complexity of our economy, new technology, and the advancement of the "new welfare state" (Calvi, 2017). The more the government does, the more those practices must be regulated. So, Congress, in establishing administrative agencies, has also authorized these agencies and executive officials to act on its behalf. Because we want to balance the needs of agency efficiency with fairness to the people, administrative law has arisen in response to this desire. Administrative law concerns itself with the prevention of arbitrary action at the hands of public administrators. It is concerned with the abuse of official power and the overstepping of official authority. Administrative law checks the exercise of discretion by public administrators and attempts to balance the rights of citizens with the rights of government (Calvi, 2017).

Like criminal law, administrative law is based mainly on published regulations and statutes. For example, eligibility for Social Security benefits is controlled by the language of the United States Code, 42 U.S.C. 1382, and the Code of Federal Regulations § 416.202. The language of the statute and regulation control who is eligible, and like the elements of a criminal statute, an applicant must be able to demonstrate that he or she meets the requirement of the code. In administrative procedures, the expert witness is typically addressing the elements of disability required by the code, and whether the individual meets the definition under the code.

Procedural Law

Procedural law is equally important and relates to "how" a case is prosecuted. Procedural law governs the process of the law and is determined primarily by codes, promulgated by legislative and administrative bodies as rules by which attorneys and litigants must operate. This "due process of law" is guaranteed in the Constitution, and while most often associated with criminal trials, is applicable across all legal disciplines. The goal of procedural law is to ensure, as best as the system can, the fundamental fairness of any legal proceeding. All types of law have their own procedural aspects, from the criminal procedure and civil procedure to the regulations and procedures associated with administrative law. However, all procedures are governed both by published rules (i.e., Federal Rules of Civil Procedure, Social Security Administration regulations) and a court's interpretation of the application of the rules (i.e., case law) (Calvi, 2017).

From the perspective of an expert witness, perhaps the most significant rule, to be discussed later in this chapter, is Federal Rule of Evidence 702, which governs the admissibility of expert testimony. However, other rules and court practices that might be considered more specifically "procedural" are also salient for the expert witness. Experts should have at least a solid working knowledge of "how" the case in which they are involved is to be conducted in order to better prepare themselves and conduct their practice.

Although we will focus our discussion on the Federal Rules of Civil Procedure and the Federal Rules of Evidence, when considering procedural law, it is important to remember again that while many states model their practices on the Federal Rules, not all follow them in either text or application. Therefore, every expert must be cognizant of the rules of the state in which their case is venued. This is typically first and foremost the job of the attorney, to advise the expert and educate them as to rules and practice. However, once educated, it is up to the expert to mind the procedural rules for the duration of the case and, when appropriate, discuss the application of the rules to a particular circumstance before proceeding.

The Federal Rules of Civil Procedure most applicable to expert practice concern discovery. The purpose of the Federal Rules is "to secure the just, speedy, and inexpensive determination of every action and proceeding" (Fed. R. Civ. P. 1., 2019). The rules governing discovery are

designed to serve these purposes, advancing the determination of relevant evidence and potential resolution of issues before a case ever sees the inside of a courtroom. Although the Federal
Rules of Criminal Procedure differ in detail, the major reason for expert discovery in both civil
and criminal matters is to allow the parties to evaluate the evidence to be provided by an expert
at trial, and "test" that evidence, through their own expert evidence or by the opposing attorney
having the opportunity to adequately prepare his cross-examination of the expert's testimony
(*Moenssens et al.*, 1995).

A full discussion of expert discovery is beyond the scope of this chapter—indeed entire
books and treatises have been dedicated to the subject. Moreover, it is the obligation of the
attorney to be fully versed in the discovery rules and educate his expert witness accordingly.
However, from a practical perspective, it is important to understand that courts have a bias
toward openness, and that discovery is designed to expedite the litigation process. Therefore,
there are a few "rules of the road" of which all experts should be aware. For civil matters, expert
disclosures and discovery are governed by Rule 26, which states that experts whom a party may
use to present evidence at trial must be disclosed. In addition to disclosing the identity of the
expert, the parties must disclose a report, prepared and signed by the expert witness. The report
must include the following information:

i. a complete statement of all opinions the witness will express and the basis and reasons for
   them;
ii. the facts or data considered by the witness in forming them;
iii. any exhibits that will be used to summarize or support them;
iv. the witness's qualifications, including a list of all publications authored in the previous
    10 years;
v. a list of all other cases in which, during the previous 4 years, the witness testified as an
   expert at trial or by deposition; and
vi. a statement of the compensation to be paid for the study and testimony in the case.

(Fed. R. Civ. P. 26[a] 2[B] [i–vi])

For most experts, the disclosures required under Rule 26 are typically not burdensome and
include their signed report, a copy of their curriculum vitae (CV), fee schedule, and a list of
testimony given over the past four years. Experts are advised to routinely update their testimony
list in order to be prepared for a Rule 26 disclosure request, which is authorized or required not
only in federal court but in many states as well.

It should be noted that experts who are hired only as consultants, retained for the purposes of
trial preparation assistance, and not expected to testify at trial are generally not subject to disclosure, except under certain circumstances (*Fed. R. Civ. P. 26 [B][4][D]*). The Federal Rules
also protect against disclosure of draft reports, as well as communications between the expert
witness and the attorney, except for communications regarding compensation, communications
of facts or data supplied by the attorney to the expert which the expert considered in forming
their opinions, and assumptions provided by an attorney which the expert relied upon in forming
their opinion (*Fed. R. Civ. P. 26 [b][3][A] and [B]*). Despite the Federal Rules, some states have
moved away from the broadest view of what is generally known as work product protections.
Some states permit the discovery of communications between attorneys and experts that might
otherwise be considered work product (*see Barbierri v. Pitney Bowes, Inc.*, 2014 Conn. Super.
LEXIS 2627 [Conn. Super. Ct. 2014], concluding that Connecticut jurisprudence indicates that
attorney-expert communications in preparation for expert testimony should be discoverable).
Additionally, Rule 26, as noted earlier, was revised to include materials "considered" by the

expert, not just those "relied upon" in forming an opinion, arguably opening the door to broader discovery. Finally, commentators have argued that giving parties on both sides access to "full disclosure" of all communications between hiring attorneys and expert witnesses, as well as all items considered by expert witnesses, will allow the jury to make a more informed decision as to the issue of bias. Bias is not unrecognizable, and will eventually reveal itself during court proceedings (Sanders, 2007). Again, while it is the attorney's job to educate the expert as to the vagaries of the discovery rules in a particular state, an expert who doesn't wish to have his laundry hung out to dry will learn the rules and confirm his practices accordingly.

In addition to their Rule 26 obligations, the other discovery tool with which experts are most often confronted is the request for deposition testimony. Depositions are another method by which the parties gather information relevant to their case as part of the discovery process. A deposition is a witness's sworn out-of-court testimony, taken before a court reporter and in the presence of the attorneys. No judge is present, and in discovery depositions attorneys are limited in their ability to object to questions posed to the expert during the deposition. For this reason, experts may spend as much, if not more, time preparing for a deposition than they do actually being deposed. Again, it is the obligation of the attorney to prepare the expert for the deposition, including regard to the scope of questioning permitted, types of responses to avoid (e.g., answering more than is asked), and the bases of the expert opinion, including all facts of the case related to that opinion (American Bar Association, 2013). For the attorney taking the deposition of an expert, the ultimate goal might be to gather enough evidence to have the expert's testimony excluded at trial, but more likely the effort will be directed at chipping away at the application or weight of the expert's testimony. Asking questions to limit the scope of an expert's testimony, demonstrating that an expert failed to consider facts relevant to the case, or otherwise identifying areas where an expert's opinion is on shaky ground or otherwise inconsistent are all ways in which an attorney can undermine the power of expert testimony to affect the result of a case (Hochstadt, 2016).

Once discovery is complete, the parties may avail themselves of motion practice prior to trial. With regard to expert testimony, this typically takes the form of a *Daubert* motion, usually presented as a motion *in limine*. In Latin, *in limine* means "at the threshold" or "at the beginning". The purpose of a motion *in limine* is to prevent evidence from being presented to the jury that is considered too prejudicial or otherwise in violation of the Federal Rules of Evidence. While motions *in limine* are typically filed before a trial, they may also be filed during a trial, but before potentially prejudicial evidence is heard by the jury (Ryskamp, 2020). A *Daubert* motion is a specific type of motion *in limine* raised before or during a trial to exclude the testimony of an expert witness on the grounds that the *Daubert* requirements are not met. Although typically the party filing a motion bears the burden of proving the basis for the relief requested, once a *Daubert* motion is filed, the party *seeking to admit the testimony* bears the burden of proof, and they must demonstrate that their expert's testimony will meet the criteria set forth by *Daubert* (Cappellino, 2021). Occasionally, when an attorney feels that the exclusion of inadequate expert testimony would result in a case being dismissed entirely, they may bring a motion for summary judgment based on a *Daubert* challenge—essentially alleging that once the expert testimony fails the *Daubert* test, a key element of the other party's case also fails, and therefore summary judgment is warranted.

As a result of a motion challenging expert testimony, the parties must file legal briefs in support of, or opposition to, the motion, and based on the record of evidence developed during discovery. Under normal circumstances, a court may resolve a *Daubert* motion without holding a hearing (*Nelson v. Tenn Gas Pipeline Co.*, 243 F.3d 244 [6th Cir., 2001]; Cappellino, 2021). When the parties brief the admissibility of experts' testimony and develop an extensive record that includes depositions, a hearing may be unnecessary. The judge has the discretion to determine whether a hearing is necessary or may resolve the question on the record presented to him. Any method of review is permitted, so long as the court performs an evaluation with a sufficient record that can be reviewed on appeal and in its ruling articulates the reasons for its determination (Cappellino, 2021; Calvi, 2017).

If a *Daubert* hearing is ordered and an expert is called to testify at the hearing, what is important to remember is that there is a presumption of admissibility when it comes to relevant evidence. The ruling in *Daubert* was in response to the Court's recognition that the more limiting "general acceptance" standard previously established by the *Frye* ruling was "at odds with the 'liberal thrust' of the Federal Rules of Evidence and their 'general approach of relaxing the traditional barriers to opinion testimony'" (*Daubert*, at 588). Factual disputes alone are not sufficient to preclude expert testimony via a *Daubert* motion, and if called to testify at a *Daubert* hearing, experts whose practices meet the standards of *Daubert* have little to fear (Edwards & Edwards, 2020).

Administrative law again presents its own set of rules for procedural law. Typically, these proceedings are designed to be informal, and procedural devices such as the exhaustion of administrative remedies doctrine, the primary jurisdiction doctrine, and the substantial evidence rule tend to keep cases in administrative court (Calvi, 2017). At the most formal adjudication, decisions are made by an administrative law judge, taking into consideration evidence, including expert testimony, presented by the petitioner and administrative agency. Controlling case law for these proceedings is *Goldberg v. Kelly* (1970). Goldberg factors include, among others, the right to present evidence, the right to present oral arguments, the right to retain an attorney, disclosure of opposing evidence (what was relied on to deny benefits), and the right to an impartial decision maker. It is not the case, however, that every administrative court has adopted all the Goldberg factors in its procedure. Moreover, in *Richardson v. Perales*, (1971), the Supreme Court reaffirmed the "informal, non-adversarial manner" of disability hearings. Some commentators have noted that despite the pretense of informality, administrative proceedings are the functional equivalent of civil non-jury trials and that more formal rules of procedure and evidence should apply (Glicksman, 1999). The argument is that the application of the Federal Rules of Evidence would provide predictability, keep bad evidence (including unreliable hearsay) from being considered, and assure fairness while still providing a viable alternative to general jurisdiction courts.

This argument has not gained any traction, however. The Supreme Court recently confirmed the deference to be provided to administrative rulings, as well as the refusal to apply more formal evidentiary rules to administrative proceedings. In *Biestek v. Berryhill* (2019), the court ruled that a vocational expert did not have to provide specific data underlying her conclusions, since her testimony met the "substantial evidence rule" applicable in administrative proceedings. The Court noted that "substantial evidence" is a term of art in administrative law, requiring only "sufficient evidence" to support the agency's factual determinations. The Court went on to note that the word "substantial" should not be construed as requiring anything more than "such relevant evidence as a reasonable mind might accept as adequate to support a conclusion". While the Court acknowledged that experts willing to share all the data on which they base their conclusions provided a stronger basis for their testimony and could be considered as engaging in "best practices", the Court refused to adopt a rule that an expert's testimony must be excluded as unreliable absent disclosure of the data.

Therefore, with regard to administrative proceedings, experts are not bound by the same procedural rules or case law such as *Daubert* and instead must look to the agency publications and applicable administrative law precedents relevant to the requirements of testimony (see Social Security Administration, *Vocational Expert Handbook* [2017]).

Expert Testimony: *Frye*, the Federal Rules of Evidence, *Daubert*, and Its Progeny

As mentioned at the start of the chapter, experts have become ubiquitous in today's legal system. While we accept this as inevitable, given the complex nature of our society and therefore its legal disputes, it is worthwhile to be reminded of the problem posed by expert testimony as expressed more than 100 years by Learned Hand and more recently noted by the Supreme Court in *Kumho Tire v. Carmichael*—that while expert testimony is welcomed because of the knowledge and skills possessed by experts which allow them to draw inferences beyond the competence of lay jurors, it is precise because of this lack of competence that jurors may be unable to properly evaluate the expert's testimony (Hand, 1901). Additionally, judges are also routinely asked to assess evidence in cases based on principles of science about which they know little. As observed by Justice Breyer, judges tend to be "generalists", dealing with a wide variety of cases and seeking mainly to reach fair decisions in a timely manner. The fact that those decisions often rest on specific facts and evidence, including expert scientific testimony, means that "the law must seek decisions that fall within the boundaries of sound scientific knowledge" (Breyer, 2011).

So, if lay jurors may be too "swayed" by expert testimony because they can't adequately examine it, then what is the solution? Since we have previously discussed the general preference of the law for openness and admissibility of relevant evidence, it makes sense that the evolution of rules governing expert witness testimony would begin with the threshold issue of admissibility. In 1923, the D.C. Circuit Court returned its decision in the matter of *Frye v. United States* (1923). *Frye* involved the use of what was at the time the equivalent of a lie detector test. At the time, the standard for admission of expert testimony was based on whether the legal determination to be made "does not lie within the range of common experience . . . but requires special experience or special knowledge" (*Frye* at 1014). If this was found to be the case, then expert opinion testimony would be admitted. As has been observed by commentators, this liberal and arguably unquestioning acceptance of expert testimony in American law resulted in a cottage industry of experts for hire; by the end of the 19th century, the "sale" of expert testimony had become so widespread that there was a tendency to distrust it entirely (Matthiesen, 2020). *Frye* took the previously established rule for admission and clarified a further requirement. In holding that the expert testimony about the "blood pressure deception test" was inadmissible, the court held that expert testimony must be based on scientific principles that are "sufficiently established to have gained general acceptance in the particular field in which it belongs" (*Frye*, at 1014). Thus, the *Frye* rule or "general acceptance test" became the standard to determine the admissibility of expert testimony. Testimony that was based on scientific methods that were generally accepted was admissible, and scientific methods that were on the fringe, or not "sufficiently established" were not.

Frye remained the standard until the U.S. Supreme Court handed down its decision in *Daubert v. Merrell Dow Pharmaceuticals, Inc.*, 509 U.S. 579 (1993). Prior to the *Daubert* decision, the Federal Rules of Evidence were promulgated by Congress and adopted by the Supreme Court and initially published in 1973. At the outset in *Daubert*, the Court noted that Rule 402 provided a baseline for admissibility, in that "All relevant evidence is admissible, except as otherwise provided . . . by these rules". The Court then referred to the requirements of Rule 401 and described relevant evidence as that "which has any tendency to make the existence of any fact that is of consequence to the determination of the action more probable or less probable than it would be without the evidence" (*Daubert* at 582). The Court thus concluded that the basic standard of relevancy was a liberal one, with a tendency to favor admissibility. With regard to expert testimony, Rule 702 of the Federal Rules provides:

> If scientific, technical, or other specialized knowledge will assist the trier of fact to understand the evidence or to determine a fact in issue, a witness qualified as an expert by knowledge,

skill, experience, training, or education, may testify thereto in the form of an opinion or otherwise.

The Court then noted that nothing in Rule 702 mentioned a "general acceptance" standard, and in fact made no mention of *Frye*, either in the comments or the drafting history. The Court concluded that *Frye* had been superseded by the Federal Rules of Evidence and should not be applied in federal trials.

The court went on to delineate the role of the judge in considering expert testimony, recognizing the trial judge as a "gatekeeper" who must evaluate proffered expert testimony. As a gatekeeper, the judge was responsible to determine that the expert testimony was "not only relevant but reliable" (*Daubert*, at 589). In order to satisfy the standard of evidentiary reliability, the *Daubert* court identified a number of factors that a judge may consider when making the inquiry "envisioned by Rule 702". These factors include (a) whether the theory or technique in question can be and has been tested; (b) whether it has been subjected to peer review and publication; (c) its known or potential error rate; (d) the existence and maintenance of standards controlling its operation; and (e) whether it has attracted widespread acceptance within a relevant scientific community. The court emphasized that a *Daubert* inquiry was designed to be a flexible standard and not a definitive checklist (*Daubert* at 593–594). Since the decision in *Daubert*, the Federal Rules of Evidence have been amended to reflect the substance of the ruling, and in its most recent iteration Rule 702 reads:

A witness who is qualified as an expert by knowledge, skill, experience, training, or education may testify in the form of an opinion or otherwise if:

(a) the expert's scientific, technical, or other specialized knowledge will help the trier of fact to understand the evidence or to determine a fact in issue;
(b) the testimony is based on sufficient facts or data;
(c) the testimony is the product of reliable principles and methods; and
(d) the expert has reliably applied the principles and methods to the facts of the case (Fed. R. Evid. 702). The "factors" set forth by the Court in *Daubert* continue to be the touchstones by which expert testimony is judged.

The Court's ruling in *Daubert* led to a proliferation of *Daubert* motions and *Daubert* hearings, all designed to test whether expert testimony could satisfy the new requirements. This led to two additional rulings which further clarified the Court's original ruling in *Daubert*. The first case, *General Electric Co. v. Joiner*, 522 U.S. 136 (1997), dealt with a trial court's exclusion of expert testimony regarding animal studies and the effects of exposure to polychlorinated biphenyls (PCBs), which the expert then extrapolated to support the plaintiff's allegation of PCB exposure as the cause of his lung cancer. The trial court applied the *Daubert* criteria, excluded the testimony of the plaintiff's experts, and granted the defendant's motion for summary judgment (*Joiner v. Gen. Elec. Co.*, 864 F.Supp. 1310 [N.D. Ga. 1994]). The 11th Circuit Court of Appeals reversed, stating "[b]ecause the Federal Rules of Evidence governing expert testimony display a preference for admissibility, we apply a particularly stringent standard of review to the trial judge's exclusion of expert testimony" (*Joiner v. Gen. Elec. Co.*, 78 F.3d 524, 529 [11th Cir. 1996]). The Supreme Court was unanimous in its rejection of the 11th Circuit's ruling. The court stated that the correct standard for an appellate court to apply in reviewing a district court's evidentiary ruling, regardless of whether the ruling allowed or excluded expert testimony, is the abuse of discretion standard (*Joiner*, at 141–143). Additionally, rather than remand the case the Court went further and conducted its own examination of the proffered expert evidence and concluded that the experts had been properly excluded. The Court noted that the plaintiff never attempted to connect the animal studies to the plaintiff's exposure and that the trial court was within its discretion to find that the limited epidemiological studies cited by the plaintiff were insufficient to support the expert's conclusions. Moreover, the Court rejected the plaintiff's position that a *Daubert* inquiry must be limited to principles and methods, not conclusions, and that as long as the scientific methods used to reach a conclusion were reliable, then it is erroneous to exclude an expert's conclusions. In rejecting the argument, the Court stated that

> conclusions and methodology are not entirely distinct from one another . . . nothing . . . requires a district court to admit opinion evidence which is connected to existing data only by the *ipse dixit* of the expert. A court may conclude that there is simply too great an analytical gap between the data and the opinion proffered.
>
> (*Joiner*, at 146)

The third case in the trilogy was decided less than a year later. In *Kumho Tire Co. v Carmichael*, 526 U.S. 137 (1999), the Court ruled that the trial judge's obligations under *Daubert* extend to all forms of expert testimony, not just "scientific evidence". In *Kumho*, the plaintiffs relied on an expert in tire failure analysis, who performed a visual inspection of a tire that had blown out, causing an accident resulting in the plaintiffs' injuries. The trial court excluded the plaintiffs' experts following the defendant's motion which alleged that the expert's testimony did not meet the criteria set forth in *Daubert*. On appeal, the plaintiffs argued that their expert had performed a "technical analysis", based on his experience and skill, and was therefore not subject to *Daubert*. The 11th Circuit reversed the trial court, concluding that the testimony of the plaintiff's expert was "non-scientific" and opining that *Daubert* applies only to scientific opinion (*Carmichael v. Samyang Tire, Inc.*, 131 F.3d 1433, 1435 [11th Cir. 1997]).

The Supreme Court reversed the 11th Circuit, finding that Federal Rule of Evidence 702 "makes no relevant distinction between 'scientific' knowledge and 'technical' or 'other specialized' knowledge" and that the reliability standard must be applied to all expert testimony (*Kumho* at 148). The Court observed that experts were likely to "draw [conclusions] from a set of observations based on extensive and specialized experience" (*Kumho* at 156) but that did not excuse the trial court from making a complete determination regarding admissibility. The *Kumho* opinion stressed a flexible approach to expert testimony, stressing "the particular circumstances of the particular case at issue", and demanding that an expert observe and apply the same standard of "intellectual rigor" in testifying as he or she would employ in similar matters outside the courtroom (*Kumho* at 150, 152). Perhaps most importantly, the Kumho court noted that, in making the type of "flexible" inquiry demanded by the Federal Rules, "Daubert's list of specific factors neither necessarily nor exclusively applies to all experts or in every case. Rather, the law grants a district court the same broad latitude when it decides how to determine reliability as it enjoys in respect to its ultimate reliability determination" (*Kumho* at 141–142).

The Application of *Daubert*

At the outset, it should be noted that while *Daubert* is strictly applied to all cases in federal court, it has not been universally adopted by the states. There are some states that still adhere to the *Frye* standard, and it is up to the expert witness to know the standard particular to the state in which he or she finds themselves testifying (*see* Matthiesen, 2020, for a state-by-state list of

Daubert and *Frye* applications). We are of the professional opinion that if an expert can meet the *Daubert* standard, they can meet the *Frye* standard, and therefore we will limit our discussion in this section to the *Daubert* criteria. Moreover, even in jurisdictions that still profess adherence to *Frye*, court decisions reflect a "creeping" influence of the *Daubert* factors when considering expert testimony (see *In re Accutane Litigation*, 191 A.3d 560 [2018], and Pehush et al., [2019]).

The qualification of an expert witness is the threshold matter in any *Daubert* inquiry. Rule 702 specifically provides an expert must have "skill, experience, training or education" to be qualified. A proposed expert must also have "knowledge" relevant to the testimony he or she will provide (Berger, 2011). An expert's qualifications are not typically defined by the court, but rather by the discipline in which that expert practices. Depending on the discipline, there may be licensure requirements put forth by a state, such as a state board of medicine. Professional organizations may define the qualifications for certification, such as the American Board of Vocational Experts. Additionally, some experts are qualified based on regulations provided by the agency or tribunal in which they will be offering an expert opinion. For example, the Social Security Administration has specific criteria for qualifying vocational experts who may testify before an administrative law judge (Social Security Administration, 2017). In addition to education, licensure, or certification, an expert should be qualified to offer testimony on the specific subject matter at issue in the case. For example, a physician should limit their testimony to only those areas in which they have appropriate training and recent, substantive experience and knowledge (American Medical Association, Code of Medical Ethics Opinion 9.7.1). Physicians or other health professionals who are multiply "boarded" or certified may be asked to testify to a wider scope of issues, given their broader expertise, although the "recent, substantive experience" requirement also gives opposing counsel an avenue to challenge testimony that strays too far.

If we assume, which seems fair to do, that most practitioners who decide to become expert witnesses are otherwise qualified in their field, why does the law concern itself with qualifying experts as a threshold matter? If we accept that the ultimate usefulness of expert testimony is assisting the trier of fact, then the test for admitting expert testimony must start with the qualifications of the expert and whether they possess the type of specialized understanding of the subject involved in the case. If not, then their testimony would be "unhelpful, superfluous, and would fail the relevancy requirement of all evidence" (Advisory Committee Notes, Federal Rule of Evidence 702). Moreover, because the rules of evidence permit experts to use otherwise inadmissible evidence (e.g., hearsay) as a basis for their opinion, the law is obligated to perform this gatekeeping duty in an initial effort to preclude the presentation of bad evidence to the jury.

It should be noted that challenges to qualifications, even for experts who have routinely accepted by courts in the past, should always be expected. Challenges must be expected not only to a witness's qualifications and expertise generally but also to specific details regarding their opinion and testimony. A recent case in the Pennsylvania Superior Court reviewed the disqualification of a life care planner who testified regarding the long-term care required for a patient with kidney failure. The defense argued at trial that the life care planner, a nurse with experience in cardiac care patients and children with cerebral palsy, was unqualified to estimate costs associated with kidney transplant patients. The trial court excluded the testimony. On appeal, the plaintiff's counsel noted that requiring life care planners to have specialized knowledge regarding all types of injury was excessive. However, the defense counsel noted that no medical expert testimony had been offered regarding future care for kidney failure, only past costs, and that therefore the life care planner had exceeded the scope of her qualifications in estimating the costs. While the appellate court ultimately rejected the defense's argument, it is reasonable to assume that similar "micro" arguments as to a particular life care planner's expertise may be presented in other cases or jurisdictions, and therefore should be considered and prepared for in advance (*Povrzenich v. Ripepi* et al., 2021 WL 1047363; "The fact that [the life care planner] had little experience with kidney transplant patients did not disqualify her from using her skills and experience to analyze the costs . . . [a]ny lack of experience with kidney transplants, in particular, went to the weight of her testimony, not to its admissibility", p. 7).

Once an expert is accepted as qualified, then the analysis shifts to the testimony and whether it meets the criteria set forth by the *Daubert* trilogy. At all times, it is important to keep in mind that the *Daubert* factors are neither exclusive nor dispositive and that not all factors apply to every expert. What courts are looking for is "reliable" evidence—reliability may be demonstrated in a variety of ways. It should also be reiterated that the application of the *Daubert* standard is a liberal one, with a preference for admitting evidence and leaving it to the fact-finder to assign the appropriate weight at trial. For physicians, life care planners, vocational experts, and disability analysts, reliability may be less based on things like published error rates and more concerned with indicia of clinical reliability—such as peer-reviewed research, standards of practice, and acceptance of the methods generally in one's field. The expert must then be able to connect their methodology to their conclusions—thereby avoiding the *ipse dixit* exclusion delineated in *Joiner*, where conclusions too loosely associated with the method are considered unreliable and inadmissible.

With regard to expert testimony, the lesson for physicians must be that substantiated, competent, and reliable evidence comes down to traditional scientific foundations—biological plausibility and prior evidence, and consistent repeated findings. Physicians applying the basic concepts of diagnostic reasoning and clinical decision-making using these traditional scientific foundations should find themselves on solid ground in the courtroom (Wong et al., 2011). When performing an evaluation of a patient, for litigation or otherwise, physicians rely on their clinical experience. However, when it comes to presenting expert testimony, that experience alone is considered insufficient under the *Daubert* criteria. Conclusions based solely on experience and anecdote may be fairly regarded as suspect in their application to other patients and other circumstances (Mangrum & Mangrum, 2019). Federal courts have agreed that clinical experience alone may not be enough—"an anecdotal account of one expert's experience, however extensive or impressive the numbers it encompasses, does not by itself equate to a methodology, let alone one generally accepted by the relevant professional community" *(Berk v. St. Vincent's Hosp. and Medical Center*, 380 F.Supp.2d 334 [SDNY 2005]). Employing additional, generally acceptable methods—SOAP (subjective complaints, objective tests, analysis through differential diagnosis, plan of treatment), differential diagnosis, and differential etiology (establishing or refuting causation between an external cause and a plaintiff's condition)—is more consistent with reliable expert testimony and more likely to survive a *Daubert* challenge (Wong et al., 2011).

Commentators have observed that physicians employing an evidence-based approach to medicine can more easily pass the *Daubert* test. Evidence-based medicine expects physicians, when making a diagnosis, to move past individual case reports up the ladder of reliability to consideration of randomized trials and case-controlled studies to systematic reviews of peer-reviewed studies. This comprehensive approach thus provides the level of reliability upon which expert testimony and the verdicts it produces can solidly rest (Mangrum & Mangrum, 2019). Reliable expert testimony from physicians comes from the quality/integrity of the witness and the application of the best evidence that compliments the witness' expertise and formulated on systematic research (Wong et al., 2011).

Courts have not shied away from excluding physician evidence that does not meet reliability standards set forth in *Daubert*. In *Maurer v. Trustees of the University of Pennsylvania et al.*, 614 A.2d 754 (Pa. Super. Ct., 1992), the Pennsylvania Superior Court ruled that a physician's testimony should have been excluded because his conclusions were based on his own personal standard of care and not the standard of medical care generally. The physician was further unable to cite any research studies that supported his standard of care (administration of a drug to prevent heterotopic ossification). The court concluded not only should his testimony have been excluded, but went so far as to enter judgment n.o.v. for the defendant's hospital, an extraordinary remedy. In *Heller v. Shaw Industries*, 167 F.3d 146 (3d. Cir., 1999), the Third Circuit ruled that a physician's testimony regarding causation in a toxic tort claim was insufficient. The court noted that although the physician used differential diagnosis in reaching his conclusions, he failed to provide any evidence of research or studies supporting his conclusions. Specifically, while the physician "ruled out" other causes of the plaintiff's symptoms, he failed to "rule in" exposure to the toxic substance as the specific cause of the plaintiff's symptoms and therefore her injuries. Summary judgment was granted in favor of the defendant. Despite its ruling in *Heller*, the Third Circuit took pains to note that physicians are not always required to cite published studies in support of their conclusions and that other methodologies accepted as reliable in the profession (i.e., experience with numerous patients, thorough examinations, discussions with peers) may suffice as sufficient to meet the *Daubert* standard (*Heller*, at 155). Finally, physicians may find themselves facing a *Daubert* challenge when their expertise lies outside the subject matter of the case. Although the American Medical Association (AMA) has promulgated ethical guidelines that call for physicians to testify "only in areas in which they have appropriate training and recent, substantive experience and knowledge", there is nothing in the law that specifically compels them to do so, other than a successful *Daubert* challenge (see *Pipitone v. Biomatrix, Inc.,* 288 F.3d 239 [5th Cir., 2002]).

For life care planners, disability analysts, and vocational experts, the lessons are much the same. Expert testimony must be supported by reliable, demonstrable methodologies, reach appropriate conclusions based on those methodologies, and experts should practice within their specialty. Those whose testimonies are excluded by the court fail to meet these standards. In *Queen v. WIC Inc.*, the U.S. District Court for the Southern District of Illinois excluded the testimony of a physiatrist life care planner, determining that his report and opinions failed to satisfy the *Daubert* standard. The court noted that the life care planner set forth his conclusions and recommendations for future care based on a severely limited record and made no attempts to corroborate his findings or conclusions with the plaintiff's treating providers. Moreover, the court observed that the life care planner, himself a physiatrist, was operating outside his area of expertise in making recommendations regarding future orthopedic and surgical care (*Queen v. W.I.C., Inc.*, Case No. 14-CV-519-DRH-SCW, [S.D. Ill. September 5, 2017]). Unfortunately, because the life care planner's testimony was excluded, the court also excluded the testimony of the plaintiff's economic expert, which relied on the life care planner's report, thereby vitiating the bulk of the plaintiff's case on damages. In a more recent case not involving but instructive for life care planners, an Illinois appellate court excluded the testimony of a medical billing expert after rejecting her methodology for determining the costs of future medical care. The court determined that the expert's reliance on a database to determine reasonable medical costs, without corroborating her numbers using other sources like providers in the plaintiff's area, or a treating physician's actual charges, rendered her testimony unreliable. In examining the reliability of the database used by the expert, the court found that it was not applicable to the issue of the plaintiff's future medical costs, and thus excluded the testimony (*Verci v. High et al.*, 2019 IL App [3d] 190106-B [December 18, 2019]). Vocational experts have also been excluded where their qualifications or methodologies have failed *Daubert* scrutiny (*see Gibson v. Smithkline*, [S.D. Miss. 2016]). For example, vocational expert testimony was excluded due to unfounded and speculative methods and insufficient basis in the record for conclusions; *Williams v. Baker*, (W.D. Pa., 2016). A vocational expert was excluded due to marginal qualifications, unreliable methodology, and speculative conclusions; *Elcock v. Kmart* (3rd. Cir. 2000). And a case was remanded for a *Daubert* hearing after the court's determination that a vocational expert's marginal qualifications, coupled with his questionable methods, could not support the verdict for the plaintiff.

Even if an expert is otherwise qualified and adheres to the standard and accepted methodologies, there are other areas where an opposing counsel can attack testimony, succeeding in having all or part of the testimony excluded. Federal Rule of Evidence 703 provides the acceptable bases for expert testimony as follows:

> An expert may base an opinion on facts or data in the case that the expert has been made aware of or personally observed. If experts in the particular field would reasonably rely on those kinds of facts or data in forming an opinion on the subject, they need not be admissible for the opinion to be admitted. But if the facts or data would otherwise be inadmissible, the proponent of the opinion may disclose them to the jury only if their probative value in helping the jury evaluate the opinion substantially outweighs their prejudicial effect.
>
> (U.S. District Court for the District of New Hampshire)

One of the ways expert testimonies can be challenged is with regard to the use of hearsay evidence by the expert. The Federal Rules of Evidence forbid the use of hearsay testimony at trial, with some exceptions. Generally speaking, Rule 801 describes hearsay as a statement made by a witness, not while testifying in the current hearing, offered as evidence of the truth of the matter stated. For the purposes of this chapter, an example of hearsay would be when a life care planner calls a doctor and asks what treatment a patient requires. If that doctor will not be testifying himself about the recommendations, then the life care planner's testimony about what the doctor said would be considered hearsay. However, there are exceptions to hearsay, and experts have generally been given further latitude, with courts permitting hearsay testimony if it reflects the type of information "generally relied upon" by experts in the field as provided in Rule 703. Additionally, records used by life care planners, physicians, and other experts, such as medical records, likely fall under exceptions to the hearsay rules and may be introduced as evidence to substantiate expert testimony.

Despite this leeway, courts in some jurisdictions have tightened hearsay rules, while others have strictly construed hearsay testimony by expert witnesses to ensure its reliability and applicability. Most significantly, in *The People v. Sanchez*, 63 Cal.4th 665 (2016), the California Supreme Court held that while an expert could still rely on hearsay testimony in forming his opinion, he could no longer present the hearsay testimony as true, case-specific facts, unless they were independently proven evidence or covered by a hearsay exception (*Sanchez*, at 24). Thus, a life care planner seeking to testify regarding future medical costs based on a phone call to a vendor or other provider may be excluded from doing so, based on the *Sanchez's* limitations on hearsay. To date, the ruling has not been significantly extended or adopted in other jurisdictions, although it has been argued against a life care planner in New Jersey. In *Morales-Hurtado v. Reinoso et al.* 230 A.3d 241 (2020), the New Jersey Supreme Court found the exclusion of an expert life care planner's testimony based on hearsay to be a reversible error. The court noted that the expert was entitled to rely on the statements of another expert, provided it met the "typically relied upon" exception. The court did not comment on the sufficiency of the life care planner's testimony and remanded the case for a new trial.

Attorneys may also choose to attack pieces of an expert's testimony in order to whittle away at any determinations in the opposing party's favor. For example, in *Cowher v. Kodali* (2021), the Pennsylvania Superior Court rejected the portion of an expert's testimony regarding pain and suffering as inadmissible. In *Cowher*, the expert physician offered an opinion regarding the plaintiff's pain and suffering during a heart attack. The opinion was based solely on the statement of a witness who had testified that she saw the plaintiff while he was having the heart attack, and he appeared to be in pain. The court noted that the physician did not apply his medical expertise to the issue of pain and suffering, but merely adopted the neighbor's fact testimony as his own. The court ruled that the testimony was therefore nothing more than the expert's personal opinion and not admissible as expert testimony. The court further noted that the admission of improper expert testimony has the significant potential for prejudicial effect, since jurors may assign more weight or credibility to expert testimony. Based on its findings, the court awarded a new trial on the issue of pain and suffering damages (*Cowher v. Kodali*, 2021).

Additionally, with the expansion of limited tort laws and statutes regarding medical malpractice claims, there have been attempts across jurisdictions to limit expert testimony regarding damages. These cases relate generally to the application of the collateral source rule, which typically excludes testimony regarding what part of medical damages might be covered by a plaintiff's insurance, and therefore should arguably not be recoverable. Particularly since the enactment of the Affordable Care Act (ACA), some jurisdictions have changed the rules with regard to expert testimony about past and future medical costs. In a pair of cases, *Howell v. Hamilton Meats & Provisions, Inc.* (2011) and *Cuevas v. Contra Costa County* (2017), courts in California ruled that injured plaintiffs are limited in their recovery of medical expenses to the amount that would be paid by an insurer to satisfy medical bills. The rule was extended to future medical costs in *Corenbaum v. Lampkin* (2013) which ruled that "evidence of the full amount billed for past medical services . . . cannot support an expert opinion on the reasonable value of future medical services" (*Corenbaum* at 1326). By limiting recovery to the amounts payable by insurance, rather than the full amount billed (i.e. "cash value") of medical care, a plaintiff's recovery is significantly reduced. The argument has evolved that, in light of the ACA's mandate regarding insurance coverage, any estimates regarding medical costs must be discounted to "insurance rates" since insurance coverage should be universal. Although affirmed in California, this line of reasoning has not been fully adopted by other states, (*see Bernheisel v. Mikaya*, 2016 WL 4211897 [M.D. PA., 2016], holding the ACA could not be used to exclude testimony as to future medical expenses as it would violate the collateral source rule). With this area of the law currently in flux, experts, particularly life care planners, must seek guidance from attorneys on how to tailor the basis for their damages testimony in order to meet the applicable jurisdictional standard.

Generally speaking, there is liberal acceptance in the courts of testimony by physicians, life care planners, vocational experts, and disability analysts. Although any of these experts risk exclusion if they deviate from the standard practices and accepted methodologies of their respective professions, those who stick to the *Kumho* rule of employing "the same level of intellectual rigor [in the courtroom] that characterizes the practice of an expert in the relevant field", will find that admissibility is a hurdle that should be routinely cleared. In fact, exclusion may never be an issue raised at all. Rather, opposing counsel may choose to attack the expert's testimony via the more traditional methods of the adversarial system. Vigorous cross-examination, presentation of contrary evidence, and careful instruction on the burden of proof are the traditional and appropriate means of attacking shaky but admissible evidence. This goes to the weight of the evidence, rather than barring it as inadmissible (Advisory Committee on Evidence Rules, 2018). At trial, each party bears the responsibility of persuading the trier of fact to accept its version of the case, based on the evidence it presents. This is referred to as the "weight" of the evidence—it is the combination of (a) credibility of the statement and (b) amount of influence the evidence has on the final verdict (Imwinkelried, 2020).

Testifying—Practical Considerations

Whether it is during a *Daubert* hearing, during direct or cross-examination at deposition, or trial, the expert's goal when testifying should be primarily to educate, rather than advocate. Leave the advocacy to the attorneys. While experts may be influenced by the adversarial nature of litigation, this is no reason to alter their standards of practice. If you would not make a conclusion or otherwise offer an opinion in your professional role, there is no justification for making the same conclusion or opinion in an advocacy role (Sanders, 2007). That being said, the wise expert will spend significant time working with the attorney who hired him or her to review case materials and facts, develop an understanding of the case, and deliver an opinion that addresses the controversy at hand. It is the attorney's job to educate the expert about the requirements of the case according to the governing law. The attorney must help the expert understand legal terminology, such as "reasonable medical certainty" or "reasonable medical probability" which are legal terms of art with no practical meaning to the practicing physician. Additionally, attorneys must explain statutory definitions (i.e., "permanent total disability"), which are borrowed from medical terminology but have no specific meaning except as provided by statute or judicial interpretation. Although the courts have acknowledged that there are no universal magic words an expert must use when testifying (*Maurer*, 1992), it is the attorney's job to make sure the testimony meets the evidentiary proofs required for the particular cause of action. So, physicians and other experts must necessarily rely on the lawyers or judges to define the terms for them and then shape the form and content of their testimony in a manner that serves the legal inquiry (Wong et al., 2011).

Once the legal terms of art are mastered and applied, the responsibility for education shifts to the expert. We may agree with the premise argued by Professor Ronald Allen that one simple rule should apply: "Expert testimony must be presented in a comprehensible manner" (Allen, 2018). Professor Allen argues that bad science—with its flaws, inconsistencies, lack of support, and incredible assumptions—can never be made comprehensible, and thus using his simple rule is unlikely to be admitted at trial. While we might not share his optimism on this count, we do believe and recommend that expert testimony be presented in a way that allows a judge and jury to *understand it*. This will first benefit the judge in making an informed decision as to the admissibility of the evidence, and subsequently the jury to assign its proper weight when considering their verdict in the case.

Prior to any testimony, the key is always to be prepared with the attorney on the case. Most attorneys have a standard practice when it comes to questioning experts and tailor it to the facts at hand. Often, experts will have developed their own set of questions regarding their field of practice, qualifications, etc., that they may provide for the attorney's use. As mentioned earlier with regard to depositions, the preparation will certainly take longer than the testimony, and it should. Effective direct examination is key for most plaintiffs in winning their cases. By presenting compelling expert testimony on direct examination, the attorney scores his first opportunity to make a significant impression on the jury (Seckinger, 1991). A typical roadmap for direct examination will include a review of the expert's credentials, as well as exploring the fact that the expert is being compensated for their time, *not* their opinion. The jury knows an expert is being paid—on direct examination, the key is to demonstrate that this is common practice and that all experts are paid, including the defendant's experts. Then, the examination will delve into the methodology the expert used—examining both the data he or she collected personally (i.e., evaluating the plaintiff) and other information he or she relied on (medical records, research, reference materials, clinical experience). The goal is always to keep it simple and clear and educate the jury on your process and basis for each fact and the rationale underlying your opinion. The attorney will then solicit your opinion, having built a foundation upon which it can solidly rest. Stating their opinion provides the expert a second opportunity to educate the jury—draw the connections from your investigation, to each piece of data, to the method you used to interpret that data, to how that method led you to your conclusion (opinion) (Seckinger, 1991).

Although courtroom dramas frequently highlight the dramatic cross-examination, the well-prepared expert can expect a standard menu of questioning designed to undermine their methods and conclusions. Experts may rest easy knowing one fact—"[r]arely if ever will the cross-examining attorney know more about a subject than the expert witness being confronted" (Epstein, 2018). Assuming that the expert otherwise meets the standards set forth in *Daubert*, then cross-examination, while never pleasant, should be bearable and potentially an opportunity to reinforce the jury's perception regarding the strength of that expert's opinions. Typically, cross-examination will re-explore an expert's credentials, focusing particularly on what might be missing (board certification, limited practical experience) and whether certain credentials are inflated ("ego" boards or certifications, where all that is required is the payment of a fee and not based on any performance standard or evaluation). The cross-examining attorney will then probe for weaknesses in the validity of the expert's methods and the quality of the expert's conclusions. Undoubtedly, questions regarding bias will come up, and experts should be prepared to answer questions about their fees, their relationship with hiring counsel (i.e., repeated use as an expert), and "positional bias" (whether the expert typically testifies on behalf of one side vs. the other) (Epstein, 2018). Again, a competent expert will spend time preparing for cross-examination, and as noted earlier, has a better understanding of the subject than the attorney questioning him. Most attorneys live by the maxim, "Never ask a question to which you don't know the answer", and so they may be wary about exploring too far into the details of the expert's opinion. The main goal is to remain calm, respond to the question asked, and if an objection is raised, wait until the ruling before responding.

While Daubert sets forth the metrics by which a judge must determine admissibility, this is only the first step that qualifies an expert's knowledge. Daubert requires relevance and a good "fit" of the evidence for the case in order to be deemed helpful to the trier of fact (Allen, 2018). When it comes to testimony, if the attorney and expert are able to effectively educate their audience—first the judge to determine the admissibility, and then the jury in order that they may assign the proper weight to the expert's testimony—then the testimony is likely to contribute to a successful outcome. Imwinkelried (2020) noted that jurors must understand the the testimony submitted to them upon retiring for discussion and verdict. It remains up to the judge to fully understand and establish the relevant application of the evidence to the case in terms of admissibility. Imwinkelried added that there is no guarantee of verdict outcomes in spite of the evidence fit to the case, but a good fit at least increases the probability of rational fact findings.

Ethical Considerations

The American Academy of Psychiatry & the Law (1995) recognizes that the Anglo-American Legal process has an adversarial focus among litigating parties that can present specific hazards to the Academy's psychiatrists. This adversarial relationship evolves by the retaining of a psychiatrist member by an attorney representing either the plaintiff or defense, which could lead the potential medical witness to a bias or distortion of the medical case fact. In essence, the psychiatrist's perceived responsibilities can be overshadowed by aggressive cross examination or fear of poor testimony performance.

Caveats like this can be found in the published ethical guidelines of almost every professional organization. A good example of ensuring good, ethical and unbiased testimony from its members is the American Association of Orthopaedic Surgeons (2005). This association's tenet regarding testimony directs their member surgeons to enter expert witness practice with an assurance that their testimony will uphold the standards of their membership association through their provision of unbiased and nonpartisan, scientific and clinically accurate testimony. Similarly, life care planners and vocational experts are required by their associations to provide opinions that are based on sound methodology, without advocation of their retaining party, or the person with a disability in question (ABVE, 2020). Beyond these basic rules, professional organizations provide additional guidance, all designed to promote responsible, reliable expert testimony. In its guidelines for forensic psychologists, the American Psychological Association outlines numerous areas of concern, including competency, integrity, the nature of the relationships involved in forensic practice, and the importance of validity of methods and accuracy in reporting (APA, 2013). Understanding and adherence to the ethical guidelines of one's profession is a requirement of good experts, and a comprehensive review of all the applicable rules is beyond the scope of this chapter. We rely on our colleagues to be thoroughly acquainted with the applicable codes and use them in their forensic practice, and we will confine our discussion to the general concerns regarding ethical expert testimony.

As a general rule, experts behave unethically when they hold themselves out as having knowledge upon which others can rely but are unable to justify their opinions. It is irresponsible, or unethical, to assert knowledge without adequate justification. "In the absence of appropriate justification, what we have is mere opinion" (Sanders, 2007). And as has been reiterated throughout this chapter, "mere opinion" is never sufficient to meet the legal standards for expert testimony. This being said, we know that an expert may hold an opinion with more or less justification, as long as he is able to meet the standards set forth in the law. We return to the test set forth by *Kumho*, that an expert must employ the "same intellectual rigor" in providing opinion testimony as he does in his regular work. There is no one standard for this across all scientific disciplines—each expert must act according to the norms of his area of expertise, using the methods, instruments, and interpretations that are otherwise accepted (Sanders, 2007). The price of failing to do so is not just having testimony excluded in court. Once an expert's testimony is excluded, it is likely that one party's case fails, and that failure may not be easily corrected. The Supreme Court held in *Weisgram v. Marley* (2000) that litigants have essentially one bite at the apple when presenting expert testimony. "Since *Daubert* . . . parties relying on expert testimony have had notice of the exacting standards of reliability such evidence must meet. . . . It is implausible to suggest, post-*Daubert*, that parties will initially present less than their best expert evidence in the expectation of a second chance should their first trial fail" (528 U.S. 440, 445).

Attorneys share ethical responsibilities with regard to the presentation of expert testimony, and it is important that they play their role in seeking, vetting, and presenting a valid expert opinion.

Saks (2001) questioned how or why an attorney could not be obligated to ensure that the witness retained has the skills, knowledge base, expertise, and the integrity of presenting evidence in a fact-based explanation and response to questioning. However, careless expert testimony happens, and while the presentation of frankly fraudulent expert testimony is not only unethical but illegal, this is the least subtle and rarest challenge faced in most cases. The greatest concern is with expert evidence that lacks sufficient foundation to truly assist the trier of fact, and given the preference for admission that has been discussed throughout this chapter, even keeping in mind the *Daubert* hurdles, the fact that such evidence is routinely admitted cannot be disputed. How then, can unethical expert behavior be addressed? The greatest sanctioning influence on experts comes from admissibility decisions written by judges in *Daubert* and *Frye* hearings that "out" bad experts. Sanctions may be produced by other means—attorneys may refuse to hire experts whose testimony can't be reliably admitted. Juries may choose to disregard testimony they perceive as insufficient or unreliable. More likely, experts whose work is shoddy will face increasing scrutiny by opposing counsel, with attacks on their work focused on demonstrating its inadequacies at the early stages of discovery, again potentially making them less likely to be hired in the future. In the absence of judicial admonition in a published opinion, one only needs to look to posts in professional network LISTSERVs on the internet for examples of how an expert, once excluded based on a *Daubert* challenge, may be identified and subsequently viewed as inherently less hirable for future matters.

Other sanctions may include adverse action by a professional agency or a lawsuit by a hiring attorney. While these are not the norm, they should serve as cautionary tales. Dr. Donald Austin, a neurosurgeon who testified against another neurosurgeon in a medical malpractice suit, was suspended by the American Association of Neurological Surgeons (AANS) following its disciplinary determination that he had provided "entirely false" testimony. Austin sued AANS alleging that their actions cost him significant business as an expert. In granting summary judgment for AANS, the court observed that AANS did not act in bad faith and had reasonable grounds for its actions (*Austin v. AANS*, 2000). More recently, we have seen a case of a law firm suing a life care planner for failure to deliver a defensible plan. One of the most frequent defense challenges to life care plans is that they are "cookie cutter" and not designed for the particular plaintiff (Hurney, 2017). A Houston law firm filed suit this year against a nurse life care planner on this basis and others, alleging that the plans for different plaintiffs were "almost identical" and that both were "incomprehensible". Because of the expert's failure to deliver usable life care plans, a mediation fell through. According to the plaintiff's law firm, the life care plans provided "absolutely no benefit" to the cases (Curley, 2021).

Ultimately, ethical expert testimony bears all the same hallmarks as admissible expert testimony, and ethical experts have all the same characteristics as ethical professionals in their respective disciplines. Experts who are able to reliably and responsibly uphold their ethical obligations are likely to remain in demand.

Conclusion

As noted at the outset of this chapter, the history of expert testimony is long, and the legal and professional literature on the topic is both wide and deep. It is beyond the scope of this chapter to address each profession, each legal decision, or each jurisdiction. Indeed, multiple articles, books, and treatises have been dedicated to this subject, and it has been written about or commented on for more than 100 years, by people with far greater experience and intellect than ours. One needs only to read any of the case opinions cited in this article to get an idea of the lengthy analyses courts have undertaken when meeting their "gatekeeping" duties regarding expert evidence and the standards that it must meet to be admissible in each unique case.

Despite its lengthy and complex history, when it comes to expert testimony, we still believe that the best lesson is a simple one; an expert who uses the best practices of his profession in all endeavors, including forensic work, is likely to be successful. The expert who takes care to meet the standards of his profession with regard to methods can collaborate effectively with attorneys in knowing and meeting the standards set by the law and has the ability to cogently communicate their expertise and the conclusions that flow from that knowledge—and will be a welcome participant in any case or courtroom.

References

Allen, R. J. (2018). Fiddling while Rome burns: The story of the federal rules and experts. *Fordham Law Review, 86*(4), 1551–1557

American Academy of Psychiatry & the Law. (1995). *Ethical guidelines for the practice of forensic psychiatry*. www.aapl.org/ethics.htm.

American Bar Association (2013). *How to prepare your expert witness for deposition*. http://clecenter.com/assets/pgm_3361/library/abacle_How_to_Prepare_Your_Expert_Witness_CET13HPE_materials.pdf

Austin v. AANS, 120 F.Supp.2d 151 (N.D. Ill. 2000).

Berger, M. (2011). The admissibility of expert testimony. In National Research Council, *Reference manual on scientific evidence: Third edition* (pp. 11–36). Washington, DC. https://doi.org/10.17226/13163

Bernheisel v. Mikaya, 2016 WL 4211897 (M.D. Pa. August 9, 2016).

Best v. Lowe's Home Centers, Inc., 563 F.3d 171 (6th Cir. 2009).

Biestek v. Berryhill, 587 U.S. __ (2019).

Breyer, S. (2011). Introduction. In National Research Council, *Reference manual on scientific evidence: Third edition* (pp. 1–9). https://doi.org/10.17226/13163

Calvi, J., & Coleman, S. (2017). *American law and legal systems* (8th ed.). Routledge.

Cappellino, A. (2021). *The Daubert standard: A guide to motions, hearings, and rulings*. www.expertinstitute.com/resources/insights/the-daubert-standard-a-guide-to-motions-hearings-and-rulings/

Commonwealth vs. Pestinikas, 617 A.2d 1339 (Pa. 1992).

Corenbaum v. Lampkin, 215 Cal.App.4th 1308 (2013).

Cowher v. Kodali, J-A27035–20 (Pa. Super. Ct. February 8, 2021).

Cuevas v. Contra Costa County, 11 Cal.App.5th 163 (2017).

Curley, M. (2021). *Houston firm sues life care planner over failed mediation*. www.law360.com/articles/1351276/print?section=commercialcontracts

Daubert v. Merrell Dow Pharmaceuticals, Inc., 509 U.S. 579 (1993).

Dawn VERCI, Plaintiff-Appellee, v. Michael HIGH and International Union of Operating Engineers, Local No. 649, Defendants-Appellants, 2019 IL Appeal No. 3-19-0106 (December 18, 2019).

Edwards, T. & Edwards J. (2020). The Daubert Expert Standard: A Primer for Florida Judges and Lawyers. *The Florida Bar Journal, 94*(2), https://www.floridabar.org/the-florida-bar-journal/the-daubert-expert-standard-a-primer-for-florida-judges-and-lawyers/

Epstein, J. (Fall, 2018). Impeaching the Adverse Witness. MASTERS OF LITIGATION: The Second Annual Joint Seminar Program Presented by Temple University Beasley School of Law And The American College Of Trial Lawyers. https://www.mytlawconnection.com/s/706/images/editor_documents/masters_of_litigation/masters_of_litigation_cle_materials_fall_2018_10-26-18.pdf?sessionid=2b670f6c-5be3-42fd-ac81-3b6cc5d4e3da&cc=1

Erstad, W. (2018). Civil law vs. criminal law: Breaking down the differences. *Rasmussen University: Justice Studies Blog*. www.rasmussen.edu/degrees/justice-studies/blog/civil-law-versus-criminal-law/

Freytag v. Commissioner, 501 U.S. 868 (1991).

Frye v. United States, 293 F. 1013 (D.C. Cir. 1923).

General Electric Co. v. Joiner, 522 U.S. 136 (1997).

Glicksman, E. B. (1999). The modern hearsay rule should find administrative law application. *Nebraska Law Review, 78*(1), 135–146.

Hand, L. (1901). Historical and practical considerations regarding expert testimony. *Harvard Law Review, 15*, 40–58.

Heller v. Shaw Industries, 167 F.3d 146 (3d. Cir. 1999).

Hochstadt, E. (2016). *Four goals for taking an effective expert deposition*. American Bar Association Practice Points. www.americanbar.org/groups/litigation/committees/expert-witnesses/practice/2016/4-goals-for-taking-effective-expert-deposition/.

Howell v. Hamilton Meats & Provisions, Inc., 52 Ca.4th 541 (2011).

Hurd v. Yaeger, No. 3:06cv1927 (M.D. Pa. August 13, 2009).

Hurney, T. J. & Miller, S. P. (2017). Songs You Know by Heart: Defending Against Life Care Plans. *Medical Liability and Health Care Law*, 1–18.

Imwinkelried, E. J. (2020). Improving the presentation of expert testimony to the trier of fact: An epistemological insight in search of an evidentiary theory. *Arizona State Law Journal, 52*, 49–73.

In re Accutane Litigation, 191 A.3d 560 (2018).

Kulich, R. J., Driscoll, J., Prescott, J. C., Jr., Pelletier, N. J., Driscoll, S., Cooke, W., Correa, L., & Mehta, N. R. (2003). The Daubert Standard, A primer for pain specialists. *Pain Medicine, 4*(1), 75–80. https://doi.org/10.1046/j.1526-4637.2003.03007.x

Kumho Tire Co. v. Carmichael, 526 U.S. 137 (1999).

Mangrum, W., & Mangrum, R. C. (2019). Evidence-based medicine in expert testimony. *Liberty University Law Review, 13*(2), 337–385.

Matthiesen, W., & Lehrer, S. C. (2020, October 27). *Admissibility of Expert Testimony in All 50 States*. https://www.mwl-law.com/wp-content/uploads/2018/02/ADMISSIBILITY-OF-EXPERT-TESTIMONY.pdf

Maurer v. Trustees of the University of Pennsylvania et al., 614 A.2d 754 (Pa. Super. Ct. 1992).

Moenssens, A., Starrs, J., Henderson, C., & Inbau, F. (1995). *Scientific evidence in civil and criminal cases*. Westbury, NY.

Morales-Hurtado v. Reinoso et al., 230 A.3d 241 (NJ Supreme Ct. 2020).

Nelson v. Tennessee Gas Pipeline Co., 243 F.3d 244 (6th Cir. 2001).

Nolan, A., & Thompson, R. M. (2014). *Congressional Power to Create Federal Courts: A Legal Overview*. Congressional Research Service (Washington, D.C.) https://fas.org/sgp/crs/misc/R43746.pdf

Pipitone v. Biomatrix, Inc., 288 F.3d 239 (5th Cir. 2002).

Povrzenich v. Ripepi et al., 2021 WL 1047363 (Pa.Super. 2021).

Queen v. W.I.C., Inc., Case No. 14-CV-519-DRH-SCW (S.D. Ill. September 5, 2017).

Rabutino v. Freedom State Realty Co., Inc., 809 A.2d 933 (Pa. Super.2002).

Richardson v. Perales, 402 U.S. 389 (1971).

Ryskamp, D. A. (2020). *Motions in limine: The complete guide*. www.expertinstitute.com/resources/insights/motions-in-limine-the-complete-guide/

Saks, M. (2001). Scientific evidence and the ethical obligations of attorneys. *Cleveland State Law Review, 49*, 421–437.

Sanders, J. (2007). Expert witness ethics. *Fordham Law Review, 76*, 1539–1584.

Seckinger, J. (1991) Presenting Expert Testimony. *American Journal of Trial Advocacy, 15*, 215–268.

Social Security Administration (2017). *Vocational expert handbook*. www.ssa.gov/appeals/public_experts/Vocational_Experts_(VE)_Handbook-508.pdf.

Staples v. United States, 511 US 600 (1994).

The People v. Sanchez, 63 Cal.4th 665 (2016).

Unified Judicial System of Pennsylvania (2020). *Legal glossary*. www.pacourts.us/learn/legal-glossary.

United States v. Aguilar, 515 U.S. 593 (1995).

U.S. District Court for the District of New Hampshire. *Federal rule of evidence 703—expert testimony based on inadmissible evidence*. www.nhd.uscourts.gov/pdf/Experts_FRE_703.pdf.

Weisgram v. Marley, 528 U.S. 440 (2000).

Wong, J. B., Gostin, L. O., & Cabrera, O. A. (2011). Reference guide on medical testimony. In National Research Council, *Reference manual on scientific evidence: Third edition* (pp. 687–745). Washington, DC. https://doi.org/10.17226/13163

22 The International Commission on Health Care Certification

Certification and Accreditation in Life Care Planning

Kathleen Kenney May and Virgil Robert May III

The International Commission on Health Care Certification (ICHCC) is the premier certifying agency in the United States and Canada for life care planners, offering the Certified Life Care Planner (CLCP) and the Canadian Certified Life Care Planner (CCLCP) credentials. The ICHCC offers multiple certifications to health care practitioners that include in addition to the CLCP/CCLCP credentials, Medicare Set-aside Certified Consultant (MSCC), the Certified Medical Cost Projection Specialist (CMCPS), and the Certified Geriatric Care Manager (CGCM) credentials. Due to the focus of this book, we will focus on the CLCP credential, and those readers interested in learning more about the other credentials will find their descriptors and required qualifications on the ICHCC website: www.ichcc.org.

The ICHCC began certifying health care practitioners in 1994 with the CDE credential. It wasn't until 1995 that the ICHCC was requested by the University of Florida to develop a certification credential for participants in its new on-campus training program in life care planning. The ICHCC offered its first administration of the CLCP examination in March 1996 to 80 qualified health care practitioners; 40 practitioners assembled in Atlanta, Georgia, and 40 practitioners assembled in San Francisco, California, for group testing. The ICHCC has never grandfathered practitioners in its certification offerings, and passing scores at that time were determined through standard deviation score-placement levels.

With the request by the University of Florida for a certifying credential for its life care planning training program, it became apparent to the ICHCC that this health care service delivery system (life care planning) was going to expand and grow immensely, with health care practitioners of all specialty areas seeking an alternative practice in their career health care specialty fields. What attracted and continues to attract practitioners to life care planning certification is best realized through a review of the certification process: its definition(s), its advantages, and the reasoning of practitioners to obtain certification in this health care specialty area.

Definitions

Certification

Simply put, certification is an outcome of an evaluation process; it is not a product that one can hold or to display in one's office. At best, there is a certificate that can be framed expressing that the holder has met certain qualifications and holds specific knowledge and skills within the health care specialty area of examination. More specifically, certification can be regarded as an "item of intellectual property that is leased to individuals who have met and continue to meet the required standards" as identified by the certifying agency (Brauer, 2011, p. 2).

DOI: 10.4324/b23293-22

Certification has been defined as a process by which an individual has mastered skills and competencies (knowledge) within the field of examination by a credentialing entity (McDavid & Huse, 2015). This definition is applied to the certification process when tests/certification examinations are involved and required. Other definitions focus on a process by which an external agency recognizes the competence of individual practitioners or grants recognition to a person who has met predetermined qualifications specified by the respective certifying agency (Arslan, 2018; Gilley & Galbraith, 1986).

Accreditation

Accreditation is defined as a process whereby the accrediting agency grants public recognition that a certifying entity has met certain predetermined qualifications or standards set forth by the accrediting agency (Gilley & Galbraith, 1986). It is a process by which an independent third party sets standards for and evaluates the respective certifying agency's compliance with those standards (Brauer, 2011). There are five major accrediting agencies in the health care industry. These include:

- American National Standards Institute National Accreditation Board (ANAB)
- National Commission for Certifying Agencies (NCCA)
- Council of Engineering and Scientific Specialty Boards CESB)
- American Board of Medical Specialties (ABMS)
- American Board of Nursing Specialties (ABNS)

The ICHCC was finishing its application to ANAB for its accreditation at the time this book was published. ANAB accreditation standards are known as ISO)/IEC 17024—Certification of Persons, and these standards are recognized in more than 85 countries. The ICHCC chose ANAB over the NCCA because NCCA's accreditation stops at the U.S. borders, while ANAB's standards cross accepting borderlines and the ICHCC will hold accreditation rights in all 85 countries to date that accept the ANAB standards. Thus, the ICHCC will hold accreditation rights internationally as well as its certificants.

The reader needs to understand the differences between the ANAB and NCCA accreditation agencies. The NCCA is very popular in the health care service delivery systems, whereas ANAB is less known for its accreditation services. Both agencies address many of the same health care service delivery matters. While the NCCA standards are somewhat stronger on examination and psychometric matters, ANAB's quality management systems are the strength of the ANSI/ISO/IEC 17024 standards. The following is a comparison of the agencies' accreditation policies:

- *Site Visit*: ANAB's ANSI/ISO/IEC 17024 procedures require site visits by the ANAB audit panel. The NCAA does not visit a certification organization. ANAB requires one site visit during the application process, and once approved for accreditation, there is a mid-cycle site visit during the five-year accreditation cycle. During a site visit, ANAB panel members may interview any member, not just senior members, of the certification organization's staff. The interviews verify whether the rules, standards, procedures, and processes in place reflect what appeared in the application materials.
- *Focus on Management Systems*: The greatest difference is the emphasis on ANAB/ISO/IEC 17024 on quality management systems. ANAB panel members expect an organization to have detailed, written management procedures. There is the assumption of ANAB that an

organization follows its written procedures. ANAB requires the organization to audit its procedures. ANAB expects the certifying agency to audit its written procedures, and the certifying agency must demonstrate with supporting documentation that it follows its management systems in detail.

- *Costs*: The fees for ANAB/ISO/IEC 17024 are higher than those of the NCCA. There is an application fee, and the certification agency seeking accreditation will pay the expenses (travel per diem and time) of the evaluation panel. There is a fee for the annual report as well. The major unforeseen costs involve setting up and operating formal quality management systems. The level of detail needed will likely require additional staff.

Key contractors that have any role in decisions about who gets certified must undergo regular evaluations by the certification organization. Contractors, such as those providing psychometric advice, examination delivery and scoring, evaluation of qualifications, etc., must undergo periodic evaluation. The certification agency must audit any organization with access to confidential information, including contractors that handle applications, mail examination results, etc. (Brauer, 2011, pp. 185–189).

Certification Concept

Brauer (2011) noted that many professional health care providers look upon certification as a very simple concept:

- The agency (owner with board) sets standards
- Candidates are tested/evaluated against those standards
- The agency awards a certificate to denote that the individual has met the standards and authorized the certificate holder to use the certification title

This sounds fairly simple and without complications, stress, or much preparation work. But in reality, the certification process requires more than putting items on paper, calling the item collection an examination, and administering it to unsuspecting candidates as a bona fide, valid examination of life care planning service delivery systems. There is so much required of a certifying agency's staff and board volunteers in terms of office management, examination management, and management of the certificants. The ICHCC is well couched in the tasks that Brauer suggested, takes its responsibilities to the field of stakeholders extremely seriously, and includes but is not limited to:

- Good business management that maintains the solvency of the business and this, in turn, protects the stakeholders' credential
- The owner and board of commissioners have a thorough understanding of the domain of practice that they serve
- Employees that are skilled and knowledgeable of the practice that the credential serves
- An administrative, as well as the board of commissioners, focus on individual CLCP certificants' certification needs
- Sound psychometrics to demonstrate reliability in test item scores as well as the validity of those items to ensure certification candidates take an examination with items that are valid and apply directly to the knowledge domains and subfactors of the life care planning process
- Effective financial planning and management
- Net revenue is required to invest in continued growth and improvements

- The software and technology to ensure timely examination administration as well as fairly written and structured items
- Collaboration with preapproved training programs to ensure training and examination content meet the standards the agency has set for life care planning
- Continued mapping of the certification process and constantly revisiting it to ensure that it works smoothly
- Address procrastinators, provide for fairness, and ensure due process on decisions
- Require a continual focus on improvement and overall quality of examination product and policy

Certification Advantages

The standing premise in certification is that certification candidates have undergone additional education and training in their desire to expand upon their career practices in health care. Additionally, certified candidates have met specific qualifications that allow them access to the certification examination in addition to having appropriate backgrounds, education, and training to meet the acceptance criterium. The advantages are numerous and well documented in the rehabilitation literature. Shackman (2015) surmised that persons certified should have more in-depth professional preparation in performing the essential functions (methodology) of their field of expertise and better strategies when addressing client problems than those colleagues who are not certified/credentialled.

The advantages of credentialling in one's area of professional training are well-documented in the rehabilitation literature. Morra Imas (cited in Shackman, 2015) reviewed the development and use of competencies for program evaluators, which she included in a table in her review article. Her table documented reasons supporting certification that include:

- Certification shows that one has successfully demonstrated knowledge, skills, training, and experience to an independent board and that one abides by a code of ethics.
- Certification provides prestige.
- Certification provides incentives by enhancing marketability and salaries.
- Certification provides a basis for disciplining those who do not follow ethical codes or who misrepresent their capabilities and/or experience.
- Certification avoids narrow competency definitions that may be self-serving to specific organizations.
- Certification helps prevent poorly qualified persons practicing the profession from undermining the public trust and confidence.

Shackman's applications were more concise in his notations of the advantages of certification. His observations were more tied to the practitioner and included:

- Increasing the credibility of the [life care planning service delivery system] and enhancing the recognition of [life care planners] as professionals
- Improving consistency and methodological rigor
- Increasing availability of training
- Demonstrating acquisition of knowledge/experience
- Providing a means of identifying those who don't have the requisite background

Ridge (2008) exemplified the advantages of certification as noting that certification is perceived by the public as influencing accountability, professional accomplishment and growth, and specialized knowledge in a particular health care specialty service. Ridge also noted that certified practitioners who pursue a national specialty certification perceived themselves as having a high level of commitment to their profession.

May (2020) accounted for the benefits of certification as applied to the client as well as to the practitioner. He conveyed the following:

- *Existence of Governing Board to Oversee Consumer Concerns/Complaints*
  Health care certifying agencies have overseeing boards responsible for monitoring certification practice applications as related to the certification credential. One area of concern is how services are delivered to clients and if they were properly administered according to ethical and methodology standards of the certifying agency. If clients receiving services feel that they have not been offered appropriate services delivery, they can file a complaint to the agency's overseeing board.
- *Existence of Governing Board to Oversee Peer Concerns/Complaints*
  The overseeing boards also address complaints from current certified credential holders regarding a peer credential holder's improper service delivery, improper marketing behaviors, or unethical practices.
- *Disciplinary Action May be Implemented on Behalf of Consumer by the Board*
  The boards of certifying agencies have the authority to review all complaints from the field and to determine the validity of the respective complaints.

Disciplinary procedures may include but are not limited to:

- *Cease and Desist Order*: Require the accused to cease and desist the challenged behavior.
- *Reprimand:* Reprimand when the committee has determined that there has been an ethics violation but there has been no damage to another person.
- *Censure:* Censure when the committee has determined that there has been an ethics violation, but the damage done to another person is not sufficient to warrant more serious action.
- *Supervision Requirement:* Require that the accused receive supervision.
- *Rehabilitation, Education, Training, or Counseling:* The accused may be required to undergo rehabilitative counseling/therapy, additional education, training, or personal counseling.
- *Probation:* Requires that the accused be placed on probation.
  Probation is defined as the relation that the **ICHCC** has with the accused when the **ICHCC** undertakes actively and systematically to monitor, for a specific length of time, the degree to which the accused complies with the ethics committee's requirements.
- *Referral:* Referral to a relevant association or state board of examiners for action.
- *Revocation:* The CLCP/CCLCP credential can be suspended or revoked based on a majority vote of the ethics board.

Specific to the practitioner, there are many advantages to being certified that can be conveyed to a potential referral source. These may include but are not limited to:

- CLCP professionals agree to be peer reviewed.
  The Certified Life Care Planner and the Canadian Certified Life Care Planner are required to submit a work sample for review by either their 120-hour required training program or by the ICHCC's administration prior to sitting for the CLCP/CCLCP examinations. Although the certification candidate may have met all background, education, and experience and completed the 120-life care planning training program, they must pass the work-sample life care plan review before having access to the examination.

- CLCP professional agrees to adhere to a set of practice standards and ethical guidelines.

  All CLCP/CCLCP practitioners must adhere to the ethical principles established by the ICHCC. Ethical principles regarding their other certifications or membership organizations are not considered for review by the ICHCC of any submitted complaint from a client, peer, or referral source.
- CLCP professional is willing to be scrutinized by a governing board regarding his or her practice behaviors

  CLCP and CCLPC practitioners are expected to accept any review of ethical principles and fully cooperate with the ICHCC regarding any alleged infraction(s).
- CLCP professionals agree to be disciplined

  The CLCP/CCLCP practitioner is expected to accept any disciplinary recommendation made by the ICHCC ethical review board. Any refusal by the practitioner to accept and abide by the disciplinary recommendations will have their credential permanently revoked/ suspended.

Tests

One of the ICHCC's primary obligations to the stakeholders of the CLCP/CCLCP credentials is to ensure that the examination items are valid and reliability has been established and maintained in the 100-item multiple choice exam. We use the Angoff method for rating the items using subject matter experts (SMEs), who determine the validity of each item in our item pool, resulting in the establishment of the validity of the examination. Reliability is established using statistical components and measures that include Cronbach's alpha, KR-20 (Kuder-Richardson), and decision consistency among item raters. One statistic that the ICHCC uses is the percentage of the pool of candidates selecting the correct answer and each of the three distractors. The chance rate for a four-choice item is 25%, and items that 90% or more of the candidates get right are considered "not performing well" as an item. Items with such high percentages of either right or wrong fail to differentiate among the test-takers, and the preferred range for the correct answer is between 35% and 90%.

Another statistic that the ICHCC uses is the point-biserial correlation statistic. This statistic measures the correlation between getting the item correct and scoring well on the examination. The point-biserial statistic has a range between -1.0 and 1.0. A high positive value for the point-biserial correlation means the candidates who correctly answered the item also had high total scores. Conversely, a low positive value means that those who correctly answered the item scored low on the examination. A negative value means that those who scored well on the examination got the item wrong.

The ICHCC Mission, Structure, and Ethical Principles

History

The ICHCC was established originally as the Commission on Disability Examiner Certification (CDEC) in 1994 in response to the health care industry's need for certified clinical examiners in impairment and disability rating practices. The CDEC expanded rapidly over its first 8 years such that its name was updated in the spring of 2002 to that of the International Commission on Health Care Certification. The name change was necessary since the CDEC was offering certifications into other specialty areas of rehabilitation by 2001, and a more generic reference was required under which each of its three certification credentials as well as future credentials could be classified. Credentialing in the specialty area of impairment rating and disability examination evolved as a result of meetings with allied health care providers around the country in the early 1990s. Issues were discussed that focused primarily on clinical examiner credentials, validity and reliability of rating protocol, and the establishment of a testing board to oversee the impairment rating and disability examining credentialing process. The resulting credential was the Certified Disability Evaluator (CDE) with three levels that allow for the inclusion of all professionals who are involved in measuring functional performance of persons reporting impairment or disability. The ICHSS awarded the Certified Disability Examiner I, II, and/or III (CDE I, II, III) credential to persons who had satisfied the educational program requirements and training standards established by the National Association of Disability Evaluating Professionals (NADEP), with all classroom instruction offered at regional locations around the country.

The commission broadened its influence in the medical and rehabilitation marketplace through its research and development of a certification program in life care planning and related catastrophic case management. Currently, comprehensive training programs in life care planning have evolved to respond to this need for life care planning services as applied to catastrophic cases. Vocational/medical rehabilitation case managers and rehabilitation nurses have established themselves as consultants and case managers in these catastrophic cases and often detail the medical and rehabilitation needs of catastrophically disabled persons. Thus, the commission developed the Certified Life Care Planner (CLCP) credential in response to the rapid growth and influence of case management in catastrophic disabilities and managed care in today's health care insurance industry. Subsequent to the development of the CLCP credential, the Canadian Certified Life Care Planner (CCLCP) was established to assist in the growth of this field in Canada as more Canadian nurses, occupational therapists, and rehabilitation counselors traveled to the United States for training in this specialty health care service delivery system.

Validity and reliability research of the CLCP credential was completed through Southern Illinois University and is based specifically on the roles and function of case managers, rehabilitation counselors, vocational rehabilitation counselors, and rehabilitation nurses who provide this service as part of their case management structure. The most recent update of life care planners' roles and functions was completed in 2020 by the ICHCC (May & Moradirekabdarkolaee, 2020). Currently, there is ample literature in the professional journals that addresses life care planning, and the commission's research goals of identifying and establishing the background, education, and experience criteria required to competently develop life care plans have been achieved. However, there is always more research required of a dynamic service delivery system in health care such as life care planning.

The third credential to be developed by the ICHCC is the Medicare Set-aside Certified Consultant (MSCC). This credential evolved out of the need for the Medicare benefit system of the United States to project the amount of monies needed to be set aside while the disabled worker utilized the benefits offered by the individual's respective state workers' compensation benefit system. After the disabled worker expends the respective disability schedule of the diagnosis/injury, Medicare benefits are awarded to continue the care routine required of the disabled individual. The MSCC is for those health care, legal, and insurance professionals who consult with the Medicare benefit program regarding the categories of need required of the disabled individual through his or her remaining life span and what costs are associated with each category.

The fourth credential to be developed by the ICHCC is the Certified Geriatric Care Manager (CGCM). This credential evolved out of the need for regulating the sudden growth of this field as a direct result of the aging of the "baby boomer" generation, to include the parents of this emerging elderly population. More elderly people are in need of case management services as nursing homes and senior living centers evolve to serve this growing population. To address this need, more case managers have added geriatric care and case management to their businesses, thus requiring regulation of geriatric care managers for the protection of the consumer. The CGCM credential ensures the consumer of services that the Certified Geriatric Care Manager has demonstrated an understanding and competency in applying geriatric care and case management standards to the disability evaluation and management process.

The ICHCC's most recent credential is the Certified Medical Cost Projection Specialist (CMCPS). This credential evolved from the observation of the CLCP board members as well as from CLCP practitioners that they were receiving referrals from attorneys requesting only the cost analysis of the needs of the client, and they were instructed not to present a full life care plan content. In essence, the referral sources were only interested in the projected costs of the equipment, medication, medical treatment, and rehabilitative services.

Mission Statement

Specific to the focus of this book, the ICHCC oversees the examination of health care providers and professionals in the specialty rehabilitative area of life care planning. The ICHCC's ongoing actions in support of this mission include:

- Developing, reviewing, and researching standards for life care planning, Medicare Set-aside allocation, functional capacity and disability evaluations, medical cost projections, and geriatric care management service delivery systems for post-graduate training in these respective areas.
- Developing, reviewing, and researching standards of practice for life care planning, Medicare Set-aside allocation, functional capacity and disability evaluations, and geriatric care management
- Developing and administering examinations that assess the knowledge and skills that comprise the essential functions required of life care planners, Medicare Set-aside allocators, functional capacity and disability evaluations, and geriatric care managers service delivery systems

Goals and Objectives

The ICHCC is dedicated to the development and administration of well-researched, standardized tests designed to measure health care provider certification applicants' working knowledge and skills of the respective health care service delivery system to which they apply for certification. To achieve its mission, the ICHCC established the following goals:

- Develop national and international tests that measure the health care provider applicant's working knowledge of disability, medical systems, associated disabilities, and treatment/ maintenance protocol required to sustain life within an acceptable comfort level.
- Conduct ongoing research in terms of test-item validity and reliability. Such research ensures that tests measure what they purport to measure and that the items are a fair representation of the respective credential's subject matter and required knowledge base.
- Procure qualified commissioners to sit on the board of commissioners to represent all ICHCC credentialed candidates and certified professionals.
- Establish and monitor recertification policies to measure continued competence and/or to enhance the continued competence of all certified health care professionals under the ICHCC.

The ICHCC recognizes that certain objectives must be met in order to achieve these goals. The objectives are detailed as follows:

- To appoint qualified health care practitioners as commissioners to sit on the board of commissioners specific to each credential offered by the ICHCC. The represented specialty areas may include but are not limited to vocational rehabilitation evaluators/counselors, medical physicians, nurses, occupational therapists, physical therapists, attorneys, social work professionals, psychologists, and physician assistants as applied to health care settings.
- To solicit the assistance of commissioners in researching the validity and reliability of the examinations, incorporating appropriate research design and statistics.

CLCP/CCLCP Qualification Requirements

The ICHCC offers certifications with reference to field experience, specialty areas of training, and a candidate's achieved degree level. The ICHCC requires the following criteria to be met by all CLCP/CCLCP candidates in order to qualify to sit for any of the ICHCC's examinations:

1. Each non-nurse candidate for the CLCP/CCLCP credentials must have at the minimum a bachelor's degree. Nurse candidates must have at the minimum a diploma in nursing.
2. Each CLCP and CCLCP candidate must have at least 120 hours of training from an ICHCC-approved training program for the respective credential. A listing of these programs can be found on the ICHCC website at www.ichcc.org. Required in the 120 hours are 16 hours dedicated to orientation, methodology, and standards of practice in life care planning or geriatric care management.
3. Applicants for the CLCP/CCLCP credentials should have a minimum of 3 years of field experience in a health care–related profession within the 5 years preceding application for certification. Applicants for the final approval of any application with ambiguity regarding training and/or experience will be left to the discretion of the ICHCC following a thorough review of the respective application. The opinion of the ICHCC is final.
4. ICHCC approved training programs completed over a time frame of 7 years from the date of application are counted as valid for consideration. Documentation of such coursework and participation verification is required in the form of attendance verification forms and/or curriculum documentation from the training agency. Each candidate must meet the minimum academic requirements for their designated health care–related profession. They must be certified, licensed, or meet the legal mandates of their respective state or province that allow him or her to practice service delivery within the definition of his or her designated health care–related profession. Those health care professionals who hold a master's degree in a health-related field are exempt from being required to have a primary certification. However, final approval of any application with ambiguity regarding training and/or experience will be left to the discretion of the ICHCC following a thorough review of the respective applications. The opinion of the ICHCC is final.

Qualified Health Care Professional Mandate

The CLCP and CCLCP credentials require the certification candidate to meet the criteria set forth in the designation of a *qualified health care professional* established by the ICHSS. This is due to the case management emphasis that typifies the life care planning credentials.

The designation of a health care professional must be specific to the care, treatment, and/or rehabilitation of individuals with significant disabilities and does not include such professions as attorney, generic educators, general administrators, etc., but does include such professions as counseling and special education with appropriate qualifications.

This designation of qualified health care professional is based on a background of education, training, and practice qualifications. A background of only experience and/or designated job title is not accepted as defining a qualified health care professional. Completion of training in the respective credential's focus area, experience, or being qualified in the court system as an expert witness do not necessarily meet the definition of a qualified health care professional under the ICHCC standards. This definition can only be met when all educational, training, and practice qualification components are reviewed and met.

Due to their unregulated professional status that varies among states or provinces, the following is offered as clarification for meeting the qualified health care professional status regarding the following professionals who do not hold a master's degree:

* Rehabilitation Counselor—CDMS, CCM, CRC
* Case Manager—Minimum Nursing Degree (Diploma)—CCM, CRC, LPC
* Counselor—Bachelor's Degree—NCC, CDMS, or State License or State Mandate to Practice
* Social Worker—State License in Social Work or meets State Mandate to Practice
* Special Education Teacher—Licensed

Persons holding licensure designations as "technicians" or "assistants", to include but are not limited to physical therapy assistants (PTA), occupational therapy assistants (OTA), dental hygienists, emergency medical technicians (EMT), nursing assistants or certified nursing assistants, massage therapists, and licensed practical nurses (LPNs), are excluded from qualifying to sit for the CLCP and CCLCP credentials. However, physician assistants are qualified to sit for the life care planning credentials. Additionally, any person meeting the previous definition of a health care professional but who also carries a "technician/assistant" title will be eligible to sit for the examination (e.g., an EMT who is a licensed RN).

Specific Credential Qualifications

The CLCP/CCLCP credentials are dedicated to those health care professionals who are adept in collecting and assimilating medical, rehabilitative, and environmental data for persons who have sustained significant to catastrophic injury to one or multiple body systems. The life care planning service delivery system requires the practitioner to not only collect current medical, rehabilitative, and environmental data but also to project the need for such associated services and the costs of services, equipment, supplies, and medical/rehabilitative resources over the remaining life span of the disabled individual. The focus of life care planning service delivery is for the consulting CLCP/CCLCP to develop a plan that outlines the needs of the individual such that their current post-injury functional capabilities and comfort can progress to as close to their premorbid function and comfort levels as possible.

Test Administration and Scoring Standards

As noted earlier, test development and scoring are complex processes that required astute knowledge of psychometrics and statistics. The CLCP/CCLCP certification examinations are composed of multiple-choice case scenarios which contain three distracters and one correct choice. All test answers are referenced within current professional literature from the medical, insurance, and rehabilitation professions. The certification candidate has two options for test administration:

1. All credential examinations are administered "online", thus requiring proctoring from an online proctoring service, Prov Exams.
2. National sites are designated by the ICHCC for test administration on an annual basis. Dates and locations of the national sites may be obtained from the ICHCC office.

All test results are scored by the testing software programs of Prov Exam and are sent directly to the corporate office of the ICHCC. The CLCP examination's cutoff score was determined using the Angoff method (modified) (Arrasmith & Hambleton, 1988; Ashby, 2001; Biddle, 1993; Bowers & Shindoll, 1989; Kara & Cetin, 2020; Tiratira, 2009). The ICHCC test committee meets periodically to review the test-item pool, rate the items using criteria gleaned from the knowledge domains from the most recent role and function study, and determine the cutoff test score using the criterion-referenced model. The specific model the ICHCC uses for validation is the modified Angoff method in which rating participants discuss the characteristics of a borderline certification candidate, and a consensus is reached as to the specific characteristics to consider when reviewing each individual item. The raters were asked, "Would a borderline candidate be able to answer the item correctly?" The items that the committee felt would be answered correctly by the borderline certification candidate were assigned a 1 = yes. Items that the committee felt that the borderline candidate would more than likely mark a wrong answer were assigned a 0 = no. A follow-up meeting of the test committee is then conducted at which time all items are reviewed and rated a second time. The analysis of ratings for the current examination at the time of publication for this book places the cutoff scores for the CLCP/CCLCP examinations was held to a score of 79.

Confidentiality

Test scores of all certification candidates are held in strict confidence within the ICHCC corporate office. Specific test scores are not released to any certification candidate; only their pass or fail status as determined statistically through the standard score protocol is released. Scores are held in confidence by the ICHCC as a means to avoid the promotion of competitive embarrassment among life care planners seeking to gain a market edge over their peers and to avoid low test score applicants from being penalized through the referral process favoring those who scored higher on the examination. Test scores are not released to the public under any circumstances except through legal subpoena. Candidates are prohibited from sharing information that may involve discussing, documenting, and in any way revealing test content, particular items, or item choices that include the correct answer and the associated distractors.

Testing Aids and Prep Courses

The ICHCC offers a review course for the CLCP/CCLCP credential and includes a review textbook to those persons who are first-time candidates or for those persons who elect to retake the examination for renewal purposes. The textbook is the primary text used in the review course offered by the ICHCC specific to the CLCP/CCLCP credentials. The CLCP/CCLCP Exam Review Webinar dates and registration forms can be found on the ICHCC.org website under "About Us" in the top horizontal menu bar. Orders for the CLCP or the CCLCP Exam Review Guide can be made online at the ICHCC website.

The review textbook does not in any way address specific test items. The book is divided into five primary disability groups of which general instruction is based. There is a voluminous amount of information contained within the textbook that is discussed over the 7-hour course period. The certification candidates are advised that while the actual test may address some of the content of the text, the textbook in and of itself by no means addresses any specific test item.

Certification Maintenance and Renewal

The ICHSS asserts that certified professionals should maintain a high level of skills and knowledge through development of professional skills and continuing education. Requirements for certification renewal are designed to encourage the continuation of professional development, which will aid in the effective delivery of health care services. Goals include but are not limited to:

- Exploration of valid and reliable testing protocols.
- Enhancement of one's skills in their area of concentration and certification.
- Developing informational resources for their area of concentration.
- Enhancement of professional assessment and processing skills.
- Exploration of new strategies for problem solving in their areas of concentration.
- Acquiring knowledge in specific areas of disabilities, vocational applications, case management, technology, public and private insurance benefit programs, legislation, and legal implications.

Code of Ethics

The ICHCC code of ethics applies to all of its credentials. The code is rather expansive, and the reader is directed to the ICHCC website at www.ichcc.org to open the *ICHCC Practice Standards and Guidelines* to review the specific principles and rules.

The preamble to the code of ethics states that CLCPs and CCLCPs are expected to make fair and impartial assessments regarding the functional capabilities and needs of the referred individual, whether that individual is considered to be catastrophically injured or adventitiously injured with a manageable orthopedic, neurological, or other system diagnoses. The CLCP/CCLCP credentialed health care practitioners are required to be thorough with competent research conducted for each identified category of need, and opinions and conclusions structured without regard for personal reimbursement resources.

CLCPs are required at a minimum to assess the client's medical and independent living service needs, assess their vocational feasibility and options, and provide consulting services to the legal system. But above all, the certified professionals of the ICHCC must demonstrate adherence to ethical standards and must ensure that the standards are enforced. The code of professional ethics is designed to serve as a reference for professionals who carry ICHCC certification credentials, thus ensuring that acceptable behavior and conduct are clarified, defined, and maintained. The basic objective of the code of professional ethics is to promote the welfare of service recipients by specifying and enforcing ethical behaviors expected of CLCPs and CCLCPs. The primary obligation of the certified health care professionals under the ICHCC is to the disabled person in question. Only when the certified health care professional (CLCP/CCLCP) is requested to perform an independent medical examination does the obligation of the disability examiner shift to that of the referring party, since there is no physician/patient relationship. The same principle applies when the certified individual is approached by the third-party funding source to critique a previously written report/care plan developed per the request of the opposing legal representative. The certified professional is obligated to communicate to the third-party referral source any discoveries which may benefit the disabled person in question regarding additional rehabilitation or vocational options.

the code of professional ethics consists of two types of standards: principles and rules of professional conduct. The principles are general standards that provide a definition of the category under which specific rules are assigned. While the principles are general in concept, the rules are exacting standards which provide guidance in specific circumstances.

Certified health care providers who violate the professional code of ethics are subject to disciplinary action. A rule violation is interpreted as a violation of the applicable principle and any one of its rules of professional conduct. The ICHCC considers the use of any of its certification's acronyms in a signature line and in one's curricula vitae a privilege and reserves unto itself the power to suspend or to revoke the privilege or to approve other penalties for a rule violation. Disciplinary penalties are imposed as warranted by the severity of the offense and circumstances. All disciplinary actions are undertaken in accordance with published procedures and penalties designed to assure the proper enforcement of the code of professional ethics within the framework of due process and equal protection of the laws.

When there is reason to question the ethical propriety of specific behaviors, persons are encouraged to refrain from engaging in such behaviors until the matter has been clarified by the ICHCC ethics committee. Persons credentialed under the ICHCC who need assistance in interpreting the code should request in writing an advisory opinion from the ICHCC.

Summary

It is clear the establishing of a certifying agency or creating a new certification for an established certifying agency is more complex than just putting items on a page, scanning it to the internet, and advertising it as a certification exam for a health care specialty service. It requires the development of *institutional memory* that requires the collection of documented information used to operate the certification agency and the certification credential (Brauer, 2011). In essence, institutional memory consists of charts and descriptions, written operating procedures containing the collection of policies, procedures, decision documentation, examination contents, records related to individual certificants, instructions for governance, administrators, volunteer board members, staff, and information regarding the domain of practice and practitioners involved in the health care field of examination (Bauer, 2011).

Writing test items and picking items that will comprise the test requires a wealth of knowledge of the domain being tested, how items are validated, and how reliability is established and applied to the examination. The ICHCC takes this program component extremely seriously, as it feels it is the fiduciary responsibility of the administration to ensure that the stakeholders (certificants) and the candidates for testing that their test is a valid representation of the practice domain as applied to the field of examination and that current certificants know that their certifying agency continues administering test items that meet the agency's validation and reliability criteria.

There is no doubt that an individual practitioner certified in life care planning holds a special commitment to the life care planning service industry, having achieved additional training and education to qualify to sit for the examination and the feeling of accomplishment when the certificate of certification is awarded. There is a special feeling of respect for certified peer groups among themselves and among the referral sources as well. Certification of a specialty health care service adds to the professionalism of the field and provides a baseline for growth of the certifying agency in its effort to ensure only qualified health care practitioners become certified and incompetent practitioners remain separated from certified credential holders. Additionally, it remains crucial to the field and to those seeking certification that the certification exams maintain validity and reliability that result in the true measure of the examination to the health care knowledge domain that is being examined.

References

Arrasmith, D., & Hambleton, R. K. (1988). Steps for setting standards with the Angoff method. *ERIC Document—ED299326*, 1–26.

Arslan, Ü. (2018). The historical development of professional counseling and an overview of vocational standards in the United States. *International Journal of Eurasia Social Sciences, 34*(9), 2524–2533.

Ashby, D. J. (2001). The CFPTM Certification Examination process: A discussion of the modified Angoff scoring method. *Financial Service Review, 10*, 187–195.

Biddle, R. (1993). How to set cutoff scores for knowledge tests in promotion, training, certification, and licensing. *Public Personnel Management, 22*(1), 63–79. https://doi.org/10.1177/009102609302200105

Bowers, J., & Shindoll, R. (1989). *A comparison of the Angoff, Beuk, and Hofstee Methods for setting a Passing Score*. ACT Research Report Series -89-2. The American College Testing Program, Iowa City, Iowa.

Brauer, R. (2011). *Exceptional certification: Principles, concepts, and ideas for achieving credentialing excellence* (pp. 2–263). Premier Print Group.

Gilley, J. W., & Galbraith, M. W. (1986). Examining professional certification. *Training & Development Journal, 40*(6), 60–61.

Kara, H., & Çetin, S. (2020). Comparison of Passing Scores Determined by The Angoff Method in Different Item Samples. *International Journal of Assessment Tools in Education, 7*(1), 80–97. https://doi.org/10.21449/ijate.699479

May, V. R. (2020). *A review webinar for the CLCP and CCLCP examinations* [Webinar]. The International Commission on Health Care Certification.

May, V. R., & Moradirekabdarkolaee, H. (2020). The International Commission on Health Care Certification life care planner role and function investigation. *Journal of Life Care Planning, 18*(2), 3–67.

McDavid, J. C., & Huse, I. (2015). How does accreditation fit into the picture? In J. W. Altschuld & M. Engle (Eds.), Accreditation, certification, and credentialing: Relevant concerns for U.S. evaluators. *New Directions for Evaluation, 145*, 53–69.

Ridge, R. (2008). Nursing certification as a workforce strategy. *Nursing Management (Springhouse), 39*(8), 50–52. https://doi.org/10.1097/01.NUMA.00003337825.80733.64.

Shackman, G. (2015). Accreditation, certification, credentialing: Does it help? In James Altschuld and Molly Engle (Editors), *Special Issue: Accreditation, Certification, and Credentialing: Relevant Concerns for U.S. Evaluators. 145*, 103–113. https://doi.org/10.1002/ev.20114

Tiratira, N. (2009). Cutoff scores: The basic Angoff method and the item response theory method. *The International Journal of Education and Psychological Assessment, 1*(1), 27–35.

Index

Note: Page numbers in *italic* indicate a figure and page numbers in **bold** indicate a table on the corresponding page.

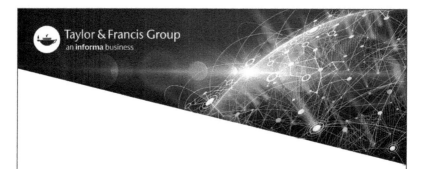